Evidence-Based Emergency Care

T0256511

Website: Evidence-Based Medicine Series

The Evidence-Based Medicine Series has a website at:

www.evidencebasedseries.com

Where you can find:

- Links to companion websites with additional resources and updates for books in the series
- Details of all new and forthcoming titles
- Links to more Evidence-Based products: including the Cochrane Library, Essential Evidence Plus, and EBM Guidelines.

How to access the companion sites with additional resources and updates:

- Go to the Evidence-Based Series site:
  www.evidencebasedseries.com
- Select your book from the list of titles shown on the site
- If your book has a website with supplementary material, it will show an icon [Companion Website] next to the title
- Click on the icon to access the website

Evidence-Based Emergency Care

Diagnostic Testing and Clinical Decision Rules

Third Edition

Edited by

Jesse M. Pines, MD, MBA, MSCE
US Acute Care Solutions,
Canton, OH, USA
Department of Emergency Medicine,
Drexel University, Philadelphia, PA, USA

Fernanda Bellolio, MD, MSC
Department of Emergency Medicine,
Mayo Clinic, Rochester, MN, USA

Christopher R. Carpenter, MD, MSC
Department of Emergency Medicine,
Washington University School of Medicine, St. Louis, MO, USA

Ali S. Raja, MD, MBA, MPH
Department of Emergency Medicine,
Massachusetts General Hospital, Harvard Medical School,
Boston, MA, USA

WILEY Blackwell

To my wife Lori and my children Asher, Molly, and Oren for all their love and support

– Jesse M. Pines

To Daniel, my husband, colleague, and greatest cheerleader, and to Matilde and Javier for filling my life with fun and wisdom

– Fernanda Bellolio

To Panechanh, Cameron, and Kayla for continually inspiring me to learn and adapt

– Christopher R. Carpenter

To my wife and sons, for always being willing to put up with my crazy

– Ali S. Raja

Contents

Section 8: Miscellaneous: Hematology Ophthalmology Pulmonology Rheumatology and Geriatrics

About the Editors

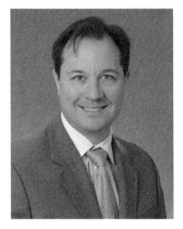

Jesse M. Pines, MD, MBA, MSCE is National Director of Clinical Innovation at US Acute Care Solutions and a Professor of Emergency Medicine at Drexel University. He is a board-certified emergency physician and practices at Allegheny General Hospital in Pittsburgh, PA. Dr. Pines previously held faculty positions at the George Washington University and the University of Pennsylvania. He previously served as the Director of Center for Healthcare Innovation and Policy Research (CHIPR) at George Washington University and prior to that served as the Director of the Center for Health Care Quality in the GW School of Public Health. Dr. Pines has served as a Senior Advisor at the U.S. Center for Medicare and Medicaid Services (CMS) Innovation Center, and a Visiting Scholar at the Brookings Institution. He has been a consultant to the National Quality Forum for >10 years. Dr. Pines holds a bachelor of arts and a master of science in clinical epidemiology from the University of Pennsylvania, and a medical degree and master of business administration from Georgetown University. He completed an emergency medicine residency at the University of Virginia, and a research fellowship at Penn. He is the author of more than 350 peer-reviewed manuscripts with a focus on emergency department quality of care, crowding, diagnostic testing, and economics. He lives in Arlington, Virginia with his wife Lori and his three children Asher, Molly, and Oren.

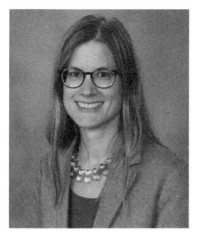

Fernanda Bellolio, MD, MS is a Professor of Emergency Medicine and Health Sciences Research at Mayo Clinic. She has a Master's in Clinical Research and Translational Sciences and completed a three-year post-doctoral program on Healthcare Delivery dedicated to secondary data analysis, research methodology, and evidence-based medicine at the Mayo Clinic Robert D. and Patricia E. Kern Center for the Science of Health Care Delivery. Dr. Bellolio is originally from Chile, and she was transplanted to Minnesota for the past 16 years (Winter season included). She has served in several financial, operational, and academic leadership roles within Mayo Clinic enterprise. She has experience in conducting observational and interventional studies, including studies on shared decision-making, diagnostic errors, claims data, and use of artificial intelligence-enhanced tools in the emergency department. Her current research is along the topics of geriatric care, delirium, outcomes prediction, pain management, and data synthesis for clinical practice guidelines.

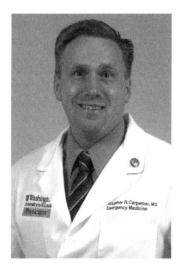

Christopher R. Carpenter, MD, MSc is a Professor of Emergency Medicine at Washington University in St. Louis. Dr. Carpenter holds a bachelor of science in Chemistry from Hope College and a master of science in clinical investigation from Washington University, and a medical degree from Wayne State University. After serving as a Diving Medical Office and General Medical Officer in the U.S. Navy, he completed a combined internal medicine-emergency medicine residency at Allegheny General Hospital. He is Deputy Editor-in-Chief of *Academic Emergency Medicine* and Associate Editor of the *Journal of the*

American Geriatrics Society and *Annals of Internal Medicine's* ACP Journal Club. At *Academic Emergency Medicine* he created the Evidence-Based Diagnostics series, as well as Guidelines for Reasonable and Appropriate Care in the Emergency Department (GRACE). He serves on the American College of Emergency Physician's Clinical Policy Committee and Clinician–Scientist in Transdisciplinary Aging Research Leadership Core. He is the author of more than 225 peer-reviewed manuscripts with a focus on geriatric emergency care, diagnostic testing, implementation science, and clinical practice guidelines. He lives in Missouri with his wife Panechanh, son Cameron, and daughter Kayla.

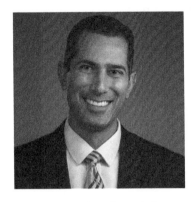

Ali S. Raja, MD, MBA, MPH is the Executive Vice Chair and the Mooney-Reed Endowed Chair in the Department of Emergency Medicine at Massachusetts General Hospital, as well as a Professor at Harvard Medical School. Dr. Raja received his MPH from Harvard, holds MD and MBA degrees from Duke and, after training in emergency medicine at the University of Cincinnati, completed a research fellowship at Brigham and Women's Hospital. He is board certified in emergency medicine and clinical informatics and is appointed to both the Departments of Emergency Medicine and Radiology at HMS.

A practicing emergency physician and author of over 250 publications, his research focuses on improving the appropriateness of resource utilization in emergency medicine. He serves on the Board of the Massachusetts Chapter of the American College of Healthcare Executives as President-Elect as well as the Boards of the Society for Academic Emergency Medicine and Boston MedFlight.

Dr. Raja is also an expert on the management of critically ill patients in the emergency department and prehospital arenas. He has served as a critical care air transport team commander for the US Air Force, a civilian flight physician, a tactical physician for a number of local, state, and federal agencies, and a physician with MA-1 DMAT.

List of Contributors

Jana L. Anderson, MD
Department of Emergency Medicine
Mayo Clinic, Rochester, MN, USA

John Bedolla, MD
Department of Surgery and Perioperative Care
Dell Medical School
University of Texas
Austin, TX, USA

Fernanda Bellolio, MD, MSc
Department of Emergency Medicine
Mayo Clinic, Rochester, MN, USA

W. Mason Bonner, PA
Department of Emergency Medicine
Mayo Clinic, Jacksonville, FL, USA

Christopher R. Carpenter, MD, MSc
Department of Emergency Medicine
Washington University School of Medicine
St. Louis, MO, USA

Brendan M. Carr, MD, MS
Department of Emergency Medicine
Mayo Clinic, Rochester, MN, USA

Ian T. Ferguson, MD, MPH
Department of Emergency Medicine
Washington University School of Medicine
St. Louis, MO, USA

Marianna M. Fischmann, MD
Department of Surgery
Pontifical Catholic University of Rio Grande do Sul
Porto Alegre, Brazil

Marc A. Probst, MD
Department of Emergency Medicine
Columbia University Irving Medical Center
New York, NY, USA

Amr Gharib, MD
Department of Emergency Medicine
University of Pittsburgh Medical Center, Harrisburg, PA, USA

Erik P. Hess
Vanderbilt University
Nashville, TN, USA

Lucas Oliveira Junqueira e Silva, MD, MSc
Department of Emergency Medicine
Hospital de Clínicas de Porto Alegre
Porto Alegre, Brazil

Department of Emergency Medicine
Mayo Clinic, Rochester, MN, USA

Jesse M. Pines, MD, MBA, MSCE
US Acute Care Solutions, Canton, OH, USA

Department of Emergency Medicine
Drexel University, Philadelphia, PA, USA

Ali S. Raja, MD, MBA, MPH
Department of Emergency Medicine
Massachusetts General Hospital
Harvard Medical School, Boston, MA, USA

Jonathan Sheele, MD, MHS, MPH
Department of Emergency Medicine
Mayo Clinic, Jacksonville, FL, USA

Lauren Westafer, DO, MPH
Department of Emergency Medicine
University of Massachusetts Chan Medical School – Baystate
Springfield, MA, USA

Foreword

Thank you to Dr. Jesse M. Pines, Dr. Fernanda Bellolio, Dr. Christopher R. Carpenter, and Dr. Ali S. Raja for this third edition of your excellent book *Evidence-Based Emergency Care: Diagnostic Testing and Clinical Decision Rules*. It is an honor and privilege to be writing the foreword.

Emergency physicians are many things, but one of the most important things we try to be is great diagnosticians. Every shift we use limited information in a busy, chaotic environment to make decisions. Sometimes, those decisions can mean life or death and need to be made quickly. We strive to be the best at exercising this important responsibility. This is the book that can help clinicians achieve that goal.

The first and second edition of *Evidence-Based Emergency Care: Diagnostic Testing and Clinical Decision Rules* is a resource I have used regularly throughout my career. It has made me a better diagnostician and better physician. Questions come up on every shift as to what evidence supports our actions. This fantastic book provides answers to those questions in a brief and helpful way. I am often accessing it for my own needs and as an educational resource for students.

The third edition contains the foundational elements of providing excellent evidence-based medicine (EBM) care. The authors start by discussing diagnostic testing in the emergency department (ED). They explain the epidemiology and statistics behind diagnostic testing. They appropriately emphasize that clinical decision instruments are tools to guide care, not rules to dictate care. They touch upon the additional responsibility of being good stewards given the realities of limited resources. They also provide a chapter to help clinicians understand the direction of bias in diagnostic research.

The third edition covers dozens of common and deadly conditions clinicians are faced with in the ED. This includes chapters on pediatrics, geriatrics, cardiac, neurological, surgical, trauma, infectious disease, and other conditions.

There are four new chapters in the latest edition of the book: Skin and Soft Tissue Infection, Shared Decision Making, Cognitive Bias, and Telemedicine

Diagnosis. There are all wonderful additions to the book. My favorite new chapter is the one discussing Shared Decision Making (SDM).

SDM goes beyond informed consent and recognizes the autonomy and agency of patients. We are making important decisions that must consider patients' values and preferences. This is one of the three pillars of EBM. While we may be the experts in clinical medicine, patients are experts in their own personal experiences. There are many examples where SDM can be utilized in the ED in my clinical experience to enrich the therapeutic patient–physician alliance.

If you want to provide patients the best care, based on contemporary evidence then this is your book.

Ken Milne, MD, MSc
Professor of Emergency Medicine
University of Western Ontario
London, Ontario, Canada

Acknowledgments

We would like to thank Susan Kirk in the Department of Emergency Medicine at Mayo Clinic for all her work in helping coordinate permissions for the third edition and other administrative support.

Jesse M. Pines,
Fernanda Bellolio,
Christopher R. Carpenter,
and Ali S. Raja

SECTION 1
The Science of Diagnostic Testing and Clinical Decision Rules

Chapter 1 **Diagnostic Testing in Emergency Care**

Jesse M. Pines[1,2] and Christopher R. Carpenter[3]

[1] US Acute Care Solutions, Canton, OH, USA
[2] Department of Emergency Medicine, Drexel University, Philadelphia, PA, USA
[3] Department of Emergency Medicine, Washington University School of Medicine, St. Louis, MO, USA

Highlights

- Emergency physicians are experts in diagnostic testing
- The choice of ED-based testing depends on the resources of the hospital
- Validated clinical decision rules can help guide ED testing decisions
- Pauker and Kassirer test-treatment thresholds are a helpful tool in determining the use and value of diagnostic tests

---

As emergency department (ED) physicians, we spend a good deal of our time ordering, interpreting, and waiting for the results of diagnostic tests. ED physicians are the experts when it comes to determining who needs a test to rule out a potentially life-threatening condition. There are several reasons for this expertise. First and foremost, we see a lot of patients with undifferentiated symptoms in a decision-dense and time-constrained environment. Especially for those working in busy hospitals, the expectation is to see everyone in a timely way, provide quality care, and ensure patients have a good experience. Some patients and consultants value lab or imaging tests more than the history and physical exam tests that formulate clinical intuition, a phenomenon called "technological tenesmus."[1] However, if we order time-consuming tests on everyone, ED crowding and inefficiency will worsen, costs of care will go

---

Evidence-Based Emergency Care: Diagnostic Testing and Clinical Decision Rules, Third Edition.
Edited by Jesse M. Pines, Fernanda Bellolio, Christopher R. Carpenter, and Ali S. Raja.
© 2023 John Wiley & Sons Ltd. Published 2023 by John Wiley & Sons Ltd.

up, and patients will experience even longer waits than they already do. In addition, there is increased pressure to carefully choose who needs and who does not need tests in an evidence-based manner, particularly as costs of care have risen so dramatically in recent years particularly in the United States.[2,3]

Differentiating which patients will benefit from ED testing is a complex process. Over the past 40 years, science and research in ED diagnostic testing and clinical decision rules have advanced considerably. Today, there is a greater understanding of test performance, specifically the reliability, sensitivity, specificity, and overall accuracy of tests. Validated clinical decision rules exist to provide objective criteria to help distinguish who does and does not need a test. Serious, potentially life-threatening conditions such as intracranial bleeding and cervical spine (C-spine) fractures can be safely ruled out based on clinical grounds alone, with acceptable accuracy and precision. There are also accurate risk stratification tools to estimate the probability for conditions like pulmonary embolism (PE) before any tests are even ordered. Since the second edition of this textbook, *Academic Emergency Medicine* created the "Evidence-Based Diagnostics" series to synthesize the ever-expanding volume of emergency medicine-specific research around history, physical exam, labs, and imaging for common diagnoses like subarachnoid hemorrhage, congestive heart failure, urinary tract infection, and mesenteric ischemia.[4,5] Similarly, the Society for Academic Emergency Medicine launched Guidelines for Reasonable and Appropriate Care to provide emergency medicine's first Grading of Recommendations Assessment Development and Evaluation (GRADE)-based diagnostic recommendations that contemplate issues like costs and health inequities.[6-8] This third edition will summarize the key recommendations from these two new resources.

How do we decide who to test and who not to test? There are some patients who clearly need tests, such as the head-injured patient who has altered mental status and who may have a head bleed. In such a case, the outcome may be dependent upon how quickly the bleeding can be detected with a computed tomography (CT) scan. There are also patients who obviously do not need tests at an individual point in time, such as patients with a simple toothache or a mild headache without concerning features. Finally, there is a large group of patients in the middle for whom testing decisions can sometimes be challenging. This group of patients may leave you feeling "on the fence" about testing. In this large middle category, it may not be clear whether to order a test or even how to interpret a test once you have the results. And when unexpected test results come back, it may not be clear how best to use those results to guide patient care.

Let us give some examples of how diagnostic testing can be a challenge in the ED. You are starting your shift and are signed out a patient for whom your colleague has ordered a D-dimer assay (a test for PE). She is 83 years old and developed acute shortness of breath, chest pain, and hypoxia (room air oxygen saturation = 89%). She has a history of a prior PE and her physical examination is unremarkable, except for mild left anterior chest wall tenderness and notably clear lung sounds. The D-dimer comes back negative. Has PE been satisfactorily ruled out? Should you order a CT scan of the chest, or maybe even consider a ventilation–perfusion (V/Q) scan? Was D-dimer the right test for her to begin with?

Let's consider a different scenario. Consider a positive D-dimer assay in a 22-year-old male with atypical chest pain, no risk factors, and normal physical examination including a heart rate of 70 beats per minute and an oxygen saturation of 100% on room air. What do you do then? Would he benefit from a CT scan of the chest to further evaluate the possibility of PE? What are the potential harms of liberally obtaining CT on every patient in whom the physician or the patient is concerned about PE just to be absolutely certain? Or is he so low risk that he's probably fine anyway? Of course, you might wonder, if he was so low risk, why was the D-dimer ordered in the first place?

As a third example, you are evaluating a 77-year-old female who has fallen down, has acute hip pain, and is unable to ambulate. The hip radiograph is negative. Should you pursue CT or magnetic resonance imaging (MRI) for a radiographically occult hip fracture? While you contemplate time-consuming advanced imaging, you also consider that regardless of whether or not CT or MRI demonstrates no fracture will she be able to go home?

These are examples of when test results may not confirm you're *a priori* clinical suspicion. What do you do in those cases? Should you believe the test result or believe your clinical judgment before ordering the test? Were these the optimal tests in the first place? Remember back to conversations with your professors in emergency medicine on diagnostic testing. Didn't they always ask, "How will a test result change your management?" and "What will you do if it's positive, negative, or indeterminate?"

The purpose of diagnostic testing is to reach a state where we are adequately convinced of the presence or absence of a condition. Test results must be interpreted in the context of the prevalence of the suspected disease state: your clinical suspicion of the presence or absence of disease in the individual patient. For example, coronary artery disease is common. However, if we look for coronary disease in a young healthy population, we are unlikely to find it because it is not common in young people. There are also times when your clinical suspicion is so high that you do not need objective testing. In certain patients, you can proceed with treatment. For example, some emergency physicians may choose to treat a dislocated shoulder based on the clinical examination rather than first obtaining a radiograph, particularly in patients with a history of prior dislocations. However, testing is often needed to confirm a diagnosis or to rule out more severe, life-threatening diseases.

The choice over whether to test or not test in the ED also depends upon the resources of the hospital and of the patient. Most hospitals allow easy access to radiographic testing and laboratory testing. In other hospitals, obtaining a diagnostic test may not be as easy. Some hospitals may not have the staff available for certain types of tests at night or on weekends (like MRIs and ultrasounds). Sometimes patients may not need a test if you believe that they are reliable to return if symptoms worsen. For others, you may believe that a patient's emergency presentation may be the only time he or she will have access to diagnostic testing. For example, saying to a patient, "Follow up with your doctor this week for a stress test" may be impractical if the patient does not have a primary doctor or does not have good access to medical care. Many clinicians practice in environments where they cannot order a lot of tests (like developing countries). You also may practice in an office environment that simply does not have easy access to testing. However, regardless of the reason why we order tests in the ED or other acute settings, what is certain is that the use of diagnostic testing in many cases can change how you manage a patient's care.

Sometimes, you may question your choice of whether to test, to not test, or to involve a specialist early. Should you get a CT scan first or just call a surgeon in for a young male with right lower quadrant pain, fever, nausea, and possible appendicitis? How many cases have you seen where the CT scan has changed your management? What if the patient is a young, nonpregnant female? Does that change your plan? What is the differential diagnosis for these symptoms in your patient and how likely are each possible diagnosis? How knowledgeable are your consultants about the additive value (or lack thereof) for the different test options and multidisciplinary consensus recommendations?[9]

How about using clinical decision rules in practice? By determining if patients meet specific clinical criteria, we can choose not to test some patients if they are low risk. Do all patients with ankle sprains need X-rays? Can you use the Ottawa ankle rules in children? What are the limits of clinical decision rules? Is it possible to apply the Canadian C-spine rules to a 70-year-old female? What is sufficiently "low risk"? These questions come up daily in the practice of emergency medicine. In fact, a major source of variability among physicians is whether or not they order tests. Remember back to your training when you were getting ready to present a patient to the attending physician. Weren't you trying to think to yourself, "What would she do in this case? What tests would she order?"

Access to test results helps us decide whether to treat a disease, initiate even more testing, or no longer worry about a condition. The cognitive psychology of clinical decision-making also has evolved rapidly over the last several decades. As ED physicians, we gain confidence in this process with experience. Much of the empirical science and mathematics behind testing that are described in this book become instinctive and intuitive the longer you practice emergency medicine. Sometimes, we may think a patient does not need to be tested because the last hundred patients who had similar presentations all had negative tests. Maybe you or your colleagues were "burned" once when a subtle clinical presentation of a life-threatening condition was missed (like a subarachnoid hemorrhage). The next patient who presents with those symptoms is probably more likely to get a head CT followed by a lumbar puncture. Is this evidence based? Recognizing our individual diagnostic biases is one way to decrease the likelihood of erroneous decision-making while increasing efficiency and effectiveness. This is discussed later in Chapter 60 on Cognitive Bias in more detail, which is new to the third edition of the book.

Step back for a moment and think about what we do when ordering a test. After evaluating a patient, we come away with a differential diagnosis of both the most common and the most life-threatening possibilities. The following approach to medical decision-making was derived by Pauker and Kassirer in 1980.[10] Imagine diagnostic testing as two separate thresholds, each denoted as "I" (for *indeterminate*). The scale at the bottom of Figure 1.1 denotes pretest probability, which is the probability of the disease in question before any testing is employed. In practice, it is often a challenge to come up with a pretest probability, and frequently opinions on pretest probability differ considerably between experienced physicians. However, for the moment, assume that pretest probability is a known quantity.

In Figure 1.1, the threshold between "don't test" and "test" is known as the *testing threshold*. The threshold between "test" and "treat" is known as the *test–treatment threshold*. In this schema, treatment should be withheld if the pretest probability of disease is smaller than the testing threshold, and no testing should be performed. Treatment should be given without testing if the pretest probability of disease is above the test–treatment threshold. And, when our pretest probability lies between the testing and test–treatment

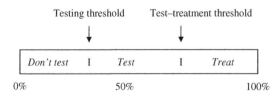

Figure 1.1 Pretest probability of disease. (Data from Pauker and Kassirer [10].)

thresholds, the test should be performed and the patients treated according to the test results.

Calculation of the testing threshold and the test–treatment threshold include seven variables:

1. $P_{pos/d}$ – The probability of a positive test in patients with disease (i.e., sensitivity)
2. $P_{neg/d}$ – The probability of a negative test in patients with disease (1-sensitivity)
3. $P_{pos/nd}$ – Probability of a positive test result in patients without disease (1-specificity)
4. $P_{neg/nd}$ – Probability of a negative test result in patients without disease (i.e., specificity)
5. B_{rx} – The benefit of treatment in patients with disease
6. R_{rx} – The risk of treatment in patients with disease
7. R_t – The risk of the diagnostic test.

Using these variables together, Figure 1.2 demonstrates the formula for the testing and test–treatment thresholds.

The *Academic Emergency Medicine* "Evidence-Based Diagnostics" series described above provides estimates of pretest probability for common diagnoses based on a synthesis of ED research and then presents an interactive test–treatment threshold calculator based on this Pauker–Kassirer theory.

But now let us make this more clinically relevant. Sometimes the disease is clinically apparent, and we do not need confirmatory testing before proceeding with treatment. If you are evaluating a patient with an obvious cellulitis, you may choose to give antibiotics before initiating any testing. How about a 50-year-old male with acute chest pain who on his electrocardiogram (ECG) has large inferior "tombstone" ST-segment elevations consistent with acute myocardial infarction (AMI)? Cardiac markers will not be very helpful in the acute management of this patient. This is an example of a situation in which it is important to treat the patient first: give the patient aspirin and/or other antiplatelet agents, anticoagulation, and other resuscitative treatments and send him off to the cardiac catheterization lab if your hospital has one, arrange for transfer, or provide intravenous thrombolysis if cardiac catheterization is not readily available. Well, now imagine that the patient has a history of Marfan's syndrome and you think he is having an AMI, but you

$$T_t \text{ (testing threshold)} = (P_{pos/nd}) \times (R_{rx}) + R_t \ / \ (P_{pos/nd}) \times (R_{rx}) + (P_{pos/d}) \times (B_{rx})$$

$$T_{trx} \text{ (test-treatment threshold)} = (P_{neg/nd}) \times (R_{rx}) - R_t \ / \ (P_{neg/nd}) \times (R_{rx}) + (P_{neg/d}) \times (B_{rx})$$

Figure 1.2 The formulas for the testing and test–treatment threshold. (Adapted from Pauker and Kassirer [10].)

want to get a chest X-ray or even a CT scan to make sure he does not have an aortic dissection before you anticoagulate him. That might put you on the "test" side of the line.

Now imagine the scenario of the potential use for tissue plasminogen activator (tPA) in stroke, a situation frequently encountered in the ED. When a patient comes to the ED within the first few hours of the onset of her stroke symptoms, you rush to get her to the CT scanner. Why? The primary reason is to differentiate between ischemic and hemorrhagic stroke, which will make a major difference in whether or not the patient is even eligible to receive tPA.

Now imagine cases that fall below the testing threshold. You have a 32-year-old male with what sounds like musculoskeletal chest pain. Many would argue that the patient does not need any emergency tests at all if he is otherwise healthy and the physical examination is normal. Others might get a chest X-ray and an ECG to rule out occult things like pneumothorax and heart disease, while some others may even get a D-dimer to rule out PE. What is the right way to manage the patient? Is there any evidence behind that decision, or is it just the physician's preference? In some patients, at the end of the ED evaluation, you may not have a definitive answer. Imagine a 45-year-old female with atypical chest pain, a normal ECG, and normal cardiac markers, who you are evaluating at a hospital that does not perform stress testing from the ED. Does she need a hospital admission or observation to rule out AMI and a stress test?

The way that Pauker and Kassirer designed the test–treatment thresholds more than 40 years ago did not account for the proliferation of "confirmatory" diagnostic testing in hospitals. While the lower bound testing threshold is certainly lower than it has ever been, the upper bound threshold has also increased to the point where we are sometimes loath to treat before testing, even when the diagnosis seems apparent. The reason for this is that Occam's razor often does not hold true in emergency medicine. What is Occam's razor? Fourteenth-century philosopher William of Occam stated, "Plurality must not be posited without necessity," which has been interpreted to mean, "Among competing hypotheses, favor the simplest one."[11] When applied to test–treatment thresholds, what we find is that a patient with objective findings for what might seem like pneumonia (e.g., hypoxia, infiltrates, and a history of cough) likely does have pneumonia, and should be treated empirically, but may also have a PE. While finding that parsimony of diagnosis is important, often the principle of test–treatment thresholds means that if you're above the test–treatment threshold, then you should certainly treat the patient but also consider testing more, particularly in patients with objective signs of additional disease.

Think about how trauma surgeons practice. In the multi-injured trauma patient, is not their approach to test, test, test? In a seriously injured patient trauma surgeons often default to scanning everything (aka the *pan-scan*) despite evidence demonstrating no patient-centric benefit.[12] Some surgeons order CT scans of areas in which the patient has no complaints. They argue that this approach is not illogical. When a patient has been in a major car accident and has a broken left femur, a broken left radius, and mild abdominal tenderness, do they need more CT scans to rule out intra-abdominal injuries and intracranial injuries? Where Occam's razor dulls is that while the most parsimonious diagnosis (just radial and femoral fractures) is possible, patients with multiple traumatic injuries tend to have not only the obvious ones but also occult injuries. This may necessitate a diagnostic search for the occult intra-abdominal, intrathoracic, and intracranial injuries in a patient with an obviously broken arm and leg, but the balance between careful trauma imaging and over-testing harms continues to be defined.[13]

Risk tolerance refers to the posttest probability at which we are comfortable with excluding or confirming a disease. That is, risk tolerance is where we are comfortable setting our own testing and test–treatment thresholds; it guides where we draw these thresholds and how much we do or do not search for the occult.[14,15] When deciding on care plans, we develop our own risk tolerance based on our training, clinical expertise, and experiences, as well as local standard practice and the attitudes of the patient, family, or other physicians caring for the patient.

For example, consider possible acute coronary syndrome.[16] After your ED evaluation with cardiac markers, an ECG, and a chest X-ray, you estimate that your patient has a 2% risk of having an unexpected cardiac event within 30 days if he is sent home without additional testing. Is it OK to send him home with this level of risk? Isn't 2% the published rate for missed AMI?[17] What if the risk is 1%, or 0.5%, or 0.1%? If you send someone home with a HEART score less than 3, what is their actual risk of a major adverse cardiovascular event within 6 weeks?[18] Does that differ if their HEART score is zero or if it's 3?

How do you make the decision about when to order a test or just treat? How do you assign a pretest probability? How do you apply test results to an individual patient and communicate our clinical impression, level of certainty, and subsequent management options with those patients?[19] This is where research and the practice of evidence-based medicine (EBM) can influence practice by taking the best evidence in the literature about diagnostic testing or clinical decision rules and using that information to make an informed decision about how to care for patients. Chapters 2 and 3 provide an updated overview of the process of EBM as well as examples of the application of EBM to individual patients in the ED, levels of evidence, and how to evaluate a body of literature on diagnostic testing. Chapter 4 is a revised discussion of how we derive, validate, and study the impact of clinical decision rules in practice. Chapter 5, a new chapter in the second edition of this book, reviews recent trends in health policy that may force us to reduce test ordering and use clinical decision rules. Chapter 6 describes various forms of bias that can skew estimates of diagnostic accuracy in research settings. Chapter 59 is a new chapter that explores the science and potential of shared decision-making in ED settings.

Understanding the evidence behind diagnostic testing and using clinical decision rules to decide when not to test is at the core of emergency medicine practice. Think back to your last shift in the ED: how many tests did you order?

The purpose of this book is to demystify the evidence behind diagnostic testing and clinical decision rules in emergency care by carefully evaluating the evidence behind our everyday decision-making in the ED. This book is written to provide objective information on the evidence behind these questions through the lens of seasoned ED clinicians who are also diagnostic testing researchers, while providing our opinion on how we manage our patients with specific clinical problems given the best available evidence. It should be noted that we are writing this from the perspective of academic emergency physicians. We all work in mostly academic EDs or well-resourced community EDs with abundant (although not always quick) access to consultants, state-of-the-art laboratories, and high-resolution imaging tests. As you read this, realize that not all emergency medicine practice is the same and you should interpret the literature yourself in the context of your own clinical practice environment.

We have designed each chapter around clinical questions that come up in everyday emergency medicine practice. In the third edition of the book, we have added more chapters and updated all of the old chapters to include new and relevant studies or insights that have emerged in the literature since the second edition was published in 2013. For each question, we present the objective data from published studies and then provide our "expert" comments on how we use these tests in our practice. While we try to provide insight into how we interpret the literature for each testing approach, again, our comments should not be interpreted as the standard of care in emergency medicine. Standard of care is based on practice guidelines and local practice patterns. Instead, these chapters should serve as a forum or basis for discussion. If you are a researcher, you can also think of this book as a roadmap to what is really "known" or "not known" with regard to diagnostic testing in emergency medicine and what needs further study. Finally, rigorous and sound research often takes months to years to accomplish, and sometimes longer to publish. Therefore, the discussions we present are likely to change as newer, larger, more comprehensive studies are published, as new prediction or decision rules are validated and replicated, and as newer diagnostic technology is introduced.

References

1. Fatovich DM. The inverted U curve and emergency medicine: Overdiagnosis and the law of unintended consequences. *Emergency Medicine Australasia.* 2016; 28(4): 480–2.

2. Carpenter CR, Raja AS, Brown MD. Overtesting and the downstream consequences of overtreatment: Implications of "preventing overdiagnosis" for emergency medicine. *Academic Emergency Medicine.* 2015; 22(12): 1484–92.

3. Venkatesh AK, Scofi JE, Rothenberg C et al. Choosing wisely in emergency medicine: Early results and insights from the ACEP emergency quality network (E-QUAL). *The American Journal of Emergency Medicine.* 2021; 39: 102–8.

4. Carpenter CR, Hussain AM, Ward MJ et al. Spontaneous subarachnoid hemorrhage: A systematic review and meta-analysis describing the diagnostic accuracy of history, physical examination, imaging, and lumbar puncture with an exploration of test thresholds. *Academic Emergency Medicine.* 2016; 23(9): 963–1003.

5. Martindale JL, Wakai A, Collins SP et al. Diagnosing acute heart failure in the emergency department: A systematic review and meta-analysis. *Academic Emergency Medicine.* 2016; 23(3): 223–42.

6. Musey PI Jr, Bellolio F, Upadhye S et al. Guidelines for reasonable and appropriate care in the emergency department (GRACE): Recurrent, low-risk chest pain in the emergency department. *Academic Emergency Medicine.* 2021; 28(7): 718–44.

7. Schünemann HJ, Oxman AD, Brozek J et al. GRADE Working Group. Grading quality of evidence and strength of recommendations for diagnostic tests and strategies. *BMJ.* 2008; 336(7653): 1106–10.

8. Carpenter CR, Bellolio MF, Upadhye S, Kline JA. Navigating uncertainty with GRACE: Society for Academic Emergency Medicine's guidelines for reasonable and appropriate care in the emergency department. *Academic Emergency Medicine.* 2021; 28(7): 821–5.

9. Moore CL, Carpenter CR, Heilbrun ME et al. Imaging in suspected renal colic: Systematic review of the literature and multispecialty consensus. *Annals of Emergency Medicine.* 2019; 74(3): 391–9.

10. Pauker SG, Kassirer JP. The threshold approach to clinical decision making. *New England Journal of Medicine.* 1980; 302: 1109–17.

11. Drachman DA. Occam's razor, geriatric syndromes, and the dizzy patient. *Annals of Internal Medicine.* 2000; 132(5): 403–4.

12. Sierink JC, Treskes K, Edwards MJ et al. REACT-2 study group. Immediate total-body CT scanning versus conventional imaging and selective CT scanning in patients with severe trauma (REACT-2): A randomised controlled trial. *Lancet.* 2016; 388(10045): 673–83.

13. Hoffman JR, Carpenter CR. Guarding against overtesting, overdiagnosis, and overtreatment of older adults: Thinking beyond imaging and injuries to weigh harms and benefits. *Journal of the American Geriatrics Society.* 2017; 65(5): 903–5.

14. Pines JM, Szyld D. Risk tolerance for the exclusion of potentially life-threatening diseases in the ED. *The American Journal of Emergency Medicine.* 2007; 25(5): 540–4.

15. Pines JM, Hollander JE, Isserman JA *et al.* The association between physician risk tolerance and imaging use in abdominal pain. *The American Journal of Emergency Medicine.* 2009; 27(5): 552–7.

16. Pines JM, Isserman JA, Szyld D, Dean AJ, McCusker CM, Hollander JE. The effect of physician risk tolerance and the presence of an observation unit on decision making for ED patients with chest pain. *The American Journal of Emergency Medicine.* 2010; 28(7): 771–9.

17. Schull MJ, Vermeulen MJ, Stukel TA. The risk of missed diagnosis of acute myocardial infarction associated with emergency department volume. *Annals of Emergency Medicine.* 2006; 48(6): 647–55.

18. Fernando SM, Tran A, Cheng W *et al.* Prognostic accuracy of the HEART score for prediction of major adverse cardiac events in patients presenting with chest pain: A systematic review and meta-analysis. *Academic Emergency Medicine.* 2019; 26(2): 140–51.

19. Hess EP, Grudzen CR, Thomson R, Raja AS, Carpenter CR. Shared decision-making in the emergency department: Respecting patient autonomy when seconds count. *Academic Emergency Medicine.* 2015; 22(7): 856–64.

Chapter 2 **Evidence-Based Medicine: The Process**

Ali S. Raja[1] and Jesse M. Pines[2,3]

[1] Department of Emergency Medicine, Massachusetts General Hospital, Harvard Medical School, Boston, MA, USA
[2] US Acute Care Solutions, Canton, OH, USA
[3] Department of Emergency Medicine, Drexel University, Philadelphia, PA, USA

The process we use in this book has been termed evidence-based medicine (EBM). The first question is "What is EBM?" EBM has been defined as "the conscientious, explicit and judicious use of current best evidence in making decisions about the care of patients."[1] However, evidence alone does not define EBM. Instead, EBM occurs within the context of clinical expertise and incorporates each patient's unique circumstances and preferences. The best way to describe EBM in the emergency department (ED) is as a process by which we: (i) ask relevant, focused clinical questions to answer (ii) search for literature to answer this question, (iii) critically appraise the literature and make conclusions with an understanding of the strength of evidence behind particular recommendations, and (iv) apply the evidence to the way that individual patients in the ED are managed. In this book, we use the process of EBM to answer important and relevant clinical questions regarding the use of diagnostic testing and clinical decision rules in the ED. Most of the questions we ask and attempt to answer have to do with how to use, when to use, and how much to trust diagnostic testing and clinical decision rules, followed by how to apply published knowledge to individual patients. However, EBM can also be used for other applications in emergency medicine outside of diagnostic testing, such as the determination of which treatment is best for an individual patient.

Evidence-Based Emergency Care: Diagnostic Testing and Clinical Decision Rules, Third Edition.
Edited by Jesse M. Pines, Fernanda Bellolio, Christopher R. Carpenter, and Ali S. Raja.
© 2023 John Wiley & Sons Ltd. Published 2023 by John Wiley & Sons Ltd.

Table 2.1 The steps in practicing and applying evidence-based medicine (EBM) to diagnostic testing in the ED

Step 1: Formulate a clear question from a patient's problem. Does this patient need a test? Which test does she need? For example, does a patient with atypical chest pain who is otherwise low risk need a troponin? You may ask yourself, "How accurate is troponin I as a screening test for acute coronary syndrome in ED patients?" Ask yourself, "Is this an answerable question?"

Step 2: Search the literature for clinical articles that have addressed this question. Ideally, the sample will include ED patients with a similar complaint or disease process (i.e., patients with chest pain who are at low risk for acute coronary syndrome where troponin has been studied). You might start by doing searches on patients with chest pain in the ED and then narrow your search to articles that deal with the use of cardiac biomarkers.

Step 3: Read and critically appraise the articles for validity and applicability to the individual patient. That is, you can ask yourself, "Would the patient have met the inclusion criteria for this study?" or "Is this patient similar to patients who were included in the study?"

Step 4: Use the study findings and apply them to the care of an individual patient (e.g., does this patient need a troponin I? How should I approach the use of cardiac troponins in the ED?).

The purpose of this chapter is to review the steps of EBM in detail and to discuss how to use EBM in the practice of emergency medicine with regard to diagnostic testing. The practice of EBM is a process that follows four simple steps (see Table 2.1).

EBM queries can be broken down into two categories: (i) general medical questions (e.g., what is the sensitivity of urine dipstick testing in diagnosing urinary tract infections?) and (ii) specific patient-based questions (e.g., in a 45-year-old female without risk factors with atypical chest pain and nonspecific electrocardiogram (ECG) changes, what is the value of a negative troponin?). In general, throughout this book, we ask the former: general medical questions. We recommend that you use our presentation of the literature as a model, from which you can use this same process to answer specific questions and apply your own interpretation of the literature to guide diagnostic plans within the context of your clinical environment.

The acronym PICO has been used to define the four elements of an answerable question regarding a diagnostic test.[2] PICO refers to (P) patient or population, (I) investigation, (C) comparison (i.e., what is the criterion standard?), and (O) outcome of interest. In our prior example, P = women in their 40s without cardiac risk factors, I = troponin I measurement, C = cardiac catheterization or possible coronary angiogram, and O = identification of an intervenable coronary artery lesion or the presence of coronary artery disease (for risk stratification).

Once you have come up with a clinical question that is answerable, the search begins. For those with access to online databases (such as MEDLINE or others), it is probably best to start there because you can enter specific search criteria and narrow your search as appropriate. Websites such as PubMed (www.pubmed.com) allow free access to abstracts and some full-text articles; sometimes hospitals and universities will allow a greater level of access to full-text articles through institutional memberships. You may also choose to use other resources such as UpToDate, which examines the latest literature on a particular topic, and sometimes makes evidence-based treatment recommendations. Other resources include EMBASE, LILACS, CINAHL, the Cochrane Collaboration, and others. There are many other sources to use to search for medical information, and one way to get an idea of what your hospital or school offers is to sit down with a reference librarian in your local medical library and get a tour of all the resources. This is a rapidly evolving area, and it is important that twenty-first-century providers are aware of current diagnostic and treatment technologies, as well as the latest electronic search engines to best access information about EBM.

OK, you are logged on to a MEDLINE database. What now? You can either search by using a specific set of search criteria like *troponin* and *chest pain* or use a more rigorous approach such as using the medical subject headings (MeSH) system. MeSH is a vocabulary that is used to index articles in MEDLINE and PubMed. It is probably a more consistent way to search because sometimes different terminology is used for the same topic. Just as what the Brits call the *boot* is what Americans call a *trunk*, these differences are even more common in medical terminology. For example, you may want to know about shortness of breath, but papers may use other terms such as respiratory distress, dyspnea, or breathlessness. Another way to search PubMed more efficiently is by using a "Clinical Query," which allows the user to search for clinical research by study category: therapy, etiology, diagnosis, prognosis, or clinical prediction guide.[3] Another common trick to use is imposing "Limits" on your search, which allows you to search for articles by a specific type only, such as a systematic review article, or to limit searches to specific age ranges, gender, publication dates, and language of publication. After finding the best evidence you can identify on a clinical topic, then conduct your own critical appraisal of the literature. Traditionally, assessment of the literature surrounding a clinical topic is good fodder for group discussion in either a conference or a residency journal club, but you can also go directly to the literature to answer important and relevant clinical questions.

Assessment of studies about diagnostic tests involves four critical steps,[4] detailed in Table 2.2. Assessing studies on clinical decision rules is similar and also involves four steps, which are detailed in Table 2.3.[5]

Table 2.2 The steps in assessing studies on diagnostic testing

Step 1: Was there an independent, blind comparison with a criterion standard (i.e., gold standard) for diagnosis? Examples of relevant criterion standards in emergency medicine include surgical evaluation or biopsy results for patients with appendicitis, cardiac catheterization results for patients with possible acute coronary syndrome, and pulmonary angiogram results for patients with potential pulmonary embolism. There may also be other ways to incompletely measure a criterion standard, as in pulmonary embolism, the use of a negative chest CT scan followed by negative leg ultrasounds.

Step 2: Was the diagnostic test under question evaluated in the same population of patients as the patient in question? You can stratify this question by age, gender, location (e.g., were they ED patients?), or presenting symptoms (e.g., patients with chest pain). That is, when I read that the sensitivity for D-dimer is 95% in a meta-analysis, is my patient similar to those who were included in the studies?

Step 3: Did all patients have the reference standard test or follow-up whereby you can be convinced that the test was either positive or negative? An example of this is: if we perform the criterion standard test only on patients with positive tests, this may skew the results of our assessment of sensitivity. For example, if we do temporal artery biopsies only on patients with positive erythrocyte sedimentation rates (ESRs), we may miss some patients who had a negative ESR and would have had a positive biopsy. This is called *verification bias*.

Step 4: Has the test been validated in another independent group of patients? This is particularly concerning when the test is derived and validated in a specific population. For example, if a diagnostic test works well in Canada, does that mean it will have the same test characteristics in the United States?

Source: Data from [4].

Table 2.3 The steps in assessing studies on clinical decision rules

Step 1: Were the patients chosen in an unbiased fashion, and do the study patients represent a wide spectrum of severity of disease? For example, did the enrollment criteria for assessing the Canadian head CT rule include patients ranging from those with minor bumps with a brief loss of consciousness to those with major head injuries?

Step 2: Was there a blinded assessment of the criterion standard for all patients? That is, e.g., did all patients who were enrolled in the study have CT scans?

Step 3: Was there an explicit and accurate interpretation of the predictor variables and the actual rule without knowledge of the outcome? (e.g., were the study forms filled out before the physicians had knowledge of the CT results?) Was there an assessment of interrater reliability?

Step 4: Was follow-up obtained for 100% of patients who were enrolled? For example, for patients who were discharged, were they followed up to ensure that they did not have pain, any positive head CT, or poor outcome in a specific time period?

Source: Data from [5].

If you read a study or series of studies about a test or a clinical decision rule that do not meet the criteria detailed in either Table 2.2 or 2.3, you should be appropriately skeptical. However, in actual practice and as we found in writing this book, topics with research sufficient to fulfill all these specifications are the exception rather than the norm. In that case, what we need to do is interpret the literature while cognizant of potential weaknesses and do our best to apply the results to how we practice medicine. Certainly, for some tests, there may be a huge literature from which we can make strong recommendations (e.g., for D-dimer or the Ottawa ankle rules). For others, like using erythrocyte sedimentation rates (ESRs) to rule out temporal arteritis, there may be no literature that meets all of these requirements.

The next step is to use these findings by applying them to individual patients. Chapter 3 describes in detail the terms *sensitivity, specificity, likelihood ratios*, and *Bayesian analysis* while illustrating the mathematics behind the practical application of what we learn from studies to individual patients. By determining a specific pretest probability (or prevalence) of the disease in a particular patient, we are then able to not only calculate a posttest probability but also decide whether we need to perform the test at all.

The purpose of diagnostic testing in the ED is not necessarily to reach 100% certainty. Instead, we are trying to reduce the level of uncertainty to allow us to optimize medical decision-making. In order to move between the test and test–treatment thresholds, we need to remember back to Chapter 1 and only order tests that ultimately change patient management by moving us over a specific threshold.

Potential pitfalls exist in applying EBM to diagnostic testing and clinical decision rules. The first is trying to describe the "P" component (patient or population) of the PICO question without being too exclusive. Let us say we are trying to determine the sensitivity for troponin I in a 45-year-old woman with atypical chest pain and a nondiagnostic ECG. There is likely not any specific study that describes sensitivity of troponin only in 45-year-old women with that exact description. On the other hand, if we are too vague in how we choose the "P" component, it can become similarly frustrating. For example, let us say we wanted to determine the test sensitivity for this patient by using a study that includes patients of different ages with all sorts of complaints. This would probably be too general to apply to a specific patient.

The "I" component (investigation) is generally fairly straightforward, but clinicians need to be aware that there is sometimes poor standardization in diagnostic testing. We need to be aware of which test our lab uses. Does your hospital use the D-dimer enzyme-linked immunosorbent assay (ELISA) or the immunoassay? This is important because the sensitivities for the two tests are actually different. Performance of a published assay is not necessarily identical to what your hospital uses.

The "C" component is the comparison. A comparison is typically a criterion standard test for whatever you might be interested in studying. The criterion standard is the most definitive test there is. For example, for appendicitis, the criterion standard would be a histologic diagnosis of inflammation of the appendix in a surgical specimen. In some studies, criterion standard tests may not be ordered on all patients because the tests may have high risks of complications (like pulmonary angiogram for pulmonary embolism). In addition, for diseases like pelvic inflammatory disease, we may never get the criterion standard, which would be a positive culture for the right bacteria on an intraperitoneal lesion biopsied during laparoscopy. Because the criterion standard is not available, we need to use clinical findings to guide our treatment decisions in the ED. Researchers can also use a follow-up evaluation for patients who have not had the criterion standard, such as a 14-day follow-up phone call for patients with potential C-spine fractures. If they are not having pain at 14 days, they likely did not have a fracture.

The "O" component is the outcome. Outcomes should be objective and clear. For example, was the patient alive at 30 days? If the data were obtained in a valid way, survival is an outcome that is difficult to dispute. Some outcomes are not ideal in the emergency medicine literature, such as whether a patient was admitted or not. Because some admission decisions can be subjective, you should be skeptical of studies that use subjective outcomes where there is the possibility of interrater variability in assessing the key outcome.

Once a question has been framed using PICO, literature searching is also straightforward. Care should be given to use "Limit" searches appropriately: for example, if you're studying children, use the age limits. When you are studying older adults, limiting the age to an upper bound can sometimes result in the exclusion of important studies.[6]

Once you've found potentially relevant studies, it is important to place them in the appropriate place in the "evidence pyramid" shown in Figure 2.1. Let us start at the top of the pyramid, with meta-analyses. *Meta-analyses* collect valid studies on a particular topic and use statistical methodology to test the studies together as if they were all from one large study. Systematic reviews focus on a clinical topic with a focused question and are conducted using a methodologically sound, extensive literature review. Included studies are then reviewed and assessed, and the results are summarized. The Cochrane Collaboration has done considerable numbers of systematic reviews that can be found at www.cochrane.org.

Next down on the evidence pyramid are randomized clinical trials, which are projects that study the effect of a therapy (or, in the case of this book, a

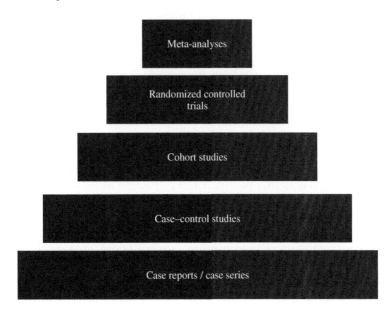

Figure 2.1 The evidence pyramid.

diagnostic test or clinical decision rule) on real patients. The level of rand-omization may be at the level of the patient (e.g., every patient is randomized to receive test 1 versus test 2), or it may be at the level of the group (e.g., a hospital is randomized to a clinical decision rule intervention) or healthcare provider (e.g., one physician is randomized to use the decision aid, while another randomized to usual care). Randomization reduces the potential for bias and allows comparison between treatment (or test or clinical decision rule) and control groups where unmeasured confounders are balanced in the two study groups. Studies that examine the efficacy of a diagnostic test typi-cally compare the test to a criterion standard study. For example, exercise stress testing may be compared to the results of cardiac catheterization (a criterion standard).

Cohort studies typically follow a large population of patients without a disease over a period of time and then examine the probability of develop-ing a condition based on an exposure to a particular treatment or circum-stances. Cohort studies are "observational" and generally are not considered to be as high quality as randomized controlled studies, because the two groups can differ in measured and unmeasured ways. Measured differ-ences can be controlled for in multivariable analyses, while unmeasured differences cannot.

Case–control studies compare a group of patients who have a specific condition to another group of people who do not, and then assess the impact of a particular exposure in the two groups. They often rely on medical record review, or patient recall of a specific exposure (which can be subject to bias because often at the time of the study, patients may know whether they do or do not have the condition in question). For example, if you have brain cancer, you may be more likely to report having a specific exposure (like daily cell phone use) than if you do not have brain cancer. Case–control studies are usually seen as less reliable than randomized controlled trials and cohort studies.

Case reports and case series are either single reports or a series of reports on the treatment of an individual or group of patients. They both report cases and do not use control groups, so they have no statistical testing or comparisons.

In conclusion, understanding the process of EBM can allow you to apply our answers to the general medical questions in this book to the patients you see in the ED. Understanding the pitfalls of EBM is important, as is sitting down and practicing clinical scenarios to see if you can make this process work for you. It is important to recognize the limitations of the literature and where studies sit on the evidence pyramid and to consider the limitations of the body of evidence on the literature surrounding a diagnostic test when determining conclusions both for clinical practice and in clinical guidelines.

References

1. Sackett DL, Rosenberg WM, Gray JA, Haynes RB, Richardson WS. Evidence based medicine: What it is and what it isn't. *British Medical Journal.* 1996; 312: 71–2.
2. Sackett DL *et al.* How to Form Clinical Questions. In: *Evidence based medicine: How to practice & teach EBM.* Chapter 1.2. Edinburgh: Churchill Livingstone; 1998.
3. Haynes RB, Wilczynski NL. Optimal search strategies for retrieving scientifically strong studies of diagnosis from Medline: Analytical survey. *BMJ.* 2004; 328(7447): 1040.
4. Jaeschke R, Guyatt G, Sackett DL. How to use an article about a diagnostic test. A. Are the results of the study valid? *Journal of the American Medical Association.* 1994; 271: 389–91.
5. Richardson WS, Detsky AS. How to use a clinical decision analysis. A. Are the results of the study valid? *Journal of the American Medical Association.* 1995; 273: 1292–5.
6. Leeflang MM, Scholten RJ, Rutjes AW, Reitsma JB, Bossuyt PM. Use of methodological search filters to identify diagnostic accuracy studies can lead to the omission of relevant studies. *Journal of Clinical Epidemiology.* 2006; 59(3): 234–40.

Additional Reading

Carpenter CR, Keim SM, Worster A, Rosen P. Brain natriuretic peptide in the evaluation of emergency department dyspnea: Is there a role? *Journal of Emergency Medicine.* 2012; 42: 489–95.

Corrall CJ, Wyer PC, Zick LS, Bockrath CR. How to find evidence when you need it part I: Databases, search programs, and strategies. *Annals of Emergency Medicine.* 2002; 39: 302–6.

Lijmer JG, Bossuyt PMM. Various randomized designs can be used to evaluate medical tests. *Journal of Clinical Epidemiology.* 2009; 62: 364–73.

Lijmer JG, Mol BW, Heisterkamp S *et al.* Empirical evidence of design-related bias in studies of diagnostic tests. *Journal of the American Medical Association.* 1999; 282: 1061–6.

Lord SJ, Irwig L, Simes RJ. When is measuring sensitivity and specificity sufficient to evaluate a diagnostic test, and when do we need randomized trials? *Annals of Internal Medicine.* 2006; 144: 850–5.

Mower WR. Evaluating bias and variability in diagnostic test reports. *Annals of Emergency Medicine.* 1999; 33: 85–91.

Newman TB, Kohn MA. *Evidence-based diagnosis (practical guide to biostatistics and epidemiology).* Cambridge: Cambridge University Press; 2009.

Chapter 3 **The Epidemiology and Statistics of Diagnostic Testing**

Jesse M. Pines[1,2], Fernanda Bellolio[3], and Lucas Oliveira Junqueira e Silva[3,4]

[1] US Acute Care Solutions, Canton, OH, USA
[2] Department of Emergency Medicine, Drexel University, Philadelphia, PA, USA
[3] Department of Emergency Medicine, Mayo Clinic, Rochester, MN, USA
[4] Department of Emergency Medicine, Hospital de Clínicas de Porto Alegre, Porto Alegre, Brazil

---

Highlights

- Sensitivity is the ability of a test to detect a disease when it is present, and specificity identifies the absence of disease.
- Prevalence is the proportion of people who have a disease within a population at one time point, and incidence refers to new cases of a disease over a certain period. Prevalence can be used interchangeably with the pretest probability of disease.
- Positive predictive value is the probability that the disease is present if the test is positive, and negative predictive value is the probability that the disease is absent if the test is negative.
- Odds are the ratio of the probability of occurrence to that of nonoccurrence. Odds ratio is a measure of the size of the difference between odds and is a ratio of the odds of an event or outcome in one group to the odds of an event or outcome in another group.
- Likelihood ratio is the proportion of patients with disease who have a specific finding divided by the proportion of patients without disease who have the same finding. LRs incorporate sensitivity and specificity and provide a direct estimate of how much a test result will change the odds of having a disease.

Evidence-Based Emergency Care: Diagnostic Testing and Clinical Decision Rules, Third Edition.
Edited by Jesse M. Pines, Fernanda Bellolio, Christopher R. Carpenter, and Ali S. Raja.
© 2023 John Wiley & Sons Ltd. Published 2023 by John Wiley & Sons Ltd.

Throughout much of this book, we refer to diagnostic test characteristics including sensitivity, specificity, negative predictive value, positive predictive value, and likelihood ratios (LRs). There are also references to common epidemiological terms such as *incidence* and *prevalence*. Terms that denote risk are *odds* and *probability*. The odds ratio (OR) is commonly used in the literature to denote comparative risk among populations. Confidence intervals (CIs) are also a frequently used but sometimes misunderstood concept. Two other more complex statistics that we will describe, because they are frequently used in diagnostic testing, are the receiver operator curve (ROC) and the interval LR. This chapter will provide explanations of these terms that we use in this book and will offer examples of how they can be used in clinical practice in the emergency department (ED).

The 2 × 2 table

Throughout this chapter and in other areas of this book, we will be using the following 2 × 2 table that you may remember (and tried to forget) from your biostatistics class in medical school:

		Disease		
		+	–	Total
Test	+			
	–			
	Total			

On the top of the table, the "disease" is listed; and on the left side of the table, the "test" is listed. An easy way to remember the structure of the 2 × 2 table is to recall that "the truth is in the heavens," so the criterion standard "truth" should always be on the top. Both "disease" and "test" are further broken down into "+" and "–" and "Total." For "disease," a "+" means that the disease is present (based upon the predefined criterion standard) and a "–" means the disease is absent; similarly for the "test," a "+" denotes a positive test and a "–" denotes a negative test.

Using information in these cells, all the common test characteristics, including sensitivity, specificity, positive predictive value, negative predictive value, and LRs, can be calculated. We can also take a pretest probability (probability that a patient has a specific condition before a test is applied) of disease, apply known sensitivity and specificity, and calculate a posttest probability. These 2 × 2 tables can be very helpful in the ED if you know how to use them properly. Their thorough understanding can allow you to apply "real-time" evidence-based medicine (EBM) as discussed in Chapter 2. First calculate a pretest probability, either based on a validated risk stratification tool or based on your own clinical judgment. Accurately assigning a pretest probability is both an art and a science. You have to think about the overall prevalence of disease. Is it common or rare? Then think about how prevalent the disease might be in the individual patient under question. However, aside from certain widely studied diseases like pulmonary embolism (PE) and acute coronary syndrome (ACS), it is often difficult to know if the pretest probability that you are assigning is correct. Often you must guess, which seems rather arbitrary given the calculations that ensue from this choice. A good way to determine how much variation there is in pretest probability is to do a simple experiment next time you are working a shift. After you and another team member (such as a nurse, resident, or medical student) evaluate a patient and decide upon a diagnostic testing plan, ask them what the probability is on a 0–100% scale that the patient will have the disease in question. Try this for 3–4 patients and what you will see is that even experienced providers often will have dramatically different assessments of pretest probability after evaluating the same patient. You'll see that this will sometimes vary 10- to 20-fold. For example, some providers may think "low risk" is 20%, while others may think "low risk" is 1%. Different assessments in pretest probability become a real challenge when one is applying evidence-based test characteristics such as sensitivity and specificity because, depending on how "off" your initial assessment is, this can give you a posttest probability that is similarly flawed. What you may see is that for certain diseases, particularly where there is better evidence, assessment of pretest probability is more similar among providers.

After you have determined your pretest probability (although it is probably imperfect), the next step is to apply diagnostic test characteristics including sensitivity and specificity. From that, we can establish what the posttest probability is (i.e., the probability that a patient has a specific condition after test results are known). Using a posttest probability, we can then decide how to proceed with the care of an individual patient. Now, that is EBM in practice!

Sensitivity and specificity

Sensitivity refers to the ability of a test to detect a disease when it is actually present. A common acronym that has been used to remember sensitivity is PID (for *positive in disease*). Intuitively, sensitivity is an illogical marker of diagnostic accuracy since the test result can be interpreted only in a population of individuals known to have the disease. In other words, if we know the patient's disease status, why would we need the test? In the 2×2 table, sensitivity can be demonstrated as follows:

		Disease		
		+	−	Total
Test	+	85		
	−	15		
	Total	100		

In this example, of 100 people with a disease, 85 of them will have a positive test and 15 will have a negative test (also known as *false negatives*). The sensitivity of the test will therefore be 85/100, or 85%.

By contrast, **specificity** correctly identifies the absence of disease. That is, in people who do not have the disease, specificity denotes the percentage of those who will have a negative test. This can be easily remembered by the acronym NIH (for *negative in health*). Again, specificity can be interpreted only in a population known not to have the disease. In the 2×2 table, specificity can be demonstrated:

		Disease		
		+	−	Total
Test	+		20	
	−		80	
	Total		100	

In this case, of the 100 people without disease, 80% of those will test negative for the disease while 20% of patients will test positive (also known as *false positives*). The test specificity is therefore 80/100, or 80%.

Another problem with sensitivity and specificity is that they require data to be dichotomized, but many lab tests (e.g., D-dimer and brain natriuretic peptide (BNP)) are continuous data ranging from zero to infinity. Splitting continuous data into groups loses valuable diagnostic accuracy detail. This problem is eliminated by using interval LRs, which assign a specific value to each level of an abnormal test result, allowing the calculation of a disease's posttest probability based on the specific test result.

Incidence and prevalence

The **prevalence** of disease is defined as the proportion of people who have a disease within a population at one time point. **Incidence** is related to prevalence but differs in that it refers to new cases of a disease over a certain period of time. For example, assuming that we have a healthy population of 1000 people on January 1, and five had developed a specific disease by December 31, the disease incidence would be five per 1000 per year.

But when it comes to diagnostic testing, prevalence is the more important property. Prevalence can be used interchangeably with the pretest probability of disease. In using our 2×2 table, we can demonstrate the concept of prevalence (or pretest probability) in the following way:

		Disease		
		+	−	Total
Test	+			
	−			
	Total	100	100	200

Of the total population of 200 people, 100 people have the disease (disease positive) and 100 people do not have the disease (disease negative). In this population, the overall prevalence is 100/200, or 50%. Sensitivity and specificity are independent of the prevalence of disease in the population, as you can see from the following table:

		Disease		
		+	−	Total
	+	85	20	105
Test	−	15	80	95
	Total	100	100	200

That is to say, sensitivity and specificity do not change when the prevalence changes. Predictive values, in contrast, always vary with prevalence.

Predictive values

Positive predictive value is the probability that the disease is present if the test is positive.

		Disease		
		+	−	Total
	+	85	20	105
Test	−			
	Total			

In this case, of the 105 people with positive tests, 85 actually have the disease; therefore, the positive predictive value is 85/105, or 81%.

The **negative predictive value** is the probability that the disease is absent if the test is negative. Of the 95 people with negative tests, 80 do not have the disease. Therefore, the negative predictive value is 80/95, or 84%.

		Disease		
		+	−	Total
	+			
Test	−	15	80	95
	Total			

Integrating concepts

Another way to integrate sensitivity and specificity with predictive values is the use of mnemonics. The mnemonics "Sn*out*" for sensitivity (to rule *out* disease) and "Sp*in*" for specificity (to "rule *in*" disease) have been proposed. When you want to rule out something (as in a clinical decision rule or a diagnostic test) for a low-risk patient, the ideal test should have near-perfect sensitivity. This will result in a correspondingly high negative predictive value (i.e., the disease is ruled out). Conversely, when you are trying to rule in something, ideal tests have near-perfect specificity that will correspond to a high positive predictive value (i.e., the disease will be ruled in).

Using 2 × 2 tables: an example

In contrast to sensitivity and specificity, positive and negative predictive values do change with changing disease prevalence. As an example, you go see a patient and based on your initial assessment, there is a high pretest probability of disease. Let us set the pretest probability estimate at 80%. If we take the same test characteristics that we had in the prior example, where sensitivity = 85% and specificity is 80%, what happens to the predictive values?

First, we start with the disease prevalence = 80%, wherein a hypothetical population of 200 people, 160 have the disease and 40 do not.

		Disease		
		+	−	Total
	+			
Test	−			
	Total	160	40	200

We then add the known sensitivity = 85% and specificity = 80%. The number of true positives will be 136, false positives 8, true negatives 32, and false negatives 24:

		Disease		
		+	–	Total
	+	136	8	144
Test	–	24	32	56
	Total	160	40	200

Now, if we have a positive test in this population, the positive predictive value is 136/144 = 94% (which is higher than when the prevalence = 50%) and the negative predictive value is 32/56 = 57% (which is lower than it was if the prevalence = 50%). What tends to happen is that as your prevalence goes up, a positive test is *more* likely to be a true positive and a negative test is *less* likely to be a true negative.

How does this work if the disease prevalence is low? Let us assume a prevalence of 10%:

		Disease		
		+	–	Total
	+			
Test	–			
	Total	20	180	200

Now, if we apply the same test characteristics where sensitivity = 85% and specificity = 80:

		Disease		
		+	–	Total
	+	17	36	53
Test	–	3	144	147
	Total	20	180	200

In this case, the positive predictive value is 17/53 = 32% (which is less than it was when the population prevalence was 50%) and the negative predictive value is 144/147 = 98% (which is higher than when the population prevalence was 50%). In this case, because the prevalence is low, a positive test is less likely to be true positive and a negative test is more likely to be a true negative.

As a general principle, as your disease prevalence goes up, positive predictive value increases. As disease prevalence goes down, your negative predictive value increases. In other words, if you are worried about a patient and you think she is at high risk for the disease, if the test is positive, it has a good chance of being a true positive. And, conversely, if a patient is probably OK and you're ordering an imperfect test (like an electrocardiogram to rule out ACS in a 25-year-old), and the results are normal, the likelihood that it is a true negative is very high.

As described in this chapter, the other way to think about prevalence in a study setting is as the pretest probability for the disease in question. After you evaluate a patient, the prevalence is equal to the pretest probability for that individual patient. If you see 100 patients with the same presentation, what percentage will have the disease? In other words, clinicians can extrapolate the disease "+/−/Total" boxes to estimate pretest probability and to determine the predictive values for an individual patient.

Let us use an example of a specific patient to illustrate how we can use EBM at the bedside in emergency medicine. Imagine you are evaluating a 55-year-old female who presents with intermittent, sharp, right-sided chest pain and shortness of breath for one week. She has no traditional risk factors for PE or coronary artery disease. She has a normal physical examination except for tenderness to palpation over the right side of the chest. Vitals are within normal limits except for a heart rate of 110 beats per minute that is regular.

You are considering the diagnosis of PE in this patient, and you want to determine this patient's risk of PE. You pose your clinical question, you search the literature, and then you evaluate a study on the Wells criteria and decide to use it. The Wells criteria are a way to determine the pretest probability of disease in the case of PE (Table 3.1).[1,2]

According to the Wells criteria, you assign based upon your clinical judgment 1.5 points for a heart rate of >100 beats per minute. This assigns her to a "low-risk" category, and *a priori* before any testing, based on the Wells criteria, you assign her a pretest probability of 3.6%, which was the prevalence of PE in that category in the original study. While this is likely not exactly her specific pretest probability, you do agree that she is at relatively low risk for PE.

Because she is low risk, you decide to order a D-dimer assay on her. You think back to one of two key questions, "What will you do if it's positive?" or "What if it's negative?" Let us go to the 2 × 2 tables to see. You first start by entering her pretest probability. Of every 200 patients you see who are identical to this one, roughly seven will have the disease.

Table 3.1 The Wells criteria for pulmonary embolism

	Points
Clinical symptoms or signs of deep vein thrombosis (DVT)	3
PE more likely than other diagnosis	3
Heart rate >100 beats per minute	1.5
Immobilization or surgery within last 4 weeks	1.5
History of DVT or pulmonary embolism (PE)	1.5
Hemoptysis	1
Malignancy	1

Clinical probability of PE	Points	Probability of disease (%)
Low	<2	3.6
Moderate	2–5	20.5
High	>5	66.7

		Disease		
		+	−	Total
Test	+			
	−			
	Total	7	193	200

Now, let us look up the sensitivity and specificity for D-dimer. We find a review article on MEDLINE that shows that in a meta-analysis, D-dimer sensitivity = 94% and the specificity = 45%.[3] Our hospital just so happens to use the same D-dimer assay that was studied in this meta-analysis. How convenient.

Let us enter the numbers and see what we get:

		Disease		
		+	−	Total
Test	+	6	106	112
	−	1	87	88
	Total	7	193	200

Well, it is not perfect, but let us say for simplicity that D-dimer will pick up 6/7 (85%) of the patients with disease to make the numbers fit.

OK, our test is positive, so what is the positive predictive value? We can calculate that 6/112 = 5.4%. This is not very good – with a positive D-dimer, we have moved from our pretest probability of 3.5% (7/200) to a posttest probability of 5.4%. This certainly does not push us over any treatment threshold. That is, we do not want to anticoagulate people with a 5.4% chance of having the disease because of the potential side effects of those medications. What if the test is negative? Well, then our negative predictive value = 87/88 = 98.9%. That's a pretty good negative predictive value. So, given a negative test, we have moved from a pretest probability of 3.6% to a posttest probability of 1.2%. With a posttest probability of 1.2%, it may be reasonable to say that a diagnosis has been mostly excluded. As we can see from this example, D-dimer is a good rule-out test because the sensitivity is high. Remember: "Snout."

Odds, probability, and the odds ratio

We will be using two related terms that denote risk in this book: *odds* and *probability*. While people often use *odds* and *probability* interchangeably, they actually mean different things. To some, probability makes more intuitive sense than odds, but often in statistics, an OR is typically used to represent the likelihood that one group will have the outcome in question over another group.

Let us start with probability because this is the easiest to understand. The probability is the expected number over the total number. An easy example is to use six-sided dice. The probability of rolling a "6" on any individual roll is 1/6 = 16.7%. Using a hypothetical clinical example, the probability that a 50-year-old male who has risk factors for coronary disease, acute chest pain, and new electrocardiographic changes is having an ACS is high (let us say 80% as an estimate). That means that out of 100 identical patients, 80 will have ACS.

Odds are related but different. Odds are the ratio of the probability of occurrence to that of nonoccurrence. Using the same example, the odds that you will roll a "6" are 1:5, while the odds that the 50-year old male will have ACS are 4:1. You can convert odds to probabilities using the following formulas:

$$\text{Odds} = \frac{\text{Probability}}{\left(1 - \text{Probability}\right)} \text{Odds} = \frac{\text{Probability}}{\left(1 - \text{Probability}\right)}$$

$$\text{Probability} = \frac{\text{Odds}}{\left(1 + \text{Odds}\right)} \text{Probability} = \frac{\text{Odds}}{\left(1 + \text{Odds}\right)}$$

An OR is a measure of the size of the difference between odds and is commonly used in the medical literature to denote risk. It is defined as a ratio of the odds of an event or outcome in one group to the odds of an event or outcome in another group. These groups are traditionally a dichotomous classification, like older people (≥65 years old) versus younger people (<65 years old) or men versus women. It can also be the difference between a treatment group and a control group. When the OR is equal to 1, this indicates that the event or outcome is equally likely in both groups. When it is greater than 1, the condition or outcome is more likely in the first group. Finally, when it is less than 1, it is less likely in the first group.

In an OR, p is the probability of the outcome in group 1 and q is the probability of the outcome in group 2. As mentioned in this chapter, we can use the formula for odds to calculate an OR in terms of probabilities:

$$\text{Odds Ratio}(\text{OR}) = \frac{\left(\dfrac{p}{1-p}\right)}{\left(\dfrac{q}{1-q}\right)}$$

As a clinical example, suppose that we have a sample of 100 male and 100 female ED patients with acute chest pain. This is only a theoretical example to demonstrate how to calculate an OR and is not based on any studies. Of the 100 patients, 20 males and 10 females will have a serious cause for their pain. The odds of a male having a serious cause for this pain are 20–80 or 1:4, while the odds of a female having a serious cause for this pain are 10–90 or 1:9. Using the above formula, we can calculate the OR:

$$\text{Odds Ratio}(\text{OR}) = \frac{\dfrac{0.20}{(1-0.20)}}{\dfrac{0.10}{(1-0.10)}} = 2.25$$

This calculation can be interpreted to mean that men have a 2.25 times higher odds of having a serious cause for their chest pain than women. This also illustrates how an OR can be larger than the difference in probability. While men are two times more likely (in terms of probability), the OR is higher (2.25).

Likelihood ratios and interval likelihood ratios

LR is defined as the proportion of patients with disease who have a specific finding divided by the proportion of patients without disease who have the same finding. LRs are a different way to incorporate sensitivity and specificity and provide a direct estimate of how much a test result (positive or negative) will change the odds of having a disease. It is a rapid and simple way to estimate posttest odds and probabilities in the emergency setting given its intuitiveness when compared to using sensitivity and specificity alone. The LR for a positive result (LR+) tells you how much the odds of the disease increase when a dichotomous test is positive. The LR for a negative result (LR−) tells you how much the odds of the disease decrease when a dichotomous test is negative.

In order to use LRs, you need to specify the pretest odds. The pretest odds are the likelihood that the patient would have a specific disease prior to any testing. Pretest odds are related to the prevalence of disease and may be adjusted upward or downward depending on the characteristics of your overall patient pool (is the disease likely in your community?) or of the individual patient (is the disease likely in the individual patient?).

In order to calculate LRs, you can use the following formulas:

$$LR+ = \frac{Sensitivity}{\left(1 - Specificity\right)}$$

$$LR- = \frac{\left(1 - Sensitivity\right)}{Specificity}$$

$$Odds\,post = Odds\,pre \times LR + \left(a\,positive\,test\right)$$

$$Odds\,post = Odds\,pre \times LR - \left(a\,negative\,test\right)$$

As a general rule of thumb, LRs >10 or <0.1 generate sizeable changes in posttest disease probability, while LRs of 0.5–2.0 have little effect. To make the use of LRs even easier, emergency physicians may *estimate* changes in probability by memorizing the LRs 2, 5, and 10 and the first 3 multiples of 15 (i.e., 15, 30, 45). It is then possible to approximate probabilities (LR 2 = +15%, LR 5 = +30%, and LR 10 = +45%). Simultaneously, LRs reciprocals of 2, 5, and 10 (i.e., 0.5, 0.2, and 0.1) decrease probability by 15%, 30%, and 45%, respectively (Figure 3.1). It is also possible to use LRs when considering a sequence of independent tests (e.g., electrocardiogram followed by troponin I testing for potential ACS). LRs can be multiplied in series.

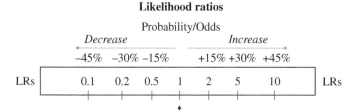

Figure 3.1 Practical use of likelihood ratios through estimation of changes in probability. Note: Likelihood ratios >10 or <0.1 usually generate clinically significant changes in posttest probabilities. (Adapted from reference [5].)

Presenting continuous data as dichotomous results neglect and oversimplify valuable diagnostic detail. One advantage of LRs over sensitivity and specificity is that interval LRs can be computed for continuous data, whereas sensitivity and specificity are always reported as dichotomous "+" or "–" results. Stratifying continuous data into ranges of results captures additional diagnostic information for clinicians to more appropriately interpret test results. See "Receiver Operator Characteristic (ROC) Curves" section in this chapter for information on calculating interval LRs. Unfortunately, most research manuscripts do not report interval LRs.

Using odds, probabilities, and likelihood ratios: an example

The best way to describe odds, probabilities, and LRs is by using a clinical example. Using D-dimer as an example, let us assume that the sensitivity = 94% and the specificity = 45%.

We can calculate the LR+ = 1.71 by the following calculation: $(0.94)/(1 - 0.45)$; and the LR– = 0.13 through the following formula: $(1 - 0.94)/(0.45)$. Now let us go through the math.

Start with a pretest probability of 10%. The next step is to convert that to an odds of $(0.10)/(1 - 0.10) = 0.1111$. So our pretest odds are 0.1111. If we want to apply LRs, we need to know our test results. If the test is positive, given a LR+ of 1.71, we can calculate a posttest odds given a positive test = $(1.71)(0.1111) = 0.1899$. If the test is negative, we can apply a LR– of 0.13. So posttest odds given a negative test = $(0.13)(0.1111) = 0.0144$. Now, we need to convert these back to probabilities. An odds of 0.1899 is equal to a probability of $(0.1899)/(1 + 0.1899) = 16.0\%$. An odds of 0.0144 is equal to a probability of $(0.0144)/(1 + 0.0144) = 1.4\%$.

Translated into English: given a pretest probability of 10%, if you have a positive D-dimer, your posttest probability = 16%. Your posttest probability is also your positive predictive value. If you have a negative test, your posttest probability is 1.4%. Another way of expressing a posttest probability when there is a negative test is a negative predictive value. In this case, your negative predictive value is (1 – posttest probability) = (1 – 0.014) = 98.6%.

An even simpler way to work from a pretest probability, modified by a LR, to a posttest probability is to use a LR nomogram (Figure 3.2). Using a ruler, start from the pretest probability in the left column and intersect the LR value in the middle column. The nomogram can be used as a point-of-care tool to rapidly estimate posttest probabilities without going through complex calculations. This is likely the best approach to use odds, probabilities, and LRs in the ED.

Extending the straight line from those two points out to the right-hand column results in the new posttest probability.

Bayes theorem

To make things even more complicated, in order to calculate a posttest probability given a pretest probability and known sensitivity and specificity, you can use the Bayes theorem and do it all in one step.

In the case of a positive test, you can calculate your posttest probability (or your positive predictive value) using the following formula:

$$\text{Posttest probability} = \frac{\left(\text{Pretest probability} \times \text{Sensitivity}\right)}{\left[\begin{array}{l}\left(\text{Pretest probability} \times \text{Sensitivity}\right) + \\ \left(1 - \text{Pretest probability}\right) \times \left(1 - \text{Specificity}\right)\end{array}\right]}$$

In the case of a negative test, you can calculate your posttest probability (or one minus your negative predictive value) using the following formula:

$$\text{Posttest probability} = \frac{\left(1 - \text{Pretest probability}\right) \times \text{Specificity}}{\left\{\begin{array}{l}\left[\left(1 - \text{Pretest probability}\right) \times \text{specificity}\right] + \\ \left[\text{Pretest probability} \times \left(1 - \text{Sensitivity}\right)\right]\end{array}\right\}}$$

Let us go back to Chapter 1, when we mentioned the 83-year-old female with shortness of breath, chest pain, a history of PE, and a negative D-dimer. Given that her pretest probability for PE is 85%, we can calculate

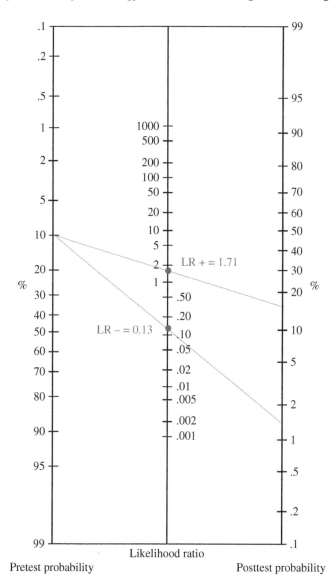

Figure 3.2 Likelihood ratio nomogram. Note: Using a straight edge (such as a ruler), it is possible to move from pretest probability to posttest probability using the likelihood ratio of the test.

our posttest probability (and also our negative predictive value) using the Bayes theorem:

$$\text{Posttest probability} = \frac{\left(1-0.85\right) \times 0.45}{\left\{\left[\left(1-0.85\right) \times 0.45\right] + \left[0.85 \times \left(1-0.94\right)\right]\right\}}$$

And after calculating it out, we get a posttest probability of 61.3% and our negative predictive value is $(1-0.613) = 38.7\%$. Given that her chance of PE is 61.3% after a negative test result, we have not safely ruled out PE. Therefore, she needs further testing such as a chest computed tomography (CT) or ventilation–perfusion (V/Q) scan, or possibly even a pulmonary angiogram. Also, given that the pretest probability was so high, you could make an argument to just treat her. But given that anticoagulation is not without potential adverse effects, if you can order a confirmatory test, it is probably reasonable to do so.

So should we have ordered a D-dimer in the first place? The answer is probably not. In the case of a negative test, it did not help us because it did not move us over the test–treatment threshold.

Confidence intervals

Throughout this book, we make reference to CIs. We will abbreviate 95% confidence intervals as CI. CIs are commonly used in statistics to give an estimated range of values that is likely to include a population parameter (like an OR or a population mean) that is unknown. As an easy example, say we are trying to estimate the average age of everyone living in your county of 50,000 people. In order to do this, we randomly choose 100 houses and go door to door to ask people what their ages are, for a total sample of 322 people. From that, we find that the average age is 32 years old. But how certain are we that 32 is the real average for the population? Instead of saying that 32 is the average, what we can do is give a CI. So we plug our numbers into our statistics program and what we find is that the average is indeed 32 but the 95% CI is from 26 to 42 years old. What we can say is that we are 95% sure that whatever the real value is (if we sampled all 50,000) lies between 26 and 42. Intervals are usually reported with 95% confidence, but if we want to be really sure, we can report wider intervals such as 99% CIs.

Let us use a clinical example. Like before, we want to know the odds of a male having a serious cause for chest pain compared to the odds for a female. What we would go out and do is collect sample data to answer the question by studying males and females with chest pain and estimating the OR based on the sample data. Based on the data, we calculate an OR of 2.25 with a 95%

CI of 1.5–3.5. Therefore, what we can say is that we are 95% confident that the real difference between men and women falls between 1.5 and 3.5. Since the lower bound of the CI is greater than one, we can say that men are significantly at higher risk of having their chest pain be due to a serious cause than women.

CI width gives an idea about how uncertain we are about this unknown parameter. For example, if we reported an OR of 2.3 (95% CI 2.0–2.5), we could be fairly confident in our estimate. However, if we reported 2.3 (95% CI 0.3–10.0), we would be less confident. A wide interval indicates that nothing very definite can be said about the parameter. As a rule of thumb, a parameter estimate with a small CI is more reliable than a result with a large CI.

Receiver operator characteristic (ROC) curves

Determination of sensitivity and specificity for a specific diagnostic test depends on the test values we define as "abnormal." The threshold value for an abnormal test that we set will determine the number of true positives, true negatives, false positives, and false negatives. For example, say that a patient with an abnormal D-dimer test is at a specific threshold, such as 500 ng/dL. If we were to set the cutoff at a higher level (e.g., 2000 ng/L), then the number of true positives would likely increase, but the number of false negatives would also increase. The purpose of ROC curves is to find the test cutoff that maximizes both sensitivity and specificity so that tests can be used and interpreted in clinically meaningful ways. Figure 3.3 shows an ROC curve.

ROC curves are a way to plot test sensitivity and specificity at different value thresholds for what defines a positive and negative test. Traditionally an ROC curve is a plot of the true positive rate (sensitivity) compared with the false positive rate (1 – specificity). The accuracy of a test is dependent on how well the test distinguishes the group being tested into those with and without the disease. Test accuracy can be measured by the area under the ROC curve. If the area is 1, then the test is perfect. An area of 0.5 is a worthless test. Table 3.2 provides a rough guide for classifying the accuracy of a diagnostic test using the area under the ROC curve.

Another way of describing the area under the ROC curve is test discrimination. It measures the ability of a test to correctly classify those with and without disease. Imagine a situation where we have two sets of patients, one with occult bacteremia and one without. If we were to randomly pick one patient from the group with bacteremia and one from the group without bacteremia and get a white blood cell (WBC) count on both, then compare the results for these two patients, the patient with the higher WBCs should be the one from the group with occult bacteremia. The area under the ROC curve is

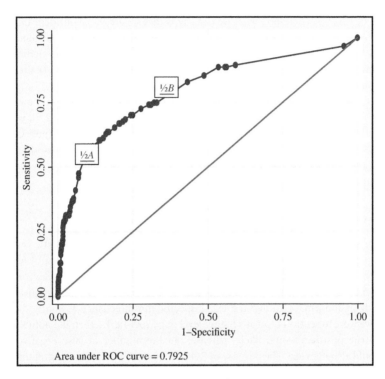

Area under ROC curve = 0.7925

Figure 3.3 Receiver operator characteristic (ROC) curve. Note: A and B are two specific points on the ROC curve. The slope of the line between the two is the interval likelihood ratio.

Table 3.2 Determining the accuracy of a diagnostic test using the area under the ROC

Value	Accuracy
0.90–1.00	Excellent
0.80–0.90	Good
0.70–0.80	Fair
0.60–0.70	Poor

the percentage of randomly drawn pairs for which this is true (i.e., the test correctly classifies the two patients in the random pair). Throughout this book, we make reference to studies that use ROC curves.

Another way of using the ROC curve is to determine interval LRs. In Figure 3.3, the interval LR for the test result between A and B is the slope of the line between those two points [$(Y_2 - Y_1)/(X_2 - X_1)$ or $(B_{sen} - A_{sen})/(B_{1-spec} - A_{1-spec})$]. The interval LR can be determined between any two values of a diagnostic test. Whereas the dichotomous LRs are labeled *positive* or *negative*, the interval LR is simply one value representing the probability of the diagnostic test yielding a value within this range among those who have disease, divided by the probability of the same test demonstrating a value within this range among those who do not have the disease. Computing posttest probabilities from the pretest probability is performed in the same fashion as described in this chapter for dichotomous LRs.

In conclusion, learning how to use diagnostic test characteristics (sensitivity, specificity, predictive values, and LRs), determine appropriate cutoff and accuracy of tests (ROC curves), and report results (ORs and CIs), can be helpful in the practice of EBM in the ED. Thorough understanding of both the power and limitations of testing can aid in diagnosis and medical decision-making. It is also important to note that although diagnostic strategies are often implemented based only on their test characteristics, patient-centered outcome should also be evaluated. With that said, an accurate diagnostic test does not necessarily translate into better outcomes for patients.[4] Emergency physicians should be careful before adopting new diagnostic strategies as often the implementation process does not look at benefits focusing on patient outcomes.[5]

References

1. Ramzi DW, Leeper KV. DVT and pulmonary embolism: Part I. Diagnosis. *American Family Physician*. 2004; 69: 2829–36.
2. Wolf SJ, McCubbin TR, Feldhaus KM, Faragher JP, Adcock DM. Prospective validation of Wells criteria in the evaluation of patients with suspected pulmonary embolism. *Annals of Emergency Medicine*. 2004; 44: 503–10.
3. Brown MD, Rowe BH, Reeves MJ et al. The accuracy of the enzyme-linked immunosorbent assay D-dimer test in the diagnosis of pulmonary embolism: A meta-analysis. *Annals of Emergency Medicine*. 2002; 40: 133–44.
4. El Dib R, Tikkinen KAO, Akl EA et al. Systematic survey of randomized trials evaluating the impact of alternative diagnostic strategies on patient-important outcomes. *Journal of Clinical Epidemiology*. 2017; 84: 61–9.
5. McGee SR. *Evidence-based physical diagnosis*. 4th ed. Philadelphia (PA): Elsevier; 2018.

Additional Reading

Brown MD, Reeves MJ. Evidence-based emergency medicine skills for evidence-based emergency care. Interval likelihood ratios: Another advantage for the evidence-based diagnostician. *Annals of Emergency Medicine*. 2003; 42: 292–7.
Gallagher EJ. Evidence-based emergency medicine editorial: The problem with sensitivity and specificity. *Annals of Emergency Medicine*. 2003; 42: 298–303.

Hayden SR, Brown MD. Likelihood ratio: A powerful tool for incorporating the results of a diagnostic test into clinical decision making. *Annals of Emergency Medicine.* 1999; 33(5): 575–80.

Pewsner D, Battaglia M, Minder C *et al.* Ruling a diagnosis in or out with "SpPin" and "SnNout": A note of caution. *BMJ.* 2004; 329: 209–13.

Phelps MA, Levitt MA. Pretest probability estimates: A pitfall to the clinical utility of evidence-based medicine? *Academic Emergency Medicine.* 2004; 11: 692–4.

Smith C, Mensah A, Mal S, Worster A. Is pretest probability assessment on emergency department patients with suspected venous thromboembolism documented before SimpliRED D-dimer testing? *CJEM.* 2008; 10: 519–23.

Chapter 4 **Clinical Decision Rules**

Jesse M. Pines[1,2] and Christopher R. Carpenter[3]

[1] US Acute Care Solutions, Canton, OH, USA
[2] Department of Emergency Medicine, Drexel University, Philadelphia, PA, USA
[3] Department of Emergency Medicine, Washington University School of Medicine, Saint Louis, MO, USA

Highlights

- Clinical decision rules (CDR) are helpful, practical tools that assist in whether a diagnostic test is needed or another clinical action is necessary
- CDRs are derived from a rigorous research and development process
- CDRs need to derived and validated, ideally externally from the site where they were developed before they are put into widespread use

---

Clinical decision rules (CDRs) are practical tools intended to assist in deciding whether a diagnostic test is needed or another clinical action should be taken such as hospital admission, or what the likelihood is for the presence or absence of a particular disease or condition. Some prefer the term Clinical Decision Instruments or decision aids, since CDRs are not actually "rules" that dictate actions or appropriateness and do not replace experienced clinical expertise. CDRs are designed to be simple and provide a practical decision-making guide to differentiate patients who require testing or treatment from those who do not. CDRs typically include at least three elements from the patient's history, a physical exam, and simple ancillary tests that can be a guide at the bedside in the emergency department (ED) or in the office.[1] CDRs are derived using a series of research studies on a specific clinical question. They then must be validated in different populations. Each step in the derivation, validation, and external testing of a decision rule involves specific

---

Evidence-Based Emergency Care: Diagnostic Testing and Clinical Decision Rules, Third Edition.
Edited by Jesse M. Pines, Fernanda Bellolio, Christopher R. Carpenter, and Ali S. Raja.
© 2023 John Wiley & Sons Ltd. Published 2023 by John Wiley & Sons Ltd.

study designs and statistical analyses. At each stage in the development process, aspects of exactly how the study was conducted (i.e., the patient population tested and specific outcomes) impact how the rule should be interpreted and used in clinical practice. In this chapter, we describe the steps researchers take to derive (generate) and validate (show that it works) CDRs.

The genesis of a CDR starts with a specific research question. When related to diagnostic testing, it traditionally starts with a question like "*XYZ* is a disease that we often suspect but it has a low positive testing rate. Is there a way to clinically differentiate cases with negative tests where there is a risk for *XYZ*, so that *XYZ* can be ruled out clinically without ordering any tests?" *XYZ* may refer to common diseases that we want to exclude but that have a low prevalence of positives on test results, like intracranial bleeds, fractures, or infections. Decision aids have also been developed to risk-stratify patients for short-term adverse outcomes with presenting symptom complexes like chest pain, transient ischemic attack (TIA), and syncope of which many are reviewed in this textbook. It is important to recognize that there are limitations for when a CDR can and should be used.[2,3] For instance, consider the inclusion criteria for a rule. If the derivation and validation of a CDR regarding whether a blunt trauma patient should get a noncontrast head computed tomography (CT) scan to rule out intracranial pathology only included adult patients over the age of 18 years, then the results cannot be applied confidently to similarly injured pediatric patients unless the rule is validated in that specific population.

CDRs are intended to include elements of the history, physical exam, or diagnostic tests that are reproducible and readily available at the bedside without special training or equipment. Elements of CDRs are also ideally binary (yes or no) or at least discrete with unambiguous options. We want to eliminate subjectivity as much as possible and maximize interrater reliability. This means that when two separate people assess an element of a rule, they have a high chance of agreeing on the results of that element. For example, consider a 72-year-old patient. Few would argue that the patient is 72 years old. If the criterion is "Is the patient 65 and older?", then there would likely be perfect agreement when two individuals assess this element. However, when we start using physical examination findings in a rule, such as "Does the patient have point tenderness over either malleolus of the ankle?", there is a greater chance for disagreement. This becomes further muddied when we try to use more subjective findings such as "Is there rebound or guarding on an abdominal examination?" This is where clinicians may have a high likelihood of obtaining different physical exam ("test") results, depending on the way they conduct physical examinations or interpret clinical signs. CDRs also frequently do not take into context other intangible elements of the clinical setting. That is to say, CDRs are not perfect. In the Canadian head CT rule, a rule that determines whether or not patients require head CT scans after blunt head trauma, one of the elements includes a failure to reach a Glasgow coma scale (GCS) of 15 within 2 hours. When assessing an individual with a GCS of 15 who is behaving strangely 30 minutes after a blunt head trauma, you probably should not wait the 2 hours to see whether she normalizes and should consider ordering a head CT scan early. CDRs often guide whether the likelihood of a disease is low enough to warrant the test. However, they are not perfect nor should they be binding or used to unequivocally define appropriateness or justify reimbursement.[4] Even though CDRs are designed to be theoretically 100% sensitive, when tested in real-life practice, they are almost always less than 100% sensitive. Clinical experience and gestalt are valuable assets in emergency medicine but are part of the intangible components that cannot be incorporated into CDRs. Unfortunately, CDRs are rarely compared to clinical gestalt.[5]

Over the past 30 years, many CDRs have been introduced in emergency medicine. The most notable and likely the most widely known are the sets of rules called the Ottawa rules (originally knee, ankle, cervical spine, and head injury rules and more recently TIA, subarachnoid hemorrhage, and congestive heart failure CDRs), which are discussed later in this book. Dr. Ian Stiell and his research colleagues in Ottawa, Canada, have made a career of taking common clinical conditions where testing is frequently employed and positive tests are relatively rare and then trying to figure out who needs tests and who doesn't. By asking very simple and straightforward questions, Dr. Stiell's research has aimed to reduce diagnostic variability via the elimination of unnecessary testing by deriving decision rules to identify low-risk patients who are unlikely to benefit from such tests. Other theoretical benefits of eliminating unnecessary testing using CDRs include (i) reductions of time in the ED for the patients, (ii) reduced exposure to radiation (for imaging), and (iii) reduced costs to both patients and the health care system overall.

The clinical decision rule development process

The first step in creating a rule is to consider a clinical situation that is common enough to warrant a CDR. Is there a discrete and finite clinical question? For instance, does every patient with ankle pain need an X-ray? How frequently are tests positive? Ankle injuries are common and widespread complaints presenting to EDs around the world, and ankle X-rays are frequently negative. Therefore, a rule that can identify low-risk criteria to reduce unnecessary ankle radiography would be clinically helpful. The clinical question is "Is there a fractured bone or not?" The practical question becomes "Is an X-ray needed?"

How do you go about creating a CDR? The rest of this chapter will summarize the approach by describing the essential steps that researchers must undertake to develop a rule that is useful in practice. Several articles describing and discussing the methods for these components are available for those who want additional details.[1-3] As astute readers of the medical literature, developing a working understanding of each of these steps in order to determine if you should use the decision rule for your patients is essential.

The first step is *defining the outcome*. The outcome should be explicitly described and clinically relevant to the condition under study. Is there a fracture of either malleolus of the ankle? Does the patient have an acute appendicitis or a cervical spine (C-spine) fracture? All of these are discrete conditions with a binary yes or no answer. In describing the condition or test being examined, researchers also must define the patient population for the rule. Defining the outcome and the appropriate target patient population is essential because this determines the patient population to whom the rule can be applied. The outcome should be defined by incorporating a global perspective that extends beyond the emergency physician to include pertinent specialists and patient-centric outcomes. For example, the Canadian head CT rule queried over 100 emergency and neurosurgery physicians to settle on the outcome of intracranial injury necessitating surgical management.[6] Some clinicians discard the validated Canadian head CT rule based on this outcome because these physicians believe that even clinically inconsequential intracranial injuries should be identified with CT scans whenever possible even if such knowledge does not alter neurosurgical approach, disposition decisions, or patient outcomes.

Next, what are considered the most relevant and logical factors that might be used to predict an outcome or diagnosis? It is from the initial pool of *predictor variables* that the final decision rule is derived. The predictor variables usually include demographic factors, medical history, circumstances surrounding the patient's injury (mechanism of injury, or timing), physical exam findings, and sometimes blood test results, electrocardiogram findings, or results from imaging studies. Accurately and consistently determining the presence of the predictor variables is vital in determining which variables should be ultimately included in the decision rule. Both intra-observer agreement (between repeated measurements by the same clinician) and inter-observer agreement (in between measurements by different clinicians) should be high for inclusion in a decision rule. In terms of statistical measurement, researchers need to show that the predictor variables they are considering have sufficiently *high reproducibility*, in the form of a kappa statistic (κ). A κ statistic is a number from -1 to 1 where 0 indicates no agreement, -1 indicates perfect disagreement, and 1 indicates perfect agreement. Variables that are too subjective and have low κ values (<0.6) should not be included in the decision rule.

If the goal is to reliably exclude a fracture based on the history and physical exam findings of a patient with ankle pain, the predictor variables should be determined before knowledge of the X-ray results.[7] Similarly, the X-ray results should not be interpreted with the knowledge of the history and physical exam findings of the patient. *Blinded assessment of the predictor variables and outcomes* from the imaging study ensures there is no observer or ascertainment bias on the validity of the findings. For instance, let us say we have examined a patient and know there is point tenderness over the medial malleolus. We may review an X-ray more carefully over the area of concern looking for a fracture in that specific area and may be more likely to call any irregularity a fracture. This is in contrast to a radiologist who is reading the similar X-ray but without knowledge or influence of the physical exam and who determines there is no fracture present.

The *derivation phase* of a decision rule is the process of collecting the data in a standardized way, including the predictor variables; assessing the reliability of those data; and determining the outcome(s) being studied (in the ankle examples, the outcome is fracture).[8] Researchers then use statistical methods to distill the predictor variable down to those that are the most predictive of the outcome. The two most common methods are recursive partitioning and logistic regression analysis.[9] Recursive partitioning takes patients and divides them sequentially into groups with a particular outcome. Subsets of patients are created with that particular outcome that have common predictor variables associated with the outcomes. Logistic regression analysis generates a model that predicts the outcome, which has to be binary (fracture or no fracture), by using the best statistical combination of predictor variables. Functionally, this type of analysis creates odds of the outcome event based on the presence or absence of the predictor variables. The end result of both methods is a set of best predictor variables that comprise the CDR.

The next phase following the derivation stage is the *validation phase*.[8] During the validation phase, the actual CDR is applied to the patients for whom it is intended, and the outcomes are determined in a blinded fashion. The elements of the decision rule are assessed and recorded in a blinded format separate from the determination of the ultimate clinical outcome. The researchers then compare the performance of the CDR with the outcome.

Validation usually takes the form of a 2 × 2 table (similar to the one we saw in Chapter 3) showing the results of the rule (rule positive or rule negative) compared to the outcome of the study (X-ray positive or X-ray negative).

	Outcome event (+)	Outcome event (−)
Clinical decision rule (+)	a	b
Clinical decision rule (−)	c	d

The results of the validation study should be clearly presented. When arranged in this format, we can then calculate the sensitivity and specificity for a rule.

Sensitivity, specificity, and likelihood ratios are performance characteristics of the rule or test being examined and are not influenced by the prevalence of the outcome event. Predictive values, both positive and negative, in contrast, change with the prevalence of the disease or outcome being studied, and therefore can and will change when the decision rule is applied to different populations or different settings. Statistical confidence in the results of the test performance should also be explicitly shown, usually in the format of 95% confidence intervals (CIs) as described in Chapter 3.

Some studies combine data collection for the derivation and validation phases in order to streamline the process. In these studies, roughly half of the patient data are used to derive the best predictor variables to create a decision rule. The remaining patient data are then used to validate the decision rule. This split-sampling validation is acceptable, but it yields a CDR with a greater potential for bias which may limit its accuracy when used with other populations. Stiell *et al.* have therefore suggested a hierarchy of CDR validation levels (Table 4.1).

Issues of usability and practicality of the final rule also need to be taken into account. The ease of use of a CDR will be linked to its acceptance and use in clinical practice. Therefore, rules that have too many elements, are complicated to interpret or apply, or have vague or subjective variables are less likely to be widely accepted. In addition, with the recent development of smartphone-based applications and electronic health record generated rules, this may help facilitate the use of more complex CDRs using more data elements.

The final steps in the CDR evolution are assessing the impact, acceptability, sustainability, portability, and cost-effectiveness of the rule in actual clinical practice.[11-15] Reports of the impact of a CDR are described in implementation studies. They reveal if the use of the CDR results in changes in clinical practice and behavior patterns. Sometimes the same CDR can safely reduce testing in some settings while increasing testing in others.[16] Once effectiveness can be demonstrated, the economic effect can then be assessed. Demonstrating that

Table 4.1 Clinical decision rule hierarchy

Level 1: Rules that are useful in a variety of settings with confidence that they change clinical behavior and improve outcomes. This includes prospectively validated rules in one or more different populations, and an impact analysis that demonstrates beneficial changes in clinical behavior

Level 2: Rules that are useful in various settings and that have been validated by a demonstration of accuracy either in a large prospective study with a broad spectrum of patients and doctors or in several small different settings

Level 3: Rules that clinicians may consider using with caution if study patients are similar to those in the clinician's setting. This may include studies that are validated in a single, narrowly defined prospective sample

Level 4: Rules that need further evaluation before clinical application. These include rules that are derived or validated in split samples, in retrospective databases, or by using statistical techniques

---

Source: Adapted from McGinn *et al.* [10] ©2000, American Medical Association, All Rights Reserved.

resources are conserved, health savings are incurred, efficiencies are found, or, optimally, all of the above can determine the success or failure of a decision rule. These trials constitute Level 1 criteria for CDRs. The trial design for an "impact analysis" is often a cluster-randomized trial whereby entire hospitals are randomized to use or not use the CDR via various educational and real-time prompting methods. An example of a well-done impact analysis was conducted across 12 sites to test the impact of the implementation of the Canadian C-spine rule.[17] In the study, six sites were randomized to use active strategies to implement the Canadian C-spine rule (e.g., education, policy, and real-time reminders), while six sites were randomized to use no intervention. The study demonstrated a positive impact, in that the intervention group had a relative reduction of 13% (CI 9–16%) in imaging, while the control group had a 13% (CI 7–18%) increase in imaging rates. No adverse events occurred at any site. The process from concept to final decision rule often takes several years. The derivation and validation phases often are published separately. Implementation and cost-effectiveness studies on a CDR add additional years to a rule's long road to acceptance and use in clinical practice. Indeed, few decision rules have undergone these latter steps of testing rendering the patient-centric value of a CDR undefined or purely theoretical.[18] There is often a temptation to apply the results of a derivation study for a promising new CDR based on the derivation study alone. We explicitly recommend this should not be done, no matter how great the results appear. The initial validation and derivation studies often employ highly trained research personnel to record and elicit the data used in these studies and are, in effect, efficacy studies. That is, under ideal clinical research terms and settings, can a rule be created and applied? This is different and distinct from effectiveness studies that examine how the rule works under regular routine clinical situations that are not study settings. The promising new decision rule should be examined critically and with caution. We should be sure to wait for external validation studies that replicate the findings in new or different settings from the initial sets of derivation and validation studies before incorporating a new CDRs into practice.

The future of CDRs

Few of the chapters in this book have the ideal series of derivation, validation, external validation, implementation, and cost-effectiveness studies to describe and discuss. Instead, many of the common clinical question CDRs have been only partially evaluated or are in the formative stages of evaluation. Since the first edition of this book was published in 2008, the science of CDRs has advanced. Researchers now have instruments to evaluate the acceptability of hypothetical CDRs before spending a decade deriving and validating them.[19] Concurrently, ED content experts continue to prioritize CDR topics that would be mostly highly valued by clinicians.[20] Shared decision-making advocates increasingly collaborate with researchers to align patient preferences with the additive information provided by CDRs in devising testing decisions.[21] Finally, multidisciplinary acceptability of CDRs to guide decision-making is rapidly accelerating. For example, the Pediatric Emergency Care Applied Research Network (PECARN) is developing an increasing number of CDRs and pediatric neurosurgeons have started to develop postimaging decision aids to more accurately align disposition decisions with traumatic brain injury patients most likely to benefit from higher levels of care.[22-24] However, as evidenced by numerous American College of Emergency Physician Clinical Policies and the recent Society for Academic Emergency Medicine Guidelines for Reasonable and Appropriate Care in Emergency Medicine, the majority of common clinical presentations lack a (or any) valid and well-accepted CDR. Our goal is for these discussions to fuel new exploration of clinically relevant questions and the development of new, innovative CDRs.

References

1. Laupacis A, Sekar N, Stiell IG. Clinical prediction rules: A review and suggested modifications of methodological standards. *Journal of the American Medical Association.* 1997; 277(6): 488–94.
2. Reilly BM, Evans AT. Translating clinical research into clinical practice: Impact of using prediction to make decisions. *Annals of Internal Medicine.* 2006; 144(3): 201–9.

3. Carmelli G, Grock A, Picart E, Mason J. The nitty-gritty of clinical decision rules. *Annals of Emergency Medicine.* 2018; 71(6): 711–3.

4. Klang E, Beytelman A, Greenberg D *et al.* Overuse of head CT examinations for the investigation of minor head trauma: Analysis of contributing factors. *Journal of the American College of Radiology.* 2017; 14(2): 171–6.

5. Schriger DL, Elder JW, Cooper RJ. Structured clinical decision aids are seldom compared with subjective physician judgment, and are seldom superior. *Annals of Emergency Medicine.* 2017; 70(3): 338–44.e3.

6. Stiell IG, Lesiuk H, Vandemheen K *et al.* Obtaining consensus for the definition of 'clinically important' brain injury in the CCC Study [abstract]. *Academic Emergency Medicine.* 2000; 7: 572.

7. Stiell IG, Greenberg GH, McKnight RD, Nair RC, McDowell I, Worthington JR. A study to develop clinical decision rules for the use of radiography in acute ankle injuries. *Annals of Emergency Medicine.* 1992; 21(4): 384–90.

8. Stiell IG, Greenberg GH, McKnight RD *et al.* Decision rules for the use of radiography in acute ankle injuries. Refinement and prospective validation. *Journal of the American Medical Association.* 1993; 269(9): 1127–32.

9. Hunter B, Carpenter CR. The development of clinical prediction rules. In: Wilson MP, Guluma KZ, Hayden S, editors. *Doing research in emergency and acute care: Making order out of chaos.* Hoboken, NJ: Wiley; 2016: 139–47.

10. McGinn TG, Guyatt GH, Wyer PC *et al.* Users' guides to the medical literature XXII: How to use articles about clinical decision rules. *JAMA.* 2000; 284(1): 79–84.

11. Stiell IG, McKnight RD, Greenberg GH *et al.* Implementation of the Ottawa ankle rules. *Journal of the American Medical Association.* 1994; 271(11): 827–32.

12. Graham ID, Stiell IG, Laupacis A, O'Connor AM, Wells GA. Emergency physicians' attitudes toward and use of clinical decision rules for radiography. *Academic Emergency Medicine.* 1998; 5(2): 134–40.

13. Verbeek PR, Stiell IG, Hebert G, Sellens C. Ankle radiograph utilization after learning a decision rule: A 12-month follow-up. *Academic Emergency Medicine.* 1997; 4(8): 776–9.

14. Graham ID, Stiell IG, Laupacis A *et al.* Awareness and use of the Ottawa ankle and knee rules in 5 countries: Can publication alone be enough to change practice? *Annals of Emergency Medicine.* 2001; 37(3): 259–66.

15. Anis AH, Stiell IG, Stewart DG, Laupacis A. Cost-effectiveness analysis of the Ottawa ankle rules. *Annals of Emergency Medicine.* 1995; 26(4): 422–8.

16. Stiell IG, Clement CM, Grimshaw JM *et al.* A prospective cluster-randomized trial to implement the Canadian CT head rule in emergency departments. *CMAJ.* 2010; 182(14): 1527–32.

17. Stiell IG, Wells GA. Methodological standards for the development of clinical decision rules in emergency medicine. *Annals of Internal Medicine.* 1999; 33(4): 437–47.

18. Green SM. When do clinical decision rules improve patient care? *Annals of Emergency Medicine.* 2013; 62(2): 132–5.

19. Brehaut JC, Graham ID, Wood TJ *et al.* Measuring acceptability of clinical decision rules: Validation of the Ottawa acceptability of decision rules instrument (OADRI) in four countries. *Medical Decision Making.* 2010; 30(3): 398–408.

20. Finnerty NM, Rodriguez RM, Carpenter CR *et al.* Clinical decision rules for diagnostic imaging in the emergency department: A research agenda. *Academic Emergency Medicine.* 2015; 22(12): 1406–16.

21. Hess EP, Knoedler MA, Shah ND *et al.* The chest pain choice decision aid: A randomized trial. *Circulation. Cardiovascular Quality and Outcomes.* 2012; 5(3): 251–9.

22. Klassen TP, Dalziel SR, Babl FE *et al.* The Pediatric Emergency Research Network (PERN): A decade of global research cooperation in paediatric emergency care. *Emergency Medicine Australasia.* 2021; 33(5): 900–10.

23. Greenberg JK, Yan Y, Carpenter CR *et al.* Development and internal validation of a clinical risk score for treating children with mild head trauma and intracranial injury. *JAMA Pediatrics.* 2017; 171(4): 342–9.

24. Greenberg JK, Yan Y, Carpenter CR *et al.* Development of the CIDSS2 score for children with mild head trauma without intracranial injury. *Journal of Neurotrauma.* 2018; 35(22): 2699–707.

Chapter 5 Appropriate Testing in an Era of Limited Resources: Practice and Policy Considerations

Fernanda Bellolio[1] and Christopher R. Carpenter[2]

[1] Department of Emergency Medicine, Mayo Clinic, Rochester, MN, USA
[2] Department of Emergency Medicine, Washington University School of Medicine, St. Louis, MO, USA

Highlights

- United States spends more on health care than any other country. Spending is not associated with improved population health care outcomes.
- Diagnostic testing accounts for a significant and rising proportion of national health expenditures.
- As a proportion of diagnostic tests are inappropriate and potentially avoidable, there is potential to reduce the direct cost of diagnostic testing. Downstream costs associated with incidental findings on unnecessary tests should also be considered.
- The overuse of diagnostic tests is multifactorial, and an important culprit is the quest for diagnostic certainty.
- Individual clinicians can take steps to improve the appropriateness of their diagnostic test ordering, learning and applying the best evidence to decisions around diagnostic testing.
- In the appropriate situations, shared decision making has been proposed as a way to decrease diagnostic testing.

Evidence-Based Emergency Care: Diagnostic Testing and Clinical Decision Rules, Third Edition.
Edited by Jesse M. Pines, Fernanda Bellolio, Christopher R. Carpenter, and Ali S. Raja.
© 2023 John Wiley & Sons Ltd. Published 2023 by John Wiley & Sons Ltd.

This chapter will focus on the United States, which spends more on health care than any other country. In 2016, the United States spent 18% of its gross domestic product (GDP) on health care, while spending in other high-income nations were 9.6% in Australia, 10.3% in Canada, 10.9% in Japan, and 12.4% in Switzerland.[1] Despite the highest spending, the United States has the lowest proportion of the population with health insurance at 90% compared to other high-income countries at 99.8–100%.[1]

Papanicolas et al. report that this spending was not associated with improved population health care outcomes, and contrary to some explanations for high spending, social spending, and health care utilization in the United States does not differ substantially from other high-income nations. Pharmaceuticals, devices, and administrative costs appeared to be the main drivers of the differences in spending. Specifically, administrative costs of care including scheduling, planning, regulating, and managing health systems and services accounted for 8% in the United States versus a range of 1–3% in the other countries. For pharmaceutical costs, spending per capita was $1443 in the United States compared to a range of $466–$939 in other countries.[1]

Understanding medical expenditures within the context of healthcare resource stewardship and sustainable spending has increased the focus on eliminating low-value care and reducing waste.[2] Proposed solutions include single-payer systems,[3] payment reform (including accountable care organizations, bundled payments, and value-based care instead of volume-based), and more reliably effective care delivery (including care coordination, decreased physician variability in care, at-home medical care, and partnership for patients U.S. Center for Medicare and Medicaid Services [CMS]-initiative).[4] We have created a very complex medical system, and there has been an attempt to reduce the time the physician spends in issues related to insurance, reporting to quality agencies, and medical billing-related paperwork.[5, 6] As an example, there has been an increase in the use of medical scribes to help the administrative tasks of documentation during the medical visit, or use of intermediaries to navigate medical records. Strategies to improve physician efficiency and the increasing administrative demands have been associated with increased rates of physician burnout.[7]

Shrank et al.[4] identified six waste domains including failure of care delivery, failure of care coordination, overtreatment or low-value care, pricing failure, fraud and abuse, and administrative complexity. A call for evidence-based strategies to reduce waste has been proposed. In this context, emergency departments (EDs) play a central role in US healthcare delivery, with 130 million visits in 2018.[8] Increases in ED visit rates have outpaced population growth, until recently with lower visits related to the coronavirus disease

(COVID-19) pandemic. Yet, there has been an increase in intensity of care which means more extensive, costly, and time consuming workup including diagnostic imaging and laboratory tests, causing ED overcrowding.[9] ED care is often fragmented and more costly than in other settings; as a result, EDs are a target for reforms. The adoption of alternative payment models to improve patient outcomes and reduce costs have been proposed. Accountable care organizations and other financial risk-bearing entities primarily focus on reducing ED visits rather than engaging with EDs improving quality of care delivery.[9]

What role does physician decision-making around the use of diagnostic tests play in the debate around the rising cost of healthcare? Diagnostic testing makes up a significant and growing proportion of national healthcare expenditures. When ordered appropriately, diagnostic tests, such as computed tomography (CT) for abdominal pain, can help reduce resource use by identifying patients who do not need hospitalization or further interventions. Yet, in our search for certainty, we sometimes order tests that are unlikely to affect our medical decision-making. Many tests add no information and do not affect decision-making (e.g., "routine bloodwork" for the adult with gastroenteritis). Worse yet, out of tradition, habit, the request of other services, or lack of access to previous results, we repeat tests that have been recently performed and are unlikely to have changed.[10, 11] Diagnostic tests that do not add useful information are a clear form of medical waste – directly visible to and controllable by clinicians. Less visible to emergency clinicians, but more important from a cost perspective, are the downstream costs of diagnostic testing. Unnecessary tests could also yield false-positive results requiring follow-up tests or treatments to ensure the patient does not have conditions not initially suspected, for example an elevated potassium may reflect a hemolyzed sample. Despite the overwhelming evidence that many diagnostic tests are of little or no value, changing practice is difficult. For example, routine preoperative testing of healthy adults is the norm across the United States despite strong evidence that it provides no value.[12, 13] We believe that improving the appropriateness of diagnostic testing is one way that medical professionals can reduce costs and improve value, as it can be done while improving the quality of patient care. Unfortunately, to date, many physicians have shown little interest or ability to do this. This is our challenge – apply the best evidence at the bedside and build systems to support us, before insurance and government regulators build them for us.

In this chapter, we discuss the role of diagnostic testing on healthcare costs, identify practice changes that physicians can implement to help improve the appropriateness of testing, and discuss policy approaches to reducing the use of testing.

Impact of diagnostic testing on healthcare expenditures

Healthcare spending is rising across the world at rates above the rate of economic growth or the willingness of societies to increase taxation. The US national healthcare spending in 2019 was $3.8 trillion, or $11,582 per person, accounting for 17.7% of GDP.[14]

As healthcare is the single largest component of current and future deficit spending, rising costs are leading to political conflict and gridlock affecting many other areas. At the individual level, as healthcare costs rise, fewer people have access to care and more people suffer when they get sick, due to events such as medical bankruptcy.[15] In this environment, healthcare providers should expect stable or shrinking resources and significant pressure to cut costs. If providers do not lead with solutions, politicians and businesses will be forced to implement controls. Political solutions to rising costs are unlikely to reflect the best available scientific evidence.

Diagnostic testing accounts for a significant and rising proportion of national health expenditures. Exact calculations of spending on diagnostic testing are difficult, as testing can appear in several different categories of health expenditures (e.g., hospital care, physician services, and other professional services) and is sometimes bundled with other costs, such as during hospitalization. The cost of diagnostic imaging has risen dramatically over the years. Spending on the physician services associated with imaging, just one component of imaging costs was $10.4 billion in 2018.[16] The US imaging services market size was valued at $128.1 billion in 2019 and is anticipated to grow at a compound annual growth rate (CAGR) of 4.6% from 2020 to 2027.[17]

Imaging has been argued to be cost-effective in reducing hospital admissions and invasive procedures, and therefore has the potential to reduce total healthcare costs. Interestingly, some studies have found that providers that perform more tests and use more ED resources are also more likely to admit patients,[18] and one study reported no significant test-ordering differences between ED physicians versus advanced practice providers caring for patients with chest pain or abdominal pain.[19]

Downstream costs of diagnostic testing

As a proportion of diagnostic tests are inappropriate and potentially avoidable, there is great potential to reduce the direct cost of diagnostic testing. Equally important as the direct costs of diagnostic tests are the downstream costs associated with incidental findings on unnecessary tests. While we should order diagnostic tests to answer a specific question, the results sometimes do not answer the question specifically. Instead, they provide a range of information that can influence the probability of disease and help with risk stratification. They may also provide additional information to other questions that we did not wish to ask. A false-positive test result may not be in concordance with the rest of our thinking, yet still requires further downstream workup. For example, consider a patient admitted to the hospital from the ED with community-acquired pneumonia and blood cultures that yield Gram-positive cocci in clusters, ultimately revealing *Staphylococcus aureus*. The blood culture may generate downstream testing such as repeat blood cultures and an echocardiogram. Studies have estimated that false-positive blood cultures add tens of thousands of dollars to the overall hospital costs.[20] Additionally, the diagnostic test may give answers to questions we did not wish to ask. For example, when ordering a pulmonary angiogram CT to evaluate a patient for pulmonary embolism, the scan will often reveal incidental findings in the thorax and upper abdomen such as pulmonary nodules or renal masses. Standard medical practice requires appropriate follow-up for these incidental findings, which usually involves repeat imaging and may require biopsies and eventual treatment. Thus, indirect costs of the original test include workup and treatment of false positives and incidental findings.

Variation in testing and inappropriate testing

There is evidence that a significant proportion of diagnostic tests performed in the United States are potentially avoidable based on the patient's clinical condition and the best available evidence.[21] One way to look at this is to look at the indications for specific tests. Retrospective studies of diagnostic test services show that a significant proportion of diagnostic tests do not have evidence to support their use in the patient. Studies of geographic variation also illustrate this.[22] For example, patients in some areas of the United States are more likely to undergo cardiac catheterization for stable angina or after an acute myocardial infarction (MI) than patients in other regions, regardless of the appropriateness of the procedure. Similar patterns have been shown with the use of laboratory tests and other diagnostic tests like magnetic resonance imaging (MRI), CT, and cardiac stress test.[23] Such variation also exists within hospitals, departments, and practices, even after adjustment for a patient's clinical condition and comorbidities. Such variation is reasonable for some diagnostic tests where there is little definitive evidence, such as abdominal CT for undifferentiated abdominal pain. It is hard to justify for conditions that have been well studied and for which validated clinical decision rules are available, such as ankle X-rays (Chapter 12) or D-dimer for pulmonary embolism[24] (Chapter 52).

There are variations in testing not explained by variations in practice or hospital settings, for example within the same institution some clinicians will test more than others.[25] Variations in testing are also dependent on the population or area of practice. EDs represent a safety net for several patients without access to primary care or outpatient clinics. Some patients who could be eligible for a conservative (e.g., wait and watch) approach might not have the opportunity to seek or access outpatient care. Also penalizing providers for patients' return visits to the ED might increase the desire for diagnostic certainty with the idea of reducing such returns. Having primary care access has been demonstrated to influence the rate of imaging. In one study, the rate of CT utilization was higher among patients without a primary care physician compared to those that had access to outpatient primary care.[26] Increased availability of primary care, particularly for follow-up from the ED, could reduce ED resource utilization and therefore decrease costs, ED lengths of stay, and radiation exposure.

Causes of inappropriate testing

Inappropriate use of diagnostic tests can be classified into the categories of underuse, overuse, and misuse. *Underuse* refers to the failure to provide a healthcare service when there is evidence that it would have produced a favorable outcome for the patient, like delay in diagnosis or treatment. *Overuse* occurs when a test or treatment is used without medical justification – a diagnostic test without evidence to support its use in the condition, patient, or setting. *Misuse* of preference-sensitive care refers to situations in which there are significant trade-offs among the available options (such as the choice between CT and observation in a young woman with an atypical presentation for early appendicitis). Choices should be based on the patient's own values, but often they are not.[27] Misuse results from the failure to accurately communicate the alternative's risks and benefits, and the failure to base the choice of diagnostic test on the patient's values and preferences. In this chapter, we focus on overuse and misuse of diagnostic tests, as they are an important focus in the ongoing discussion of cost control in healthcare. In Chapter 60 we discuss shared decision-making with examples of cases of equipoise and balance of available evidence and patients' values and preferences. Table 5.1 illustrates the types of overuse and misuse of diagnostic testing.

The overuse of diagnostic tests in the United States is multifactorial, and an important culprit is the quest for diagnostic certainty. Clinicians give many reasons why they order diagnostic tests that they acknowledge have little or no value, including fear of missing diagnoses (defensive medicine),

Table 5.1 Categories of misuse and overuse of diagnostic testing in emergency medicine

Category	Rationale	Examples
Bad test	Evidence does not support the use of the diagnostic test for the clinical indication	• Erythrocyte sedimentation rate (ESR) and C-reactive protein (CRP) to evaluate for septic arthritis[28] • Abdominal X-rays (KUB) for abdominal pain
Good test but wrong patient	Evidence does not support the use of the diagnostic test in the patient population	• Blood culture for non-critically ill cases of community-acquired pneumonia • X-ray for atraumatic low back pain without red flags • D-dimer for patients at very low clinical risk of pulmonary embolism (PERC rule negative)
Good test but wrong time or setting	Evidence does not support the use of the diagnostic test at the time of the encounter	• Lyme disease serology testing at the time of tick identification and removal • Screening labs for a patient with known psychiatric disease presenting with symptom exacerbation[29]
Lack of additive information in context to other tests being ordered	The test does not add information beyond other tests being performed	• Creatinine kinase in addition to troponin to evaluate for acute myocardial infarction (MI) (excluding recent MI) • Amylase in addition to lipase to evaluate for pancreatitis
Misuse of diagnostic test	The test is not appropriate based on available alternatives and the patient's preferences	• Routine use of CT abdomen and pelvis in young women with early presentation of right lower quadrant pain that could be early appendicitis, when ultrasound or observation is preferred

avoiding diagnostic errors, lack of clear guidelines on the specific encounter, lack of awareness or adoption of clinical decision rules, lack of awareness of the cost, patient's requests, other physicians or consulting services' requests, increased complexity of emergency care, and incentives to decrease hospital admissions.[30, 31] Additionally, there are financial incentives to encourage inappropriate testing, such as the fee-for-service medical system. Specifically, in emergency medicine in the United States, physician reimbursement is determined by the complexity of the visit. Ordering and interpretation of diagnostic tests are key determinants of complexity. For example, evaluating a patient with a mild traumatic head injury by routinely ordering a CT will generate a larger bill than using a clinical decision rule and not ordering a CT. While each of these plays a role in over-ordering diagnostic tests, none is as important as our cultural search for medical certainty. According to Sir William Osler, medicine at its heart is an art and science of uncertainty.

A systematic review found that diagnostic testing did not reduce illness concern, symptom persistence, or anxiety when compared with no testing. Furthermore, diagnostic testing did not influence the frequency of return visits among patients with low probability of serious disease.[32]

Advances in diagnostic testing have dramatically improved our ability to reduce uncertainty, reduce unnecessary invasive procedures and hospitalizations, but uncertainty will never be eliminated. In the United States, we have built a culture that expects diagnostic certainty, despite our knowledge of Bayesian theory and the limitations of specific diagnostic tests. This is reflected in our clinical language, such as "this test will rule out that diagnosis," our systems, such as having single cutoffs for normal and abnormal on continuous tests, our medical culture, such as morbidity and mortality conferences, and our legal system. A major casualty of this quest for diagnostic certainty is an appreciation and use of clinical evidence at the bedside. If diagnostic certainty is valued above all else, there is little incentive for physicians to learn and apply the available evidence when ordering tests. Unsurprisingly clinicians do not routinely apply the best evidence to the decision to order diagnostic tests – leading to inappropriate testing.[33, 34]

Medical liability and the fear of getting sued might lead physicians to order more diagnostic tests, but these are not the main causes of inappropriate testing.[35] In fact, significant tort reform across three states between 1997 and 2011 was not associated with reductions in CT or MRI ordering – image ordering actually increased when adjusted for ED volumes.[36] It is worth noting that ordering tests that are not supported by medical evidence is unlikely to protect a practitioner from liability. Furthermore, inappropriate testing exposes clinicians to additional liability such as having incongruent and unexplained lab results (e.g., an elevated white blood cell (WBC) count in a patient without other signs of infection) and incidental findings requiring outpatient follow-up.[37] While limiting medical liability could influence our quest for diagnostic certainty, it would not stop inappropriate testing by itself. We have trained patients and family members to expect diagnostic certainty. Reducing inappropriate testing will require us to acknowledge uncertainty with each other and our patients and build systems that allow clinicians to apply the best evidence to diagnostic decisions at the bedside. We hope this book is one step in that direction.

Improving appropriateness in diagnostic testing: practice considerations

Individual clinicians can take steps to improve the appropriateness of their diagnostic test ordering. Primarily, they can attempt to learn and apply the best evidence to their frequent decisions around diagnostic testing. This includes identifying good sources of information around diagnostic testing, regular reading, and applying the knowledge at the bedside. The use of handbooks such as this and websites like www.mdcalc.com will help in busy clinical situations.

Physician practices, including EDs, should implement systems to improve the appropriateness of test ordering. These systems include standardized pathways and guidelines, clinical decision support (CDS), and auditing practice with feedback to providers including data on the cost of testing. Ideally, the systems and decision support facilitate workload and do not increase the currently overloaded clinicians. Table 5.2 lists approach to improving appropriateness.

Standardized clinical pathways and guidelines are widely published[38] but have had little effect on individual clinicians' practice behavior.[39] The practice of medicine has been taught as an individual art with emphasis on provider autonomy and exceptionalism. Standardization of practice, such as through guidelines, is often seen as anathema to physician autonomy. Clinicians can overcome these barriers and successfully implement practice guidelines if they follow several steps. First, the guideline should be developed using the best available evidence. Second, the guidelines need to be adapted or modified locally, so it addresses local practice patterns and concerns, and includes stakeholder's input. Third, clinical decision leaders need to endorse and promote the guideline. Fourth, clinical systems need to be modified so that the practice guideline is integrated into the clinical workflow. Finally, practitioners need to receive data on their performance relative to the guideline of the group. Some practices have been able to demonstrate reduced utilization of tests, shorter lengths of stay, decrease costs, and

Table 5.2 Practice improvements to address inappropriate diagnostic testing

Intervention
Improved provider knowledge • Better evidence: comparative effectiveness studies, systematic reviews, and evidence-based clinical guidelines • Provider awareness: journal clubs, required reading, continuous professional development activities • Awareness of costs
Availability of evidence at the time of ordering • Tailoring guidelines to local practice, specific patients, and clinical situations • Posters and pocket cards • Decision aids and user-friendly clinical prediction rules • Computerized decision support systems
Performance monitoring and feedback • Use of pretest probability, diagnostic testing, and diagnostic yield • Real-time feedback on appropriateness of diagnostic testing • Cost of diagnostic testing

improved quality through the development and integration of guidelines into local clinical culture, information systems, and practices.[40] Yet, it is not easy work, and clinicians will need tools to support this practice change. Educational outreach visits and audit and feedback interventions for clinical practice guideline implementation were shown to be effective in improving the process of care and clinical outcomes; results for reminders and provider incentives showed mixed or ineffective results in one study.[41]

A review on barriers and facilitators for de-implementation of low-value care found several articles focused on diagnostic tests including 11 studies for imaging and 11 for laboratory tests. Provider level factors included beliefs and opinions of healthcare providers, fear of medical errors, practicing defensive medicine, and desire to meet patient's expectations. Facilitators for change included ownership of the problem and a desire to restrict unnecessary care. It was noted that even if a provider has the knowledge of low-value care, behaviors are difficult to change secondary to routines and habits. The review reported that provider–patient communication was a key skill for de-implementation and should be part of a multifaceted de-implementation strategy to reduce low-value care.[42] Other studies evaluating interventions for decreasing low-value care included providing timely feedback to providers. A study proposed to display the mean abnormal result rate as metric for benchmarking selectivity in laboratory test ordering.[43] Another study failed to demonstrate a reduction of inappropriate laboratory use when imposing co-pay fees for patients and test restrictions for emergency providers.[44]

To support implementation and reduce work duplication, the American College of Emergency Physicians (ACEP) has endorsed clinical policies from outside organizations including, for example, guidelines for ventilation-perfusion imaging in pulmonary embolism[45] and appropriate utilization of cardiovascular imaging in ED patients with chest pain.[46]

In recent years, there has been an exponential use of CDS integrated into the electronic medical record. CDS uses patient data to generate case-specific clinical advice. For example, a radiology ordering system's decision support would include validated clinical decision rules, and clinicians would be required to complete them prior to ordering tests (e.g., Wells criteria for pulmonary embolus). When clinicians want to order a test outside of the guideline, the system can impose varying degrees of interference, from a requirement that the clinician document the reason for deviation to a hard stop requiring a conversation with a supervisory physician. Decision support systems have been shown to improve appropriateness of test ordering and to decrease utilization of diagnostic testing in some studies.[47] One variation on decision support is to actively provide the cost of diagnostic tests to providers at the time of ordering. This makes the cost of testing visible and has been shown to reduce use and improve appropriateness of testing. Leveraging the electronic health record in a way that is acceptable to clinicians will become the basis of interventions that may help to combat the compulsion to "do more." Such interventions might include default options, accountable justification alerts, or peer comparison.[48]

The Choosing Wisely initiative in the United States specifically addresses issues related to imaging in the ED including avoid CT scans of the head in ED patients with minor head injury who are at low risk based on validated decision rules; avoid CT of the head in patients with syncope, insignificant trauma and a normal neurological evaluation; avoid CT pulmonary angiography patients with a low pretest probability of pulmonary embolism and either a negative pulmonary embolism rule out criteria (PERC) or a negative D-dimer; avoid lumbar spine imaging for adults with nontraumatic back pain unless the patient has severe or progressive neurologic deficits or is suspected of having a serious underlying condition (such as vertebral infection or bony metastasis); avoid ordering CT of the abdomen and pelvis in young otherwise healthy patients (age < 50) with known histories of kidney stones, or ureterolithiasis, presenting with symptoms consistent with uncomplicated renal colic.[49] Guidelines with a combination of evidence and multispecialty consensus and stakeholder engagement, including patients, are needed to help appropriate testing. For example, Moore *et al.* attained consensus between Urologists, Radiologists, and Emergency Medicine representatives by synthesizing diagnostic accuracy and impact evidence around ultrasonography or no further imaging in specific clinical scenarios for patients with renal colic or reduced-radiation-dose CT when CT is recommended for patients with suspected renal colic.[50] More multidisciplinary, vignette-based approaches to illustrate the application of evidence to specific diagnostic testing scenarios are required in emergency medicine.

When clinicians are faced with a diagnostic challenge, shared decision-making has been proposed as a way to decrease diagnostic testing. A qualitative study on factors influencing variation in investigations after a negative CT brain in suspected subarachnoid hemorrhage demonstrated patient interaction was at the forefront of the identified factors. Specifically, how the clinician communicates the benefits and harms of the diagnostic options. Patient risk profile, clinical evidence and practice guidelines, providers experience, requests for consulting services, practice location, and work processes also influenced variation in testing.[51]

Health policy considerations

In response to rising US healthcare costs, payers and policy makers are implementing measures to improve the efficiency of the acute care system through payment reform and delivery innovation. Alternative payment models that move away from traditional fee-for-service payment often have explicit goals to reduce utilization.[9] Examples include funding comparative effectiveness research, publishing guidelines, implementing performance measures for public reporting and incentive-based compensation ("pay-for-performance"), and requiring preauthorization prior to ordering diagnostic tests. If physicians and hospitals cannot control the rising cost of diagnostic testing, we should be prepared for government and external payers to impose external controls upon us.

Full and partially capitated models create incentives for longitudinal and episodic ED providers and payers to unite to create interventions to reduce costs. However, prospective attribution remains a challenge for EDs because of exogenous demand, which makes it important for EDs to be one of the components of capitated payment along with longitudinal providers who can exert greater control on overall care demands.[9] Improved availability of electronic health information across settings, evidence generated from developing and testing acute care-specific payment models, and engaging acute care providers directly in reform efforts will help meet these goals.[9]

Government and private payers are trying to improve the quality of evidence available to clinicians regarding diagnostic tests. It has long been noted that the majority of government research funding for healthcare goes into basic sciences and the development of new tests and treatments, the primary aims of the National Institutes of Health. Research on how to effectively apply available tests and treatments is funded at only a fraction of this level, primarily through the Agency for Healthcare Research and Quality and Patient-Centered Outcomes Research (PCORI). However, most of this currently available funding does not align with acute ED care.

Public and private payers are developing and implementing performance measures of diagnostic testing for public reporting and pay-for-performance programs. These performance measures, also known as *quality measures*, aim to measure utilization or appropriateness of diagnostic testing.[52, 53] Utilization measures are easiest to develop and calculate, as they can be calculated from a large administrative database, such as Medicare claims. Alternatively, appropriateness measures attempt to use clinical information to determine if the diagnostic test was appropriate for the patient for whom it was ordered. Appropriateness measures require electronic medical records or chart review and are therefore more time-consuming and costly to implement. Payers and providers are at odds over the accuracy of utilization measures calculated from administrative claims – a debate that will intensify as the pressure over costs grows. An example is Medicare's measure "OP-15: Use of brain CT in the ED for atraumatic headache." This measure uses Medicare claims to determine the appropriateness of brain CT scans performed in patients with headaches but providers are concerned that it does not accurately account for patients' clinical condition.[54]

The most direct way to control diagnostic test utilization is to require prior authorization. Private payers have increasingly implemented such authorizations for expensive tests and treatments. They are nearly universal for high-cost imaging tests such as CT and MRI. Although EDs were initially excluded, they are being increasingly required to obtain prior authorization or are subject to retroactive denials. Table 5.3 lists several policy and regulatory approaches to reducing diagnostic testing in the United States.

Table 5.3 Policy and regulatory approaches to reducing utilization of testing in the United States

Regulations on ordering of tests	Preauthorization requirements for imaging
Cost-sharing by patients	Co-pays for high-cost diagnostic tests (e.g., MRI)
Pay-for-performance programs around diagnostic testing	Medicare measures of imaging efficiency Head CT for atraumatic headache in the ED MRI for low back pain prior to conservative therapy

The Centers for Medicare & Medicaid Services is implementing the program and requires following the Appropriate Use Criteria through approved CDS mechanisms prior to ordering advanced imaging services like CTs, MRI, or nuclear medicine images. In 2014, the Protecting Access to Medicare Act (PAMA) created the Appropriate Use Criteria program, which will require specific steps for providers ordering advanced imaging for Medicare patients. PAMA exempts emergency services ordered for an individual with an emergency medical condition, and this includes individuals with a suspected emergency. The American College of Radiology (ACR) defines the appropriateness criteria as evidence-based guidelines to assist health providers in selecting the most appropriate imaging for a specific clinical condition. It includes acute pathology like syncope, chest pain, and pelvic pain, among others. The ACR's practice parameters report that these standards are not inflexible rules or requirements of practice and are not intended, nor should they be used, to establish a legal standard of care. The report establishes that certain imaging might be appropriate depending on the clinical condition of the patient, limitations of available resources, or advances in knowledge or technology subsequent to publication of the guidelines.[55]

Preventing overdiagnoses in emergency medicine include the following policy priorities: (i) Review and revise all specialist-directed guidelines using the grading of recommendations assessment development and evaluation (GRADE) to explicitly recognize, describe, and quantify the potential harms of overdiagnosis and consequential overtreatment.[38, 56] (ii) Derive mutually agreeable measures of overuse, overtesting, overdiagnosis, and overtreatment. (iii) Dissociate physician payments from test ordering. (iv) Provide incentives for "appropriate" testing. (v) Regulate direct-to-consumer advertising.[57–59] Other policy recommendations included the development of widely accepted measures across specialties and stakeholders for overtesting, and ensuring that guideline developers include a representative voice and standardized terms.[59]

Transitioning to a state of health care delivery that prioritizes value over volume will require balancing policies and work to affect local cultural change. Such an approach involves implementing de-adoption strategies tailored to address the behavioral and organizational factors that drive the provision of low-value care within a local health care ecosystem, whether it is an individual practice or a tertiary referral center.[48] Proposed de-adoption approaches include: (i) Validated and readily applicable approaches to measure low-value care across the spectrum of health services. (ii) A roadmap to guide de-adoption efforts and develop embedded research agendas in which the measurement of low-value care becomes a standard component of quality measurement. (iii) Policies and interventions intended to mitigate the delivery of low-value care must align with the motivations of patients and clinicians at the time a health service is ordered. (iv) A bottom-up approach to targeting low-value care necessitates the development of new interventions that focus on shared heuristics, cognitive biases, and attitudes. For example, poor numeracy and framing could lead physicians and patients to systematically overestimate potential benefits and underestimate potential harms of low-value services.[48]

Comment

More testing does not translate to better outcomes, and several studies suggest higher spending and increased testing linked to worse outcomes and overtreatment.[59] With the aging of the population, the number of patients with a high number of comorbidities and atypical presentations will increase furthering the financial implications of overuse of diagnostic testing.[59, 60]

Discomfort with uncertainty and fear of missing a diagnosis can drive overuse, because physicians and patients may perceive that it is better to do something rather than nothing.[61] These examples highlight implicit cognitive errors rather than extrinsically motivated overuse decisions.[48] Carpenter *et al.*[59], while referring to overtesting, reported that each condition is likely to have different diagnostic thresholds depending on perspective, which in turn may drive overdiagnosis. In this regard, patient and key stakeholder engagement, and focus on patient-centered and patient-important outcomes are required for appropriate testing. Agreement between multidisciplinary stakeholders within a healthcare system, risk management leaders, patients, payers, and policy makers will be difficult, and an intense public health campaign might be required. Communication of this message should include a summary of the evidence for overdiagnosis within the context of overtreatment, balance of harms and benefits between overtesting and undertesting, in conjunction with educating healthcare providers in graduate and postgraduate education, among others.[59] Informing practice through patient-oriented outcomes will likely provide the right balance to guard against overtesting, overdiagnosis, and overtreatment, particularly in older adults.[60]

Overtesting is a way to increase diagnostic certainty in a setting with limited time available at the patients' bedside, multiple simultaneous patients not known to the provider, and high cognitive overload. Replacing readily available imaging with more detailed clinical evaluation and close follow-up necessitates more time at the bedside, which may negatively affect ED operational flow.[59] Development of effective decision support tools at the point of care is needed, educating providers in pretest and posttest probabilities, to guide them when choosing different diagnostic testing. Further work on clinical practice guidelines in common scenarios is needed to describe reasonable approaches for diagnostic in the ED setting. Moving away from fee-for-service via payment reforms, and initiatives to address the behavioral drivers of low-value care are needed. Key to these efforts will be the reliable measurement of low-value care; incorporation of low-value care as a component of performance measurement; and the implementation of interventions that align with the motivations of patients, clinicians, and health care organizations.[48]

References

1. Papanicolas I, Woskie LR, Jha AK. Health care spending in the United States and other high-income countries. *JAMA*. 2018; 319: 1024–39.

2. Berwick DM, Hackbarth AD. Eliminating waste in US health care. *JAMA*. 2012; 307: 1513–6.

3. Woolhandler S, Himmelstein DU. Single-payer reform: The only way to fulfill the president's pledge of more coverage, better benefits, and lower costs. *Annals of Internal Medicine*. 2017; 166: 587–8.

4. Shrank WH, Rogstad TL, Parekh N. Waste in the US health care system: Estimated costs and potential for savings. *JAMA*. 2019; 322: 1501–9.

5. Casalino LP, Gans D, Weber R et al. US physician practices spend more than $15.4 billion annually to report quality measures. *Health Affairs (Millwood)*. 2016; 35: 401–6.

6. Tseng P, Kaplan RS, Richman BD, Shah MA, Schulman KA. Administrative costs associated with physician billing and insurance-related activities at an academic health care system. *JAMA*. 2018; 319: 691–7.

7. Shanafelt TD, Boone S, Tan L et al. Burnout and satisfaction with work-life balance among US physicians relative to the general US population. *Archives of Internal Medicine*. 2012; 172: 1377–85.

8. National Center for Health Statistics. Emergency Department Visits. https://www.cdc.gov/nchs/fastats/emergency-department.htm. 2018. Accessed April 1, 2021.

9. Pines JM, McStay F, George M, Wiler JL, McClellan M. Aligning payment reform and delivery innovation in emergency care. *The American Journal of Managed Care*. 2016; 22: 515–8.

10. Liepert AE, Cochran A. CT utilization in transferred trauma patients. *The Journal of Surgical Research*. 2011; 170: 309–13.

11. Griffey RT, Sodickson A. Cumulative radiation exposure and cancer risk estimates in emergency department patients undergoing repeat or multiple CT. *AJR. American Journal of Roentgenology*. 2009; 192: 887–92.

12. Mudumbai SC, Pershing S, Bowe T et al. Variability and costs of low-value preoperative testing for cataract surgery within the veterans health administration. *JAMA Network Open*. 2021; 4: e217470.

13. Matulis J, Liu S, Mecchella J, North F, Holmes A. Choosing wisely: A quality improvement initiative to decrease unnecessary preoperative testing. *BMJ Quality Improvement Reports*. 2017; 6: bmjqir.u216281.w6691.

14. National Health Expenditures. Highlights. https://www.cms.gov/Research-Statistics-Data-and-Systems/Statistics-Trends-and-Reports/NationalHealth ExpendData/NationalHealthAccountsHistorical. 2019. Accessed April 1, 2021.

15. Himmelstein DU, Thorne D, Warren E, Woolhandler S. Medical bankruptcy in the United States, 2007: Results of a national study. *The American Journal of Medicine*. 2009; 122: 741–6.

16. Medicare Payment Advisory Commission (MEDPAC). Health Care Spending and the Medicare Program. https://www.medpac.gov/wp-content/uploads/ import_data/scrape_files/docs/default-source/data-book/july2021_medpac_ databook_sec.pdf. 2020. Accessed April 1, 2021.

17. Grand View Research. U.S. Imaging Services Market Size, Share & Trends Analysis Report By Modality (X-ray, Nuclear Medicine Scans, Ultrasound, MRI Scans), By End Use (Hospitals, Diagnostic Imaging Centers), and Segment Forecasts, 2020 - 2027. https://www.grandviewresearch.com/industry-analysis/ us-imaging-services-market. 2020. Accessed April 1, 2021.

18. Hodgson NR, Saghafian S, Mi L *et al.* Are testers also admitters? Comparing emergency physician resource utilization and admitting practices. *The American Journal of Emergency Medicine*. 2018; 36: 1865–9.

19. Pines JM, Zocchi MS, Ritsema TS, Bedolla J, Venkat A, USACSR Group. Emergency physician and advanced practice provider diagnostic testing and admission decisions in chest pain and abdominal pain. *Academic Emergency Medicine*. 2021; 28: 36–45.

20. Dempsey C, Skoglund E, Muldrew KL, Garey KW. Economic health care costs of blood culture contamination: A systematic review. *American Journal of Infection Control*. 2019; 47: 963–7.

21. Waste and Inefficiency in the U.S. Health Care System. Clinical Care: A Comprehensive Analysis in Support of System-Wide Improvements. New England Healthcare Institute. https://www.nehi.net/writable/publication_files/ file/waste_clinical_care_report_final.pdf. 2008. Accessed April 1, 2021.

22. How Many More Studies Will It Take? NEHI Compendium on Overuse. https:// www.nehi.net/publications/56-how-many-more-studies-will-it-take/view. 2008. Accessed April 1, 2021.

23. Tailor TD, Choudhury KR, Tong BC, Christensen JD, Sosa JA, Rubin GD. Geographic access to CT for lung cancer screening: A census tract-level analysis of cigarette smoking in the United States and driving distance to a CT facility. *Journal of the American College of Radiology*. 2019; 16: 15–23.

24. Venkatesh AK, Kline JA, Courtney DM *et al.* Evaluation of pulmonary embolism in the emergency department and consistency with a national quality measure: Quantifying the opportunity for improvement. *Archives of Internal Medicine*. 2012; 172: 1028–32.

25. Prevedello LM, Raja AS, Ip IK, Sodickson A, Khorasani R. Does clinical decision support reduce unwarranted variation in yield of CT pulmonary angiogram? *The American Journal of Medicine*. 2013; 126: 975–81.

26. Bellolio MF, Bellew SD, Sangaralingham LR *et al.* Access to primary care and computed tomography use in the emergency department. *BMC Health Services Research*. 2018; 18: 154.

27. Dorsett M, Cooper RJ, Taira BR, Wilkes E, Hoffman JR. Bringing value, balance and humanity to the emergency department: The right care top 10 for emergency medicine. *Emergency Medicine Journal.* 2020; 37: 240–5.

28. Carpenter CR, Schuur JD, Everett WW, Pines JM. Evidence-based diagnostics: Adult septic arthritis. *Academic Emergency Medicine.* 2011; 18: 781–96.

29. Chennapan K, Mullinax S, Anderson E *et al.* Medical screening of mental health patients in the emergency department: A systematic review. *The Journal of Emergency Medicine.* 2018; 55: 799–812.

30. Litkowski PE, Smetana GW, Zeidel ML, Blanchard MS. Curbing the urge to image. *The American Journal of Medicine.* 2016; 129: 1131–5.

31. Newman-Toker DE, McDonald KM, Meltzer DO. How much diagnostic safety can we afford, and how should we decide? A health economics perspective. *BMJ Quality and Safety.* 2013; 22(Suppl 2): ii11–20.

32. Rolfe A, Burton C. Reassurance after diagnostic testing with a low pretest probability of serious disease: Systematic review and meta-analysis. *JAMA Internal Medicine.* 2013; 173: 407–16.

33. Salehi L, Phalpher P, Ossip M, Meaney C, Valani R, Mercuri M. Variability in practice patterns among emergency physicians in the evaluation of patients with a suspected diagnosis of pulmonary embolism. *Emergency Radiology.* 2020; 27: 127–34.

34. Sud R, Langfield J, Chu G. Heightened clinical suspicion of pulmonary embolism and disregard of the D-dimer assay: A contemporary trend in an era of increased access to computed tomography pulmonary angiogram? *Internal Medicine Journal.* 2013; 43: 1231–6.

35. Baicker K, Fisher ES, Chandra A. Malpractice liability costs and the practice of medicine in the medicare program. *Health Affairs (Millwood).* 2007; 26: 841–52.

36. Waxman DA, Greenberg MD, Ridgely MS, Kellermann AL, Heaton P. The effect of malpractice reform on emergency department care. *The New England Journal of Medicine.* 2014; 371: 1518–25.

37. Gale BD, Bissett-Siegel DP, Davidson SJ, Juran DC. Failure to notify reportable test results: Significance in medical malpractice. *Journal of the American College of Radiology.* 2011; 8: 776–9.

38. Musey PI Jr, Bellolio F, Upadhye S *et al.* Guidelines for reasonable and appropriate care in the emergency department (GRACE): Recurrent, low-risk chest pain in the emergency department. *Academic Emergency Medicine.* 2021; 28: 718–44.

39. Trent SA, Johnson MA, Morse EA, Havranek EP, Haukoos JS. Patient, provider, and environmental factors associated with adherence to cardiovascular and cerebrovascular clinical practice guidelines in the ED. *The American Journal of Emergency Medicine.* 2018; 36: 1397–404.

40. The New York Times Magazine. Making Health Care Better. https://www.nytimes.com/2009/11/08/magazine/08Healthcare-t.html. 2009. Accessed April 1, 2021.

41. Chan WV, Pearson TA, Bennett GC *et al.* ACC/AHA special report: Clinical practice guideline implementation strategies: A summary of systematic reviews by the NHLBI Implementation Science Work Group: A report of the American College

of Cardiology/American Heart Association Task Force on Clinical Practice Guidelines. *Circulation.* 2017; 135: e122–37.

42. van Dulmen SA, Naaktgeboren CA, Heus P *et al.* Barriers and facilitators to reduce low-value care: A qualitative evidence synthesis. *BMJ Open.* 2020; 10: e040025.

43. Naugler CT, Guo M. Mean abnormal result rate: Proof of concept of a new metric for benchmarking selectivity in laboratory test ordering. *American Journal of Clinical Pathology.* 2016; 145: 568–73.

44. Petrou P. Failed attempts to reduce inappropriate laboratory utilization in an emergency department setting in cyprus: Lessons learned. *The Journal of Emergency Medicine.* 2016; 50: 510–7.

45. Waxman AD, Bajc M, Brown M *et al.* Appropriate use criteria for ventilation-perfusion imaging in pulmonary embolism: Summary and excerpts. *Journal of Nuclear Medicine.* 2017; 58: 13N–5N.

46. Emergency Department Patients With Chest Pain Writing Panel, Rybicki FJ, Udelson JE, Peacock WF *et al.* ACR/ACC/AHA/AATS/ACEP/ASNC/NASCI/ SAEM/SCCT/SCMR/SCPC/SNMMI/STR/STS appropriate utilization of cardiovascular imaging in emergency department patients with chest pain: A joint document of the American College of Radiology Appropriateness Criteria Committee and the American College of Cardiology Appropriate Use Criteria Task Force. *Journal of the American College of Radiology.* 2015; 2016(13): e1–29.

47. Roshanov PS, You JJ, Dhaliwal J *et al.* Can computerized clinical decision support systems improve practitioners' diagnostic test ordering behavior? A decision-maker-researcher partnership systematic review. *Implementation Science.* 2011; 6: 88.

48. Oakes AH, Radomski TR. Reducing low-value care and improving health care value. *JAMA.* 2021; 325(17): 1715–6.

49. American College of Emergency Physicians. Ten Things Physicians and Patients Should Question. https://www.acep.org/globalassets/uploads/uploaded-files/ acep/membership/chapters/grants/choosing-wisley-5-things-phys.pdf. 2018. Accessed April 1, 2021.

50. Moore CL, Carpenter CR, Heilbrun ME *et al.* Imaging in suspected renal colic: Systematic review of the literature and multispecialty consensus. *Annals of Emergency Medicine.* 2019; 74: 391–9.

51. Chu K, Windsor C, Fox J *et al.* Factors influencing variation in investigations after a negative CT brain scan in suspected subarachnoid haemorrhage: A qualitative study. *Emergency Medicine Journal.* 2019; 36: 72–7.

52. Berdahl C, Schuur JD, Fisher NL, Burstin H, Pines JM. Policy measures and reimbursement for emergency medical imaging in the era of payment reform: Proceedings From a Panel Discussion of the 2015 Academic Emergency Medicine Consensus Conference. *Academic Emergency Medicine.* 2015; 22: 1393–9.

53. Kanzaria HK, Hall MK, Moore CL, Burstin H. Emergency department diagnostic imaging: The journey to quality. *Academic Emergency Medicine.* 2015; 22: 1380–4.

54. McKenna M. CMS head CT rule under fire. *Annals of Emergency Medicine.* 2012; 60: 20A–2A.

55. American College of Radiology. ACR Practice Parameters for Radiologist Coverage of Imaging Performed in Hospital Emergency Departments. https://www.acr.org/-/media/ACR/Files/Practice-Parameters/HospER.pdf. 2018. Accessed October 15, 2021.

56. Carpenter CR, Bellolio MF, Upadhye S, Kline JA. Navigating uncertainty with GRACE: Society for Academic Emergency Medicine's guidelines for reasonable and appropriate care in the emergency department. *Academic Emergency Medicine*. 2021; 28: 821–5.

57. Schunemann HJ, Mustafa R, Brozek J *et al*. GRADE guidelines: 16. GRADE evidence to decision frameworks for tests in clinical practice and public health. *Journal of Clinical Epidemiology*. 2016; 76: 89–98.

58. Schunemann HJ, Mustafa RA, Brozek J *et al*. GRADE guidelines: 22. The GRADE approach for tests and strategies-from test accuracy to patient-important outcomes and recommendations. *Journal of Clinical Epidemiology*. 2019; 111: 69–82.

59. Carpenter CR, Raja AS, Brown MD. Overtesting and the downstream consequences of overtreatment: Implications of "preventing overdiagnosis" for emergency medicine. *Academic Emergency Medicine*. 2015; 22: 1484–92.

60. Hoffman JR, Carpenter CR. Guarding against overtesting, overdiagnosis, and overtreatment of older adults: Thinking beyond imaging and injuries to weigh harms and benefits. *Journal of the American Geriatrics Society*. 2017; 65: 903–5.

61. Keijzers G, Cullen L, Egerton-Warburton D, Fatovich DM. Don't just do something, stand there! The value and art of deliberate clinical inertia. *Emergency Medicine Australasia*. 2018; 30: 273–8.

Chapter 6 **Understanding Bias in Diagnostic Research**

Christopher R. Carpenter[1] and Jesse M. Pines[2,3]

[1] Department of Emergency Medicine, Washington University School of Medicine, St. Louis, MO, USA
[2] US Acute Care Solutions, Canton, OH, USA
[3] Department of Emergency Medicine, Drexel University, Philadelphia, PA, USA

Highlights

- The Standards for Reporting of Diagnostic Accuracy Studies (STARD) criteria and Preferred Reporting Items for Systematic Review and Meta-analysis of Diagnostic Test Accuracy (PRISMA-DTA) criteria provide transparent recommendations for reporting diagnostic accuracy research.
- Subtypes of diagnostic bias include incorporation, partial verification, differential verification, imperfect gold standard, spectrum, context, interval, and cutoff biases that skew observed estimates of sensitivity and specificity in varying directions.
- A hierarchy of diagnostic evidence exists from technical efficacy, diagnostic accuracy efficacy, diagnostic thinking efficacy, therapeutic efficacy, clinical outcome efficacy, and societal efficacy.
- Diagnostic randomized controlled trials can evaluate the comparative efficacy between differing diagnostic approaches, but are not always necessary and when available often neglect patient-centered outcomes.

Chapter 2 summarizes the components and philosophy of evidence-based medicine (EBM), including methods to evaluate individual study quality before incorporating it into patient care. Attaining EBM proficiency requires mentored learning and consistent practice just like any other procedural skill in medicine.[1] Awareness of EBM concepts and resources can assist clinicians

---

Evidence-Based Emergency Care: Diagnostic Testing and Clinical Decision Rules, Third Edition.
Edited by Jesse M. Pines, Fernanda Bellolio, Christopher R. Carpenter, and Ali S. Raja.
© 2023 John Wiley & Sons Ltd. Published 2023 by John Wiley & Sons Ltd.

to assess the quality and applicability of diagnostic research evidence for individual questions.[2]

The Standards for Reporting of Diagnostic Accuracy Studies (STARD) criteria provide a systematic approach to conducting and reporting diagnostic research.[3] STARD provides a 30-item checklist of essential details that diagnostic researchers must report (Table 6.1). An extension of the original STARD reporting standards for history and physical examination also exists.[4] Although the quality of diagnostic accuracy reporting continues to improve, emergency medicine researchers frequently do not adhere to STARD, which increases the potential for unrecognized bias in the study results.[5-7]

As described in Chapter 2, systematic reviews are at the top of the evidence pyramid (i.e., one of the least biased forms of research when done methodically), but systematic review methods for diagnostic tests are relatively new.[8] Diagnostic test accuracy systematic reviews also have reporting standards called Preferred Reporting Items for Systematic Review and Meta-analysis of Diagnostic Test Accuracy (PRISMA-DTA).[9] The Quality Assessment Tool for Diagnostic Accuracy Studies (QUADAS-2) methods provide an instrument to assess four domains of bias that can skew individual trial estimates of diagnostic accuracy: patient selection, index test, criterion standard, and timing.[10] QUADAS-2 is the preferred approach to evaluate the quality of evidence in diagnostic meta-analyses. While diagnostic accuracy systematic reviews increasingly report the quality of included studies, few extrapolate the implications of the QUADAS-2 assessment into their conclusions.[11] In this chapter, we will describe the forms of bias to consider in diagnostic research and provide suggestions for incorporating this data into guidelines.

Diagnostic science is vulnerable to several forms of bias that physicians should recognize while critically appraising original research (Table 6.2).[12] For this discussion the new test being evaluated by researchers will be called the "index test" whereas the gold standard upon which the presence or absence of the disease is determined will be called the "criterion standard." The criterion standard is the most accurate method available to delineate whether a disease or condition is present or absent. For example, in appendicitis, diagnostic tests would be compared to the pathologic findings of appendiceal inflammation, which is the criterion standard for appendicitis.

Types of bias

Incorporation bias is likely when the index test is one determinant of the criterion standard. This occurs when the criterion standard involves a review of all pertinent clinical information by a panel of experts, including the index

Table 6.1 STARD 2015 criteria

Checklist item

Title
Identify manuscript as a study of diagnostic accuracy reporting at least one measure of accuracy

Abstract
Structured summary of design, methods, results, and conclusions

Introduction
Scientific/clinical background, including the intended use of the index test
Explicit statement of study objectives and hypothesis

Methods
Design
Whether data collection planned before index test and criterion standard performed (prospective) or after (retrospective)

Participants
Eligibility criteria for participants
Basis upon which participants identified (symptoms, previous test results, registry)
Where and when potentially eligible participants were identified
Whether participants formed a consecutive, random, or convenience sampling

Test methods
Index test described in sufficient detail to allow replication
Criterion standard described in sufficient detail to allow replication
Rationale for selecting the criterion standard (if alternatives exist)
Definition of and rationale for index test positivity cut-offs, distinguishing prespecified from exploratory
Definition of and rationale for criterion standard test positivity cut-offs or result categories
Whether clinical information and criterion standard were available to performers/ readers of the index test
Whether clinical information and criterion standard were available to assessors of the criterion standard

Analysis
Methods for estimating or comparing measures of diagnostic accuracy
How indeterminate index test or criterion standard results were handled
How missing data on the index test or criterion standard were handled
Any analyses of variability in diagnostic accuracy, distinguishing prespecified from exploratory
Intended sample size and how it was determined

Results
Participants
Flow of participants, using a diagram
Baseline demographic and clinical characteristics of participants
Distribution of severity of disease in those with the target condition
Distribution of alternative diagnoses in those without the target condition

(Continued)

Table 6.1 (*Continued*)

Time interval and any clinical interventions between the index test and criterion standard

Test results
Cross tabulation of the index test by the results of the criterion standard
Estimates of diagnostic accuracy and their precision (such as 95% confidence intervals)
Any adverse events from performing the index test or the criterion standard

Discussion
Study limitations, including sources of potential bias, statistical uncertainty, and generalizability
Implications for practice, including the intended use and clinical role of the index test

Other information
Registration number and name of registry
Where the full study protocol can be accessed
Sources of funding and other support with role of funders

---

test. For example, when evaluating the accuracy of B-type natriuretic peptide (BNP) for decompensated congestive heart failure (CHF) and the criterion standard is consensus of two cardiologists reviewing history, physical examination, imaging, and labs that include the BNP result, then incorporation bias occurs. The experimentally observed sensitivity and specificity of BNP will be higher than occurs in actual clinical practice. Another example of incorporation bias in emergency medicine is a study evaluating BNP that appropriately blinded two cardiologists assessing the presence or absence of CHF, which concluded "the best clinical predictor of CHF was an increased size on chest roentgenogram."[13] Since cardiologists evaluated the chest X-ray in addition to the medical history and follow-up studies, the heart size certainly influenced the decision to label a patient as CHF or not. The main problem with incorporation bias is the overestimation of both sensitivity and specificity.[14] To avoid incorporation bias, the index test cannot be a component of or reviewed to determine the criterion standard.

Partial verification bias occurs when patients with abnormal index test results are more likely to receive a subsequent criterion standard evaluation and only those with criterion standard testing are included in the study. Accurate quantification of sensitivity and specificity in research requires that all patients in whom the index test would be obtained in actual practice receive the criterion standard evaluation regardless of the index test result. Partial verification bias is particularly problematic in studying the accuracy of signs or symptoms. For example, one study quantified the sensitivity of right lower quadrant pain (RLQ) for pediatric appendicitis as 96% and

Table 6.2 Description of bias in diagnostic research

Threats to diagnostic accuracy	Alternative names or subtypes	Description	Sensitivity is falsely	Specificity is falsely
Incorporation bias	Review bias	Classification of disease status partly depends on results of the index test, including failure to blind the outcome assessor to the index test	Raised	Raised
Partial verification bias	Verification bias, work-up bias, referral bias	Positive index test cases are more likely to have criterion standard testing and only patients with criterion standard testing are included	Raised	Lowered
Differential verification bias	Double gold standard bias	Positive index test cases more likely to receive immediate invasive criterion standard, while patients with negative index test more likely to receive clinical follow-up for "disease" with bias when criterion standards give different answers	Raised Lowered	Raised for disease that can resolve spontaneously Lowered for disease that only becomes detectable during follow-up
Imperfect gold standard bias	Copper standard bias	The criterion standard determining patient's disease status misclassifies some patients	Raised Lowered	Raised if errors on the index test and copper standard are correlated Lowered if errors on the index test and the gold standard are independent
Spectrum bias, disease severity	Case-mix or subgroup bias	Spectrum of disease and nondisease differs from clinical practice. Sensitivity depends on spectrum of disease, whereas specificity depends on spectrum of nondisease that mimic disease of interest	Raised when disease skewed toward higher severity than observed in clinical practice	Raised when nondisease skewed toward healthier patients than observed in clinical practice

(Continued)

Table 6.2 (*Continued*)

Threats to diagnostic accuracy	Alternative names or subtypes	Description	Sensitivity is falsely	Specificity is falsely
Spectrum bias, exclusion of ambiguous tests		Patients with ambiguous or intermediate test results are excluded	Raised when excluded patients with disease more likely than those included to have been false negative	Raised when excluded patients without disease more likely to have been false positive

Source: Data from [12].

specificity is very low at 5%.[15] As discussed in Chapter 3, this equates to a likelihood ratio positive and negative of 1.0, implying that RLQ pain is useless in the diagnosis of pediatric appendicitis because it is so nonspecific. This study used histological findings as the criterion standard for appendicitis, yet only children with RLQ pain underwent surgery. This introduces partial verification bias because not all children had the same assessment of the criterion standard because children that were ruled out based on clinical grounds were assumed to be true negatives. Another example illustrating partial verification bias via a modified 2×2 table in Figure 6.1 uses results from a headache study. In this decades-old study, computed tomography (CT) was more likely to be obtained in patients with a headache, so studying headache as a predictor of intracranial hemorrhage demonstrates higher sensitivity and lower specificity than if headache played no role in obtaining the criterion standard CT.[16,17]

Differential verification bias occurs when researchers use different criterion standards to define the presence of absence of disease when different gold standards can give different results. As just described with pediatric appendicitis, rather than excluding patients who did not undergo surgery, another approach would be to follow nonoperative patients longitudinally to ensure that they do not develop appendicitis (and are therefore true negatives rather than early-stage or initially mild appendicitis). However, two different criterion standards for detecting the presence or absence of appendicitis then exist – one surgical and the other clinical, creating differential verification bias. Appendicitis sometimes resolves spontaneously and nonoperative management is increasingly common.[18] If a child with mild appendicitis

All patients with acute neurologic deficits receive head CT scans, regardless of whether they have complaint or recent history of headache.

Not all patients with acute neurologic deficits receive head CT scans, and a complaint or recent history of headache makes a CT more likely. (Only patients who received head CT scans are included in the study.)

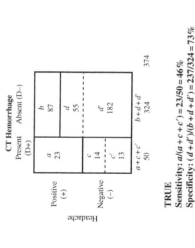

		CT Hemorrhage	
		Present (D+)	Absent (D−)
Headache	Positive (+)	a 23	b 87
	Negative (−)	c 14	d 55
		c' 13	d' 182	374
		$a+c+c'$ 50	$b+d+d'$ 324

TRUE
Sensitivity: $a/(a+c+c') = 23/50 = 46\%$
Specificity: $(d+d')/(b+d+d') = 237/324 = 73\%$

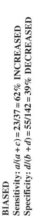

		CT Hemorrhage	
		Present (D+)	Absent (D−)
Headache	Positive (+)	a 23	b 87
	Negative (−)	c 14	d 55
		EXCLUDED	
		$a+c$ 37	$b+d$ 142	179

BIASED
Sensitivity: $a/(a+c) = 23/37 = 62\%$ INCREASED
Specificity: $d/(b+d) = 55/142 = 39\%$ DECREASED

c' = patients with hemorrhage but no headache who would not have had a CT if presence of headache influenced the decision to order a CT. These false negatives would be excluded from a study where presence of headache influenced CT ordering and only patients with CTs were included.

d' = patients without hemorrhage who do not have headache and would not have had a CT if presence of headache influenced the decision to order a CT. These true negatives would be excluded from a study where headache influenced CT ordering and only patients with CTs were included.

$c/c' > d/d'$ because patients with hemorrhage but without headache are more likely to have more severe neurologic deficits that prompt CT than patients without hemorrhage and without headache.

Figure 6.1 Partial verification bias in a study of headache as a predictor of intracranial hemorrhage. As depicted on the left, most emergency department patients with acute unilateral neurological deficits today are evaluated with a head CT regardless of the presence or absence of headache. On the other hand in 1985, CT was not readily available and patients with a neurological deficit and headache were more likely to have CT imaging. (Data from [12].)

reports RLQ pain and goes to the operating room, the inflamed appendix will be noted on histology and the presence of RLQ be recognized as a true positive. If the same child does not have RLQ pain and the clinical follow-up criterion standard is employed with spontaneous resolution of appendicitis, the absence of RLQ will be recorded as a true negative. Sensitivity and specificity will be artificially elevated if compared to a study where every patient had the same criterion standard applied regardless of the index test result. Another example involves assessment of inability to fully extend the elbow after blunt trauma as a predictor of fracture. In this study, every patient who had an abnormal elbow extension test had X-rays obtained, but only 19% of those with normal elbow extension had X-rays with the remainder evaluated by clinical follow-up.[19] Assuming that 2.4% of the 250 patients with normal elbow extension and negative follow-up would have had fracture identified if X-rays were obtained, Figure 6.2 demonstrates how partial verification bias overestimates both sensitivity and specificity.[12] Using different criterion standards dependent on the index test may be ethically or pragmatically challenging to avoid in some situations, but recognizing the artificial increases in sensitivity and specificity associated with this bias is important.[20]

Diagnostic research for emergency conditions often relies upon "copper standard" criterion standards to rule in or rule out suspected pathology because more definitive tests like biopsied histopathology are unavailable or unethical. Occasionally, multiple criterion standards are possible without a mutually acceptable gold standard.[21] *Imperfect gold standard bias* depends on whether the errors on the suboptimal "copper standard" correlate with errors on the index test. This bias often exists in patients with mild or early-stage disease when errors on the copper standard and index test correlate. For example, the accuracy of polymerase chain reaction (PCR) for *Bordetella pertussis* compared with traditional gold standard bacterial culture. PCR is more sensitive, therefore, less likely than a culture to yield false negative results when pertussis is present. Yet comparing PCR to the imperfect gold standard of cultures tends to overestimate sensitivity and underestimate specificity as demonstrated by Figure 6.3 where Strebel *et al.*[22] compared pertussis serology, PCR, and culture in patients with paroxysmal cough. Multiple approaches to adjust analyses for imperfect gold standard bias exist, including correction of accuracy estimates based on external evidence quantifying degree of imperfection of the criterion standard, re-analysis within a range of plausible error rates, or development of a construct criterion standard via panel consensus or latent class analysis.[23–25] Applying one or more of these solutions to imperfect gold standard bias in clinical research remains a challenge for clinical investigators.[26]

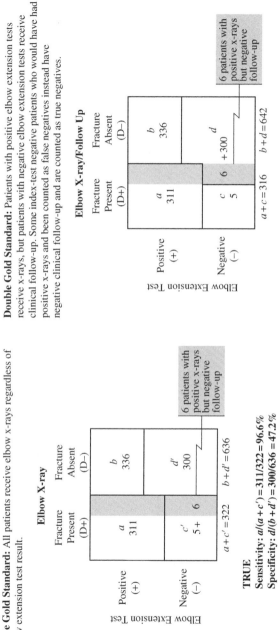

Figure 6.2 Differential verification bias also called double gold standard bias. (Data from [12].)

Apparent sensitivity and specificity of PCR relative to culture show a falsely high sensitivity and a falsely low specificity.

True pertussis status in patients presenting with cough. Pertussis culture (Cx) is positive in only 8 out of 27 (29.6%) of patients with pertussis. Polymerase Chain Reaction (PCR) has slightly better sensitivity of 10/27 (37%). Neither Cx nor PCR is falsely positive in a patient without pertussis. PCR is less likely to be falsely negative when the Cx is positive (3/8 = 38%) than when culture is negative (14/19 = 74%) or overall (17/27 = 63%). This is positive dependence for sensitivity.

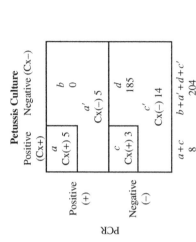

Petussis Culture

PCR	Positive (Cx+)	Negative (Cx−)
Positive (+)	a Cx(+) 5 a' Cx(−) 5	b 0
Negative (−)	c Cx(+) 3 c' Cx(−) 14	d 185
	$a+c$ 8	$b+a'+d+c'$ 204

BIASED
Sensitivity: $a/(a+c) = 5/8 = 62.5\%$ **INCREASED**
Specificity: $(d+c')/(b+a'+d+c') = 199/204 = 97.5\%$ **DECREASED**

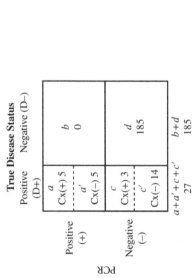

True Disease Status

PCR	Positive (D+)	Negative (D−)
Positive (+)	a Cx(+) 5 a' Cx(−) 5	b 0
Negative (−)	c Cx(+) 3 c' Cx(−) 14	d 185
	$a+a'+c+c'$ 27	$b+d$ 185

TRUE
Sensitivity: $(a+a')/(a+a'+c+c') = 10/27 = 37\%$
Specificity: $d/(b+d) = 185/185 = 100\%$

Figure 6.3 Imperfect gold standard bias. (Data from [12].)

Disease processes often occur over a range of severities from mild to severe and diagnostic test performance can vary across this range.[27] This is called *spectrum bias* or spectrum effect.[28] Spectrum bias exists in two subtypes: disease severity or exclusion of ambiguous results. As discussed in Chapter 3, positive and negative predictive values fluctuate with the prevalence of disease in the population tested. Sensitivity and specificity can also vary based upon disease prevalence since sensitivity depends on the spectrum of disease while specificity depends on the spectrum of nondisease. For example, in quantifying the accuracy of BNP for acute CHF in undifferentiated dyspnea can be caused by multiple overlying disease processed in patients with left ventricular dysfunction. Figure 6.4 depicts the observed sensitivity and specificity when researchers exclude those with left ventricular dysfunction but not acute CHF.[12]

The other subtype of spectrum bias involves the exclusion of ambiguous results. This results in limiting the study to subset of patients not representative of those tested in actual practice. The effect of exclusion of intermediate results on observed accuracy depends upon how the presence or absence of "disease" would change if those intermediate results were included. If intermediate results were stratified as "disease positive," excluding these cases biases sensitivity downward and specificity upward. On the other hand, if intermediate results tend to be stratified as "disease negative," this biases sensitivity upward and specificity downward. As demonstrated in Figure 6.5 using ventilation–perfusion (V/Q) interpretation as an example, when forcing index test interpreters to make a choice for each patient between positive or negative (rather than intermediate, indeterminate, or ambiguous), this tends to falsely increase both sensitivity and specificity. Emergency medicine physicians illustrated this subtype of spectrum bias in the evaluation of point-of-care ultrasound (POCUS) for the diagnosis of deep vein thrombosis. In two studies using a convenience sampling that excluded ambiguous POCUS studies sensitivity was 100% and specificity 92–95%,[29,30] but another study that enrolled consecutive patients demonstrated 70% sensitivity and 89% specificity.[31] One approach to handling intermediate results is to replace the standard 2×2 table with a 3×2 table in which dichotomous sensitivity and specificity do not exist.[32,33] Instead likelihood ratio positive, likelihood ratio intermediate, or likelihood ratio negative are reported. If original research authors do not report 3×2 results for intermediate results, systematic review authors recognizing this potential bias can.[34]

Other biases can also affect diagnostic accuracy research, but the direction of skew for sensitivity and specificity is less clear. *Context bias* is problematic when ambient conditions influence the outcome assessors while they are reviewing the data for the index test and the criterion standard. For example,

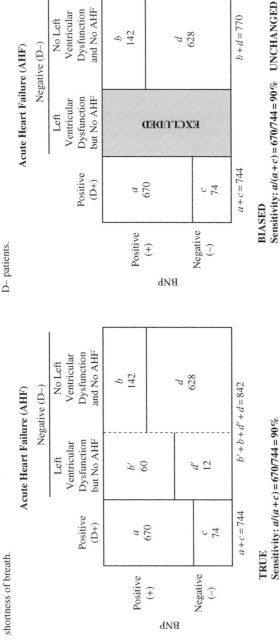

The effect of excluding the subgroup of patients with left ventricular dysfunction but no AHF creating an artificially homogeneous group of D– patients.

Acute Heart Failure (AHF)

BIASED
Sensitivity: $a/(a+c) = 670/744 = 90\%$ **UNCHANGED**
Specificity: $(d)/(b+d) = 628/770 = 82\%$ **INCREASED**

ED dyspnea patients who do not have acute heart failure (AHF) include some patients with left ventricular dysfunction but other causes for their shortness of breath.

TRUE
Sensitivity: $a/(a+c) = 670/744 = 90\%$
Specificity: $(d' + d)/(b' + b + d' + d) = 640/842 = 76\%$

Figure 6.4 Spectrum bias, disease severity subtype. (Data from [12].)

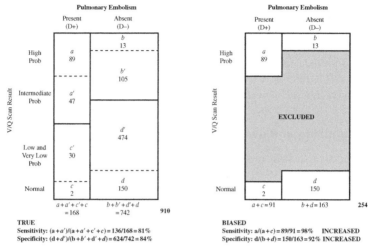

Figure 6.5 Spectrum bias, exclusion of ambiguous results subtype. In this case, excluding intermediate V/Q scan results for pulmonary embolism. (Data from [12].)

if a clinician is assessing a constellation of symptoms for influenza-like illness (ILI) during the coronavirus 2019 (COVID-19) pandemic they may be more likely to attribute malaise and fever to COVID-19 than during periods of low ILI prevalence. The radiology literature describes this form of bias, but it is difficult to detect and seldom reported.[35] *Interval bias* occurs when there is a clinically significant delay between the index test and the criterion standard, which is sufficiently long for the disease status to change. In general, this form of bias is only applicable in disease states that can change quickly over a short period of time such as infections. Chronic disease states such as dementia, by definition, do not spontaneously reverse their pathological processes. Interval bias can also affect diagnostic accuracy estimates in acute disease states, too. For example, in subarachnoid hemorrhage CT sensitivity is most sensitive immediately after the onset of a sentinel headache with reduced sensitivities noted after 6 hours.[36]

Cutoff bias occurs when different studies (or the same study) use variable and undefined thresholds to transform continuous data into dichotomous "disease present" or "disease absent" states. As described in Chapter 3, receiver operator characteristic (ROC) curves can be used to identify an optimal cutoff value for continuous data that simultaneously maximizes sensitivity and specificity, but researchers sometimes fail to explicitly state how or what cutoff values were used or they assign these thresholds after data analysis.[20] *Temporal bias* is particularly problematic in diagnostic radiology since technological advances are continually improving as is reader expertise.[37] For example, as discussed in Chapter 50 the diagnostic accuracy of CT for pulmonary embolism using first-generation scanners was 70% while the later prospective investigation of pulmonary embolism diagnosis II (PIOPED II) data demonstrated a sensitivity of 83% for newer generation scanners.[38]

Recognizing and overcoming diagnostic biases

Diagnostic systematic reviews and meta-analyses adherent to PRISMA-DTA and include QUADAS-2 evaluations of original research provide one method to assess the evidence for new tests with respect to various forms of bias.[39] Diagnostic systematic reviews from other specialties are also extremely useful to ED physicians. For example, the *Journal of the American Medical Association's* Rational Clinical Exam series provides three decades of diagnostic systematic reviews for a variety of medical and surgical topics.[40] However, other specialty diagnostic systematic reviews do not specifically focus on ED populations, clinical situations, or diagnostic strategies, so may be difficult to apply to ED patients. The Evidence-Based Diagnostics series in *Academic Emergency Medicine* has introduced a venue for ED-based systematic reviews that also provide estimates of test–treatment thresholds based on currently available emergency interventions, as well as implications for future diagnostic research.[41,42]

Assessing bias in diagnostic accuracy research is essential, but is only the first step since test accuracy is only a surrogate for patient-oriented outcomes. The implicit assumption is that if clinicians have a better idea of whether a disease is present or absent, morbidity and mortality outcomes will improve. The Grading of Recommendations Assessment, Development and Recommendations (GRADE) criteria is another approach that assesses the overall patient-centric effectiveness of diagnostic testing based upon the available evidence.[43] The GRADE approach is to assess the diagnostic accuracy and clinical effectiveness data for a diagnostic test in order to make specific "actionable" recommendations for the use of these tests in guidelines. Although the least biased study design to assess the effectiveness or additive value of an alternative diagnostic strategy would be a randomized controlled trial (RCT), such trials are not uncommon but often neglect patient-centric outcomes.[44] Most diagnostic studies are observational designs and calculate test characteristics based on convenience sampling of patients who received both the index test and a criterion standard. According to the

GRADE criteria, the most clinically relevant studies on diagnostic testing include representative and consecutive patients where diagnostic uncertainty exists. The focus has to be on the patient for whom clinicians would reasonably apply a test in the course of practice: ED patients in whom the diagnostic impression is somewhere between the test and treatment thresholds described in Chapter 1.

Although diagnostic testing RCTs are sometimes lacking, criteria exist to establish when accuracy studies alone are insufficient.[45] The first step is to assess the sensitivity of the new test in comparison to the old test(s). If the sensitivities are similar, one can assume that either test will detect the same true cases of disease. In this scenario, if the new test has superior specificity, then the potential adverse effects of additional testing or treatment of false positives will be reduced and an RCT is unnecessary. Additionally, when the new test is either cheaper or more readily available than the old test, RCTs are not needed.

If the new test is more sensitive than the old test with similar specificity, the benefit of the new test relates to the therapeutic responses of the additional true-positive cases identified as identified by RCTs of therapy. For example, CT colonography performed in the supine and prone position is more sensitive (with equal specificity) than when performed in the prone position alone.[46] Therapeutic trials demonstrate improved survival associated with early detection and treatment of colorectal polyps on a similar spectrum of disease, so diagnosticians can reasonably assume that compared with supine positioning dual positioning CT colonography will improve survival without awaiting an RCT. However, when evaluating these therapeutic RCTs clinicians need to contemplate whether the results apply to the new cases identified by the index test. Do the extra cases respond to therapy in the same manner as the cases identified by the older (less sensitive) test? For example, in the 1960s, the diagnosis of pulmonary embolism only occurred in extreme life-threatening cases using older imaging strategies (or at autopsy), whereas modern CT technology identifies small and possibly clinically inconsequential emboli with high sensitivity. Do these peripheral emboli respond to anticoagulation therapy to the same degree as the massive PEs upon which we base the therapeutic management of PE?[47] If the newly identified cases do respond to the existing therapy and the new test has no negative attributes (safety, specificity, cost) then use the new test without awaiting an RCT. If there are negative attributes such as over-diagnosis of self-resolving and otherwise clinically inconsequential "disease," carefully contemplate the tradeoffs before using the new test.[48] In the situation where the more sensitive new test identifies additional cases that may not respond to therapy and one cannot deduce whether the extra cases represent the same spectrum of disease, awaiting RCTs is warranted.[45] Various RCT designs will evaluate the effect of emerging tests and testing strategies on patient-centric outcomes.[49] These diagnostic RCTs sometimes provide surprising results for accurate tests. For example, BNP is an accurate test to discriminate CHF from other etiologies of dyspnea (see Chapter 19), but multiple ED-based RCTs have not consistently identified significant patient-centric benefits to this new diagnostic technology.[50] Similarly, high-sensitivity troponin has been adapted worldwide even though diagnostic RCTs demonstrate inconsistent beneficial impact on ED flow or downstream testing.[51–53]

One proposal is to evaluate a new test using a hierarchical approach that groups research outcomes into six categories: technical efficacy, diagnostic accuracy efficacy, diagnostic thinking efficacy, therapeutic efficacy, clinical outcome efficacy, and societal efficacy (Table 6.3).[54,55] These categories represent levels of diagnostic test assessment that progressively

Table 6.3 Hierarchical outcomes based approach to diagnostic research

Level	Domain	Considerations
1	Technical efficacy	Acceptability
		Analytic sensitivity
		Intra/interobserver reliability
		Feasibility
		Measurement inaccuracy and imprecision
		Operator dependence, training, and skill maintenance
2	Diagnostic accuracy efficacy	Area under the curve
		Likelihood ratios
		Predictive values
		Sensitivity/specificity
3	Diagnostic thinking efficacy	Confidence in diagnosis
		Cost of change in clinical diagnosis
		Differences in clinicians' posttest probability estimates before and after knowledge of test information
		Proportion of cases in which test judged to be helpful
		Proportion of cases in which test changed the final diagnosis
4	Therapeutic efficacy	Proportion of cases in which further testing was avoided
		Proportion of cases in which management changed
		Total and per patient cost with new diagnostic strategy
5	Patient outcome efficacy	Cost per unit of change in outcome variable
		Expected value of test in formation in quality adjusted life years
		Functional status
		Morbidity avoided by testing
		Mortality
6	Societal efficacy	Cost-effectiveness analysis from societal perspective

eliminate tests based upon their potential impact. Technical efficacy is the first level and serves to evaluate the operator and instrument characteristics, including reliability. The next level evaluates the diagnostic accuracy of the test using traditional measures of sensitivity, specificity, and likelihood ratios. The third level is diagnostic thinking efficacy to assess the proportion of cases in which the final diagnosis changes because of the new test. The fourth level of research, therapeutic efficacy, evaluates the proportion of cases in which management changes based on the test information. The fifth level of research, patient outcome efficacy, evaluates the impact of the new test on symptom severity, functional status, and mortality including a cost-effectiveness analysis reporting the cost per unit change for each outcome variable using quality-adjusted life year. The sixth and final level of research evaluates the costs and benefits of the new test from a societal perspective.

The integration of most diagnostic tests into clinical practice occurs after the second level of assessment in this hierarchy. In fact, the evaluation of diagnostic tests in research settings is unlikely to follow this hierarchy in a linear fashion. Instead, this process is usually a cyclic and repetitive process.[55] This book will provide quantitative estimates of diagnostic accuracy while exploring the higher levels of diagnostic research whenever it exists. However, as scientific methods for diagnostic research continues evolving, readers must remain cognizant of ongoing studies that will continue to enhance clinicians' ability to accurately identify diseases in the ED in populations most likely to benefit from such testing.

References

1. Carpenter CR. Teaching lifelong learning skills: Journal club and beyond. In: Rogers RL, Mattu A, Winters M, Martinez J, editors. *Practical teaching in emergency medicine*. 2nd ed, Chapter 11. Oxford: Wiley-Blackwell; 2012: 151–62.

2. Newman TB, Kohn MA. Critical appraisal of studies of diagnostic test accuracy. In: Newman TB, Kohn MA, editors. *Evidence-based diagnosis: An introduction to clinical epidemiology*. 2nd ed. New York: Cambridge University Press; 2020: 75–109.

3. Bossuyt PM, Reitsma JB, Bruns DE et al. STARD 2015: An updated list of essential items for reporting diagnostic accuracy studies. *BMJ*. 2015; 351: h5527.

4. Simel DL, Rennie D, Bossuyt PM. Overcoming the tower of babel in medical science by finding the "EQUATOR": Research reporting guidelines. *Journal of General Internal Medicine*. 2008; 23(6): 768–74.

5. Korevaar DA, Wang J, van Enst WA et al. Reporting diagnostic accuracy studies: Some improvements after 10 years of STARD. *Radiology*. 2015; 274(3): 781–9.

6. Gallo L, Hua N, Mercuri M, Silveira A, Worster A. Adherence to standards for reporting diagnostic accuracy in emergency medicine research. *Academic Emergency Medicine.* 2017; 24(8): 914–9.

7. Carpenter CR, Meisel ZF. Overcoming the tower of babel in medical science by finding the "EQUATOR": Research reporting guidelines. *Academic Emergency Medicine.* 2017; 24(8): 1030–3.

8. Whiting P, Rutjes AWS, Dinnes J, Reitsma JB, Bossuyt PMM, Kleijnen J. A systematic review finds that diagnostic reviews fail to incorporate quality despite available tools. *Journal of Clinical Epidemiology.* 2005; 58(1): 1–12.

9. Salameh JP, Bossuyt PM, McGrath TA *et al.* Preferred reporting items for systematic review and meta-analysis of diagnostic test accuracy studies (PRISMA-DTA): Explanation, elaboration, and checklist. *BMJ.* 2020; 370: m2632.

10. Whiting P, Rutjes AWS, Westwood ME *et al.* QUADAS-2: A revised tool for the quality assessment of diagnostic accuracy studies. *Annals of Internal Medicine.* 2011; 155(8): 529–36.

11. Ochodo EA, van Enst WA, Naaktgeboren CA *et al.* Incorporating quality assessments of primary studies in the conclusions of diagnostic accuracy reviews: A cross-sectional study. *BMC Medical Research Methodology.* 2014; 14: 33.

12. Kohn MA, Carpenter CR, Newman TB. Understanding the direction of bias in studies of diagnostic test accuracy. *Academic Emergency Medicine.* 2013; 20(11): 1194–206.

13. Maisel AS, Krishnaswamy P, Nowak RM *et al.* Rapid measurement of B-type natriuretic peptide in the emergency diagnosis of heart failure. *The New England Journal of Medicine.* 2002; 347(3): 161–7.

14. Worster A, Carpenter C. Incorporation bias in studies of diagnostic tests: How to avoid being biased about bias. *CJEM.* 2008; 10(2): 174–5.

15. Pearl RH, Hale DA, Molloy M, Schutt DC, Jaques DP. Pediatric appendectomy. *Journal of Pediatric Surgery.* 1995; 30(2): 173–8.

16. Panzer RJ, Feibel WH, Griner PF. Predicting the likelihood of hemorrhage in patients with stroke. *Archives of Internal Medicine.* 1985; 145(10): 1800–3.

17. Panzer RJ, Suchman AL, Griner PF. Workup bias in prediction research. *Medical Decision Making.* 1987; 7(2): 115–9.

18. Podda M, Gerardi C, Cillara N *et al.* Antibiotic treatment and appendectomy for uncomplicated acute appendicitis in adults and children: A systematic review and meta-analysis. *Annals of Surgery.* 2019; 270(6): 1028–40.

19. Appelboam A, Reuben AD, Benger JR *et al.* Elbow extension test to rule out elbow fracture: Multicentre, prospective validation and observational study of diagnostic accuracy in adults and children. *BMJ.* 2008; 337: a2428.

20. Begg CB. Biases in the assessment of diagnostic tests. *Statistics in Medicine.* 1987; 6(4): 411–23.

21. Naaktgeboren CA, de Groot JAH, van Smeden M, Moons KG, Reitsma JB. Evaluating diagnostic accuracy in the face of multiple reference standards. *Annals of Internal Medicine.* 2013; 159(3): 195–202.

22. Strebel P, Nordin J, Edwards K *et al.* Population-based incidence of pertussis among adolescents and adults, Minnesota, 1995-1996. *The Journal of Infectious Diseases.* 2001; 183(9): 1353–9.

23. Reitsma JB, Rutjes AW, Khan KS, Coomarasamy A, Bossuyt PM. A review of solutions for diagnostic accuracy studies with an imperfect or missing reference standard. *Journal of Clinical Epidemiology.* 2009; 62(8): 797–806.

24. Hui SL, Zhou XH. Evaluation of diagnostic tests without gold standards. *Statistical Methods in Medical Research.* 1998; 7(4): 354–70.

25. Wang C, Lin X, Nelson KP. Bayesian hierarchical latent class models for estimating diagnostic accuracy. *Statistical Methods in Medical Research.* 2020; 29(4): 1112–28.

26. Chikere CMU, Wilson K, Graziadio S, Vale L, Allen AJ. Diagnostic test evaluation methodology: A systematic review of methods employed to evaluate diagnostic tests in the absence of gold standard - An update. *PLoS One.* 2019; 14(10): e0223832.

27. Ransohoff DF, Feinstein AR. Problems of spectrum and bias in evaluating the efficacy of diagnostic tests. *The New England Journal of Medicine.* 1978; 299(17): 926–30.

28. Mulherin SA, Miller WC. Spectrum bias or spectrum effect? Subgroup variation in diagnostic test evaluation. *Annals of Internal Medicine.* 2002; 137(7): 598–602.

29. Farahmand S, Farnia M, Shahriaran S, Khashayar P. The accuracy of limited B-mode compression technique in diagnosing deep venous thrombosis in lower extremities. *The American Journal of Emergency Medicine.* 2011; 29(6): 687–90.

30. Jang T, Docherty M, Aubin C, Polites G. Resident-performed compression ultrasonography for the detection of proximal deep vein thrombosis: Fast and accurate. *Academic Emergency Medicine.* 2004; 11(3): 319–22.

31. Kline JA, O'Malley PM, Tayal VS, Snead GR, Mitchell AM. Emergency clinician-performed compression ultrasonography for deep venous thrombosis of the lower extremity. *Annals of Emergency Medicine.* 2008; 52(4): 437–45.

32. Simel DL, Feussner JR, Delong ER, Matchar DB. Intermediate, indeterminate, and uninterpretable diagnostic test results. *Medical Decision Making.* 1987; 7(2): 107–14.

33. Schuetz GM, Schlattmann P, Dewey M. Use of 3x2 tables with an intention to diagnose approach to assess clinical performance of diagnostic tests: Meta-analytical evaluation of coronary CT angiography studies. *BMJ.* 2012; 345: e6717.

34. Stickles SP, Carpenter CR, Gekle R *et al.* The diagnostic accuracy of a point-of-care ultrasound protocol for shock etiology: A systematic review and meta-analysis. *CJEM.* 2019; 21(3): 406–17.

35. Egglin TK, Feinstein AR. Context bias. A problem in diagnostic radiology. *Journal of the American Medical Association.* 1996; 276(21): 1752–5.

36. Carpenter CR, Hussain AM, Ward MJ *et al.* Spontaneous subarachnoid hemorrhage: A systematic review and meta-analysis describing the diagnostic accuracy of history, physical examination, imaging, and lumbar puncture with an exploration of test thresholds. *Academic Emergency Medicine.* 2016; 23(9): 963–1003.

37. Begg CB, McNeil BJ. Assessment of radiologic tests: control of bias and other design considerations. *Radiology.* 1988; 167(2): 565–9.

38. Stein PD, Fowler SE, Goodman LR *et al.* Multidetector computed tomography for acute pulmonary embolism. *The New England Journal of Medicine.* 2006; 354(22): 2317–27.

39. Leeflang MMG, Deeks JJ, Gatsonis C, Bossuyt PMM. Systematic reviews of diagnostic test accuracy. *Annals of Internal Medicine.* 2008; 149(12): 889–97.
40. Simel DL, Rennie D. *The rational clinical examination: Evidence-based clinical diagnosis.* New York: McGraw-Hill; 2009.
41. Carpenter CR, Schuur JD, Everett WW, Pines JM. Evidence-based diagnostics: Adult septic arthritis. *Academic Emergency Medicine.* 2011; 18(8): 781–96.
42. Lang ES, Worster A. Getting the evidence straight in emergency diagnostics. *Academic Emergency Medicine.* 2011; 18(8): 797–9.
43. Schünemann AHJ, Oxman AD, Brozek J *et al.* GRADE: Grading quality of evidence and strength of recommendations for diagnostic tests and strategies. *BMJ.* 2008; 336(7653): 1106–10.
44. El Dib R, Tikkinen KAO, Akl EA *et al.* Systematic survey of randomized trials evaluating the impact of alternative diagnostic strategies on patient-important outcomes. *Journal of Clinical Epidemiology.* 2017; 84: 61–9.
45. Lord SJ, Irwig L, Simes RJ. When is measuring sensitivity and specificity sufficient to evaluate a diagnostic test, and when do we need randomized trials? *Annals of Internal Medicine.* 2006; 144(11): 850–5.
46. Yee J, Kumar NN, Hung RK, Akerhar GA, Kumar PR, Wall SD. Comparison of supine and prone scanning separately and in combination at CT colonography. *Radiology.* 2003; 226(3): 653–61.
47. Newman DH, Schriger DL. Rethinking testing for pulmonary embolism: Less is more. *Annals of Emergency Medicine.* 2011; 57(6): 622–7.
48. Carpenter CR, Raja AS, Brown MD. Overtesting and the downstream consequences of overtreatment: Implications of "preventing overdiagnosis" for emergency medicine. *Academic Emergency Medicine.* 2015; 22(12): 1484–92.
49. Lijmer JG, Mol BW, Heisterkamp S *et al.* Empirical evidence of design-related bias in studies of diagnostic tests. *Journal of the American Medical Association.* 1999; 282(11): 1061–6.
50. Carpenter CR, Keim SM, Worster A, Rosen P. Brain natriuretic peptide in the evaluation of emergency department dyspnea: Is there a role? *The Journal of Emergency Medicine.* 2012; 42(2): 197–205.
51. Shah ASV, Anand A, Strachan FE *et al.* High-sensitivity troponin in the evaluation of patients with suspected acute coronary syndrome: A stepped-wedge, cluster-randomised controlled trial. *Lancet.* 2018; 392(10151): 919–28.
52. Chew DP, Lambrakis K, Blyth A *et al.* A randomized trial of a 1-hour troponin T protocol in suspected acute coronary syndromes: The rapid assessment of possible acute coronary syndrome in the emergency department with high-sensitivity troponin T study (RAPID-TnT). *Circulation.* 2019; 140(19): 1543–56.
53. Carlton EW, Ingram J, Taylor H *et al.* Limit of detection of troponin discharge strategy versus usual care: Randomised controlled trial. *Heart.* 2020; 106(20): 1586–94.
54. Pearl WS. A hierarchical outcomes approach to test assessment. *Annals of Emergency Medicine.* 1999; 33(1): 77–84.
55. Lijmer JG, Leeflang M, Bossuyt PMM. Proposals for a phased evaluation of medical tests. *Medical Decision Making.* 2009; 29(5): E13–21.

SECTION 2
Trauma

Chapter 7 **Cervical Spine Fractures**

Jesse M. Pines[1,2] and Fernanda Bellolio[3]

[1]US Acute Care Solutions, Canton, OH, USA
[2]Department of Emergency Medicine, Drexel University, Philadelphia, PA, USA
[3]Department of Emergency Medicine, Mayo Clinic, Rochester, MN, USA

Highlights

- The prevalence of cervical spine injuries from blunt trauma is low (approximately 2–4%) in adults, and lower in children (<1%).
- Applying either of the clinical decision rules for bluntly injured patients (the Canadian C-spine rules or NEXUS low-risk rules) safely identifies low-risk patients in the ED who do not need neck imaging.
- CT imaging of the cervical spine is more sensitive than plain-film imaging and should be the imaging modality of choice whenever available in adults.
- Some seriously ill trauma patients who are neurologically intact with persistent midline tenderness and a negative CT have disco-ligamentous injuries and warrant MRI to definitively rule out injuries. However, a systematic review demonstrated that the risk of significant injury in obtunded trauma patients with normal CT is very low and recommends C-collar removal after a negative CT scan.
- The NEXUS criteria can be used in all children but were developed from a dataset with very few injuries in children ≤8 years old. In children needing cervical spine imaging after blunt trauma, X-ray should be the modality of choice.
- If imaging is needed in children ≤8 years old, those having a head CT performed or in whom an adequate odontoid X-ray cannot be obtained should have a CT of the occiput to C3, given their higher risk for high-cervical-spine injury.

Evidence-Based Emergency Care: Diagnostic Testing and Clinical Decision Rules, Third Edition.
Edited by Jesse M. Pines, Fernanda Bellolio, Christopher R. Carpenter, and Ali S. Raja.
© 2023 John Wiley & Sons Ltd. Published 2023 by John Wiley & Sons Ltd.

- New decision rules for younger children have not yet been prospectively validated.
- Clinicians should have a low threshold for imaging the cervical spine in older adults due to anatomic and physiologic changes that are less tolerant of even minor trauma.
- The NEXUS low-risk criteria's sensitivity in the subgroup of older adults rivals its sensitivity for all patients.

Background

Of the 138.9 million US emergency department (ED) visits in 2017, 26.2 million – nearly one in five visits were for injury.[1] Injured patients commonly undergo assessment for potential injury to the cervical spine (C-spine), and a subset of patients undergo radiographic imaging (X-ray or computed tomography [CT]). The diagnostic yield of C-spine imaging is low and has been estimated at 2–4% of all imaging studies ordered.[2,3] As a result, many patients without injuries undergo negative radiographic evaluations. The development of sensitive clinical decision rules to help identify patients who are at extremely low risk of a cervical spine injury (CSI) has been exceptionally useful for clinicians who hope to reduce unnecessary imaging.

CSIs also occur, but more rarely in the pediatric blunt trauma population. Their overall prevalence is approximately 1.3%, increasing in a stepwise fashion from 0.4% in infants to 2.6% in adolescents.[4] Despite this, C-spine CT imaging of injured children continues to increase, especially outside of Level I pediatric trauma centers.[5] To minimize unnecessary ionizing radiation exposure in children and to ensure the appropriateness of C-spine imaging while also maximizing patient safety, emergency physicians need to be able to identify a subset of patients at very low risk of clinically significant injury who can have their C-spines safely cleared without imaging.

Older adults ($\geq$65 years of age) with blunt trauma are also commonly evaluated for potential CSIs. Anatomic and physiologic factors associated with these older patients, including osteopenia, osteophytes, and relative immobility, predispose them to CSIs even by low-impact or minimal-energy mechanisms. The overall 1-year mortality for older adults who sustain C-spine fractures is between 24% and 28%, necessitating that emergency physicians evaluating these patients remain acutely aware of the significance of these injuries in this population.[6,7]

Two rules have been developed using accepted clinical decision rule methodology: the National Emergency X-ray Utilization Study (NEXUS) criteria, referred to as the NEXUS low-risk rules, and the Canadian C-spine rules

(CCR).[8,9] Each rule has been derived and validated in large and diverse populations of ED patients with very high sensitivity and negative predictive values (NPVs).

There are multiple radiographic modalities available to study the C-spine, including plain films (Figure 7.1), CT scan (Figure 7.2), and magnetic resonance imaging (MRI). While CT and MRI are more sensitive and accurate

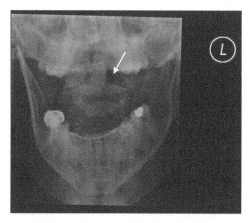

Figure 7.1 Open mouth odontoid cervical spine X-ray showing widening of the lateral pillar (arrow) of the first cervical vertebra, consistent with acute fracture.

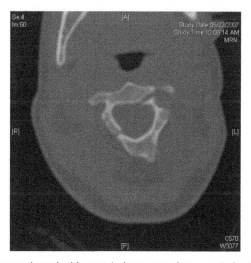

Figure 7.2 A second vertebral fracture is demonstrated on a cervical spine CT.

for fractures, plain films involve less radiation than CT. However, often plain films are inadequate because of poor patient positioning, patient body habitus, degenerative joint disease, or age-related changes (such as osteophytes). When the lateral view does not provide an adequate view of the C7–T1 space, repeat films with special (i.e., swimmer's) views are necessary to definitively rule out injuries. Instead of repeat films, physicians often perform CT scans on patients with inadequate X-rays. MRI provides additional information over the CT scan in that it can identify ligamentous and spinal cord injuries.

There is also an open question about what constitutes a "significant" CSI. The two major decision rules for CSIs were derived and validated using plain radiography, which is less sensitive than CT and MRI. Some clinicians may argue that the decision rules may not be sensitive enough and that any C-spine fracture is important information, because patients with any fracture might be treated differently from those without a fracture through a better understanding of the prognosis, the treatment in terms of immobilization, or the provision of pain control. Examples of clinically insignificant fractures as defined by the derivation and validation studies of the NEXUS and CCR include spinous process fractures, simple wedge fractures without loss of 25% or more of vertebral body height, isolated avulsion fractures without accompanying ligamentous injury, Type 1 odontoid fractures, end plate fractures, fractures of osteophytes, trabecular bone injuries, and transverse process fractures. Finally, additional open questions are whether patients should receive an MRI to rule out ligamentous or spinal cord injury following another normal test (e.g., CT or plain radiography), and whether obtunded trauma patients require MRI imaging after a negative C-spine CT.

Clinical question

Which features of the history and physical exam identify patients at very low risk for clinically significant CSIs who do not need radiography?

The NEXUS group used pilot study data and expert consensus to create a clinical decision rule that includes five elements (Table 7.1). The NEXUS

Table 7.1 NEXUS low-risk criteria

- Absence of tenderness at the posterior midline of the cervical spine
- Absence of a focal neurologic deficit
- Normal level of alertness
- No evidence of intoxication
- Absence of clinically apparent pain that would distract a patient from the pain of a cervical injury

Source: Data from [8].

criteria were assessed as present, absent, or unable to be assessed. Whenever a component of the NEXUS criteria was not able to be assessed, the patient was considered not to have met that criterion. Patients who met all five criteria were considered to be low risk for clinically significant CSI and to not require any radiography.

The initial study for the NEXUS criteria was a prospective observational study at 21 US medical centers that tested the hypothesis that blunt trauma patients who met all of the criteria would have an extremely low probability of CSI. All patients who underwent imaging of the C-spine were included unless they had penetrating trauma or underwent imaging of the C-spine for a reason unrelated to trauma. Patients underwent either standard three-view imaging of the C-spine (lateral, anteroposterior, and open-mouth views) or advanced imaging (CT or MRI). The NEXUS criteria were applied in 34,069 patients who underwent imaging of the C-spine. The prevalence of radiographically documented CSI was 2.4%. Table 7.2 shows the results of the study and the performance of the NEXUS criteria.

The criteria from this study missed a total of eight patients with documented CSIs. Only two of those injuries were clinically significant as defined by the study; however, neither required surgical intervention or had any long-term clinical consequences. With 100% sensitivity and a 100% NPV, it

Table 7.2 NEXUS low-risk criteria study results and test performance

Decision rule	Assessment result for any cervical spine injury		
	Positive	Negative	Totals
Positive	810	28,950	29,760
Negative	8	4301	4309
Totals	818	33,251	34,069
Sensitivity (CI)		99% (98–100%)	
Specificity (CI)		13% (13–13%)	
Positive likelihood ratio (LR+)		1.1	
Negative likelihood ratio (LR−)		0.08	

Decision rule	Clinically significant cervical spine injury		
	Positive	Negative	Totals
Positive	576	29,184	29,760
Negative	2	4307	4309
Totals	578	33,491	34,069
Sensitivity (CI)		100% (99–100%)	
Specificity (CI)		13% (13–13%)	
Positive likelihood ratio (LR+)		1.1	
Negative likelihood ratio (LR−)		0.03	

Source: Data from [8].

was felt that patients meeting all of the criteria could safely be considered at extremely low risk for CSI and did not need imaging.

In a similar study performed at approximately the same time in Canada, Stiell *et al.*[9] created the CCR. This decision rule was first published as a derivation study in 2001. Their goal was similar to that of the NEXUS investigators: to develop a prediction rule with extremely high sensitivity for detecting acute CSIs in stable ED patients with blunt trauma. The authors conducted a prospective cohort study in 10 Canadian EDs and derived the clinical and historical factors that would optimize the detection of a CSI. In this, they differed from the NEXUS investigators, in that the NEXUS criteria did not consider the events surrounding the injury. Patients with blunt head or neck trauma were included in the study if they were alert (defined as a Glasgow coma scale (GCS) score of 15) and stable (defined as a systolic blood pressure >90 mmHg and a respiratory rate greater than 10 but less than 24 breaths per minute). Patients were excluded if they met one of the following predefined criteria: age younger than 16 years, minor injuries not including blunt head or neck trauma (such as lacerations or abrasions), GCS <15, grossly abnormal vital signs, time since injury of greater than 48 hours, penetrating trauma, acute paralysis, known vertebral disease, return for reassessment of the same injury, or pregnancy.

Data were collected on 20 standardized clinical findings from the neurologic status, history, and physical exam. Patients underwent imaging of the C-spine at the discretion of the treating physician. Imaging of the C-spine was not mandatory; therefore, some patients did not undergo imaging. For those patients without C-spine imaging, a structured telephone follow-up was conducted to assess for missed injuries. The purpose of this hybridized criterion standard was to ensure that there were no missed injuries in patients who did not receive radiographs. Patients were considered not to have had a clinically significant CSI if, during the telephone interview at 14 days, they met all of the following criteria: (i) neck pain rated as mild or none, (ii) restriction of neck movement rated as mild or none, (iii) use of a cervical collar not required, and (iv) neck injury did not prevent return of patient to usual occupational activities.

The CCR include three sets of criteria that need to be evaluated in a stepwise manner. However, if a patient satisfies all of the criteria, the decision rule indicates a low risk of CSI, and radiography can be avoided. Table 7.3 lists the criteria that must be fulfilled to safely avoid imaging according to the CCR.

For the derivation study, a total of 12,782 patients were eligible for the study; of those, 3281 patients were not enrolled and another 577 patients were excluded because they did not undergo imaging and could not be

Table 7.3 The Canadian C-spine rules

- Criterion 1: Is there any high-risk factor that mandates radiography?
  - Age 65 years or older
  - Paresthesia in any extremity
  - Dangerous mechanism of injury (fall from 1 meter or greater, axial load to the head (e.g., diving injury), motor vehicle crash at high speed (>100 km/hour), rollover or ejection, or motorized recreational vehicle or bicycle collision)?
  If yes to any of these, radiographic imaging is recommended. If no, criteria 2 and 3 are assessed.
- Criterion 2: Are there any low-risk factors that allow safe assessment of range of motion of the cervical spine? Low-risk factors: simple rear-end motor vehicle crash (excludes being pushed into oncoming traffic, hit by a bus or large truck, or hit by a high-speed vehicle, as well as rollovers), sitting position in the ED, ambulatory at any time, delayed onset of neck pain (defined as not immediate onset of neck pain), or absence of midline cervical spine tenderness? If none of these are present, radiographic imaging is recommended. If any one of these is present, criterion 3 is assessed.
- Criterion 3: Is the patient able to actively rotate his or her neck 45° to the left and right? If not, radiographic imaging is recommended. If yes, the patient meets all of the criteria to safely forgo imaging of the cervical spine.

Source: Adapted from [9].

Table 7.4 Canadian C-spine rules study results and test performance

Decision rule	Radiographically documented injury		
	Positive	Negative	Totals
Positive	151	5041	5192
Negative	0	3732	3732
Totals	151	8773	8924
Sensitivity (CI)	100% (98–100%)		
Specificity (CI)	43% (40–44%)		
Positive likelihood ratio (LR+)	1.8		
Negative likelihood ratio (LR−)	0		

Source: Data from [9].

reached for follow-up. A total of 8924 patients were included in the final study group and had either radiographic imaging or the proxy 14-day telephone follow-up. The prevalence of documented CSI in the study was 2%. Table 7.4 shows the study results and test performance. The stepwise nature of the CCR makes it more complicated than the NEXUS criteria and more difficult to remember; however, studies have shown that the rule can be used by paramedics in the field.[10]

Stiell *et al.*[11] also compared both sets of rules in a large prospective study in the same EDs that participated in the derivation study for the CCR. The study aimed to compare the performances of the two rules (CCR versus NEXUS) to determine which was more specific, and also to validate the CCR. The methodologies for applying the clinical decision rules were the same as outlined in the original studies, but the inclusion and exclusion criteria of the CCR derivation study were used and not all patients underwent imaging (consistent with the CCR study but in contrast to the NEXUS study). Criteria for both sets of rules were prospectively determined and recorded prior to C-spine imaging. The authors achieved their objective of validating the CCR. Among the 8283 patients enrolled, 7438 had complete data from both sets of rules and underwent either C-spine imaging or the 14-day telephone proxy instrument. The incidence of CSI in this study was 2%. Table 7.5 shows the test results and test characteristics. In comparing the performances of the NEXUS and the CCR, the authors found the CCR to have a higher sensitivity, NPV, and specificity. Table 7.6 shows the results and performances of the NEXUS criteria.

Table 7.5 Validation results of the Canadian C-spine rule and test performance

| Decision rule | Radiographically documented injury | | |
	Positive	Negative	Totals
Positive	161	3995	4156
Negative	1	3281	3282
Totals	162	7276	7438
Sensitivity (CI)		99% (96–100%)	
Specificity (CI)		45% (44–46%)	
Positive likelihood ratio (LR+)		1.8	
Negative likelihood ratio (LR−)		0.01	

Source: Data from [11].

Table 7.6 NEXUS low-risk criteria test performance

| Decision rule | Radiographically documented injury | | |
	Positive	Negative	Totals
Positive	147	4599	4746
Negative	15	2677	2692
Totals	162	7276	7438
Sensitivity (CI)		91% (85–94%)	
Specificity (CI)		37% (36–38%)	
Positive likelihood ratio (LR+)		1.4	
Negative likelihood ratio (LR−)		0.24	

Source: Data from [11].

Finally, in a study that assessed the effectiveness of a strategy to implement the CCR in multiple EDs using a matched-pair clustered-randomized design in 11,824 patients in 12 Canadian hospitals, patients seen at intervention sites had a relative reduction in C-spine imaging of 12.8% (confidence interval [CI] 9–16%; 61.7% versus 53.3%; p = 0.01), and the control group had a relative increase of 12.5% (CI 7–18%; 52.8% versus 58.9%; p = 0.03).[12] In addition, the changes were significant when both groups were compared directly: there were no missed fractures and no adverse outcomes in either group. The authors concluded that implementation of the CCR could lead to a significant decrease in imaging without missing injuries.

A systematic review compared the accuracy of the CCR and NEXUS criteria. Fifteen studies comprising 79,526 patients were included. CCR had a sensitivity between 90% and 100% and a specificity between 1% and 77%. Median LR– was 0.18 (interquartile range [IQR] 0.03–0.24) and median LR+ was 1.69 (IQR 1.57–1.81). NEXUS had a sensitivity between 83% and 100% and a specificity between 2% and 46%. Median LR– was 0.30 (IQR 0.19–0.41) and median LR+ was 1.44 (IQR 1.14–1.52). One study directly compared the accuracy of these rules using the same cohort and assessors and found that the CCR had better accuracy. The prevalence of clinically important spinal injury ranged from 0.4% to 6% (median 2%) and included injuries that required surgical intervention, specialist follow-up, or both. Both rules had high sensitivity which indicated that a negative test result was helpful in excluding a clinically important CSI and, therefore, the need for radiographic examination.[13]

Clinical question

How do the test performances of plain radiography and CT of the C-spine compare for identifying CSIs after blunt trauma?

The increased availability of CT technology has resulted in more widespread use for C-spine imaging. An important question is how the test performance of CT compares to that of plain films, especially given that it is sometimes difficult to obtain adequate plain film images to rule out spinal fractures. A meta-analysis in 2005 examined the English language literature from 1995 to 2004 and found seven studies in which both types of imaging were performed. Studies had to have C-spine plain imaging with at least three standard views (anteroposterior, lateral, and open-mouth odontoid) and CT scanning that extended from the occiput to the first thoracic vertebra with the distance between images of <5 mm.[14] The analysis examined 3834 patients and the criterion standards used were the final radiologist interpretation of all imaging studies for five of the studies and the CT results themselves in two of the studies. The prevalence of CSI in the studies was 12%, which is notably higher than in a general population of ED patients. Given the heterogeneity of the studies, there was no consistent definition of what constituted an injury among all the pooled studies. The pooled sensitivity of plain radiography for detecting CSI was 52% (CI 47–56%) while the pooled sensitivity of CT scanning of the C-spine was 98% (CI 96–99%) but, due to the lack of independent criterion standards in many of the studies, specificities could not be calculated for X-ray and CT.

A later study tried to further define this question by stratifying injuries into clinically significant injuries (defined as those requiring an operative procedure, halo application, or rigid cervical collar), and further defined them into high risk, moderate risk, and low risk in a single Level I trauma center, based on the type of injury.[15] Patients were included who met one or more of the NEXUS criteria. In 1505 patients, 78 (5%) had an injury on either plain C-spine radiography or C-spine CT. Of those, 50 (3% of the total) had clinically significant injuries. CT was 100% sensitive for clinically significant injuries, while C-spine radiography only detected 18, yielding a 36% sensitivity. For high-risk, moderate-risk, and low-risk CSIs, plain radiography was 46%, 37%, and 25% sensitive, respectively.

Clinical question

Which alert, neurologically intact patients with negative radiography should receive an MRI to assess for ligamentous and spinal cord injury?

A study examined this precise question, specifically to find factors associated with cervical disc or ligamentous injury found on MRI in alert trauma patients with a negative CT and persistent midline tenderness on physical examination.[16] The study was performed in one Australian hospital (a Level I trauma center) and studied patients who underwent a CT and an MRI for persistent tenderness. The outcomes in the study were the presence and extent of MRI-detected injury of the cervical ligaments, intervertebral discs, spinal cord, or associated soft tissues. In 178 patients with negative CT imaging, 78 (44%) had acute cervical injuries found on MRI. Thirty-eight patients (21% of the overall sample) required intervention: thirty-three patients with cervical collars ranging from 2 to 12 weeks and five patients with operative management, one of whom had delayed instability. Factors associated with a higher number of spinal columns injured included CT-detected advanced cervical spondylosis (odds ratio [OR] 11.6, CI 3.9–34.3%), minor isolated thoracolumbar fractures (OR 5.4, CI 1.5–19.7%), and multidirectional C-spine forces (OR 2.5, CI 1.2–5.2%).

A prospective multicenter study from the Western Trauma Association among patients that had failed NEXUS criteria and underwent CT of the

C-spine included 18 centers and 10,276 patients. These patients had a mean age of 48 years, and injury severity score of 9. There were 1.9% with a clinically significant injury requiring surgery. The sensitivity of CT was 98.5%, specificity 91.0%, and NPV 100%. There were three (0.03%) false-negative CT scans that missed a clinically significant injury, all had a focal neurologic abnormality on their index clinical examination consistent with central cord syndrome.[17] The authors recommended that in patients with abnormal neurological exam after CSI, an MRI should be performed.

Clinical question

In the obtunded adult blunt trauma patient, can the cervical collar be removed after a negative C-spine CT?

In obtunded patients who are unable to communicate whether they have neck pain or tenderness, C-spine CT is commonly used as an initial study to rule out fracture or other injuries. For patients who remain obtunded, a common practice has been to allow the C-collar to remain in place until the patient is awake and alert or to obtain additional imaging such as MRI or upright plain radiography. Keeping the C-collar in place for an extended period of time can lead to pressure injury and other morbidities.

A systematic review and management guideline published by the Eastern Association of Surgery in Trauma (EAST) addressed this question.[18] The article included adult blunt trauma patients 16 years or older, who underwent C-spine CT with axial thickness of less than 3 mm and who were obtunded using any definition. A quantitative meta-analysis due not possible due to the heterogeneity in study design. A total of five studies with complete follow-up were included, which had enrolled 1017 included subjects. Of those, none reported new neurologic changes (paraplegia or quadriplegia) after cervical collar removal. The study identified a worst-case scenario of 9% (161 of 1718 subjects in 11 studies) for stable injuries and a 91% NPV for no injury, after coupling a negative C-spine CT with MRI, upright X-rays, flexion-extension CT, and/or clinical follow-up. The study identified a best-case scenario of 0% (0 of 1718 subjects in 11 studies) incidence of unstable injuries after negative initial imaging result with a high-quality C-spine CT. Based on these results, the authors recommended cervical collar removal after a negative C-spine CT scan.

In the case of patients with intoxication secondary to alcohol or other drugs, a retrospective observational study evaluated the role of CT in ruling out clinically relevant spinal injury (defined as requiring cervical stabilization). The study included 632 adults with alcohol intoxication, who underwent C-spine CT at a Level I trauma center. There were 65 abnormal CT scans (10.3%). Among the 567 with normal CT scans, 4 (0.7%) had central cord syndrome found on initial physical examination, and 1 (0.2%) had a symptomatic unstable ligament injury abnormal on subsequent MRI. CT had a NPV of 99.2% for patients with CSI. The authors concluded that C-spine clearance based on a normal CT scan among intoxicated patients with no gross motor deficits appears to be safe and avoids prolonged and unnecessary immobilization.[19]

A prospective study for C-spine evaluation and clearance in the intoxicated patient included 17 trauma centers and 10,191 patients, 67% men, mean age 48 years, with a mean injury severity score of 11. The incidence of spine injury was 10.6%, and 30% of the patients were intoxicated (defined as alcohol or other drugs). In the intoxicated patients, CT had a sensitivity of 94%, specificity of 99.5%, and NPV of 99.5% for all CSIs. For clinically significant injuries, the NPV was 99.9%.[20]

Clinical question

Which features of the history and physical exam identify children who are at very low risk of clinically significant CSI and do not need radiography?

There is one large multicenter prospective study that examines a clinical decision rule for obtaining C-spine radiographs in pediatric patients with blunt trauma from more than 20 years ago.[21] The study was a prespecified analysis of patients enrolled in NEXUS in which the NEXUS criteria were applied to patients <18 years of age.

The NEXUS cohort comprised 34,069 patients and included 3065 pediatric patients (9% of the total study cohort).[8] The incidence of CSI in the pediatric subgroup was 1.0% ($n = 30$) and Table 7.7 shows the performance of the NEXUS criteria in children. A perfect sensitivity was achieved, but due to the

Table 7.7 Test characteristics for the NEXUS low-risk rules in children

| Decision rule | Radiographically documented injury | | |
	Positive	Negative	Totals
Positive	30	2432	2462
Negative	0	603	603
Totals	30	3035	3065
Sensitivity (CI)		100% (88–100%)	
Specificity (CI)		20% (19–21%)	
Positive likelihood ratio (LR+)		1.3	
Negative likelihood ratio (LR−)		0.08	

Source: Data from [8].

low number of actual injuries, the CIs are wide (88–100%). The authors pointed out that of the 603 (approximately 20%) patients who the NEXUS criteria classified as low risk (the decision rule was negative), no CSI occurred. They do note, however, that while 817 of the 3065 (27%) patients were 3–8 years old, only four of them (0.5%) had CSIs. Similarly, 88 (2.8%) of the 3065 patients were 0–2 years old and none of them sustained CSIs. The authors concluded that, while the NEXUS criteria can safely be used in children older than 8 years, they should be used with caution in children aged 8 years or younger, due to the low number of injuries recorded in their study population.

While NEXUS is the largest prospectively collected dataset of children at risk for CSI, two additional studies have also focused on the development of decision instruments designed to identify a subset of patients at low risk for injury. Leonard et al.[22] conducted a case–control study of children younger than 16 years who received C-spine X-rays after blunt trauma in hospitals in the Pediatric Emergency Care Applied Research Network (PECARN). They reviewed 540 patients with CSIs (defined as injuries to the cervical vertebrae, ligaments, or spinal cord as well as any spinal cord injury without radiographic association) and matched them to controls without injury, identifying eight factors associated with CSI (Table 7.8). Having one or more of the factors was 98% (CI 96–99%) sensitive and 26% (CI 23–29%) specific for CSI, with a LR+ of 1.3 and a LR− of 0.08. While the use of these factors as a decision rule needs validation, they show promise as a decision rule with discriminative ability similar to that of NEXUS.

Pieretti-Vanmarcke et al.[23] reviewed trauma registries from 22 Level I or Level II trauma centers, focusing on children <3 years old who had sustained blunt trauma. They found 12,537 patients meeting these criteria, developed a decision rule with two-thirds of this population, and then

Table 7.8 PECARN factors associated with cervical spine injury in children after blunt trauma

- Altered mental status
- Focal neurologic findings
- Neck pain
- Torticollis
- Substantial torso injury
- Conditions predisposing to cervical spine injury
- Diving
- High-risk motor vehicle crash

Source: Data from [22].

Table 7.9 Decision rule to identify children <3 years old who are at low risk for cervical spine imaging

Patients with total scores of 0 or 1 point may not need cervical spine imaging performed:

• GCS<14	(3 points)
• Motor vehicle accident	(2 points)
• GCS (eye) = 1	(2 points)
• Age>2 years	(1 point)

Source: Data from [23].

validated it on the remaining one-third. Their population contained 83 (0.66%) confirmed CSI patients (defined as any osseous or ligamentous injury to the C-spine seen on CT, radiograph, or MRI), and their decision rule (Table 7.9) had a range from 0 to 8; a score of 0 or 1 had a sensitivity of 93%, a specificity of 70%, a LR+ of 3.1, and a LR− of 0.10 for excluding CSI. While the rule was developed retrospectively from a trauma registry and needs refinement and multicenter prospective validation before it is applied, it shows promise in a younger age group that has not yet been the focus of an imaging decision rule, and which was specifically underrepresented in NEXUS.

A more recent, prospective observational study of children 0–17 years old with blunt trauma, emergency medical services (EMS) scene response, trauma evaluation, and/or cervical imaging. ED clinicians recorded, CSI risk factors.[24] In 4019 children, 74 (1.8%) had CSIs. There were 14 factors with bivariable associations with CSIs: (i) diving, (ii) axial load, (iii) clotheslining, (iv) consciousness loss, (v) neck pain, (vi) an inability to move the neck, (vii) altered mental status, (viii) signs of basilar skull fracture, (ix) torso injury, (x) thoracic injury, (xi) intubation, (xii) respiratory distress, (xiii) decreased oxygen saturation, and (xiv) neurologic deficits.

A model that included (i) high-risk motor vehicle crash, (ii) diving, (iii) predisposing condition, (iv) neck pain, (v) decreased neck mobility (report or exam), (vi) altered mental status, (vii) neurologic deficits, or (viii) torso injury was 91% (CI 84–97%) sensitive and 46% (CI 44–47%) specific for CSIs. A second model that included (i) diving, (ii) axial load, (iii) neck pain, (iv) inability to move neck, (v) altered mental status, (vi) intubation, or (vii) respiratory distress was 92% (CI 86–98%) sensitive and 50% (CI 49–52%) specific. While neither of these models have been prospectively validated, they do confirm previously known pediatric CSI risk factors that could be potentially used for future prediction rule development.

Clinical question

Which C-spine–imaging modality should be used when evaluating pediatric patients with blunt trauma who cannot be clinically cleared?

Given the increased risks of radiation exposure in children, the choice of which imaging modality to use in pediatric blunt trauma patients who cannot be clinically cleared by NEXUS is an important one.[25] Pediatric anatomy, especially increased head size in young children, places greater torque and acceleration stress higher in the C-spine than in adults, increasing the likelihood of upper CSI in these patients. To balance radiation exposure with this increased risk of high-CSI, CT imaging of the occiput to C3 is often recommended in these younger children who cannot be clinically cleared.[26]

Garton and Hammer[27] retrospectively reviewed records over a 20-year period from their institution and found 239 pediatric blunt trauma patients with final diagnoses of CSI based on billing codes, 187 (78%) of whom had adequate radiologic records. In the 157 patients aged 8 years or older, X-rays were 93% sensitive for the detection of CSIs, while the addition of occiput to C3 CT scans increased this sensitivity to 97%. In the smaller group of 33 (22%) patients younger than 8 years old, X-rays were only 75% sensitive, and sensitivity increased to 94% with the limited CT described in this chapter. While this study is limited by its retrospective nature and reliance on billing codes (since they included only patients with known diagnoses, specificities could not be calculated, and the true number of missed injuries is unknown), it is the largest set of children with blunt traumatic CSIs in the literature.

Although their study contained fewer injuries in children 8 years old or younger, Viccellio *et al.*[21] noted that all of the children were diagnosed by X-rays, and one 16-year-old girl had a C7 fracture missed by CT examination. Similarly, Hernandez *et al.*[28] performed a retrospective review of 606 children undergoing ED C-spine imaging at their institution, 459 (76%) of whom were cleared using clinical examination and X-ray findings. Of the remaining 147 patients evaluated with CT, only four (2.7%) had positive findings of fracture, dislocation, or instability, and all of them also had positive findings on their X-rays.

An Australian single-center study compared C-spine imaging rates in children applying the NEXUS, CCR, and PECARN. The data were prospectively collected, and the rules were applied post hoc. A total of 1010 children were enrolled, 41% of them had C-spine imaging (32% X-rays, 13% CT, and 3% MRI). All three rules identified the five children (0.5%) with clinically significant injury. The authors report that if the decision rules were strictly applied, projected imaging rates would be higher than what was observed clinically: NEXUS 44% (CI 41–47%), CCR 48% (CI 45–52%), and PECARN 68% (CI 65–71%).[29]

Clinical question

Are there decision rules for determining which older adult patients are at low risk for CSI?

Three studies that address the issue of a clinical decision rule to identify older adults with a low risk of CSI. Two of these examine subsets of patients from the NEXUS low-risk criteria study: one evaluates the very elderly (age ≥80 years),[30] and the other evaluates the population of older adults typically classified as elderly (age ≥65 years).[31] A third study examined patients 65 years and older in order to stratify CSI risk and guide appropriate imaging.[32]

The first of the studies is a subgroup analysis of 1070 patients from the NEXUS study who were 80 years of age or older.[30] The NEXUS low-risk criteria state that C-spine radiography can be avoided if five clinical criteria are met (Table 7.1). The predefined study objective was to test the performance of the NEXUS criteria in this very elderly patient population. In addition, the injury patterns were examined to determine how injuries sustained in this subgroup differed from those of the entire study population. Their results demonstrated that the prevalence of CSI in this patient group was 4.7%, almost twice that of the total NEXUS cohort (2.4%). Table 7.10 shows the test performance in this subgroup.

No injuries were missed in this cohort. A total of 13% of patients were correctly identified as being low risk, representing those who could have forgone cervical imaging. Injuries of the first and second cervical vertebrae accounted for nearly half of all injuries (47%), in contrast to younger patients in whom the lower C-spine was injured more frequently.

Table 7.10 Performance of the NEXUS criteria among patients 80 years and older

Decision rule	Radiographically documented injury		
	Positive	Negative	Totals
Positive	50	888	938
Negative	0	132	132
Totals	50	1020	1070
Sensitivity (CI)	100% (93–100%)		
Specificity (CI)	13% (11–15%)		
Positive likelihood ratio (LR+)	1.1		
Negative likelihood ratio (LR–)	0		

Source: Data from [31].

Table 7.11 Performance of NEXUS among patients 65 years and older

	Sensitivity, % (CI)	Specificity, % (CI)	Positive likelihood ratio (LR+)	Negative likelihood ratio (LR−)
Assessment result for any cervical injury	99% (95–100%)	15% (15–15%)	1.2	0.07
Clinically significant cervical injury	100% (97–100%)	15% (15–15%)	1.2	0

Source: Data from [30].

The second study is a subgroup analysis of the 2943 patients from the NEXUS study who were 65 years or older.[31] The prevalence of CSI in this subgroup was 4.6%, which is similar to that of the very elderly population in the first study. The authors examined the performance of the NEXUS criteria among this group and found that they had an overall sensitivity of 99% for any cervical injury and 100% for clinically significant cervical injury (Table 7.11).

CSIs occurred in a total of 135 elderly patients, with the NEXUS criteria identifying all but two injuries. Neither of the two injuries misclassified by the NEXUS criteria required surgical intervention. Analysis of the specific types of injuries occurring in this population aged 65 years or older revealed that fractures of C1 and C2 represented more than half of all cervical fractures, similar to the very elderly population noted in the first study. Among the individual NEXUS criteria not met and thus responsible for patients not being classified as low risk, midline tenderness (present in 53% of patients) and distracting injury (present in 44%) were the most frequent.

In a more recent study, performed specifically to examine C-spine fractures in elderly patients, Bub *et al.*[32] performed a case–control study among trauma registry patients in Seattle, Washington, from 1995 to 2002. Their objective was to derive and validate a clinical decision rule that identified C-spine fracture, using clinical and historical elements to guide imaging in patients aged 65 years or older.

Cases were identified for inclusion from their inpatient trauma registry. Only patients 65 years or older with nonpenetrating trauma who had confirmatory cervical imaging prior to death were eligible. Patients transferred to the trauma center were excluded in an effort to minimize referral bias. Controls were chosen from among ED patients seen between 1995 and 2002 (admitted or discharged) who were age 65 years or older, had blunt trauma with the absence of cervical fracture, and were also not transferred to the ED. Statistical methods adjusted for confounding. The prevalence of C-spine fracture was 2.6% among all the trauma registry patients meeting the inclusion criteria during the study period (n = 3958). One hundred and three cases and 107 control patients were identified and included in the analysis. The final clinical prediction rule (Figure 7.3) is able to stratify patients according to cervical fracture risk and uses the author definitions listed in Table 7.12 The authors do not give recommendations for or against imaging a particular subgroup themselves, but aimed only to develop an understanding of the risk for cervical fracture in each subgroup, allowing individual clinicians to use that risk when deciding who to image.

A recent retrospective cohort study from a tertiary-care academic ED evaluated patients ≥65 years, including dementia, after a ground-level fall. Among 1035 patients, 683 (66%) had CT of the C-spine, and 16 (1.5%) had a cervical fracture. C-spine tenderness (OR 4.7, CI 1.5–14.1), neck pain (OR 10.5, CI 3.4–32.5), altered mental status (OR 5.1, CI 1.7–15.6), and trauma above the clavicles (OR 3.8, CI 1.2–12.3) were associated with C-spine fracture. Dementia (OR 0.2, CI 0.4–0.9) was not associated with fracture. A combination of trauma above the clavicles, C-spine tenderness, and altered

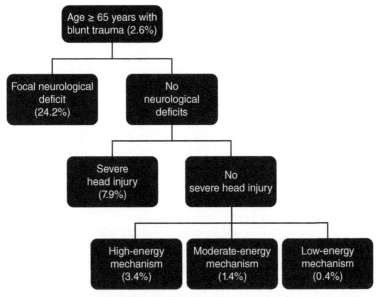

Figure 7.3 Schematic of clinical prediction rule for cervical spine fractures in elderly patients in a trauma registry. The risk of cervical spine fractures in each subgroup is shown in parentheses. (Adapted from [32]. Percentages correspond to absolute cervical fracture risk.)

Table 7.12 Definitions for clinical prediction rule

Criterion	Definition
severe head injury	• Intracranial hemorrhage • Skull fracture • Unconsciousness • All intubated patients
High-energy mechanism	• Falls from 10-foot height • Pedestrian struck by an auto • Airplane accident • High-speed motor vehicle injury ($\geq$30 mph)
Moderate-energy mechanism	• Low-speed motor vehicle injury (<30 mph) • Fall from <10 feet • Skiing accident
Low-energy mechanism	• Fall from standing or sitting position

Source: Adapted from [32].

mental status had a sensitivity of 100% and a specificity of 40.0% for detection of C-spine fracture.[33]

Comment

The NEXUS and the CCR have both been validated in large cohorts of ED patients with blunt trauma to the neck. In the validation cohorts, both have high sensitivities (>99.3%) and NPVs (>99.9%) making both decision rules safe for detecting clinically significant injuries on plain radiography. In addition, the implementation of the CCR is associated with lower use of spine radiography.

When comparing the two rules, Stiell *et al.* have concluded that the CCR performed better than the NEXUS criteria. We feel that there are sufficient differences between the two rules and the studies supporting them to make the issue not as clear-cut. Table 7.13 compares and contrasts the differences in the derivation, validation, and implementation of these rules.

Given the differences, both rules are useful for assessing the stable patient with blunt trauma. Overall, the NEXUS criteria are somewhat easier to use clinically because they are less difficult to remember. The CCR are more complex and must be employed in a stepwise fashion. In our experience, the most common reason for failure of the NEXUS criteria and for the requirement of cervical radiography is midline tenderness. The CCR are more specific than the NEXUS criteria, and patients with midline

Table 7.13 Comparison of NEXUS criteria and the Canadian C-spine rule

	NEXUS low-risk criteria	Canadian C-spine rule (CCR)	Comment
Explicit description for each criterion in the rule	Intoxication and painful distracting injury left undefined	High-risk mechanism defined by the authors	NEXUS • Authors felt that intoxication and painful distracting injury were best determined clinically and that strict definitions would limit use in clinical practice CCR • Intoxication not included as it was found in the preliminary studies to not be predictive of injury • Provided list of high-risk mechanisms, but many others exist that are not explicitly listed
Patient enrollment	Patients with blunt trauma undergoing cervical imaging	Patients with complete data (undergoing either imaging or 14-day proxy telephone survey)	NEXUS • Risk of selection bias based on whether or not at-risk patients got initial imaging, possibly limiting generalizability CCR • Not all patients had criterion standard (imaging), but proxy tool accounted for those patients without imaging
Exclusion criteria	Patients with penetrating trauma or who had cervical imaging for reasons other than blunt trauma	Excluded conditions explicitly listed	NEXUS • These are reasonable given the emphasis on blunt trauma CCR • Exclusion criteria limit generalizability

Table 7.13 (*Continued*)

	NEXUS low-risk criteria	Canadian C-spine rule (CCR)	Comment
Age criteria	No age limit	Age 16 years or older	CCR • Excluded patients <16 years, limiting generalizability
Prevalence of clinically significant injury	2%	2%	–
Study size (validation study)	>34,000 patients in 21 US medical centers	>7400 patients in nine Canadian medical centers	Diverse ED patient populations make results generalizable
Sensitivity, % (validation study)	99% (CI 98–100%)	100% (CI 96–100%)	Comparable sensitivities, with correspondingly high negative predictive values (NPVs)
Specificity, % (validation study)	13% (CI 12.8–13.0%)	45.1% (CI 44–46%)	The CCR has a significantly higher specificity and therefore fewer false positives
Decision rule usability	Five elements to determine as present or absent	A total of three sets of criteria, totaling 14 elements to determine; some dictate imaging, others dictate no imaging	NEXUS • With fewer elements and a straightforward interpretation, it is simpler to use CCR • Many elements make it cumbersome to use • Age criteria simplify approach for older patients

tenderness can be identified who do not otherwise meet the criteria for cervical radiography.

Because of the higher specificity of the CCR, we propose that the CCR criteria be applied as a first step in the ED. While both the NEXUS and the Canadian rules have roughly equal high sensitivity and high NPVs, Canadian rules will have many fewer false positives. This is not to say that the NEXUS criteria should not be used, but you should be aware that while the NPV is

116 Chapter 7: Cervical Spine Fractures

very high with both sets of rules, the very low specificity of the NEXUS criteria will lead to more unnecessary imaging (i.e., false positives in which the prediction rule indicates the patient is not low risk and therefore recommends imaging). We would point out that either rule was not designed to be used in isolation of other clinical information. If there are historical or exam findings that lead you to have a high suspicion for CSI, then you should proceed to imaging and not apply any clinical decision rule. Regarding whether or not plain films or CT C-spine should be the initial test of choice in blunt cervical trauma, it appears in the limited studies of highly selected trauma patients that CT C-spine has a higher sensitivity for detecting CSI compared to plain-film imaging. However, in these studies, the overall prevalence of CSI was much higher than is seen in everyday ED practice. In fact, it was nearly six times higher than in the NEXUS and Canadian studies. This selection bias makes it difficult to generalize the patients in these studies (patients were enrolled at primary trauma centers) to the typical patient after a minor motor vehicle crash who is seen in the ED outside of the trauma bay. Regardless, at this time, in patients suspected of CSI, our opinion is to consider CT imaging over plain radiographs, especially in high-risk cases. However, radiation exposure and cost are the two factors that have not been sufficiently explored. While there may be subgroups of patients who would benefit from CT scanning over plain radiography (such as patients with obesity, a history of degenerative joint disease, advanced age, or prior surgery), there are no good data on this topic.

Performing MRI in stable, awake trauma patients with persistent C-spine tenderness and a negative CT may detect important injuries, particularly because of the relatively high prevalence of injuries for which a different management plan may be indicated. However, it is important to understand that the referenced study was conducted in a select group of patients seen by the trauma team (i.e., already very high-risk patients). Therefore, we do not recommend performing an MRI in relatively low-risk ED patients who have midline tenderness without other injuries or neurological findings. In addition, when higher-risk patients with blunt injuries are obtunded, a CT C-spine can be used as the primary way to exclude clinically significant CSI.

With respect to children, the only prospective study examining a decision rule regarding risk determination for CSI in children with blunt trauma, Viccellio et al.[21] validated the NEXUS criteria as being highly sensitive. Exploration of their data also found no cases of spinal cord injury without radiographic abnormality (SCIWORA) in any child, which is a lingering concern in the minds of clinicians. The authors were careful to note that there were 3065 patients with only 30 CSIs, resulting in wide CIs around the test parameters, despite their having not missed any cases of CSI. They further reported that it would require a study of nearly 80,000 children to narrow the CIs to within 0.5%, making it unlikely that another study will improve on the current performance of the NEXUS criteria.

A major concern that clinicians may have is applying the NEXUS criteria to infants (0–2 years) and toddlers (2–8 years) as they may be nonverbal or it may be difficult to accurately determine whether any individual item is present or absent. While only four of the 30 CSIs occurred in patients ≤8 years old, at least one criterion was positive in each of those four patients. Until a new decision rule focusing on this younger population is developed and validated, we recommend using the NEXUS in all pediatric patients, with the caveat that the inability to obtain certain NEXUS criteria on very young patients should not imply their absence.

In children needing radiographic evaluation for CSI after blunt trauma, we recommend X-ray as the modality of choice. In patients ≤8 years old who are also obtaining head CT or in whom an odontoid view is unobtainable, we recommend a CT of the occiput to C3, given the increased incidence of high-CSIs in this population.

With respect to older adults, it is clinically intuitive that they can sustain CSIs from traumatic mechanisms that might not cause injury in younger patients, such as falling out of a chair or from standing height. Furthermore, older patients may not report symptoms or circumstances in as clear a manner as younger patients because of underlying medical illnesses or cognitive impairment. However, we would exercise caution in using the clinical prediction rule developed by Bub et al.[32] It was derived and validated in the same setting, done so retrospectively from chart review of a preselected trauma registry population, and identified only C-spine fractures rather than all types of clinically significant injury. The simple conclusion that all older patients are at risk of cervical fractures does nothing to support a more selective approach to imaging, which was the goal of both the NEXUS and Canadian C-spine studies.

In contrast to the NEXUS criteria, the CCR have an age criterion and do not allow for avoidance of imaging in patients ≥65 years old. To date, no subset analysis of elderly patients from the Canadian dataset has been published. Nevertheless, the two secondary analyses from the NEXUS study reveal that using the NEXUS criteria allows identification of patients at low risk of CSI with a very high sensitivity in both the elderly (≥65 years) and the very elderly (≥80 years). While there has been one published case report in which the application of the NEXUS criteria to a 101-year-old patient resulted in misclassification of the patient as low risk for CSI, the case (and the few others like it that remain unpublished) should not deter emergency physicians from applying the well-validated NEXUS criteria to elderly patients given the two subset analyses noted in this chapter.[31–33]

References

1. National Hospital Ambulatory Medical Care Survey: 2017 Emergency Department Summary Tables. https://www.cdc.gov/nchs/data/nhamcs/web_tables/2017_ed_web_tables-508.pdf. Accessed February 18, 2022.
2. Milby AH, Halpern CH, Guo W, Stein SC. Prevalence of cervical spinal injury in trauma. *Neurosurgical Focus.* 2008; 25(5): E10.
3. Yadollahi M, Paydar S, Ghaem H *et al.* Epidemiology of cervical spine fractures. *Trauma Monthly.* 2016; 21(3): e33608. doi: 10.5812/traumamon.33608.
4. Mohseni S, Talving P, Branco BC *et al.* Effect of age on cervical spine injury in pediatric population: a National Trauma Data Bank review. *Journal of Pediatric Surgery.* 2011; 46(9): 1771–6.
5. Mannix R, Nigrovic LE, Schutzman SA *et al.* Factors associated with the use of cervical spine computed tomography imaging in pediatric trauma patients. *Academic Emergency Medicine.* 2011; 18(9): 905–11.
6. Harris MB, Reichmann WM, Bono CM *et al.* Mortality in elderly patients after cervical spine fractures. *The Journal of Bone and Joint Surgery. American Volume.* 2010; 92(3): 567–74.
7. Damadi AA, Saxe AW, Fath JJ, Apelgren KN. Cervical spine fractures in patients 65 years or older: A 3-year experience at a level I trauma center. *The Journal of Trauma.* 2008; 64(3): 745–8. doi: 10.1097/TA.0b013e3180341fc6.
8. Hoffman JR, Mower WR, Wolfson AB, Todd KH, Zucker MI. Validity of a set of clinical criteria to rule out injury to the cervical spine in patients with blunt trauma. National Emergency X-Radiography Utilization Study Group. *The New England Journal of Medicine.* 2000; 343(2): 94–9.
9. Stiell IG, Wells GA, Vandemheen KL *et al.* The Canadian C-spine rule for radiography in alert and stable trauma patients. *Journal of the American Medical Association.* 2001; 286(15): 1841–8.
10. Vaillancourt C, Stiell IG, Beaudoin T *et al.* The out-of-hospital validation of the Canadian C-spine rule by paramedics. *Annals of Emergency Medicine.* 2009; 54(5): 663–71.e1.
11. Stiell IG, Clement CM, McKnight RD *et al.* The Canadian C-spine rule versus the NEXUS low-risk criteria in patients with trauma. *The New England Journal of Medicine.* 2003; 349(26): 2510–8.
12. Stiell IG, Clement CM, Grimshaw J *et al.* Implementation of the Canadian C-spine rule: Prospective 12 centre cluster randomised trial. *BMJ.* 2009; 29(339): b4146.
13. Michaleff ZA, Maher CG, Verhagen AP, Rebbeck T, Lin CW. Accuracy of the Canadian C-spine rule and NEXUS to screen for clinically important cervical spine injury in patients following blunt trauma: A systematic review. *CMAJ.* 2012; 184(16): E867–76.
14. Holmes JF, Akkinepalli R. Computed tomography versus plain radiography to screen for cervical spine injury: A meta-analysis. *The Journal of Trauma.* 2005; 58(5): 902–5.
15. Bailitz J, Starr F, Beecroft M *et al.* CT should replace three-view radiographs as the initial screening test in patients at high, moderate, and low risk for blunt cervical

spine injury: A prospective comparison. *The Journal of Trauma.* 2009; 66(6): 1605–9.

16. Ackland HM, Cameron PA, Varma DK *et al.* Cervical spine magnetic resonance imaging in alert, neurologically intact trauma patients with persistent midline tenderness and negative computed tomography results. *Annals of Emergency Medicine.* 2011; 58(6): 521–30.

17. Inaba K, Byerly S, Bush LD *et al.* Cervical spinal clearance: A prospective Western Trauma Association Multi-institutional Trial. *Journal of Trauma and Acute Care Surgery.* 2016; 81(6): 1122–30.

18. Patel MB, Humble SS, Cullinane DC *et al.* Cervical spine collar clearance in the obtunded adult blunt trauma patient: A systematic review and practice management guideline from the Eastern Association for the Surgery of Trauma. *Journal of Trauma and Acute Care Surgery.* 2015; 78(2): 430–41.

19. Bush L, Brookshire R, Roche B *et al.* Evaluation of cervical spine clearance by computed tomographic scan alone in intoxicated patients with blunt trauma. *JAMA Surgery.* 2016; 151(9): 807–13.

20. Martin MJ, Bush LD, Inaba K *et al.* Cervical spine evaluation and clearance in the intoxicated patient: A prospective Western Trauma Association Multi-Institutional Trial and Survey. *Journal of Trauma and Acute Care Surgery.* 2017; 83(6): 1032–40.

21. Viccellio P, Simon H, Pressman BD *et al.* A prospective multicenter study of cervical spine injury in children. *Pediatrics.* 2001; 108(2): E20.

22. Leonard JC, Kuppermann N, Olsen C *et al.* Factors associated with cervical spine injury in children after blunt trauma. *Annals of Emergency Medicine.* 2011; 58(2): 145–55.

23. Pieretti-Vanmarcke R, Velmahos GC, Nance ML *et al.* Clinical clearance of the cervical spine in blunt trauma patients younger than 3 years: A multi-center study of the American Association for the surgery of trauma. *The Journal of Trauma.* 2009; 67(3): 543–9; discussion 549–50. doi: 10.1097/TA.0b013e3181b57aa1.

24. Leonard JC, Browne LR, Ahmad FA *et al.* Cervical spine injury risk factors in children with blunt trauma. *Pediatrics.* 2019; 144(1): e20183221.

25. Brenner D, Elliston C, Hall E, Berdon W. Estimated risks of radiation-induced fatal cancer from pediatric CT. *AJR. American Journal of Roentgenology.* 2001; 176(2): 289–96.

26. Chung S, Mikrogianakis A, Wales PW *et al.* Trauma Association of Canada Pediatric Subcommittee National Pediatric Cervical Spine Evaluation Pathway: consensus guidelines. *The Journal of Trauma.* 2011; 70(4): 873–84.

27. Garton HJ, Hammer MR. Detection of pediatric cervical spine injury. *Neurosurgery.* 2008; 62(3): 700–8. discussion 700–8.

28. Hernandez JA, Chupik C, Swischuk LE. Cervical spine trauma in children under 5 years: Productivity of CT. *Emergency Radiology.* 2004; 10(4): 176–8.

29. Phillips N, Rasmussen K, McGuire S *et al.* Projected paediatric cervical spine imaging rates with application of NEXUS, Canadian C-Spine and PECARN clinical decision rules in a prospective Australian cohort. *Emergency Medicine Journal.* 2021; 38(5): 330–7.

30. Ngo B, Hoffman JR, Mower WR. Cervical spine injury in the very elderly. *Emergency Radiology.* 2000; 7(5): 287–91.
31. Touger M, Gennis P, Nathanson N *et al.* Validity of a decision rule to reduce cervical spine radiography in elderly patients with blunt trauma. *Annals of Emergency Medicine.* 2002; 40(3): 287–93.
32. Bub LD, Blackmore CC, Mann FA, Lomoschitz FM. Cervical spine fractures in patients 65 years and older: A clinical prediction rule for blunt trauma. *Radiology.* 2005; 234(1): 143–9.
33. Williams JR, Muesch AJ, Svenson JE, Clegg AW, Patterson BW, Ward MA. Utility of bedside assessment to evaluate for cervical-spine fracture post ground-level fall for patients 65 years and older. *The American Journal of Emergency Medicine.* 2022; 53: 208–14.

Chapter 8 **Blunt Abdominal Trauma**

Brendan M. Carr and Fernanda Bellolio

Department of Emergency Medicine, Mayo Clinic, Rochester, MN, USA

Highlights

- There are multiple diagnostic tests available to evaluate for the presence of intra-abdominal injury in patients with blunt abdominal trauma including CT scan, focused assessment with sonography for trauma (FAST), and diagnostic peritoneal lavage (DPL).
- FAST is highly specific and accurate in adult patients and is a useful, rapid, noninvasive adjunct in the evaluation of blunt abdominal trauma.
- High clinical suspicion in the setting of a negative FAST should prompt further evaluation by serial exams, CT imaging, or surgical exploration.
- FAST should be used with caution in pediatric trauma patients due to its lower sensitivity in this population.

Background

In the acutely injured patient with abdominal trauma, several diagnostic modalities are available in the emergency department (ED) to detect the presence of solid organ injury and intra-abdominal hemorrhage. Many studies have compared abdominal ultrasound with computed tomography (CT) scan, most of which have shown that CT is superior to ultrasound in detecting intra-abdominal injuries. A challenge often encountered with CT imaging in trauma patients, however, is that it cannot always be safely performed in unstable patients. In such patients, a diagnostic peritoneal lavage (DPL) performed at the bedside in the ED was historically the test of choice to assess for intra-abdominal injury (e.g., hemorrhage, perforated viscus) for which surgical intervention may have been needed. In DPL, a

---

Evidence-Based Emergency Care: Diagnostic Testing and Clinical Decision Rules, Third Edition.
Edited by Jesse M. Pines, Fernanda Bellolio, Christopher R. Carpenter, and Ali S. Raja.
© 2023 John Wiley & Sons Ltd. Published 2023 by John Wiley & Sons Ltd.

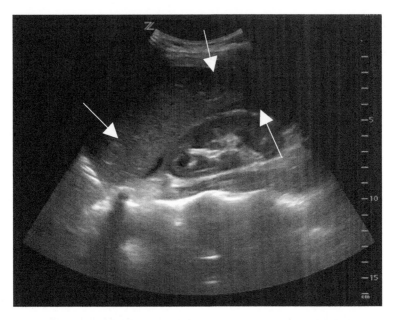

Figure 8.1 A focused assessment by sonography in trauma (FAST) reveals fluid in Morison's pouch and surrounding the caudal tip of the liver (arrows). (Courtesy of Tobias Kummer, MD.)

surgical incision is made in the abdomen which is then lavaged for the presence of blood or red blood cells. In recent years, however, diagnostic ultrasound has emerged as a safe, rapid, and noninvasive alternative to DPL, and has replaced the use of DPL in hospitals at which ED ultrasound is available (Figure 8.1). The focused assessment with sonography for trauma (FAST) exam is the best-studied and most commonly performed ultrasound protocol for trauma patients in the ED and will be the focus of discussion here. While the FAST exam is not 100% sensitive and thus cannot completely rule out the presence of intra-abdominal injuries, it can be used during the initial evaluation of trauma patients to provide early information and rule in intra-abdominal bleeding.

Clinical questions

How accurate is FAST compared to CT scan and DPL in adult patients with blunt abdominal trauma?
One of the earliest prospective studies to compare DPL, the abdominal windows of the FAST exam, and CT scan was performed in China in 1990.[1]

Table 8.1 Early study of sensitivity and specificity of test sensitivity, specificity and accuracy of computed tomography (CT) scan, diagnostic peritoneal lavage (DPL), and ultrasound in 55 patients using surgical findings as the criterion standard

	Sensitivity, %	Specificity, %	Accuracy, %
CT	97.2	94.7	96.4
DPL	100	84.2	94.5
Ultrasound	91.7	94.7	92.7

Source: Data from Liu et al. [1].

Liu *et al.* compared the accuracy of the three modalities for the detection of significant intra-abdominal injuries. Patients with stable vital signs after their initial resuscitation and who had equivocal physical examination findings underwent CT and ultrasound, followed by DPL. If any of the three exams were positive, the investigators performed a laparotomy. They compared surgical findings (the criterion standard) to the results of the diagnostic tests. For the 55 patients included in this early study, the sensitivity, specificity, and accuracy are shown in Table 8.1.

Since then, many studies have been performed evaluating the use of ultrasound in adults with blunt abdominal trauma. A systematic review in 2012 evaluated the test characteristics of bedside FAST exam for "clinically significant intra-abdominal injuries." This reported a sensitivity and specificity of 74% and 96%, respectively, when the possibility of publication bias was factored into the calculations.[2] This systematic review included 23 studies and 15,750 patients, with a prevalence (pretest probability) of intra-abdominal injury in ED patients with blunt abdominal trauma of 13%, and a prevalence of clinically significant injuries requiring surgery or embolization of 4.7%. The presence of intra-peritoneal fluid or organ injury had a LR+ 30 (CI 20–46), and a normal FAST had LR− 0.26 (CI 0.19–0.34). Furthermore, a positive FAST exam in hemodynamically unstable patients (LR+ 82) is highly indicative of intra-abdominal injury increasing a pretest probability of 13% to a posttest probability of 92%. However, a negative FAST in high-risk clinically stable patients does not sufficiently exclude intra-abdominal injury (LR− 0.33). This study included CT as one of multiple (laparotomy, DPL, clinical course, autopsy) possible reference standards. The review concluded FAST exams aid with risk stratification and its more accurate to history, physical exam, labs, X-rays, or clinician judgment, but a normal ultrasound does not rule out an intra-abdominal injury.[2] More than a dozen studies since then have continued to attempt to address this question for adult patients, most with similar results. These more recent studies are presented in Table 8.2.

Table 8.2 Sensitivity and specificity of FAST for adult patients with blunt trauma in studies published 2015–2019

Author	Year	N	Sensitivity (%)	Specificity (%)
Nixon *et al.*	2019	87	75	100
Lee *et al.*[*]	2019	4263	92.1	98.7
Do *et al.*	2019	274	51	–
Rowell *et al.*	2019	317	62	83
Carter *et al.*	2018	187	75	99.3
Christian *et al.*	2018	81	96	96
Akoglu *et al.*	2018	132	42.9	98.4
Matsushima *et al.*	2018	103	68.5	93.9
Zanobetti *et al.*	2018	–[**]	22	–
Elbaih *et al.*	2017	150	92.6	100
Dammers *et al.*	2017	421	67	99
Ghafouri *et al.*	2016	120	93.1	93.4
Kumar *et al.*	2015	50	75	96
Carter *et al.*	2015	–	56	98
Smith *et al.*	2015	–	75	96

[*]This study was a systematic review looking at FAST in the disaster setting.
[**]Data not reported.
Source: Data from references [3–17].

One of the issues with FAST is that it is operator dependent in both image acquisition and image interpretation, and most studies do not report the learning curve or training level needed to develop and maintain expertise with the FAST exam. In addition, it can be more challenging in patients with large body habitus. The available data overall suggests that an abnormal FAST exam is very specific for intra-abdominal injury in the setting of trauma. Its sensitivity varies among studies and clinical settings, however, and FAST is inferior to CT imaging in overall diagnostic accuracy. Thus, some reserve its use for the hemodynamically unstable patient for whom transport to a CT suite may not be feasible, but where sonographic evidence of intra-abdominal injury may suggest emergency surgical exploration is necessary.

Clinical question

Can FAST exclude intra-abdominal injuries in pediatric patients with blunt trauma?
Multiple studies have examined the sensitivity of FAST for the detection of intra-abdominal injuries in pediatric patients. Overall, the accuracy of FAST in pediatric patients is lower than in adults. A systematic review and meta-analysis published in 2019 reviewed eight prospective studies that included a

total of 2135 patients. Included studies were noted by the review authors, with the primary quality concern being that all studies were at risk for verification bias given that FAST results were interpreted in real time and used to guide subsequent management. Nonetheless, these studies were deemed to be of moderate quality, and this meta-analysis found an overall sensitivity and specificity of 35% and 96%, respectively.[18] This suggests the FAST exam, while still specific for intra-abdominal injury when positive, has a lower sensitivity in pediatric patients. In contrast to adults, children with blunt abdominal trauma and solid organ injury are less likely to require surgical intervention, which may further limit the ability of a positive FAST result to direct immediate management decisions. The above data support the current recommendations from the Advanced Trauma Life Support (ATLS) 10th edition textbook, which states "FAST should not be relied upon as the sole diagnostic test to rule out the presence of intra-abdominal injury [in pediatric trauma patients]."[19]

Comment

The FAST examination performs with high specificity and at least moderate sensitivity for the detection of hemoperitoneum and, therefore, has a role in the evaluation of adult patients who have experienced blunt abdominal trauma. It is less accurate than CT. It is most useful as an adjunct to CT, in cases of hemodynamic instability, or in cases where CT imaging cannot be completed. In many trauma centers, FAST has become a useful adjunct in nearly all patients with blunt abdominal trauma and is part of the evaluation process during the primary and secondary surveys. In centers where ultrasound is readily available, it has replaced DPL in unstable trauma patients with potential intra-abdominal injury. However, a negative FAST cannot be used to rule out significant intra-abdominal injury and it should not be used as a reference standard. In patients in whom a high pretest probability exists, further testing or laparotomy should be considered in consultation with a trauma surgeon.

Why adjust for publication bias?
Publication bias is when the likelihood of a study being published is affected by the findings of the study, and studies with positive findings are more likely to be published than studies with negative findings. The most common way to evaluate for publication bias is by inspecting the funnel plot. In one of the systematic reviews discussed, publication bias was detected with suspicion for missing studies of lower accuracy.[2] Publication bias in this context suggested that a negative FAST examination might have a less favorable

likelihood ratio. The impact of this bias is inferred when comparing the two studies in which the overall clinical impression was established before versus after the FAST examination. When the FAST examination was included as part of the clinical impression, the overall impression of no abdominal injury was less accurate, suggesting that physicians underestimate the possibility of a false-negative FAST examination result. Using the adjusted LR+ was more conservative (unadjusted sensibility, specificity, positive, and negative likelihood ratio were 82%, 99%, 69, and 0.18; versus after adjustment by publication bias, 74%, 96%, 30 and 0.26.)

References

1. Liu M, Lee CH, P'Eng FK. Prospective comparison of diagnostic peritoneal lavage, computed tomographic scanning, and ultrasonography for the diagnosis of blunt abdominal trauma. *The Journal of Trauma*. 1993; 35(2): 267–70.

2. Nishijima DK, Simel DL, Wisner DH, Holmes JF. Does this adult patient have a blunt intra-abdominal injury? *Journal of the American Medical Association*. 2012; 307(14): 1517–27.

3. Akoglu H, Celik OF, Celik A, Ergelen R, Onur O, Denizbasi A. Diagnostic accuracy of the extended focused abdominal sonography for trauma (E-FAST) performed by emergency physicians compared to CT. *The American Journal of Emergency Medicine*. 2018; 36(6): 1014–7.

4. Carter JW, Falco MH, Chopko MS, Flynn WJ Jr, Wiles Iii CE, Guo WA. Do we really rely on fast for decision-making in the management of blunt abdominal trauma? *Injury*. 2015; 46(5): 817–21.

5. Carter NJ, Gay D. FAST in the deployed military setting. *Journal of the Royal Army Medical Corps*. 2018; 164(5): 332–4.

6. Christian NT, Burlew CC, Moore EE et al. The FAST exam can reliably identify patients with significant Intraabdominal hemorrhage in life threatening pelvic fractures. *Journal of Trauma and Acute Care Surgery*. 2018; 84(6): 924–8.

7. Dammers D, El Moumni M, Hoogland II, Veeger N, Ter Avest E. Should we perform a FAST exam in haemodynamically stable patients presenting after blunt abdominal injury: A retrospective cohort study. *Scandinavian Journal of Trauma, Resuscitation and Emergency Medicine*. 2017; 25(1): 1.

8. Do WS, Chang R, Fox EE et al. Too fast, or not fast enough? The FAST exam in patients with non-compressible torso hemorrhage. *The American Journal of Surgery*. 2019; 217(5): 882–6.

9. Elbaih AH, Abu-Elela ST. Predictive value of focused assessment with sonography for trauma (FAST) for laparotomy in unstable polytrauma Egyptians patients. *Chinese Journal of Traumatology*. 2017; 20(6): 323–8.

10. Ghafouri HB, Zare M, Bazrafshan A, Modirian E, Farahmand S, Abazarian N. Diagnostic accuracy of emergency-performed focused assessment with sonography for trauma (FAST) in blunt abdominal trauma. *Electronic Physician*. 2016; 8(9): 2950–3.

11. Kumar S, Bansal VK, Muduly DK *et al*. Accuracy of focused assessment with sonography for trauma (FAST) in blunt trauma abdomen-a prospective study. *The Indian Journal of Surgery*. 2015; 77(Suppl 2): 393–7.

12. Lee C, Balk D, Schafer J *et al*. Accuracy of focused assessment with sonography for trauma (FAST) in disaster settings: A meta-analysis and systematic review. *Disaster Medicine and Public Health Preparedness*. 2019; 13(5–6): 1059–64.

13. Matsushima K, Khor D, Berona K *et al*. Double jeopardy in penetrating trauma: Get FAST, get it right. *World Journal of Surgery*. 2018; 42(1): 99–106.

14. Nixon G, Blattner K, Muirhead J, Kiuru S, Kerse N. Point-of-care ultrasound for FAST and AAA in rural New Zealand: Quality and impact on patient care. *Rural and Remote Health*. 2019; 19(3): 5027.

15. Rowell SE, Barbosa RR, Holcomb JB, Fox EE, Barton CA, Schreiber MA. The focused assessment with sonography in trauma (FAST) in hypotensive injured patients frequently fails to identify the need for laparotomy: A multi-institutional pragmatic study. *Trauma Surgery and Acute Care Open*. 2019; 4(1): e000207.

16. Smith IM, Naumann DN, Marsden ME, Ballard M, Bowley DM. Scanning and war: Utility of FAST and CT in the assessment of battlefield abdominal trauma. *Annals of Surgery*. 2015; 262(2): 389–96.

17. Zanobetti M, Coppa A, Nazerian P *et al*. Chest abdominal-focused assessment sonography for trauma during the primary survey in the emergency department: The CA-FAST protocol. *European Journal of Trauma and Emergency Surgery*. 2018; 44(6): 805–10.

18. Liang T, Roseman E, Gao M, Sinert R. The utility of the focused assessment with sonography in trauma examination in pediatric blunt abdominal trauma: A systematic review and meta-analysis. *Pediatric Emergency Care*. 2021; 37(2): 108–18.

19. American College of Surgeons. Chapter 10 Pediatric trauma. In: *Advanced trauma life support: ATLS student course manual*. 10th ed. Chicago (IL): American College of Surgeons; 2018: 186–212.

Chapter 9 **Acute Knee Injuries**

Jesse M. Pines[1,2] and Fernanda Bellolio[3]

[1] US Acute Care Solutions, Canton, OH, USA
[2] Department of Emergency Medicine, Drexel University, Philadelphia, PA, USA
[3] Department of Emergency Medicine, Mayo Clinic, Rochester, MN, USA

Highlights

- Acute knee fractures are identified in only a small proportion of ED patients with acute knee injuries.
- The Ottawa knee rule and Pittsburgh knee rule are highly sensitive in guiding the need for imaging in adults and children with acute knee injury.
- The prevalence of vascular and neurological injuries and resulting morbidity following acute knee dislocation is high, suggesting that imaging should be pursued to rule out vascular injuries following acute knee dislocation.

Background

Acute knee pain is a common complaint in the emergency department (ED). It is the most commonly injured joint in athletes with an estimated 2.5 million sports-related injuries presenting to EDs annually, and an overall rate of 2.29 knee injuries per 1000 population. In one study, including more than 6 million ED visits secondary to knee injuries from 1999 through 2008, patients aged 15 to 24 years had the highest injury rate (3.83 per 1000). Injuries were associated with sports and recreation in one-half of the cases. Older patients are more likely to sustain injuries after a fall.[1] Prior to the advent of clinical decision rules, plain radiographs of the knee were typically obtained to rule out a fracture after blunt knee trauma where there was any

---

Evidence-Based Emergency Care: Diagnostic Testing and Clinical Decision Rules, Third Edition.
Edited by Jesse M. Pines, Fernanda Bellolio, Christopher R. Carpenter, and Ali S. Raja.
© 2023 John Wiley & Sons Ltd. Published 2023 by John Wiley & Sons Ltd.

Table 9.1 Clinical decision rules to defer radiography in patients with blunt knee trauma

---

The Ottawa knee rule

The Ottawa knee rule recommends radiography if any of the following is present in the context of an acute knee injury:

1. Age > 55 years
2. Tenderness at the head of fibula
3. Isolated tenderness at the patella
4. Inability to flex knee to 90 degrees
5. Inability to transfer weight for four steps, both immediately after the injury and in the ED

Exclusion criteria for the Ottawa knee rule include age <18 years, superficial skin injuries, injuries more than 7 days old, reevaluation of recent injuries, altered levels of consciousness, paraplegia, or multiple injuries

The Pittsburgh knee rule

The Pittsburgh knee rule recommends radiography if:
The mechanism of injury is either blunt trauma or a fall AND either

1. Age is <12 years or >50 OR
2. There is an inability to walk four weight-bearing steps in the ED

Exclusion criteria for the Pittsburgh knee rule are knee injuries >6 days prior to presentation, only superficial lacerations and abrasions, a history of previous surgeries or fractures on the injured knee, and patients being reassessed for the same injury

---

clinical suspicion of fracture. However, similar to ankle injuries, knee fractures are identified in only a small proportion (4–7%) of knee injuries. Two clinical decision rules have been created to identify patients in whom knee radiography may be deferred in the setting of an acute knee injury: the Ottawa knee rule and the Pittsburgh knee rule. The Ottawa knee rule and the Pittsburgh knee rule are described in Table 9.1.

Clinical question

How well does the Ottawa knee rule identify patients requiring knee radiography?
A systematic review of studies on the Ottawa knee rule directly addressed this question.[2] The authors included articles that reported patient-level information to determine sensitivity and specificity. Two reviewers independently tallied data on study samples, the details about how the Ottawa knee rule was used, and methodological characteristics. Of the 11 studies identified, data were collected from six, resulting in a set of 4249 adult patients who were considered appropriate for pooled analysis. The aggregate negative likelihood ratio was 0.05 (95% confidence interval [CI] 0.02–0.23), sensitivity was

Table 9.2 Six studies reporting sensitivity and specificity of the Ottawa knee rule

References	Year	Sensitivity (%)	Specificity (%)
Steill et al.[3]	1996	100% (CI 94–100%)	50% (CI 46–53%)
Steill et al.[4]	1997	100% (CI 94–100%)	48% (CI 45–51%)
Richman et al.[5]	1997	85% (CI 65–96%)	45% (CI 39–52%)
Emparanza and Aginaga[6]	2001	100% (CI 96–100%)	52% (CI 50–55%)
Szucs et al.[7]	2001	100% (CI 63–100%)	47% (CI 36–58%)
Ketelslegers et al.[8]	2002	100% (CI 87–100%)	32% (CI 26–38%)

99% (CI 93–100%), and specificity was 49% (CI 43–51%). Given a knee fracture prevalence of 7%, a negative Ottawa knee rule resulted in a probability of knee fracture of 1.5%. Table 9.2 shows data from the six studies reviewed with reported sensitivities and specificities.

Clinical question

How does the Ottawa knee rule compare with the Pittsburgh knee rule?
A prospective study conducted at three academic centers investigated this question.[9] The decision on whether to order radiographs was made using physician judgment. All patients who underwent radiography had a three-view knee series (anterior-posterior, lateral, and obliques), with a sunrise view added in patients with suspected patellar fractures. The performance of the Ottawa knee rule and Pittsburgh knee rule was determined by using appropriate variables from the data sheets and film reports from board-certified radiologists. There were 934 patients evaluated, and the Ottawa knee rule and the Pittsburgh knee rule were applicable to 745 and 750 patients, respectively. The main results of the study are detailed in Table 9.3.

Table 9.3 Study comparing the Ottawa knee rule with the Pittsburgh knee rule

	Sensitivity	Specificity	Positive predictive value (PPV)	Negative predictive value (NPV)	LR+	LR–
Ottawa knee rule	97% (CI 90–99)	27% (CI 23–30%)	15%	99%	1.3	0.11
Pittsburgh knee rule	99% (CI 94–100%)	60% (CI 56–64%)	24%	100%	2.5	0.02

Source: Data from [9].

The difference in sensitivity was not significant; however, the Pittsburgh knee rule was considerably more specific (33% difference; CI 28–38%). With greater specificity, this means that there will be fewer false positives for the rule. The result is more people being able to defer radiography. However, two elements of this study bring into question its validity. First, the authors did not follow patients who did not undergo radiography, introducing potential bias. However, in a previous study, 357 patients with knee pain who did not have radiography were reevaluated by a formal telephone interview 2 weeks later, and none required clinical reassessment. Second, two of the three clinical sites were University of Pittsburgh-affiliated hospitals, and the physicians making the initial determination of imaging need may have already been using the Pittsburgh knee rule or the Ottawa knee rule, leading to selection bias in the population of patients enrolled in the study.

Clinical question

How well does the Ottawa knee rule work in pediatric patients?
A recent study aimed to determine the sensitivity and specificity of the Ottawa knee rule in children.[10] The authors performed a prospective, multicenter validation study, and included children aged 2 to 16 years presenting to the ED with a knee injury sustained within 7 days. Physicians ordered radiographs according to their usual practice. The outcome measure was any fracture and patients with negative films were followed for 14 days. A total of 750 were enrolled; 670 had radiography, and fewer than 10% (*n* = 70) had fractures. The Ottawa knee rule was 100% sensitive (CI 95–100%), with a specificity of 43% (CI 39–47%). The authors concluded that the Ottawa knee rule is valid for use in children.

Clinical question

What is the prevalence of vascular injury following knee dislocation?
Following an acute knee dislocation, vascular injuries can be a serious, limb-threatening complication. A variety of small studies on the prevalence of vascular and neurological injuries following knee dislocation exist in the literature, as well as how often vascular injuries require surgery. A 2014 systematic review was conducted that aimed to assess the frequency of vascular and neurological injuries, whether surgical interventions were performed, and what types of imaging modalities were used to detect the vascular injury.[11] A total of 23 papers were included in the analysis, which together identified 862 patients with knee dislocations. Of those 171 (18%) sustained vascular injuries. Of the 252 patients included in studies that also reported

nerve injuries, 75 (25%) reported a neurological injury following a knee dislocation. A total of 80% (134 of 160) of vascular injuries underwent surgical repair, and 12% (22 of 134) resulted in amputation. A variety of different types of diagnostic modalities were used to detect vascular injuries, the most common being selective angiography (61%).

Comment

Both the Pittsburgh knee rule and the Ottawa knee rule can be used (in the ED) to identify adults and children who are at very low risk of fracture and do not need X-rays following acute knee injury. The Pittsburgh knee rule is considerably more specific and includes the mechanism of injury. This is important since blunt knee trauma, including direct blows to the knee and falls, accounts for 80% of knee fractures. With this mechanism, patients are four times more likely to suffer fractures.[12] While the specificity of the Pittsburgh knee rule is higher and may therefore result in less unnecessary radiography, the sensitivity for both rules is near 100%, making them safe for use in the ED. In addition, one study validated the use of the Ottawa knee rule in children between 2 and 16 years of age. Because the prevalence of vascular and neurological injuries and resulting morbidity following acute knee dislocation is high, we recommend that imaging should be pursued to rule out vascular injuries following acute knee dislocation. Selective angiography of the limb is the most commonly used modality to rule out vascular injury.

References

1. Gage BE, McIlvain NM, Collins CL, Fields SK, Comstock RD. Epidemiology of 6.6 million knee injuries presenting to United States emergency departments from 1999 through 2008. *Academic Emergency Medicine.* 2012; 19(4): 378–85.
2. Bachmann LM, Haberzeth S, Steurer J et al. The accuracy of the Ottawa knee rule to rule out knee fractures: A systematic review. *Annals of Internal Medicine.* 2004; 140: 121–4.
3. Stiell IG, Greenberg GH, Wells GA et al. Prospective validation of a decision rule for the use of radiography in acute knee injuries. *The Journal of the American Medical Association.* 1996; 275: 611–5.
4. Stiell IG, Wells GA, Hoag RH et al. Implementation of the Ottawa knee rule for the use of radiography in acute knee injuries. *The Journal of the American Medical Association.* 1997; 278: 2075–9.
5. Richman PB, McCuskey CF, Nashed A et al. Performance of two clinical decision rules for knee radiography. *The Journal of Emergency Medicine.* 1997; 15: 459–63.

6. Emparanza JI, Aginaga JR. Validation of the Ottawa knee rules. *Annals of Emergency Medicine.* 2001; 38: 364–8.
7. Szucs PA, Richman PB, Mandell M. Triage nurse application of the Ottawa knee rule. *Academic Emergency Medicine.* 2001; 8: 112–6.
8. Ketelslegers E, Collard X, Vande Berg B *et al.* Validation of the Ottawa knee rules in an emergency teaching centre. *European Radiology.* 2002; 12: 1218–20.
9. Seaberg DC, Yealy DM, Lukens T *et al.* Multicenter comparison of two clinical decision rules for the use of radiography in acute, high-risk knee injuries. *Annals of Emergency Medicine.* 1998; 32: 8–13.
10. Bulloch B, Neto G, Plint A *et al.* Validation of the Ottawa knee rule in children: A multicenter study. *Annals of Emergency Medicine.* 2003; 42: 48–55.
11. Medina O, Arom GA, Yeranosian MG, Petrigliano FA, McAllister DR. Vascular and nerve injury after knee dislocation: A systematic review. *Clinical Orthopaedics and Related Research.* 2014; 472(9): 2621–9.
12. Dalinka MK, Alazraki NP, Daffner RH *et al. Expert panel on musculoskeletal imaging: Imaging evaluation of suspected ankle fractures.* Reston (VA): American College of Radiology (ACR); 2005.

Chapter 10 **Acute Ankle and Foot Injuries**

Jesse M. Pines[1,2] and Fernanda Bellolio[3]

[1] US Acute Care Solutions, Canton, OH, USA
[2] Department of Emergency Medicine, Drexel University, Philadelphia, PA, USA
[3] Department of Emergency Medicine, Mayo Clinic, Rochester, MN, USA

Highlights

- The prevalence of ankle fractures among ED patients with ankle sprain is approximately 15%.
- The Ottawa ankle and foot rules are widely used, well-validated clinical decision rules that accurately identify patients at low risk for fractures.
- The Ottawa ankle and foot rules are highly sensitive in children; however, they should be used only in patients who can verbally communicate and are able to ambulate prior to injury.
- The Ottawa ankle and foot rules can be safely implemented by nonphysician providers who receive training on how to conduct the assessment.

Background

Patients with acute foot and ankle injuries often present to the emergency department (ED), most commonly with injuries occurring after over-inversion of the ankle. In a 2010 study using data from the National Electronic Injury Surveillance System (NEISS), all ankle sprain injuries presenting to EDs were identified and incidence rate ratios were calculated by age, sex, and race.[1] The overall incidence rate was 2.15 per 1000 person-years in the United States, with a peak incidence in the 15–19 age cohort with an incidence of 7.2 per 1000 person-years, with males 15–24 having a substantially higher

---

Evidence-Based Emergency Care: Diagnostic Testing and Clinical Decision Rules, Third Edition.
Edited by Jesse M. Pines, Fernanda Bellolio, Christopher R. Carpenter, and Ali S. Raja.
© 2023 John Wiley & Sons Ltd. Published 2023 by John Wiley & Sons Ltd.

An ankle X-ray series is only necessary if there is pain near the malleoli and any of these findings:

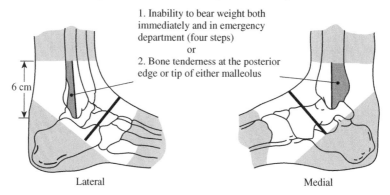

1. Inability to bear weight both immediately and in emergency department (four steps)

or

2. Bone tenderness at the posterior edge or tip of either malleolus

6 cm

Lateral   Medial

Figure 10.1 The Ottawa ankle and foot rules. (Reproduced with permission from Stiell IG, Greenberg GH, McKnight RD, *et al*. Decision Rules for the Use of Radiography in Acute Ankle Injuries: Refinement and Prospective Validation. JAMA 1993; 269 (9): 1127–1132. ©1993, American Medical Association.)

incidence compared to females, with an incidence rate ratio of 1.53. Other notable study findings were that about half of all ankle sprains occurred during athletic activity with basketball (41%), football (9%), and soccer (8%) associated with the highest prevalence of injury.

However, regardless of mechanism, ankle injuries can result in either ankle fractures (typically seen on a three-view ankle series) or foot fractures (also seen on a three-view foot series). Among ankle and foot sprains, only a small percentage will ultimately have fracture. This low overall prevalence of fractures (about 15%) led to the development of the Ottawa ankle and foot rules. The Ottawa ankle and foot rules originated nearly 30 years ago. They were derived to have a sensitivity of 100%; if the criteria for the rules (listed in Figures 10.1 and 10.2) are met, fractures can be effectively ruled out based on clinical evaluation, and radiography can be deferred. In the studies that formed the basis for the Ottawa ankle and foot rules, patients were excluded if they had a delayed presentation of injury (greater than 1 week), had altered mental status, or were pregnant.

The Ottawa ankle and foot rules are probably the best-studied decision rules in emergency medicine. The rules have been validated in multiple settings across multiple cultures. The purpose of this chapter will be to briefly review the evidence behind the Ottawa ankle and foot rules and to examine their use in children.

A foot X-ray series is only necessary if there is pain in the mid-foot and any of these findings:

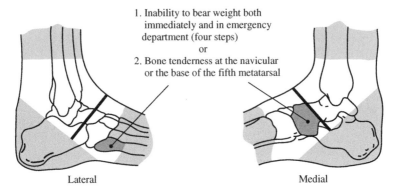

1. Inability to bear weight both immediately and in emergency department (four steps)
   or
2. Bone tenderness at the navicular or the base of the fifth metatarsal

Lateral   Medial

Figure 10.2 The Ottawa foot rules. (Reproduced with permission from Stiell IG, Greenberg GH, McKnight RD, et al. Decision Rules for the Use of Radiography in Acute Ankle Injuries: Refinement and Prospective Validation. JAMA 1993; 269 (9): 1127–1132. ©1993, American Medical Association.)

Clinical question

How strong is the evidence supporting the use of the Ottawa ankle and foot rules to clinically exclude fractures of the ankle and midfoot?

In 2003, Bachmann et al. performed a systematic review and meta-analysis of the evidence on the Ottawa ankle and foot rules.[2] They extracted data on study populations and methodologies. Their intent was to calculate a pooled sensitivity for the decision rules. A bootstrapping method for statistical analysis was performed to ensure that their estimate of the standard error was correct, they calculated and pooled negative likelihood ratios (LR−) for many subgroups, they adjusted for methodological quality, and they excluded retrospective studies and those that did not specifically blind the radiologists involved. Of the 32 studies that met the inclusion criteria, the data from 27 were pooled, resulting in an evaluation of 15,581 patients. The authors calculated a LR− of 0.08 (95% CI 0.03–0.18) for the ankle rule and 0.08 (95% CI 0.03–0.20) for the midfoot rule. In children, the pooled LR− was 0.07 (95% CI 0.03–0.18). Data were tabulated as bootstrapped sensitivities and specificities with a focus on specific populations, prevalence of fracture, and time to referral in Table 10.1 – the *n* denotes the number of studies used to calculate the point estimate for the sensitivity or the median specificity.

They calculated that applying these ratios to a population with a 15% fracture prevalence would yield a less than 1.4% probability of actual fracture and

Table 10.1 Sensitivities and specificities of the Ottawa ankle rules in pooled studies

Category	Sensitivity (95% CI)	Median specificity (interquartile range)
All studies (n = 39) type of assessment	97.6% (96.4–98.9)	31.5% (23.8–44.4%)
Ankle (n = 15)	98.0% (96.3–99.3%)	39.8% (27.9–47.7%)
Foot (n = 10)	99.0% (97.3–100%)	37.8% (24.7–70.1%)
Combined (n = 14)	96.4% (93.8–98.6%)	26.3% (19.4–34.3%)
Population		
Children (n = 7)	99.3% (98.3–100%)	26.7% (23.8–35.6%)
Adults (n = 32)	97.3% (95.7–98.6%)	36.6% (22.3–46.1%)
Prevalence of fracture		
<25th centile (n = 7)	99.0% (98.3–100%)	47.9% (42.3–77.1%)
25th–75th centile (n = 22)	97.7% (95.9–99.0%)	30.1% (23.8–40.1%)
>75th centile (n = 10)	96.7% (94.2–99.2%)	27.3% (15.5–40.0%)
Time to referral (hours)		
<48 (n = 5)	99.6% (98.2–100%)	27.9% (24.7–31.5%)
>48 (n = 34)	97.3% (95.9–98.5%)	36.6% (19.9–46.8%)

Source: Data from [2].

that the evidence supports the use of the Ottawa ankle and foot rules as accurate tools to exclude fractures of the midfoot and ankle, with an almost 100% sensitivity and low specificity.

Clinical question

Can the Ottawa ankle and foot rules be safely used in children to exclude ankle and foot fractures?

Three major considerations differentiate the use of the Ottawa ankle and foot rules in children from their safe use in adults. The first issue is that children may not be as reliable regarding the verbal histories of their injuries. Second, the most common missed fracture type, a Salter–Harris type I fracture (defined as a separation of the bone 0.3 mm through the physis) is often associated with trauma in infants and children, and point tenderness will be present only if patients are able to communicate effectively. Third, the application of the Ottawa ankle and foot rules requires that children be able to walk prior to their injuries, excluding infants and children who are not yet able to ambulate.

In addition to the high estimate for the sensitivity of the Ottawa ankle and foot rules in the seven pediatric studies in the systematic review by

Bachmann *et al.*[2], a more recent review has included more data confirming the excellent sensitivity of the Ottawa ankle and foot rules in children. With the addition of more recent data, its authors calculated an overall sensitivity of 97% (CI 93–100%) and a specificity of 29% (CI 18–40%). In all the studies examined, a prevalence of 12% was calculated. While one article in their review showed that a total of five patients who were rule negative actually had fractures yielding a sensitivity of 83% (CI 65–94%),[3] most articles had zero or one missed fracture in their pediatric populations.

Clinical question

Can the Ottawa ankle and foot rules be implemented by nonphysician providers?

Two recent studies addressed this question. One study enrolled children 5 to 17 with an acute ankle or foot injury.[4] Nonphysician providers (NPP) which included nurses and orthopedic technologists were educated on use of the rules. When NPPs applied the rule to 184 patients, the sensitivity of the foot rule was 100% (CI 56–100%) and the specificity was 17% (CI 9–29%) for clinically significant fracture. The sensitivity of the ankle portion of the rule was 88% (CI 47–99%) and the specificity was 31% (23–40%). In the study, there was one clinically significant fracture that was missed by NPPs yet later detected on physician assessment. The inter-observer agreement was $\kappa = 0.24$ for the ankle rule and $\kappa = 0.49$ for the foot rule meaning fair to moderate agreement. The authors concluded that the sensitivity was very good and that increased practice and training would likely improve inter-observer reliability.

A second study was a randomized trial of a nurse-initiated radiographic-test protocol with the Ottawa ankle and foot rules compared with usual practice.[5] The goal was to reduce potentially unnecessary ankle and foot radiographic test requests and shortening patients' length of stay in an ED by reducing their waiting time for physician reassessment. A total of 112 patients were enrolled and all participants were unblinded. The study found that the proportions of ankle and foot radiographic tests requested by triage nurses in the protocol group were lower than those requested by physicians in the usual practice group. As a result, the diagnostic yield, specifically the proportions of malleolar and midfoot fractures detected by triage nurses implementing the Ottawa ankle and foot rules in protocol group were higher than those detected by physicians. Finally, patient length of stay and waiting time from consultation to discharge in the nurse-initiated protocol group were shorter than those in the usual practice group.

Comment

Use of the Ottawa ankle and foot rules allows for the clinical exclusion of fractures in both adult and pediatric populations and has been validated in multiple settings. In applying the Ottawa ankle and foot rules to children, it is important to use the rule only in children who are able to communicate verbally and had the ability to walk prior to the injury. In the pooled studies reviewed in this chapter, a small percentage of patients who did not receive X-rays based on the Ottawa ankle and foot rules actually had fractures. However, given a prevalence of 12% in pediatric studies and 15% in adult studies, a very low percentage of patients (less than 1.4%) will fall into this category. The clinical relevance of these subtle missed ankle fractures is also unknown. Therefore, in the case of either negative or deferred (due to the Ottawa ankle and foot rules) ankle radiography in patients with significant soft tissue injury, we recommend that patients be splinted; use ice, elevation, and crutches; and obtain close follow-up and reevaluation.

In the pediatric population, missed fractures will most likely be Salter–Harris type I fractures, which typically have almost no long-term consequences. As a note of caution, because the sensitivity for the rule is not 100%, in patients in whom the rule is negative and whose pretest probability is high, clinicians should use their best judgment in the decision to order foot and ankle X-rays.

Many EDs have nonphysician providers implement the Ottawa ankle and foot rules at triage and in other parts of the ED. Studies published on this topic demonstrate that this can be done safely and that the sensitivity and specificity of the rules are similar to physicians. However, studies have ensured that NPPs require specific training in order to conduct this evaluation independently.

References

1. Waterman BR, Owens BD, Davey S, Zacchilli MA, Belmont PJ Jr. The epidemiology of ankle sprains in the United States. *The Journal of Bone and Joint Surgery. American Volume.* 2010; 92(13): 2279–84.
2. Bachmann LM, Kolb E, Koller MT *et al.* Accuracy of Ottawa ankle rules to exclude fractures of the ankle and mid-foot: Systematic review. *British Medical Journal.* 2003; 326(7386): 417.
3. Clarke KD, Tanner S. Evaluation of Ottawa ankle rules in children. *Pediatric Emergency Care.* 2003; 19: 73–8.
4. MacLellan J, Smith T, Baserman J, Dowling S. Accuracy of the Ottawa ankle rules applied by non-physician providers in a pediatric emergency department. *CJEM.* 2018; 20(5): 746–52.

5. Ho JK, Chau JP, Chan JT, Yau CH. Nurse-initiated radiographic-test protocol for ankle injuries: A randomized controlled trial. *International Emergency Nursing.* 2018; 41: 1–6.
6. Myers A, Kanty K, Nelson T. Are the Ottawa ankle rules helpful in ruling out the need for X ray examination in children? *Archives of Disease in Childhood.* 2005; 90: 1309–11.

Chapter 11 **Blunt Head Injury in Children**

Lucas Oliveira Junqueira e Silva[1,2] and Fernanda Bellolio[1]

[1] Department of Emergency Medicine, Mayo Clinic, Rochester, MN, USA
[2] Department of Emergency Medicine, Hospital de Clínicas de Porto Alegre, Porto Alegre, Brazil

Highlights

- Blunt head trauma in children is associated with significant morbidity and mortality, and the need to diagnose clinically significant intracranial injuries must be balanced with the risks of radiation exposure in children.
- Four decision rules have been derived and validated: PECARN, NEXUS II, CATCH, and CHALICE.
- The PECARN decision rules have the best performance in their internal and external validation studies. The two rules (for children < 2 years old and ≥ 2 years old) are highly sensitive for the detection of clinically important intracranial injuries in children.
- Two additional risk scores (CHIIDA and $CIDSS_2$) have been derived but not yet validated. These tools are meant to help clinicians when making decisions about admission in pediatric patients with mild traumatic brain injury either with or without intracranial injuries.
- The use of the biomarker S100B needs further validation and implementation studies before being used in the emergency setting.

Background

Traumatic brain injury is a leading cause of morbidity and mortality in children and adolescents and accounts for a significant proportion of the >1 million annual emergency department (ED) visits and hospitalizations due to trauma-related head injuries.[1] The clinical challenge when evaluating

Evidence-Based Emergency Care: Diagnostic Testing and Clinical Decision Rules, Third Edition.
Edited by Jesse M. Pines, Fernanda Bellolio, Christopher R. Carpenter, and Ali S. Raja.
© 2023 John Wiley & Sons Ltd. Published 2023 by John Wiley & Sons Ltd.

a child with head trauma is to determine the presence of an intracranial injury. Because the radiation risks of computed tomography (CT) are greater in children, North American and European investigators have developed clinical decision rules (CDRs) for imaging children with blunt head trauma. The objectives of these head injury CDRs are to identify patients who are either at low risk for injury and can thus be evaluated without imaging, or at sufficient risk for injury to require imaging.

Clinical question

Can elements of the history and physical exam identify children with minor head injury who are at low risk for intracranial injury and who therefore do not need CT imaging?

In a systematic review, Pickering *et al.*[2] found six CDRs that were developed to identify children who are at low risk of intracranial injury after a mild traumatic brain injury (mTBI). However, only four rules have been both derived and validated. The first rule to be validated and the most widely used is by Pediatric Emergency Care Applied Research Network (PECARN).[3] They enrolled 42,412 children younger than 18 years old who presented within 24 hours of blunt trauma and had Glasgow coma scale (GCS) scores of 14 or 15, and 14,969 (35%) of them had head CTs (HCTs) performed. Patients were enrolled at 25 EDs, and their outcome of clinically important traumatic brain injury (ciTBI) was defined *a priori* as death from traumatic brain injury, neurosurgery, intubation for more than 24 hours, or hospital admission for two nights or more associated with traumatic brain injury on CT. Medical records were reviewed for the outcomes, and telephone follow-up was performed between 7 and 90 days after ED visits to identify any missed injuries. The PECARN rule was derived in a population of 33,785 patients and then validated in 8627 patients by continued data collection at the same sites.

The PECARN investigators analyzed preverbal (<2 years old) and verbal (≥2 years old) children separately to account for differences in communicative ability, mechanisms, and risks for intracranial injury. Of the 8502 preverbal children in the derivation cohort, there were 73 cases (0.86%) of intracranial injuries and, of the 25,283 verbal children, there were 215 (0.85%) cases of intracranial injuries. The PECARN decision rule for children <2 years old (Table 11.1) had a sensitivity of 99%, a specificity of 54%, a positive likelihood ratio (LR+) of 2.2, and a negative likelihood ratio (LR−) of 0.02. Similarly, the rule for children ≥2 years old (Table 11.2) had a sensitivity of 97%, a specificity of 59%, a LR+ of 2.4, and a LR− of 0.05. Test characteristics were similar in the validation cohorts (Tables 11.3 and 11.4).

Table 11.1 The PECARN head CT rule for children <2 years old

CT can be avoided in children without any of the following:
- Altered mental status
- Scalp hematoma
- Loss of consciousness ($\geq$5 seconds)
- Severe mechanism of injury
- Palpable or unclear skull fracture
- Acting abnormally per parent

If none of these are present their risk of clinically significant injury is very low.
Source: Data from [3].

Table 11.2 The PECARN head CT rule for children $\geq$2 years old

CT can routinely be avoided in children without any of the following:
- Altered mental status
- Loss of consciousness
- History of vomiting
- Severe mechanism of injury
- Clinical signs of basilar skull fracture
- Severe headache

If none of these are present their risk of clinically significant injury is very low.
Source: Data from [3].

Table 11.3 Performance of the PECARN head CT rule in children <2 years old

Derivation cohort	PECARN-defined clinically important traumatic brain injury		
Decision rule	Injury	No injury	Totals
Positive	72	3901	3973
Negative	1	4528	4529
Totals	73	8429	8502
Sensitivity (95% confidence interval [CI])		99% (93–100%)	
Specificity (95% CI)		54% (53–55%)	
Positive likelihood ratio (LR+)		2.2	
Negative likelihood ratio (LR−)		0.02	
Validation cohort	PECARN-defined clinically important traumatic brain injury		
Decision rule	Injury	No injury	Totals
Positive	25	1015	1040
Negative	0	1176	1176
Totals	25	2191	2216
Sensitivity (95% CI)		100% (86–100%)	
Specificity (95% CI)		54% (52–56%)	
Positive likelihood ratio (LR+)		2.2	
Negative likelihood ratio (LR−)		0	

Source: Data from [3].

Table 11.4 Performance of the PECARN head CT rule in children ≥2 years old

Derivation cohort	PECARN-defined clinically important traumatic brain injury		
Decision rule	Injury	No injury	Totals
Positive	208	10,412	10,620
Negative	7	14,656	14,663
Totals	215	25,068	25,283
Sensitivity (95% confidence interval [CI])		97% (93–99%)	
Specificity (95% CI)		59% (58–59%)	
Positive likelihood ratio (LR+)		2.4	
Negative likelihood ratio (LR–)		0.05	
Validation cohort	PECARN-defined clinically important traumatic brain injury		
Decision rule	Injury	No injury	Totals
Positive	61	2550	2611
Negative	2	3798	3800
Totals	63	6348	6411
Sensitivity (95% CI)		97% (89–100%)	
Specificity (95% CI)		60% (59–61%)	
Positive likelihood ratio (LR+)		2.4	
Negative likelihood ratio (LR–)		0.05	

Source: Data from [3].

Aside from its original derivation and validation cohorts, several external validation and implementation studies have evaluated the performance of PECARN across different ED settings throughout the globe. In a large US-based single-center prospective cohort study, Easter et al.[4] enrolled 1009 children with minor head injury presenting within 24 hours of their injuries, and compared the PECARN rule with physician judgment and two other CDRs (Canadian Assessment of Tomography for Childhood Head injury [CATCH] and Children's Head injury ALgorithm for prediction of Clinically Important Events [CHALICE]). The authors found that only physician's practice (as defined by actual CT ordering practice) and the PECARN rule identified all ciTBIs as well as all injuries requiring neurosurgical intervention, with sensitivity of 100%.

Schonfeld et al.[5] performed a cross-sectional study to validate PECARN in two pediatric EDs in the United States and Italy. A total of 2439 children were included, of whom 373 (15%) had a CT performed, 69 (3%) had a positive

CT, and 19 (0.8%) had a ciTBI. None of the patients with ciTBI were classified as very low risk by PECARN (overall sensitivity 100%, specificity 55%, negative predictive value 100%). In a prospective cohort study in 1179 children from Singapore, Thiam et al.[6] evaluated the diagnostic performance of PECARN, CATCH, and CHALICE. There were 12 (1%) patients who underwent CT and only 6 (0.5%) who had positive findings. Although the PECARN originally used the outcome of ciTBI, this study evaluated its ability to predict a positive HCT. The sensitivity of the rule was 100% even though a different outcome was used from its original derivation and validation studies.

Lorton et al.[7] prospectively validated the PECARN rule in a French population. Among 1499 children from three EDs in France, there were 9 (0.6%) children with ciTBI, and none were classified as very low risk by the PECARN rule, obtaining a sensitivity of 100% in both cohorts of children <2 years and ≥2 years.

The Pediatric Research in Emergency Departments International Collaborative (PREDICT) performed a multicenter prospective external validation study[8] including 20,137 children in 10 Australian and New Zealand EDs, and evaluated the performance of PECARN, CATCH, and CHALICE. They enrolled all children (age < 18) with head injuries of any severity, and collected data on the inclusion and exclusion criteria of these three CDRs, as well as on their predictor variables and outcomes measures. In this cohort, 280 (1%) had ciTBI as defined by PECARN. PECARN did not miss any patients younger than 2 years but did miss one patient aged 2 years or older who did not require neurosurgery (sensitivity of 100% for <2 years and 99% for ≥2 years).

Ide et al.[9,10] validated the PECARN rule in Japan both retrospectively and prospectively. In their retrospective study,[9] among 2208 children there were 24 (1.1%) patients with ciTBI. They found a reduced sensitivity and specificity when compared to the PECARN derivation and validation cohorts. The sensitivity was 85.7% in children <2 years. There were 16 cases of physically abused children in their cohort, 10 of which were in the <2 years group. There were two cases of abused children with ciTBI that were identified as very low risk and therefore missed by the PECARN rule. When the authors analyzed the cohort excluding these cases, however, the sensitivity of the rule improved to 100%.

In the Japanese prospective study[10], Ide et al. enrolled children younger than 16 with minor head trauma (GCS ≥ 14) who presented to six participating EDs within 24 hours of their injuries. Among 6585 patients, 463 (7%) underwent a HCT and 23 (0.35%) had ciTBI. Two patients with ciTBI were classified as very low risk by PECARN, yielding an overall sensitivity of 91.3% (95% confidence interval [CI] 72–98.9%) and a negative predictive value of 99.96% (95% CI 99.86–100%).

Table 11.5 Performance of the PECARN head CT rule in external validation studies

Rule	N	Sensitivity	Specificity	NPV	PPV	LR–	LR+
Easter et al.[4] (the United States) – outcome of clinically important TBI							
PECARN*	981	21/21, 100%	361/960, 62%	100%	5.5%	0.0	2.7
Easter et al.[4] (the United States) – outcome of injury requiring neurosurgical intervention							
PECARN*	981	4/4, 100%	599/977, 61%	100%	1%	0.0	2.6
Schonfeld et al.[5] (the United States, Italy) – outcome of clinically important TBI							
PECARN<2years	959	6/6, 100%	410/950, 43.2%	100%	1.7%	0.0	1.76
PECARN≥2years	1439	13/13, 100%	705,1459, 48.3%	100%	2%	0.0	1.93
Thiam et al.[6] (Singapore) – outcome of positive head CT							
PECARN*	1179	6/6, 100%	723/1173, 61.6%	100%	1.3%	0.0	2.6
Lorton et al.[7] (France) – outcome of clinically important TBI							
PECARN<2years	421	3/3, 100%	267/418, 64%	100%	2%	0.0	2.77
PECARN≥2years	1078	6/6, 100%	774/1072, 72.2%	100%	2%	0.0	3.59
Babl et al.[8] (Australia, New Zealand) – outcome of clinically important TBI							
PECARN<2years	4011	38/38, 100%	2139/3973, 53.8%	100%	2%	0.0	2.16
PECARN≥2years	11,152	97/98, 99%	5067/11054, 45.8%	100%	1.6%	0.02	1.83
Ide et al.[9] (Japan) – outcome of clinically important TBI							
PECARN<2years	792	12/14, 85.7%	572/778, 73.5%	99.7%	5.5%	0.19	3.23
PECARN≥2years	1416	10/10, 100%	1032/1406, 73.4%	100%	2.6%	0.0	3.76
Ide et al.[10] (Japan) – outcome of clinically important TBI							
PECARN**<2years	2237	86.7%	71.1%	99.9%	2%	0.19	3
PECARN≥2years	4348	100%	79.7%	100%	0.9%	0.0	4.9

N = sample size; NPV = negative predictive value; PPV = positive predictive value; LR– = likelihood ratio for a negative test, LR+ = likelihood ratio for a positive test.

*This study did not report the performance of PECARN separated by age.

**This study did not report the raw numbers for their calculations.

The performance of PECARN across the different external validation cohorts is summarized in Table 11.5. Implementation studies of the PECARN rule were also performed and evaluated its impact on HCT rates. Three studies showed safe reductions (i.e., without missing ciTBI) with imaging rates ranging from 4% to 17%.[11-13] This is in contrast with high rates of CT imaging shown by validation studies[8] when the rule was applied alone without taking into consideration clinical judgment. This rule was not intended to be applied without clinician input to the decision-making process.

While the PECARN investigators suggest that patients at intermediate risk of ciTBI should either undergo observation or proceed with imaging, the use of shared decision-making is key. Hess et al.[14] performed a cluster randomized trial to evaluate the impact of a decision aid tool to improve parents-centered outcomes. Its use was associated with significant improvement in parent knowledge, decisional conflict, and involvement in decision-making. No changes in the rates of imaging or ciTBI were found.

The 2009 PECARN rules were the first validated CT CDRs for pediatric blunt trauma and it is the most comprehensively studied, but there are three other CDRs that were derived before the PECARN. The first of these, a pre-planned analysis of the National Emergency X-Radiography Utilization Study II (NEXUS II) investigation by Oman et al.[15] studied patients ≤18 years old to examine the performance of the NEXUS II low-risk HCT rule on this population. The NEXUS II HCT rules are shown in Table 11.6. In an adaptation suited for the study of children, only seven of the eight variables were evaluated (the age > 65 criterion was dropped). NEXUS II enrolled 1666 children, all of whom underwent HCT. The outcomes evaluated were the same as for the larger NEXUS II study: clinically important intracranial injury requiring neurosurgical intervention or likely to lead to significant long-term neurological impairment. The prevalence of clinically significant intracranial

Table 11.6 The NEXUS II low-risk head CT rule for children

Children without any of the following are at very low risk of clinically important traumatic brain injury, and CT can routinely be avoided:
• Evidence of skull fracture
• Altered level of alertness
• Neurologic deficit
• Persistent vomiting
• Presence of scalp hematoma
• Abnormal behavior
• Coagulopathy

Source: Data from [15].

Table 11.7 Performance of the NEXUS II HCT rule in children

Derivation cohort	NEXUS II head CT rule-defined clinically important intracranial injury		
Decision rule	Injury	No injury	Totals
Positive	136	1298	1434
Negative	2	230	232
Totals	138	1528	1666
Sensitivity (95% CI)		98% (95–100%)	
Specificity (95% CI)		15% (13–17%)	
Positive likelihood ratio (LR+)		1.2	
Negative likelihood ratio (LR−)		0.13	
Derivation cohort	NEXUS II head CT rule-defined clinically important intracranial injury (age < 3 years)		
Decision rule	Injury	No injury	Totals
Positive	25	269	294
Negative	0	15	15
Totals	25	284	309
Sensitivity (95% CI)		100% (86–100%)	
Specificity (95% CI)		5% (3–9%)	
Positive likelihood ratio (LR+)		1.0	
Negative likelihood ratio (LR−)		0	
Validation cohort	NEXUS II head CT rule-defined neurosurgical intervention (age < 3 years)		
Decision rule	Injury	No injury	Totals
Positive	27	661	688
Negative	0	330	330
Totals	27	991	1018
Sensitivity (95% CI)		100% (87.2–100%)	
Specificity (95% CI)		33.3% (30.3–36.3%)	
Positive likelihood ratio (LR+)		1.5	
Negative likelihood ratio (LR−)		0	

Source: Data from [15, 16].

injury was 8.3% (138/1666). The performance of the adapted NEXUS II HCT rules is shown in Table 11.7 and, given the fact that this population was a subset of the original population from which the NEXUS II rule was derived, the test characteristics (high sensitivity and low specificity) are similar to those of the rule when it was applied to the population as a whole.

Although this rule was initially derived in 2006, its validation study was recently published in 2018. Gupta *et al.*[16] performed a planned secondary analysis of the NEXUS study and enrolled 1108 children with blunt head injuries. As mentioned above, their primary outcome was neurosurgical intervention which included death due to head injury, need for craniotomy, elevation of skull fracture, intubation related to head injury, or intracranial pressure monitoring within 7 days of head injury. The rule correctly identified all patients who required neurosurgical intervention as high risk (sensitivity 100% [95% CI 87.2–100%]). Also, when considering the outcome of clinically significant head injury on CT imaging, the rule identified 48 of the 49 patients with the injuries (sensitivity of 98% [95% CI 89.1–99.9%]).

It is important to highlight that all patients included in NEXUS II derivation and validation studies underwent CT imaging. The rule was designed to be used in children who were deemed to merit imaging by clinical judgment as this population represents an opportunity to identify uninjured patients for whom imaging could be deferred.

British researchers created the CHALICE rule.[17] From 2000 to 2002, the CHALICE study examined all children <16 years old who presented to EDs in 10 hospitals in northwest England with any history or sign of head injury (not just blunt trauma). Data were collected on 40 clinical variables. The primary outcome was a composite of death from head injury, requirement for neurosurgical intervention, or marked abnormality on HCT. CT abnormalities were defined as acute, new traumatic intracranial injuries that included intracranial hematomas, cerebral contusions, cerebral edema, and depressed skull fractures. Nondepressed skull fractures were specifically excluded as they were deemed not significant injuries that do not normally require intervention or hospitalization. Similar to the Canadian CT head rule, the study did not mandate that all patients undergo CT. Patients who were admitted for inpatient stays, had a HCT or skull radiographs, or underwent neurosurgery were followed up. At the end of the study, all participating hospital radiology records were reviewed for skull radiographs and HCTs and cross-referenced with enrolled patients. The National Office of Statistics was also contacted regarding the deaths of children with head injury.

The CHALICE study, which was the largest of its kind dedicated to examining children when it was published, enrolled 22,772 patients. Only 744 patients (3.2%) underwent HCT. The prevalence of clinically significant head injuries was 1.2% (281/22,772). The CHALICE rule is shown in Table 11.8. It consists of 14 criteria, with a HCT being indicated when any item is present. In this derivation study, the clinical prediction rule for detecting any clinically significant head injury was performed with a sensitivity of 98.6% and specificity of 86.9% (Table 11.9).

Table 11.8 The Children's Head Injury Algorithm for the Prediction of Important Clinical Events (CHALICE) rule

A head computed tomography (CT) is indicated if any of the following are present:

History
- Witnessed loss of consciousness (LOC)>5 minutes
- History of amnesia>5 minutes duration
- Drowsiness
- ≥3 episodes of vomiting after injury
- Suspicion of nonaccidental injury
- Seizure after injury (in patients without epilepsy)

Exam
- Glasgow coma scale (GCS) <14 (or GCS <15 if <1-year-old)
- Suspicion of penetrating or depressed skull fracture, or bulging fontanelle
- Signs of skull base fracture
- Focal neurological finding
- Bruise, swelling, or laceration >5 cm if <1-year-old

Mechanism
- High-speed road traffic injury (>40 mph)
- Fall from >3 meters (10 feet) height
- High-speed injury from projectile or object

Source: Data from [17].

Table 11.9 Test performance of the CHALICE rule

Derivation cohort	Clinically significant head injury		
Decision rule	Injury	No injury	Totals
Positive	277	2933	3210
Negative	4	19,558	19,562
Totals	281	22,491	22,772
Sensitivity (95% CI)	99% (96–100%)		
Specificity (95% CI)	87% (87–87%)		
Positive likelihood ratio (LR+)	7.6		
Negative likelihood ratio (LR−)	0.02		

Source: Data from [17].

This United Kingdom-based rule has been externally validated in different countries such as the United States, Australia, New Zealand, and Singapore (Table 11.10). Easter et al.[4] found a decreased diagnostic accuracy when compared to the derivation cohort. Among 1009 children, the sensitivity of the rule was only 84% and the specificity of 85%; however, this was based on

Table 11.10 Performance of the CHALICE head CT rule in external validation studies

Rule	N	Sensitivity	Specificity	NPV	PPV	LR–	LR+
Easter et al.[4] **(the United States)** – outcome of clinically important TBI							
CHALICE	858	16/19, 84%	711/839, 85%	99.5%	11%	0.2	5.5
Easter et al.[4] **(the United States)** – outcome of injury requiring neurosurgical intervention							
CHALICE	858	3/4, 75%	713/854, 84%	99.8%	2%	0.3	4.5
Thiam et al.[6] **(Singapore)** – outcome of positive head CT							
CHALICE	1179	5/6, 83.3%	896/1173, 76.4%	99.9%	1.8%	0.2	3.5
Babl et al.[8] **(Australia, New Zealand)** – outcome of clinically significant intracranial injury							
CHALICE	20,029	370/401, 92.3%	15352/19655, 78.1%	99.8%	7.9%	0.1	4.2

N = sample size; NPV = negative predictive value; PPV = positive predictive value; LR– = likelihood ratio for a negative test; LR+ = likelihood ratio for a positive test.

the outcome defined by PECARN (i.e., ciTBI). In a much larger cohort of 20,029 children in Australia and New Zealand[8], the PREDICT group found that 403 (2%) had clinically significant intracranial injury as defined by CHALICE. The rule missed 31 patients, two of whom required neurosurgery (sensitivity 92.3%, specificity 78.1%). In a separate publication derived from the same Australasian cohort,[18] Babl et al. assessed the physician accuracy for the outcome of ciTBI and compared with the performance of PECARN, CATCH, and CHALICE. CHALICE missed 12 patients (sensitivity of 92.5%, specificity 78.6%), while physicians not using a CDR missed 2. In the prospective cohort study from Singapore[6] in which the outcome assessed was a positive HCT, CHALICE had worse sensitivity (83.3%) when compared to PECARN (100%) and CATCH (100%).

The most recently developed CDR for children with minor head injury, CATCH was published by the Pediatric Emergency Research Canada (PERC) Head Injury Study Group in 2010.[19] Their rule was derived in a population of children 0–16 years old enrolled consecutively at 10 Canadian pediatric teaching EDs. All patients had been injured within 24 hours of presentation, had a GCS of 14 or 15 at presentation, and had blunt trauma to the head resulting in witnessed loss of consciousness (LOC), definite amnesia, witnessed disorientation, persistent vomiting (two or more distinct episodes of vomiting 15 minutes apart), or persistent irritability in the ED (for children under 2 years of age). The primary outcome was the need for neurologic intervention, and their secondary outcome was intracranial injury on CT. Patients who did not undergo CT were followed up at 14 days with a phone call, and those who could not be reached were excluded from the final analysis.

Table 11.11 The Canadian Assessment of Tomography for Childhood Head Injury (CATCH) rule

---

A head CT is required only for children with minor head injury and any one of the following:

High-risk factors (predict need for neurological intervention):
1. Glasgow coma scale (GCS) <15 at 2 hours after injury
2. Suspected open or depressed skull fracture
3. History of worsening headache
4. Irritability on examination

Medium-risk factors (predict brain injury on computed tomography [CT] scan):
1. Any sign of basal skull fracture (e.g., hemotympanum, "raccoon" eyes, otorrhea or rhinorrhea of the cerebrospinal fluid, or Battle's sign)
2. Large, boggy hematoma of the scalp
3. Dangerous mechanism of injury (e.g., motor vehicle crash, fall from elevation ≥3 ft (≥91 cm) or five stairs, or fall from bicycle with no helmet)

Source: Data from [19].

The CATCH investigators enrolled 3866 patients, 159 (4.1%) of whom had intracranial injury. Their rule consists of four high-risk factors and three medium-risk factors (Table 11.11). The high-risk factors predict the need for neurological intervention, while the addition of the medium-risk factors to the high-risk factors predicts any brain injury on CT scan. The test's performance is described in Table 11.12.

The PERC investigators prospectively validated and refined the CATCH rule in nine Canadian pediatric EDs[20]. Among 4060 enrolled patients, 23 (0.6%) patients underwent neurosurgical intervention and 197 (4.9%) had brain injury on imaging. In this validation cohort, the original CATCH (7-item rule) had sensitivities of 91.3% for neurosurgical intervention and 97.5% for predicting brain injury. After recursive partitioning analysis, they refined the rule by adding a new variable (≥4 episodes of vomiting). The CATCH2 (8-item rule) was then performed with a sensitivity of 100% for neurosurgical intervention and 99.5% for brain injury (Table 11.13).

The original CATCH rule was also externally validated in other non-Canadian populations (Table 11.14). In a US-based cohort, Easter et al.[4] found a sensitivity of 91% and specificity of 44% for detecting ciTBI as defined by PECARN. Babl et al.[8], however, used rule-specific criteria derived from the original CATCH study and among 4957 eligible children, showed a 95.2% sensitivity for neurosurgical intervention outcome and 88.7% for predicting brain injury on CT. Thiam et al.[6] evaluated the prediction ability of CATCH to detect a positive HCT and found a sensitivity of 100% and specificity of 80.3%.

Table 11.12 Test performance of the CATCH rule

Derivation cohort	Injury requiring neurological intervention		
Decision rule	Injury	No injury	Totals
Positive	24	1144	1168
Negative	0	2698	2698
Totals	24	3842	3866
Sensitivity (95% CI)	100% (86–100%)		
Specificity (95% CI)	70% (69–72%)		
Positive likelihood ratio (LR+)	3.3		
Negative likelihood ratio (LR–)	0		
Derivation cohort	Presence of brain injury on computed tomography (CT) scan		
Decision rule	Injury	No injury	Totals
Positive	156	1851	2007
Negative	3	1856	1859
Totals	159	3707	3866
Sensitivity (95% CI)	98% (95–99%)		
Specificity (95% CI)	50% (49–52%)		
Positive likelihood ratio (LR+)	2.0		
Negative likelihood ratio (LR–)	0.04		

Source: Data from [19].

Table 11.13 Performance of CATCH and CATCH2 in their respective validation studies.

CATCH (validation cohort)	CATCH – neurosurgical intervention	CATCH – brain injury on imaging	CATCH2* – neurosurgical intervention	CATCH2* – brain injury on imaging
Sensitivity (95% CI)	91.3% (72–98.9%)	97.5% (94.2–99.2%)	100% (85.2–100%)	99.5% (97.2–100%)
Specificity (95% CI)	57.1% (55.5–58.6%)	59.6% (58–61.1%)	45.7% (44.2–47.3%)	47.8% (46.8–49.4%)

*CATCH2 was developed during the validation cohort study and it includes an additional variable (≥4 episodes of vomiting).
Source: Data from [20].

Aside from evaluating the performance of the three main CDRs (PECARN, CATCH, and CHALICE) using rule-specific criteria derived from their original studies, the PREDICT investigators created a homogeneous comparison cohort from their large Australasian prospective study.[8] A secondary analysis was performed with 18,913 children who presented within 24 hours of injury

Table 11.14 Performance of the CATCH head CT rule in external validation studies

Rule	N	Sensitivity	Specificity	NPV	PPV	LR–	LR+
Easter et al.[4] **(the United States)** – outcome of clinically important TBI							
CATCH	1002	19/21, 91%	431/981, 44%	99%	3.3%	0.2	1.6
Easter et al.[4] **(the United States)** – outcome of injury requiring neurosurgical intervention							
CATCH	1002	3/4, 75%	432/998, 43%	99%	0.5%	0.6	1.3
Thiam et al.[6] **(Singapore)** – outcome of positive head CT							
CATCH	1179	6/6, 100%	942/1173, 80.3%	100%	2.5%	0.0	5.1
Babl et al.[8] **(Australia, New Zealand)** – outcome of neurological intervention							
CATCH*	4957	20/21, 95.2%	4157/4936, 84.2%	100%	2.5%	0.05	6
Babl et al.[8] **(Australia, New Zealand)** – outcome of positive head CT							
CATCH**	4957	125/141, 88.7%	2716/4816, 56.4%	99.4%	5.6%	0.2	2.3

N = sample size; NPV = negative predictive value; PPV = positive predictive value; LR– = likelihood ratio for a negative test; LR+ = likelihood ratio for a positive test.
*Using the four high-risk predictors.
** Using the seven medium and high-risk predictors.

with mild head injuries (GCS scores 13–15 at admission). The PECARN-specific outcome of ciTBI was selected as the primary outcome for this cohort and the diagnostic performance of the three CDRs was compared across the same cohort. In this comparison cohort analysis, the PECARN performed better (higher sensitivity) than CHALICE and CATCH, however, the difference was not statistically significant (Table 11.15).

Using the same cohort but in a separate publication,[21] the PREDICT investigators performed a decision analysis model based on these 18,913 injured children and found that the usual care in the Australasian specialized pediatric hospital setting was more cost-effective than CATCH, CHALICE, and PECARN rules, meaning that these decision tools could lead to scanning more children than necessary and may miss more neurosurgical and non-neurosurgical TBIs that are likely to increase hospital costs, with a potential reduction in positive health outcomes.

Although their rule has not yet been validated, a group from Italy examined a cohort of children <16 years old with blunt head trauma presenting to pediatric EDs to determine predictors of the diagnosis of intracranial injury and death.[22] They enrolled 3806 patients from 1996 to 1997, 22 (0.58%) of whom had intracranial injuries. All patients discharged from the ED were followed up by phone after 10 days. All patients underwent routine care, but HCTs were only obtained at the discretion of the treating physician. The

Table 11.15 Performance of PECARN, CATCH, and CHALICE in a pragmatic comparison cohort

	PECARN<2 years	PECARN≥2 years	CATCH	CHALICE*
	n = 5046	n = 13,867	n = 18,913	n = 18,913
Outcome of clinically important TBI				
Sensitivity	100% (91.6–100%)	99.2% (95.4–100%)	91.9% (86.5–95.6%)	92.5% (87.3–96.1%)
Specificity	59.1% (57.7–60.5%)	52% (51.1–52.8%)	70.4% (69.7–71%)	78.6% (78–79.2%)
Outcome of positive head CT				
Sensitivity	100% (94.9–100%)	99.4% (97–100%)	87.6% (82.9–91.5%)	90.4% (86.1–93.8%)
Specificity	59.4% (58–60.8%)	52.2% (51.4–53%)	70.6% (69.9–71.3%)	78.9% (78.3–79.5%)
Outcome of neurosurgery				
Sensitivity	100% (54.1–100%)	100% (81.5–100%)	95.8% (78.9–99.9%)	91.7% (73–99%)
Specificity	58.7% (57.3–60%)	51.6% (50.7–52.4%)	69.9% (69.2–70.6%)	78.1% (77.5–78.6%)

*Using both medium-risk and high-risk predictor variables when evaluating CHALICE performance. Source: Data from [8].

seven variables included in their prediction model are listed in Table 11.16. Patients were classified as high risk for death or intracranial injury by the presence of any one of these variables, necessitating imaging. The absence of these variables classified a patient as low risk for these outcomes. The performance of the derived model is shown in Table 11.17.

Clinical question

Can risk scores identify children with minor head injury either with or without intracranial injuries who will need higher level care (either extended hospitalization or intensive care-unit [ICU])?

Going beyond the robust literature on CDRs, two new risk scores were developed to help clinicians when deciding about disposition of patients with

Table 11.16 Criteria associated with traumatic brain injuries in children with closed head trauma

Children with any of the following are at risk of intracranial injury and should have a head CT performed:
• Abnormal Glasgow coma scale
• Abnormal neurological examination
• Clinical signs of skull base fracture or of skull fracture in nonfrontal area
• Prolonged loss of consciousness
• Persistent headache
• Persistent drowsiness
• Amnesia

Source: Data from [22].

Table 11.17 Test performance of the Italian pediatric head CT rule

| Decision rule | Clinically significant intracranial injury or death | | |
	Positive	Negative	Totals
Positive	22	478	500
Negative	0	3298	3298
Totals	22	3776	3798*
Sensitivity (95% CI)	100% (84–100%)		
Specificity (95% CI)	87% (86–88%)		
Positive likelihood ratio (LR+)	7.7		
Negative likelihood ratio (LR–)	0		

*Eight children with negative outcomes had no initial evaluation and therefore were not included. Source: Data from [22].

mTBI. One score was created to help decisions among patients with mTBI and intracranial injuries (Children's Intracranial Injury Decision Aid [CHIIDA]),[23] and the other for patients with mTBI but no intracranial injuries ($CIDSS_2$).[24]

Greenberg *et al.*[23] performed a secondary analysis of the original PECARN study to identify risk factors for needing ICU level care in children with mTBI and intracranial injury. The CHIIDA score was developed to predict the need for ICU admission and included the following variables: depressed skull fracture (7 points), midline shift (7 points), epidural hematoma (5 points), GCS of 13 (5 points), GCS of 14 (2 points). The performance of this score on predicting the need for ICU level care was as follows: sensitivity of 93.2% (95% CI 84.7–97.7%) and specificity of 55.5% (95% CI 51.9–59%) for admitting at >0 points; and sensitivity of 86.3% (95% CI 76.3–93.2%) and specificity of 70.4% (95% CI 67–73.6%) for admitting at >2 points (Table 11.18). The negative predictive value of having none of the risk factors identified was 98.8%. Also, this score was found to potentially avoid ICU admission in 50–65% of children with mTBI and an intracranial injury.

The same investigators from the CHIIDA score also evaluated the risk factors for extended inpatient management (defined as hospitalization for two or more days) among children with mTBI and no intracranial injury using the same cohort.[24] The $CIDSS_2$ was created as a tool to help emergency physicians on their admission decisions; it included the following variables: GCS < 15 (1 point), drug/alcohol Intoxication (1 point),

Table 11.18 The CHIIDA score and its performance to identify the need for intensive care-unit level care in children with mild TBI and intracranial injury

Children's Intracranial Injury Decision Aid (CHIIDA) score		
Depressed skull fracture (7 points) Midline shift (7 points) Epidural hematoma (5 points) GCS of 13 (5 points) GCS of 14 (2 points)		
	Admit at >0 points	Admit at >2 points
Sensitivity (95% CI)	93% (84.7–97.7%)	86.3 (76.3–93.2%)
Specificity (95% CI)	55.5% (51.9–59%)	70.4 (67–73.6%)
PPV (95% CI)	16.6% (13.2–20.6%)	21.7 (17.1–26.9%)
NPV (95% CI)	98.8% (97.3–99.6%)	98.2% (96.7–99.1%)
LR+ (95% CI)	2.1 (1.9–2.3)	2.9 (2.5–3.4)
LR– (95% CI)	0.12 (0.02–0.23)	0.19 (0.08–0.31)

Source: Data from [23].

Table 11.19 The CIDSS$_2$ score and its performance to identify the need for extended inpatient management in children with mild TBI and no intracranial injury

CIDSS$_2$ score		
GCS 13–14 (1 point) Intoxication with alcohol/drugs suspected (1 point) Deficit (neurological) (1 point) Seizure (1 point) Skull fracture (2 points)		
	Admit ≥ 2 points	Admit ≥ 3 points
Sensitivity (95% CI)	50.5% (40.7–60.2%)	19.3% (12.3–27.9%)
Specificity (95% CI)	95.9% (95.6–96.3%)	99.4% (99.3–99.5%)
PPV (95% CI)	8.7% (6.6–11.2%)	19.6% (12.6–28.4%)
NPV (95% CI)	99.6% (99.5–99.7%)	99.4% (99.2–99.5%)
LR+ (95% CI)	12.4 (10.2–15.2)	31.8 (20.5–49.4)
LR– (95% CI)	0.52 (0.43–0.62)	0.81 (0.74–0.89)

Source: Data from [24].

neurological Deficit (1 point), Seizure (1 point), and Skull fracture (2 points). When using a threshold of ≥2 points to decide about admission, the tool had a sensitivity of 50.5% (95% CI 40.7–60.2%) and specificity of 95.9% (95% CI 95.6–96.3%), while when the cutoff was evaluated for ≥3 points, the sensitivity was 19.3% (12.3–27.9%) and the specificity was 99.4% (95% CI 99.3–99.5%). While its sensitivities were low, the negative predictive value remained high for both strategies (99.6% for ≥2 points, and 99.4% for ≥3 points) (Table 11.19).

Clinical question

Can blood markers identify children with minor head injury who are at risk for intracranial injury and who need CT imaging?

Serum biomarkers might help identify patients at risk for intracranial lesions and be used together with the CDRs described above. A meta-analysis[25] including eight prospective cohort studies which included 601 patients, was conducted to assess the accuracy of the biomarker S100B on predicting intracerebral lesions in children with mTBI. Only one out of the eight studies was deemed to have high risk of bias based on the Quality Assessment Tool for Diagnostic Accuracy Studies (QUADAS-2) tool criteria. The overall pooled sensitivity and specificity after excluding that study were 100% (95% CI 98–100%) and 34% (95% CI 30–38%), respectively. A secondary analysis performed based on 373 individual data points from four studies using the same automated assay found that the sensitivity was 97% (95% CI 84.2–99.9%) in children whose sampling time (time from injury to blood sampling) was <3 hours. Only one patient had a low S100B level and a positive CT, however, this patient did not have a clinically important injury.

Although blood testing such as S100B is not widely available in the ED setting, its use in combination with CDRs might potentially reduce the rate of unnecessary imaging in children with mTBI.

Comments

Children with head injuries present commonly to EDs, and clinicians must decide whether or not to perform HCTs, with their associated risk of ionizing radiation and costs. The prevalence of intracranial injury in the studies ranged from 0.58% to 8.3% and differs partially due to the varying definitions of intracranial injury used by the studies. In addition, the studies can be divided into two groups based on their stated goals; while PECARN and NEXUS II were derived to identify children who do not require imaging, the other studies explicitly identify those children who do. While this may seem like an academic distinction, it is not. For example, the presence of a PECARN predictor variable does not mandate CT imaging. Rather, the PECARN investigators recommend observation if certain predictor variables are present and imaging if others are present, leaving much to individual clinician discretion.[3] A later study by the PECARN group demonstrated that children with blunt trauma who undergo observation are less likely to end up receiving HCTs, suggesting that a period of ED observation might decrease HCT use.[26]

While all of these CDRs have favorable test characteristics, to date only the PECARN, NEXUS II, CHALICE, and CATCH rules have been validated. Although with different criteria and outcome measurements, the PECARN seems to be the most sensitive and reliable CDR in different population settings. We recommend its use for the identification of children with blunt head trauma who are at very low risk for intracranial injury to avoid the overuse of imaging.

Besides the robust literature about the CDRs, two new risk scores might help to make disposition decisions in patients with mTBI with either presence or absence of intracranial injuries. The CHIIDA and $CIDSS_2$ scores, however, are still to be validated. The use of the biomarker S100B in the emergency setting, although promising, might be challenging given the lack of its availability in a timely manner.

References

1. Langlois JA, Rutland-Brown W, Thomas KE. Traumatic brain injury in the United States; emergency department visits, hospitalizations, and deaths. National Center for Injury Prevention and Control (U.S.), Division of Injury Response. https://stacks.cdc.gov/view/cdc/12294. 2006. Accessed January 2006.

2. Pickering A, Harnan S, Fitzgerald P, Pandor A, Goodacre S. Clinical decision rules for children with minor head injury: A systematic review. *Archives of Disease in Childhood*. 2011; 96(5): 414–21.

3. Kuppermann N, Holmes JF, Dayan PS *et al*. Identification of children at very low risk of clinically-important brain injuries after head trauma: A prospective cohort study. *Lancet*. 2009; 374(9696): 1160–70.

4. Easter JS, Bakes K, Dhaliwal J, Miller M, Caruso E, Haukoos JS. Comparison of PECARN, CATCH, and CHALICE rules for children with minor head injury: A prospective cohort study. *Annals of Emergency Medicine*. 2014; 64(2): 145–52, 152.e1–5.

5. Schonfeld D, Bressan S, Da Dalt L, Henien MN, Winnett JA, Nigrovic LE. Pediatric Emergency Care Applied Research Network head injury clinical prediction rules are reliable in practice. *Archives of Disease in Childhood*. 2014; 99(5): 427–31.

6. Thiam DW, Yap SH, Chong SL. Clinical decision rules for paediatric minor head injury: Are CT scans a necessary evil? *Annals of the Academy of Medicine, Singapore*. 2015; 44(9): 335–41.

7. Lorton F, Poullaouec C, Legallais E *et al*. Validation of the PECARN clinical decision rule for children with minor head trauma: A French multicenter prospective study. *Scandinavian Journal of Trauma, Resuscitation and Emergency Medicine*. 2016; 24: 98.

8. Babl FE, Borland ML, Phillips N *et al*. Accuracy of PECARN, CATCH, and CHALICE head injury decision rules in children: A prospective cohort study. *Lancet*. 2017; 389(10087): 2393–402.

9. Ide K, Uematsu S, Tetsuhara K, Yoshimura S, Kato T, Kobayashi T. External validation of the PECARN head trauma prediction rules in Japan. *Academic Emergency Medicine*. 2017; 24(3): 308–14.

10. Ide K, Uematsu S, Hayano S *et al*. Validation of the PECARN head trauma prediction rules in Japan: A multicenter prospective study. *The American Journal of Emergency Medicine*. 2020; 38(8): 1599–603.

11. Dayan PS, Ballard DW, Tham E *et al*. Use of traumatic brain injury prediction rules with clinical decision support. *Pediatrics*. 2017; 139(4): e20162709.

12. Jennings RM, Burtner JJ, Pellicer JF *et al*. Reducing head CT use for children with head injuries in a community emergency department. *Pediatrics*. 2017; 139(4): e20161349.

13. Nigrovic LE, Stack AM, Mannix RC *et al*. Quality improvement effort to reduce cranial CTs for children with minor blunt head trauma. *Pediatrics*. 2015; 136(1): e227–33.

14. Hess EP, Homme JL, Kharbanda AB *et al*. Effect of the head computed tomography choice decision aid in parents of children with minor head trauma: A cluster randomized trial. *JAMA Network Open*. 2018; 1(5): e182430.

15. Oman JA, Cooper RJ, Holmes JF et al. Performance of a decision rule to predict need for computed tomography among children with blunt head trauma. *Pediatrics.* 2006; 117(2): e238–46.

16. Gupta M, Mower WR, Rodriguez RM, Hendey GW. Validation of the pediatric NEXUS II head computed tomography decision instrument for selective imaging of pediatric patients with blunt head trauma. *Academic Emergency Medicine.* 2018; 25(7): 729–37.

17. Dunning J, Daly JP, Lomas J-P, Lecky F, Batchelor J, Mackway-Jones K. Derivation of the children's head injury algorithm for the prediction of important clinical events decision rule for head injury in children. *Archives of Disease in Childhood.* 2006; 91(11): 885–91.

18. Babl FE, Oakley E, Dalziel SR et al. Accuracy of clinician practice compared with three head injury decision rules in children: A prospective cohort study. *Annals of Emergency Medicine.* 2018; 71(6): 703–10.

19. Osmond MH, Klassen TP, Wells GA et al. CATCH: A clinical decision rule for the use of computed tomography in children with minor head injury. *CMAJ.* 2010; 182(4): 341–8.

20. Osmond MH, Klassen TP, Wells GA et al. Validation and refinement of a clinical decision rule for the use of computed tomography in children with minor head injury in the emergency department. *CMAJ.* 2018; 190(27): E816–22.

21. Dalziel K, Cheek JA, Fanning L et al. A cost-effectiveness analysis comparing clinical decision rules PECARN, CATCH, and CHALICE with usual care for the management of pediatric head injury. *Annals of Emergency Medicine.* 2019; 73(5): 429–39.

22. Da Dalt L, Marchi AG, Laudizi L et al. Predictors of intracranial injuries in children after blunt head trauma. *European Journal of Pediatrics.* 2006; 165(3): 142–8.

23. Greenberg JK, Yan Y, Carpenter CR et al. Development and internal validation of a clinical risk score for treating children with mild head trauma and intracranial injury. *JAMA Pediatrics.* 2017; 171(4): 342–9.

24. Greenberg JK, Yan Y, Carpenter CR et al. Development of the CIDSS2 score for children with mild head trauma without intracranial injury. *Journal of Neurotrauma.* 2018; 35(22): 2699–707.

25. Oris C, Pereira B, Durif J et al. The biomarker S100B and mild traumatic brain injury: A meta-analysis. *Pediatrics.* 2018; 141(6): e20180037.

26. Nigrovic LE, Schunk JE, Foerster A et al. The effect of observation on cranial computed tomography utilization for children after blunt head trauma. *Pediatrics.* 2011; 127(6): 1067–73.

Chapter 12 **Adult Blunt Head Injury**

Ian T. Ferguson and Christopher R. Carpenter

Department of Emergency Medicine, Washington University School of Medicine, St. Louis, MO, USA

Highlights

- The Canadian CT head rule and the New Orleans criteria are both highly sensitive and well-validated clinical decision rules that identify patients at low risk for clinically significant head injuries and in whom noncontrast head CT can be deferred.
- The Canadian CT head rule has proven to be more specific than the New Orleans criteria, and its use will reduce inappropriate imaging to a greater extent.
- No decision rules have yet identified a population of older adults who are at low risk for intracranial injuries following head trauma.
- Biomarkers for traumatic brain injury have not yet been validated for routine use in the ED setting and their ability to reduce CT scanning has not been studied.

Background

In 2013, 2.5 million traumatic brain injury (TBI)-related emergency visits occurred in the United States with approximately 282,000 hospitalizations and 56,000 deaths.[1] Emergency department (ED) physicians must first recognize the possibility of TBI, which can be overlooked in multitrauma patients or in those who present remotely from their injury.[2] For example, older adults who have fallen often fail to report the fall or related head trauma, yet approximately 5% of these patients will have intracranial bleeding.[3] Patients with mild TBI, typically described as those having a Glasgow Coma

Evidence-Based Emergency Care: Diagnostic Testing and Clinical Decision Rules, Third Edition.
Edited by Jesse M. Pines, Fernanda Bellolio, Christopher R. Carpenter, and Ali S. Raja.
© 2023 John Wiley & Sons Ltd. Published 2023 by John Wiley & Sons Ltd.

Scale (GCS) score of 14–15 and a nonfocal neurological examination, comprise the majority of ED blunt head injury cases.[4] Evaluation for operative or otherwise significant intracranial injuries using computed tomography (CT) increases radiation exposure, healthcare costs, and the risk of over-diagnosis and over-treatment.[5]

As discussed in Chapter 5, multiple stakeholders, including payers and guideline developers, increasingly promote appropriateness criteria to justify imaging decisions for common presentations such as blunt head injury.[6,7] Adherence to appropriateness criteria varies widely between ED physicians with a skew toward over-imaging.[8] A number of clinical aids exist to standardize imaging decisions. In addition, TBI biomarker research is accelerating, although the practical application of these advances in ED settings is inconclusive.

Clinical question

Can history, physical exam, and/or decision aids accurately and reliably identify adults with blunt head injury at low risk for intracranial injury?

Based upon nine studies summarized in a 2015 meta-analysis, history and physical exam have limited accuracy to identify the severe intracranial injury.[9] In history, more than two episodes of post head injury vomiting most accurately increases the risk of severe intracranial injury, while the absence of any of these findings is inadequate to reduce the risk as summarized in Table 12.1.

The most accurate physical exam finding to increase the risk of severe intracranial injury is the presence of a skull fracture as summarized in Table 12.2. Physical exam findings concerning for a skull fracture most accurately increase the risk of severe intracranial injury, but the absence of any of these findings does not significantly decrease the risk. Specific findings suggestive of a skull fracture include a bony depression on palpation. Basilar skull fractures are suggested by the presence of Battle sign, hemotympanum, cerebrospinal fluid otorrhea, or raccoon eyes (Figure 12.1).

Three head injury decision aids exist. The New Orleans decision aid was the first one and is summarized in Table 12.3.[10] In the original derivation/validation study, inclusion criteria included: ≥3 years old who had loss of consciousness or amnesia, a normal neurological examination, GCS of 15, and a presentation within 24 hours of injury. A total of 1429 patients were enrolled and all underwent head CT, with 520 patients included in the derivation phase. The primary outcome was the presence of an acute traumatic intracranial lesion (subdural, epidural, or parenchymal hematoma; subarachnoid

Table 12.1 Accuracy of history for severe intracranial injury

Risk factor	Positive likelihood ratio	Negative likelihood ratio
Dangerous mechanism	2.1 (1.5–2.9)	0.75 (0.61–0.92)
Pedestrian struck	3.0–4.3	0.87–0.93
Age ≥ 65 years	2.3 (1.8–3.1)	0.77 (0.72–0.82)
Age ≥ 60 years	2.2 (1.6–3.2)	0.78 (0.70–0.85)
Coagulopathy	2.2 (1.0–4.2)	0.97 (0.79–1.0)
Male	1.1–1.3	0.56–0.80
Vomiting ≥2 episodes	3.6 (3.1–4.1)	0.76 (0.61–0.95)
Any vomiting	2.3 (1.8–2.8)	0.89 (0.85–0.93)
Nausea	1.4–1.9	0.84–0.94
Postinjury seizure	2.5 (1.3–4.3)	0.98 (0.95–0.99)
Anterograde amnesia	2.2 (1.6–3.1)	0.75 (0.64–0.88)
Any amnesia	1.5 (0.81–2.8)	0.55 (0.31–0.97)
Loss of consciousness	1.6 (1.1–2.1)	0.60 (0.39–0.81)
Headache	1.2 (1.0–1.5)	0.84 (0.73–0.94)

Dangerous mechanism is a pedestrian struck by a vehicle, an occupant ejected from a vehicle, or a fall from more than 5 stairs or 1 meter.
Source: Adapted from [9].

Table 12.2 Accuracy of physical exam for severe intracranial injury

Risk factor	Positive likelihood ratio	Negative likelihood ratio
Any skull fracture	16 (3.1–59)	0.85 (0.48–0.98)
Basilar skull fracture	6.0 (3.9–8.0)	0.84 (0.76–0.92)
Open skull fracture	4.6–5.0	0.90–0.91
GCS decline	3.4–16	0.76–0.80
GCS <15 at 2 hours	3.4 (1.4–8.4)	0.57 (0.34–0.96)
Initial GCS 13	4.9 (2.8–8.5)	0.88 (0.84–0.93)
Initial GCS 14	4.2 (0.85–7.6)	0.71 (0.60–0.83)
Focal neurological deficit	1.9–7.0	0.91–0.96
Trauma above clavicles	1.3 (1.1–1.5)	0.80 (0.62–1.0)

Source: Adapted from [9].

hemorrhage; cerebral contusion; or depressed skull fracture). Figure 12.2 depicts an epidural hematoma on CT. The New Orleans decision aid was then validated on a separate cohort (n = 909) and demonstrated 100% sensitivity for any of the outcomes.

In deriving the Canadian CT head decision aid (Table 12.4), investigators examined patients presenting to 10 Canadian EDs within 24 hours of blunt head trauma who had a loss of consciousness, amnesia, or disorientation and

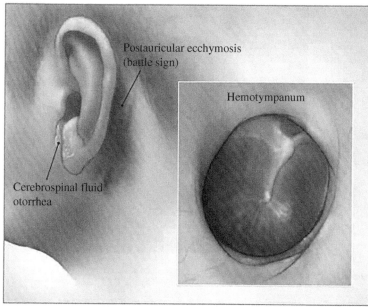

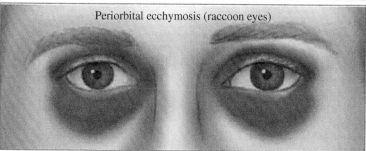

Figure 12.1 Findings suggestive of basilar skull fractures are Battle sign, hemotympanum, cerebrospinal fluid otorrhea, or raccoon eyes.

Table 12.3 The New Orleans criteria for patients with minor head injury

If none of the following are present, patients are unlikely to have a positive CT and do not need CT imaging:
- Age > 60 years old
- Vomiting
- Drug or alcohol intoxication
- Short-term memory loss
- Seizure after the injury
- Evidence of trauma above the clavicles

Source: Data from [10].

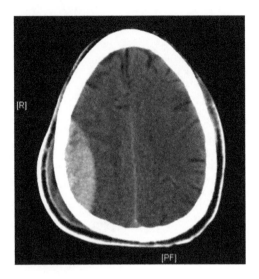

Figure 12.2 Acute epidural hematoma.

Table 12.4 The Canadian CT head rule

CT imaging is indicated if any of the following are present:

High risk (for neurosurgical intervention)
1. Glasgow Coma Scale (GCS) score <15 at 2 hours after injury
2. Suspected open or depressed skull fracture
3. Vomiting ≥2 episodes after injury
4. Any sign of basal skull fracture
5. Age ≥ 65 years old

Medium risk (for brain injury on head CT)
1. Amnesia before impact >30 minutes
2. Dangerous mechanism (pedestrian struck by motor vehicle, ejection from motor vehicle, or fall from >3 feet height or 5 stairs)

Source: Data from [11].

an initial GCS ≥13. Their primary outcomes included death, neurosurgical intervention, or clinically important brain injury requiring hospital admission and neurological follow-up.[12]

The National Emergency X-Radiography Utilization Study II (NEXUS II) group derived a third clinical decision aid in the largest derivation study to date summarized in Table 12.5.[11] A total of 13,728 patients were enrolled, including 917 (6.9%) patients with intracranial injuries, of whom 330 (2.4%)

Table 12.5 NEXUS II head CT rule

Patients without any of the following are at very low risk of clinically important traumatic brain injury, and CT can routinely be avoided for them:
- Evidence of significant skull fracture
- Scalp hematoma
- Neurological deficit
- Age ≥ 65 years old
- Altered level of consciousness
- Abnormal behavior
- Coagulopathy
- Persistent vomiting

Source: Data from [13].

Table 12.6 Accuracy of physical exam for severe intracranial injury by decision aid

Decision aid	Positive likelihood ratio	Negative likelihood ratio
Patients with loss of consciousness, amnesia, or disorientation		
Canadian	1.6 (1.5–1.8)	0.04 (0–0.65)
NEXUS-II	1.3 (1.2–1.4)	0.47 (0.30–0.73)
New Orleans	1.1 (1.1–1.2)	0.08 (0.01–0.84)
Patients with or without loss of consciousness, amnesia, or disorientation		
Canadian	1.4–1.7	0.29–0.33
New Orleans	1.0–1.2	0.26

Source: Adapted from [9].

had a GCS of 15. The accuracy of each decision aid to identify at high-risk or low-risk of severe intracranial injury is summarized in Table 12.6.[9] None of the decision aids accurately identify high-risk populations, but the Canadian and New Orleans criteria may identify low-risk subsets though the confidence intervals are quite wide.

Head-to-head comparison studies also exist. The New Orleans criteria and the Canadian CT head decision aid both have 100% sensitivity for injuries requiring neurosurgical intervention or any clinically important CT finding following blunt head injury with a GCS of 15. The Canadian CT head rule specificity was superior and was associated with a safe reduction in head CTs ordering compared with the New Orleans criteria.[14,15]

Another study compared NEXUS II to the Canadian Head CT aid across 4 EDs and 7759 patients summarized in Table 12.7.[16] Both decision aids accurately identify head injury patients at lower risk for significant intracranial injury, but neither accurately identifies a high-risk population.

Table 12.7 External validation comparing the performance of two clinical decision aids on US patients with blunt head injury

	Decision rule					
	NEXUS II			Canadian Head CT		
Need for neurosurgical intervention	Injury	No injury	Totals	Injury	No injury	Totals
Positive	111	5158	5269	108	3150	3258
Negative	0	2490	2490	3	4498	4501
Totals	111	7648	7759	111	7648	7759
Sensitivity (CI)	100%	(96.7–100%)		97.3%	(92.3–99.4%)	
Specificity (CI)	32.6%	(31.5–33.6%)		58.8%	(57.7–59.9%)	
LR+		1.5			2.36	
LR–		0			0.05	
Clinically important CT finding	Injury	No injury	Totals	Injury	No injury	Totals
Positive	299	4970	5269	301	6536	6837
Negative	7	2483	2490	5	917	922
Totals	306	7453	7759	306	7453	1336
Sensitivity (CI)	97.7%	(95.3–99.1%)		98.4%	(96.2–99.5%)	
Specificity (CI)	33.3%	(32.3–34.4%)		12.3%	(11.6–13.1%)	
LR+		1.47			1.12	
LR–		0.07			0.13	

Note: LR+ = positive likelihood ratio; LR– = negative likelihood ratio.
Source: Data from [16].

Additional mild TBI decision aids exist including the National Institute of Health and Care Excellence (NICE), Scandinavian Neurotrauma Committee (SNC) guideline, and the Neurotraumatology Committee of the World Federation of Neurosurgical Societies, but these instruments have not been studied as frequently so are not described in detail here.[9] Theoretically, the decision aid with the lowest negative likelihood ratio would most efficiently reduce imaging, but diagnostic randomized controlled trials evaluating real-world impact at actually reducing imaging for mild TBI are rare. One prospective cluster-randomized impact analysis of the Canadian CT head rule found that CT utilization at six sites increased when compared to utilization at six control sites.[17] Retrospective application of NICE and SNC would have reduced CT ordering by 9–17%, while New Orleans criteria, Canadian Head CT, and NEXUS-II would have increased imaging by 5–35%.[13]

Clinical question

Can biomarkers or imaging identify adult blunt head injury patients at risk for postconcussive syndrome or other adverse outcomes?

The ideal TBI biomarker would be highly specific for brain, released only after clinically significant tissue damage occurs, appear in serum immediately following that trauma, and reflect the extent of neurological injury.[18,19] Hundreds of biochemical markers have been evaluated to detect TBI over many decades, with S100β being the most frequently studied.[20] In 2008, the American College of Emergency Physicians (ACEP) Clinical Policy on head injuries provided a Level C recommendation (evidence from class III studies or expert consensus) for the consideration of not ordering a CT scan in patients with a S100β level of <0.1 µg/L measured within 4 hours of injury and without significant extracranial injuries.[6] A meta-analysis from 2010 reported a pooled sensitivity of 96% (95%CI 85–99) for detecting intracranial lesions on CT using a S100β cut-off of 0.1 µg/L.[21] Retrospective research suggests S100β is superior to The Canadian CT Head Rule and New Orleans Criteria with the lowest negative likelihood ratio.[22] Different S100β assays are available for ED use with variability observed between different kits.[23] Currently, TBI researchers are exploring frequent sampling of serum protein biomarkers to predict concussion or concussion severity.[24]

Other commonly reported biomarkers for TBI include glial fibrillary acidic protein (GFAP), ubiquitin C-terminal hydrolase-L1 (UCH-L1), and neuron-specific enolase (NSE).[18,25] Prior to the routine use of any biomarker, including S100β, to reduce the posttest probability of clinically significant TBI and reduce routine CT scanning a number of issues must be addressed. These include the need for available and standardized assays, further research on cost-effectiveness and safety compared with CT, and studies comparing biomarkers with existing clinical decision instruments. No biomarker currently has Food and Drug Administration (FDA) approval for clinical use in detecting brain injury.

Clinical question

Can adult blunt head injury patients with mild TBI be safely discharged home if noncontrast CT demonstrates no operative intracranial injury?

In patients without a bleeding disorder, who are not receiving anticoagulation or antiplatelet therapy, and who have not had a previous neurosurgical procedure, ACEP Clinical Policy provides a level B recommendation (moderate clinical certainty, based on evidence from one or more class II studies or strong consensus of class III studies) regarding the safety of discharge in TBI patients following a negative head CT.[6] One class I study was reported in these recommendations, which reported no complications at 3-month follow-up in patients after a negative head CT.[26] No new evidence has been published regarding this question since the 2008 guidelines,[27] but the incidence of intracranial hemorrhage in anticoagulated patients has been investigated. Based on meta-analysis of five prospective studies of anticoagulated patients (98% on vitamin K antagonists) following head injury, approximately 9% experience intracranial hemorrhage following minor head injury.[28] Notably, intracranial bleeding is not the most common consequence of head trauma. As many as 63% of discharged patients experience postconcussive symptoms at 1-month postinjury.[29] Predictors of postconcussive syndrome among ED head injury patients are beginning to emerge.[30]

Comments

The New Orleans criteria and Canadian CT head rule both demonstrate sensitivity of 100%, but the specificity of the New Orleans criteria appears to be significantly lower. Theoretically, this difference means emergency physicians using the Canadian CT head would order less imaging to evaluate for TBI, but this remains an untested theory. Definitive proof that one decision aid pragmatically and safely reduces CT ordering would likely require a diagnostic randomized controlled trial as discussed in Chapter 6.[31,32] Incorporating shared decision-making into future TBI decision aid impact research is also important.[33] Multiple factors influence whether physicians employ decision aids prior to diagnostic testing, including time constraints, malpractice concerns, confidence in the instrument, and patient preferences.[34] Some emergency physicians only apply decision aids after they have made the decision to image or not image.[35]

Acknowledging theoretical advantages for both the New Orleans criteria and the Canadian CT head rule, the ACEP Clinical Policy recommends using each for distinct patient populations. Since the New Orleans criteria specifically enrolled patients with loss of consciousness, the policy recommends using the decision rule specifically for those patients. Conversely, since the Canadian CT head rule enrolled both patients with and without loss of consciousness, the clinical policy recommends using it for patients without loss of consciousness.[9] The ACEP Clinical Policy has also been approved by the Emergency Nurses Association and the Centers for Disease Control and Prevention.

Notably, none of these decision aids identifies older adults head injury patients at low risk of intracranial injury. The New Orleans criteria (age > 60 years old), the Canadian CT head rule (≥65 years old), and the NEXUS II head CT rule (≥65 years old) each designate older adults as high risk after mild TBI. For now, imaging older adults depends upon physician intuition. Research is underway to identify anticoagulated older adults in whom brain imaging might be safely deferred after a fall.[36]

References

1. Taylor CA, Bell JM, Breiding MJ, Xu L. Traumatic brain injury-related emergency department visits, hospitalizations, and deaths - United States, 2007 and 2013. *MMWR Surveillance Summaries*. 2017; (9): 1–16.

2. Cota MR, Moses AD, Jikaria NR *et al.* Discordance between documented criteria and documented diagnosis of traumatic brain injury in the emergency department. *Journal of Neurotrauma*. 2019; 36(8): 1335–42.

3. de Wit K, Merali Z, Kagoma YK, Mercier E. Incidence of intracranial bleeding in seniors presenting to the emergency department after a fall: A systematic review. *Injury*. 2020; 51(2): 157–63.

4. Rutland-Brown W, Langlois JA, Thomas KE, Xi YL. Incidence of traumatic brain injury in the United States, 2003. *The Journal of Head Trauma Rehabilitation*. 2006; 21(6): 544–8.

5. Carpenter CR, Raja AS, Brown MD. Overtesting and the downstream consequences of overtreatment: Implications of "preventing overdiagnosis" for emergency medicine. *Academic Emergency Medicine*. 2015; 22(12): 1484–92.

6. Jagoda AS, Bazarian JJ, Bruns JJ Jr *et al.* Clinical policy: Neuroimaging and decision making in adult mild traumatic brain injury in the acute setting. *Annals of Emergency Medicine*. 2008; 52(6): 714–48.

7. Shetty VS, Reis MN, Aulino JM *et al.* ACR appropriateness criteria head trauma. *Journal of the American College of Radiology*. 2016; 13(6): 668–79.

8. DeAngelis J, Lou V, Li T *et al.* Head CT for minor head injury presenting to the emergency department in the era of choosing wisely. *The Western Journal of Emergency Medicine*. 2017; 18(5): 821–9.

9. Easter JS, Haukoos JS, Meehan WP, Novack V, Edlow JA. Will neuroimaging reveal a severe intracranial injury in this adult with minor head trauma?: The rational clinical examination systematic review. *JAMA*. 2015; 314(24): 2672–81.

10. Haydel MJ, Preston CA, Mills TJ, Luber S, Blaudeau E, DeBlieux PM. Indications for computed tomography in patients with minor head injury. *The New England Journal of Medicine*. 2000; 343(2): 100–5.

11. Mower WR, Hoffman JR, Herbert M *et al.* Developing a decision instrument to guide computed tomographic imaging of blunt head injury patients. *The Journal of Trauma*. 2005; 59(4): 954–9.

12. Stiell IG, Wells GA, Vandemheen K *et al.* The Canadian CT Head Rule for patients with minor head injury. *Lancet*. 2001; 357(9266): 1391–6.

13. Svensson S, Vedin T, Clausen L, Larsson PA, Edelhamre M. Application of NICE or SNC guidelines may reduce the need for computerized tomographies in patients with mild traumatic brain injury: A retrospective chart review and theoretical

application of five guidelines. *Scandinavian Journal of Trauma, Resuscitation and Emergency Medicine.* 2019; 27(1): 99.

14. Papa L, Stiell IG, Clement CM *et al.* Performance of the Canadian CT Head Rule and the New Orleans Criteria for predicting any traumatic intracranial injury on computed tomography in a United States level I trauma center. *Academic Emergency Medicine.* 2012; 19(1): 2–10.

15. Stiell IG, Clement CM, Rowe BH *et al.* Comparison of the Canadian CT Head Rule and the New Orleans Criteria in patients with minor head injury. *JAMA.* 2005; 294(12): 1511–8.

16. Mower WR, Gupta M, Rodriguez R, Hendey GW. Validation of the sensitivity of the National Emergency X-Radiography Utilization Study (NEXUS) Head computed tomographic (CT) decision instrument for selective imaging of blunt head injury patients: An observational study. *PLoS Medicine.* 2017; 14(7): e1002313.

17. Stiell IG, Clement CM, Grimshaw JM *et al.* A prospective cluster-randomized trial to implement the Canadian CT Head Rule in emergency departments. *CMAJ.* 2010; 182(14): 1527–32.

18. Nehar MD, Keene CN, Rich MC, Moore HB, Stahel PF. Serum biomarkers for traumatic brain injury. *Southern Medical Journal.* 2014; 107(4): 248–55.

19. Rahimian S, Potteiger S, Loynd R *et al.* The utility of S100B level in detecting mild traumatic brain injury in intoxicated patients. *The American Journal of Emergency Medicine.* 2020; 38(4): 799–805.

20. Papa L. Potential blood-based biomarkers for concussion. *Sports Medicine and Arthroscopy Review.* 2016; 24(3): 108–15.

21. Unden J, Romner B. Can low serum levels of S100B predict normal CT findings after minor head injury in adults?: An evidence-based review and meta-analysis. *The Journal of Head Trauma Rehabilitation.* 2010; 25(4): 228–40.

22. Jones CMC, Harmon C, McCann M, Gunyan H, Bazarian JJ. S100B outperforms clinical decision rules for the identification of intracranial injury on head CT scan after mild traumatic brain injury. *Brain Injury.* 2020; 34(3): 407–14.

23. Delefortrie Q, Lejeune F, Kerzmann B *et al.* Evaluation of the Roche® Elecsys and the Diasorin˙ Liaison S100 kits in the management of mild head injury in the emergency room. *Clinical Biochemistry.* 2018; 52: 123–30.

24. Thelin EP, Zeiler FA, Ercole A *et al.* Serial sampling of serum protein biomarkers for monitoring human traumatic brain injury dynamics: A systematic review. *Frontiers in Neurology.* 2017; 8: 300.

25. Anderson TN, Hwang J, Munar M *et al.* Blood-based biomarkers for prediction of intracranial hemorrhage and outcome in patients with moderate or severe traumatic brain injury. *Journal of Trauma and Acute Care Surgery.* 2020; 89(1): 80–6.

26. af Geijerstam JL, Oredsson S, Britton M, OCTOPUS Study Investigators. Medical outcome after immediate computed tomography or admission for observation in patients with mild head injury: Randomised controlled trial. *BMJ.* 2006; 333(7566): 465.

27. Manquen J, Combs T, Mazur-Mosiewicz A *et al*. A review of research efforts to address the 2008 ACEP guideline for mild traumatic brain injury. *The American Journal of Emergency Medicine*. 2019; 37(1): 73–9.

28. Minhas H, Welsher A, Turcotte M *et al*. Incidence of intracranial bleeding in anticoagulated patients with minor head injury: A systematic review and meta-analysis of prospective studies. *British Journal of Haematology*. 2018; 183(1): 119–26.

29. Cunningham J, Brison RJ, Pickett W. Concussive symptoms in emergency department patients diagnosed with minor head injury. *The Journal of Emergency Medicine*. 2011; 40(3): 262–6.

30. Varner C, Thompson C, de Wit K, Borgundvaag B, Houston R, McLeod S. Predictors of persistent concussion symptoms in adults with acute mild traumatic brain injury presenting to the emergency department. *CJEM*. 2021; 23(3): 365–73.

31. El Dib R, O'Tikkinen KAO, Akl EA *et al*. Systematic survey of randomized trials evaluating the impact of alternative diagnostic strategies on patient-important outcomes. *Journal of Clinical Epidemiology*. 2017; 84: 61–9.

32. Kanzaria HK, McCabe AM, Meisel ZM *et al*. Advancing patient-centered outcomes in emergency diagnostic imaging: A research agenda. *Academic Emergency Medicine*. 2015; 22(12): 1435–46.

33. Hess EP, Grudzen CR, Thomson R, Raja AS, Carpenter CR. Shared decision-making in the emergency department: Respecting patient autonomy when seconds count. *Academic Emergency Medicine*. 2015; 22(7): 856–64.

34. Finnerty NM, Rodriguez RM, Carpenter CR *et al*. Clinical decision rules for diagnostic imaging in the emergency department: A research agenda. *Academic Emergency Medicine*. 2015; 22(12): 1406–16.

35. Chan TM, Mercuri M, Turcotte M, Gardiner E, Sherbino J, de Wit K. Making decisions in the era of the clinical decision rule: How emergency physicians use clinical decision rules. *Academic Medicine*. 2020; 95(8): 1230–7.

36. de Wit K, Mercuri M, Clayton N *et al*. Which older emergency patients are at risk of intracranial bleeding after a fall? A protocol to derive a clinical decision rule for the emergency department. *BMJ Open*. 2021; 11(7): e044800.

Chapter 13 **Chest Trauma**

Ali S. Raja[1] and Jesse M. Pines[2,3]

[1]Department of Emergency Medicine, Massachusetts General Hospital,
Harvard Medical School, Boston, MA, USA
[2]US Acute Care Solutions, Canton, OH, USA
[3]Department of Emergency Medicine, Drexel University, Philadelphia, PA, USA

Highlights

- Potential injuries due to blunt chest trauma include cardiac contusion, pneumothorax, hemothorax, lung contusion, diaphragmatic injury, rib fracture, and injuries to the thoracic aorta.
- Chest wall tenderness, hypoxia, and chest pain are sensitive to injury. The NEXUS Chest Decision Instrument for Blunt Chest Trauma has been validated to identify patients who can receive a chest X-ray only.
- Chest CT is more sensitive than chest X-ray for significant intrathoracic injuries and should be used to evaluate severely injured patients.
- Data on the use of troponin I to detect cardiac contusion are inconclusive, with some studies reporting high sensitivity and one study reporting very low sensitivity (23%).
- Minor cardiac contusions, while detectable using troponin I, electrocardiography, and echocardiography, are associated with no adverse consequences.
- In pediatric trauma patients with blunt chest injury, one study found the prevalence of elevated troponin I was 1 in 4; however, this finding was not predictive of significant myocardial injury.

Evidence-Based Emergency Care: Diagnostic Testing and Clinical Decision Rules, Third Edition.
Edited by Jesse M. Pines, Fernanda Bellolio, Christopher R. Carpenter, and Ali S. Raja.
© 2023 John Wiley & Sons Ltd. Published 2023 by John Wiley & Sons Ltd.

Background

Patients with blunt chest trauma in the emergency department (ED) often require diagnostic testing to exclude potential injuries such as cardiac or pulmonary contusion, pneumothorax, hemothorax, diaphragmatic injury, rib fracture, and injury to the thoracic aorta. For patients with severe thoracic trauma, criterion standard imaging (i.e., computed tomography [CT] angiography) is often performed because, in 70–90% of cases, multiple injuries are present.

There is a clinical divide between multitrauma patients and ambulatory patients with histories of blunt chest trauma and chest pain. While both groups typically receive screening chest radiography (Figure 13.1), the probabilities of clinically significant injuries in each are considerably different. When a patient is ambulatory or not severely injured, he or she can receive upright posterior–anterior and lateral chest X-rays (CXRs). In contrast, multitrauma patients typically receive an initial supine anterior–posterior CXR because their presumed critical injuries preclude their receiving upright X-rays safely. The initial screening supine X-ray is less sensitive than an upright CXR for the detection of thoracic injuries, but both can be useful in guiding the initial management of patients with blunt chest trauma. Most patients in the United States with severe blunt chest trauma will receive CT scans.

Clinical question

Which ED patients need diagnostic CXRs following blunt chest trauma?
A 2006 study enrolled 507 patients with blunt chest trauma.[1] The investigators' objective was to derive a clinical decision rule able to identify

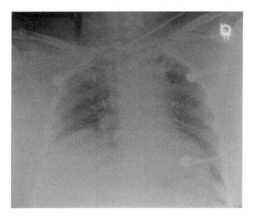

Figure 13.1 Chest X-ray from a patient with a traumatic aortic injury demonstrating a wide mediastinum, blurring of the aortic arch, left apical cap, and deviation of the nasogastric tube.

blunt chest trauma patients at low risk for intrathoracic injury. The authors excluded patients <15-years-old and those with penetrating trauma, trauma that occurred greater than 72 hours before presentation, isolated head trauma, and Glasgow coma scale scores <14. Providers filled out surveys prior to viewing radiographic results and documented the mechanism of injury, vital signs (including oxygen saturation), patient symptoms, intoxication, distracting injuries, and the presence of visible chest wall injury, chest tenderness, pain on lateral chest compression, crepitus, and abnormal chest auscultation. Significant intrathoracic injuries were defined as pneumothoraces, hemothoraces, aortic injuries, two or more rib fractures, sternal fractures, or pulmonary contusions on blinded plain chest radiography. The prevalence of significant intrathoracic injury was 6% (31 of the 492 who had complete data). Tenderness to palpation and chest pain had the highest sensitivity (90%) as individual criterion to predict significant injuries, and hypoxia (defined as an O_2 saturation <95% on room air) was the most specific (97%). The combination of tenderness to palpation and hypoxia identified all significant injuries: sensitivity 100% (confidence interval [CI] 91–100%), specificity 50% (CI 45–54%), positive predictive value 12% (CI 9–17%), and negative predictive value 100% (CI 99–100%).

In a follow-up study, the authors derived a decision rule to identify patients with blunt chest trauma with very low risk of significant intrathoracic injury who therefore do not require any chest imaging.[2] The authors conducted a study at a single Level I trauma center and enrolled patients aged 15 or older with blunt chest trauma. They used the same definition of significant intrathoracic injury as in the earlier study, with the only addition being diaphragmatic rupture. In 2628 subjects, 271 (10.3%) had a total of 462 significant intrathoracic injuries, with rib fractures (73%), pneumothoraces (38%), and pulmonary contusions (29%) being the most common. Once again, the clinical factors with the highest sensitivities for significant injury were chest pain and chest wall tenderness. Additional high-risk factors in the decision rule included painful distracting injury, intoxication, age >60 years, rapid deceleration, and altered alertness or mental status. If all factors were absent, the proposed rule had a sensitivity of 99% (CI 97–100%), a specificity of 14% (CI 13–15%), a negative predictive value of 99% (CI 98–100%), and positive predictive value of 12% (CI 11–13%). When the seven criteria were assessed for interrater reliability (i.e., whether two raters would agree on a factor being present or absent), there was reasonable interrater reliability for all variables, with a κ range of 0.51–0.81. From this, the authors proposed the National Emergency X-ray Utilization Study (NEXUS) Chest Decision Instrument for Blunt Chest Trauma in Figure 13.2.

In a validation study of the NEXUS Chest Decision Instrument in 9905 patients, thoracic injury was seen on chest imaging seen in 1478 (15%)

Criteria	Point value
Age > 60 years	+1
Rapid deceleration mechanism (fall > 20 ft or MVC > 40 mph)	+1
Chest pain	+1
Intoxication	+1
Altered mental status	+1
Distracting painful injury	+1
Tenderness to chest wall palpation	+1

If NEXUS ≥1:

In well-appearing patients with no evidence of multitrauma, consider CXR only without CT. In ill-appearing patients and/or those receive workups for other serious injury, consider adding chest CT.

Figure 13.2 NEXUS Chest Decision Instrument for Blunt Chest Trauma.

patients.[3] Of those, 363 (25%) were of major clinical significance, 1079 (73%) minor clinical significance, and 36 (2%) no clinical significance. The NEXUS Chest had a sensitivity of 98.8% (95% CI, 98.1–99.3%), a negative predictive value of 98.5% (95% CI, 97.6–99.1%), and a specificity of 13.3% (95% CI, 12.6–14.1%). The sensitivity and negative predictive value with clinically major injury were 99.7% (95% CI, 98.2–100.0%) and 99.9% (95% CI, 99.4–100.0%).

Clinical question

How does CXR compare to CT scan in excluding thoracic injuries in patients with blunt chest trauma?

Most studies addressing this question have been small and retrospective, involving trauma registries, and including only severely injured trauma patients seen at large trauma centers. One study of 112 patients with blunt chest trauma found that four of the nine patients with acute aortic rupture had a normal mediastinum on the initial supine CXR, while helical CT scan was diagnostic in eight of nine and suggestive in one patient who had a brachiocephalic injury.[4] A study from Australia involved a 2-year retrospective survey of 141 patients with injury severity scores (ISS) >15 (i.e., multitrauma patients) and blunt trauma to the chest.[5] Patients had both a supine CXR and a CT of the chest. In patients with chest wall tenderness, the authors found that the CT was more likely to provide additional diagnostic information compared to plain radiography (odds ratio [OR] 6.7, CI 2.6–17.7). Similarly, CT was more likely to add clinical information about patients with reduced air entry (OR 4.5, CI 1.3–15.0) and abnormal respiratory effort (OR 4.1, CI 1.3–12.7). They also found that CT scan was more effective than routine CXR at detecting lung contusions, pneumothoraces, mediastinal injuries, hematomas, and fractures (of the ribs, scapulae, sternums, and vertebrae).

A prospective study of 103 patients with chest trauma and a mean ISS of 30 (severely injured trauma patients) found that, in 67 patients (65%), CT scan detected major chest trauma complications that were missed on CXR; of those, 33 were lung contusions, 27 were pneumothoraces (including seven residual pneumothoraces after tube thoracostomy), 21 were hemothoraces, five were displaced chest tubes, two were diaphragmatic ruptures, and one was a myocardial rupture.[6] In 11 patients, minor additional findings were visualized on CT scan, and in only 14 of the 103 patients did CXR and CT scan show the same results.

Another study followed 93 consecutive trauma patients with blunt chest trauma, all of whom had anterior–posterior chest radiographs and helical chest CTs.[7] Chest radiography was abnormal in 73% of patients. In 13 of the 25 patients with normal radiography (52%), CT demonstrated multiple injuries, including two aortic lacerations and one pericardial effusion.

Clinical question

What is the role of troponin I (TnI) in excluding myocardial injury in blunt chest trauma?

Patients with blunt chest trauma can sustain myocardial injuries. In severe cases, this can be dramatic, involving hemodynamic instability. In minor cases, however, blunt cardiac injury can be an occult event producing mild symptoms that may be misattributed to musculoskeletal trauma. CT and X-ray are often unhelpful in diagnosing cardiac contusions, unless there is associated great-vessel or other intrathoracic injury. The limited role of CT and X-ray has led to the use of laboratory testing, electrocardiogram (ECG), and echocardiogram to detect these injuries. While creatine kinase (CK) levels can be used, their use in the detection of cardiac injury in patients with blunt chest trauma can be difficult because creatine kinase-MB (CK-MB) can be elevated from skeletal muscle injury. Thus, TnI has emerged as a potential indicator of cardiac contusion.

One study followed 44 patients with blunt chest trauma and suspected cardiac contusion who underwent serial echocardiograms and TnI testing.[8] Six out of 44 (14%) had evidence of cardiac injury by echocardiography, and all had elevations of CK-MB and TnI. There was one patient with elevations of both CK-MB and TnI found to have a pericardial effusion.

Another study followed 32 patients admitted with signs of acute blunt chest trauma.[9] All patients underwent transesophageal echocardiography within 24 hours of injury and had serial TnI measured. A total of 17 (53%) patients had abnormal TnI (>0.4 ng/mL) levels, and 10 had levels of greater than 1 ng/mL. In six out of the 10 with elevated troponins greater than 1 ng/mL, there were segmental wall motion abnormalities consistent with myocardial contusion. None of the patients with troponins between 0.4 and 1 ng/mL had abnormal echocardiograms.

Another study followed 96 patients with blunt chest trauma admitted to a trauma center for evaluation.[10] A total of 24/96 (28%) had myocardial contusion diagnosed on echocardiogram, ECG, or both. Notably, all of the patients survived to admission and were hemodynamically stable. No patients died or had severe in-hospital cardiac complications. There were no differences in the percentage of patients with elevated CK (CK-MB/total CK) ratio, or CK-MB mass concentration among patients with and without cardiac contusion. In patients with cardiac contusion, the percentage of patients with elevated circulating TnI and troponin T (defined as greater than or equal to 0.1 µg/L) was higher in patients with myocardial contusion (23% versus 3%). The respective sensitivity, specificity, and negative and positive predictive values of TnI and troponin T in predicting a myocardial contusion in blunt trauma patients were 23%, 97%, 77%, and 75% (for TnI), and 12%, 100%, 74%, and 100% (for troponin T), respectively. The patients were followed for up to 18 months, and 88% had complete follow-up. There were no deaths from cardiac complications, and no patients had any long-term cardiac complications or myocardial failure related to blunt chest trauma.

A recent study examined this question in pediatric patients.[11] It specifically assessed the prevalence of elevated cardiac TnI in pediatric trauma patients to determine if elevated TnI correlated with clinically significant myocardial injury, defined as the presence of abnormalities on echocardiogram or ECG. The authors studied a small sample of 59 pediatric trauma patients with an ISS > 12. Both TnI and CK-MB were measured at admission and then serially until the TnI had normalized. Patients who had elevated TnI levels had echocardiograms within 24 hours of admission and underwent daily ECGs. Elevated TnI was found in 16 patients (27%); all cases had an associated elevated CK-MB. There were abnormal echocardiograms in four out of the 16 patients with elevated TnI; however, peak TnI values were not correlated with any echocardiogram abnormality. There was only one patient with a clinically significant reduction in cardiac function. In this small study, all ECGs were normal. The authors concluded that TnI was a reflection of the severity of illness of the patient and that it was frequently elevated with associated clinically significant injuries to the myocardium. However, they cautioned that larger-scale studies are needed prior to making any definitive conclusions.

Comment

In ED patients with blunt chest trauma, the prevalence of clinically significant injuries is relatively low (6%). In these trauma patients, clinical factors such as the presence of chest wall tenderness and chest pain increase the likelihood of injury suggesting the need for chest radiography. In deciding which patients need a CXR as compared with CT, the NEXUS Chest Decision Instrument for Blunt Chest Trauma is a validated tool that is 99% sensitive. In patients with severe chest trauma or a high index of suspicion for intrathoracic injury, CT scan is the study of choice given the high miss rate (50%) of CXR in severely injured patients.

The data on myocardial contusion are inconclusive. While some studies have concluded that TnI is a sensitive marker for myocardial injury, in another study its sensitivity was only 23%. An interesting finding was that in patients with these minor contusions (without any hemodynamic instability) there were no clinical complications. Therefore, whether minor contusions are detected electrocardiographically or through laboratory testing, these contusions are not clinically significant. This was confirmed in a recent study on pediatric patients. Certainly, a larger study is needed before concluding that objective findings of cardiac contusion are clinically benign.

References

1. Rodriguez RM, Hendey GM, Marek G *et al.* A pilot study to derive clinical variables for selective chest radiography in blunt trauma patients. *Annals of Emergency Medicine.* 2006; 47: 415–8.
2. Rodriguez RM, Hendey GW, Mower W *et al.* Derivation of a decision instrument for selective chest radiography in blunt trauma. *Journal of Trauma.* 2011; 71: 549–53.
3. Rodriguez RM, Anglin D, Langdorf MI *et al.* NEXUS chest: Validation of a decision instrument for selective chest imaging in blunt trauma. *JAMA Surgery.* 2013; 148(10): 940–6.
4. Demetriades D, Gomez H, Velmahos GC *et al.* Routine helical computed tomographic evaluation of the mediastinum in high-risk blunt trauma patients. *Archives of Surgery.* 1998; 133: 1084–8.
5. Traub M, Stevenson M, McEvoy S *et al.* The use of chest computed tomography versus chest X-ray in patients with major blunt trauma. *Injury.* 2007; 38: 43–7.
6. Trupka A, Waydas C, Hallfeldt KK *et al.* Value of thoracic computed tomography in the first assessment of severely injured patients with blunt chest trauma: Results of a prospective study. *Journal of Trauma.* 1997; 43: 405–11.
7. Exadaktylos AK, Sclabas G, Schmid SW. Do we really need routine computed tomographic scanning in the primary evaluation of blunt chest trauma in patients with "normal" chest radiograph? *Journal of Trauma.* 2001; 51: 1173–6.

8. Adams JE, Davila-Roman VG, Bessey PQ *et al.* Improved detection of cardiac contusion with cardiac troponin I. *American Heart Journal.* 1996; 131(2): 308–12.

9. Mori F, Zuppiroli A, Ognibene A *et al.* Cardiac contusion in blunt chest trauma: A combined study of transesophageal echocardiography and cardiac troponin I determination. *Italian Heart Journal.* 2001; 2: 222–7.

10. Bertinchant JP, Polge A, Mohty D *et al.* Evaluation of incidence, clinical significance, and prognostic value of circulating cardiac troponin I and T elevation in hemodynamically stable patients with suspected myocardial contusion after blunt chest trauma. *Journal of Trauma.* 2000; 48: 924–31.

11. Sangha GS, Pepelassis D, Buffo-Sequeira I, Seabrook JA, Fraser DD. Serum troponin-I as an indicator of clinically significant myocardial injury in paediatric trauma patients. *Injury.* 2012; 43(12): 2046–50.

Chapter 14 **Occult Hip Fracture**

Ali S. Raja[1] and Jesse M. Pines[2,3]

[1] Department of Emergency Medicine, Massachusetts General Hospital, Harvard Medical School, Boston, MA, USA
[2] US Acute Care Solutions, Canton, OH, USA
[3] Department of Emergency Medicine, Drexel University, Philadelphia, PA, USA

Highlights

- Hip fractures will be missed by plain radiography in up to 10% of patients with hip pain after falls or trauma. Severe pain or the inability to bear weight should increase suspicion of occult fracture.
- Advanced imaging (MRI or CT) should be used in cases of suspected occult fracture. MRI is the study of choice if it is available and there are no contraindications.

Background

Hip fractures are common in geriatric adults, and the incidence is increasing with aging global populations. It is estimated that the incidence of hip fracture will rise from 1.66 million in 1990 to 6.26 million by 2050, with incidence varying significantly by country.[1,2] Many patients with hip fractures will present to the emergency department (ED) for evaluation and treatment, typically following a fall or other acute traumatic injury. The diagnosis of hip fracture is typically not a diagnostic dilemma because plain radiographs are often diagnostic, particularly in patients with classic anatomic deformities (Figure 14.1). However, a small proportion of patients with hip fracture (2–9%) will have initially negative plain films.[3] These occult hip fractures are more common in the elderly because of the high prevalence of osteoporosis in this age group.[4] Delayed surgical treatment has been associated with

---

Evidence-Based Emergency Care: Diagnostic Testing and Clinical Decision Rules, Third Edition.
Edited by Jesse M. Pines, Fernanda Bellolio, Christopher R. Carpenter, and Ali S. Raja.
© 2023 John Wiley & Sons Ltd. Published 2023 by John Wiley & Sons Ltd.

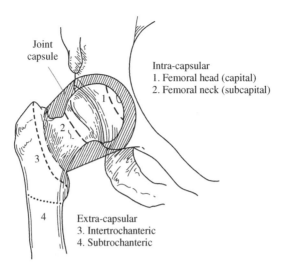

Joint capsule

Intra-capsular
1. Femoral head (capital)
2. Femoral neck (subcapital)

Extra-capsular
3. Intertrochanteric
4. Subtrochanteric

Figure 14.1 Hip fractures. This illustration depicts the different types of proximal hip fractures. (Knoop *et al.* Atlas of Emergency Medicine 2nd edition, 2002).

increased mortality, suggesting that delays in diagnosis may worsen outcomes.[5] Emergency physicians, therefore, face a diagnostic dilemma when treating a patient in whom they have a high suspicion for hip fracture based on physical examination or history but whose plain radiographs are negative or equivocal. The classic case is an older adult patient who has fallen, has hip tenderness, and cannot bear weight on the affected leg. A missed diagnosis of hip fracture can place older adults at substantial risk of fracture displacement, avascular necrosis, and the need for more involved surgical procedures.

Approaches to the diagnosis of occult hip fractures have evolved over the last several decades. Previously, repeat plain films or bone scans were recommended. Bone scans will typically become positive after 24–72 hours following an acute fracture. More recently, clinicians have increasingly used computed tomography (CT) or magnetic resonance imaging (MRI) in this setting (Figure 14.2).[6] Certain historical factors can predict the presence of hip fractures in patients with acute traumatic hip pain, such as the inability to ambulate. Patients whose ambulatory status cannot be assessed require further imaging to exclude occult hip fracture. MRI has been advocated as the test of choice due to its extremely high sensitivity. However, this modality is frequently unavailable in acute settings or limited by contraindications to MRI in older adults with implanted devices such as pacemakers, or behavioral

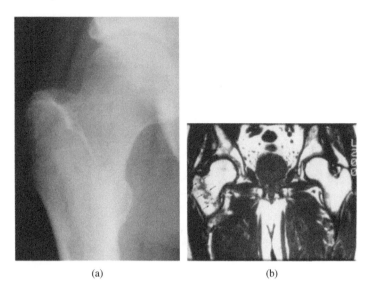

(a)   (b)

Figure 14.2 Occult hip fracture. (a) Anteroposterior radiograph of a 65-year-old patient on steroids who had right hip pain after a fall. No fracture is evident. (b) A T1-weighted coronal MRI of the same hip clearly demonstrates a nondisplaced hip fracture (thin arrows). (Reproduced from Tintanelli *et al.* (2004), with permission of McGraw Hill Education, Inc.)

issues such as dementia. Clinicians will often be faced with the dilemma of which advanced imaging modality to obtain: CT or MRI?

Clinical question

In patients with hip injury and normal X-ray, can the clinical exam reliably exclude significant fractures?

One small retrospective single-center study attempted to examine the value of various clinical signs in relation to this question.[7] Of 57 patients over 6 years who had an MRI for suspected hip fracture and also had normal initial X-rays, 35 had occult fractures. Both pain on axial loading of the limb and prefracture restricted mobility were associated with fractures ($p < 0.005$), with similar positive predictive (76%) and negative predictive (69%) values. Nonetheless, posttest probabilities of disease given a negative clinical test were high at 30%. Predictive values were the same when both factors were combined. Patients who were mobile prior to the fall and without pain upon axial loading of the leg were less likely to have fractures; however, these signs alone or in combination were not sufficient to exclude fractures. This study was limited by its design of including only those patients who clinicians already felt had high enough suspicion of occult hip fracture to undergo MRI. Patellar-pubic percussion auscultation tests have shown variable performance as a screening test to rule out occult hip fracture and are likely subject to operator-dependent performance.[8,9]

In summary, clinical signs are insufficient to reliably exclude occult hip fracture. Up to 22% of patients with hip pain and inability to bear weight despite negative radiographs have an occult fracture.[10] Additionally, patients sustaining blunt force trauma who have persistent hip pain after negative radiographs frequently are found to have other associated injuries such as pelvic or sacral fractures, or muscle injuries associated with hip fractures.[11,12] Due to the high risk of occult fracture and associated injuries despite negative plain radiographs, advanced imaging is recommended for all patients with signs of occult hip fracture.

Clinical question

What is the accuracy and cost-effectiveness of CT or MRI for the diagnosis of hip fracture not evident on plain radiography?
Once the decision to evaluate a patient for an occult hip fracture has been made, the clinician is faced with the choice of either MRI or CT (Figure 14.3). Early cohort studies showed that MRI has extremely high sensitivity compared to clinical follow-up. Thus, MRI has been advocated as the ideal imaging test and is frequently used as a reference standard in research.[12–14]

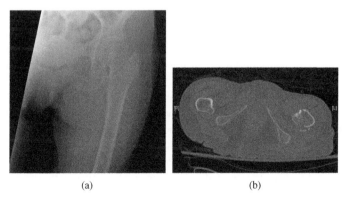

(a)   (b)

Figure 14.3 Intertrochanteric fracture (a) was suspected on the left hip plain X-ray and (b) was confirmed with a noncontrast CT scan.

A systematic review and meta-analysis of 13 retrospective cohort studies found that CT scan has 96% sensitivity and 100% specificity for occult hip fracture compared to reference standard of MRI or clinical follow-up.[15] This review was limited by the weaknesses of the included studies – most used the imperfect reference standard, clinical follow-up. Another study prospectively compared CT and MRI directly in studies of 67 hips with reported sensitivity of 87% though wide confidence intervals leave uncertainty as to the true accuracy.[10]

Pragmatic considerations including the availability of imaging modalities will impact the choice of CT or MRI. A retrospective study of 218 patients with suspected occult hip fracture undergoing CT or MRI found that MRI was associated with significantly longer time in the ED (70 minutes) with no benefit in diagnostic efficiency. This study also reported that 26% of patients had contraindications to MRI scan.[16]

Significant delays in diagnosing occult fractures have associated harms and MRI is associated with increased costs, particularly if a facility transfer is needed to obtain MRI. A cost-effectiveness analysis found that an MRI-first compared to CT-first strategy would be the most cost-effective, resulting in 0.05 quality-adjusted life years for an incremental cost of $1227. If MRI is not available, transferring a patient for MRI without first obtaining a CT would only be cost-effective if transfer was less than $1227. If CT is negative, transfer for MRI would be cost-effective only if transfer was less than about $4000.[17] Though limited by the quality of published data and best assumptions regarding benefits, harms, and costs, this analysis supports an MRI-first approach if available.

Comment

There is a high rate of occult hip fracture in older adults with hip pain after trauma and apparently negative radiographs. Clinicians should maintain a high index of suspicion for occult fracture in patients with severe pain or inability to bear weight. High-quality randomized trials that directly compare the performance of CT to MRI for diagnosis of occult hip fracture are lacking.[18] Meta-analysis of multiple cohort studies and retrospective reviews suggest high rates of diagnostic accuracy with both modalities, though CT infrequently will miss a fracture that is evident on MRI. MRI also has the advantage of identifying alternative diagnoses such as hematoma, muscle tear, degenerative disease, and osteonecrosis.[11,12] A pragmatic diagnostic approach recognizes that MRI is not routinely available in all settings and some patients may have contraindications to MRI. The accuracy of CT scan and resulting posttest probability makes this a reasonable alternative option in most instances. In cases when there is persistent concern for occult hip fracture after negative CT scan, consider MRI.

A reasonable algorithm has been proposed as an approach to the evaluation of patients with suspected hip fractures.[4] The first step in ED care should include pain control, assessing comorbid conditions, and X-ray imaging. If a fracture is identified on X-ray, then initiate appropriate fracture care. If not, the patient should be tested for safe weight bearing. If the patient can safely bear weight, then discharge the patient home if there is no other reason to admit. If the patient is unable to weight bear or complains of severe pain, then MRI or CT should be obtained based on the availability and acceptability of the test for the patient.

References

1. Cheng SY, Levy AR, Lefaivre KA, Guy P, Kuramoto L, Sobolev B. Geographic trends in incidence of hip fractures: A comprehensive literature review. *Osteoporosis International*. 2011; 22(10): 2575–86.

2. Dhanwal DK, Dennison EM, Harvey NC *et al.* Epidemiology of hip fracture: Worldwide geographic variation. *Indian Journal of Orthopaedics*. 2011; 45(1): 15–22.

3. Dominguez S, Liu P, Roberts C *et al.* Prevalence of traumatic hip and pelvic fractures in patients with suspected hip fracture and negative initial standard radiographs: A study of emergency department patients. *Academic Emergency Medicine*. 2005; 12: 366–9.

4. Carpenter CR, Stern ME. Emergency orthogeriatrics: Concepts and therapeutic alternatives. *Emergency Medicine Clinics of North America*. 2010; 28: 927–49.

5. Bottle A, Aylin P. Mortality associated with delay in operation after hip fracture: Observational study. *British Medical Journal*. 2006; 332: 947–51.

6. Pejic A, Hansson S, Rogmark C. Magnetic resonance imaging for verifying hip fracture diagnosis why, when and how? *Injury*. 2017; 48: 687–91.

7. Hossain M, Barwick C, Sinha AK, Andrew JG. Is magnetic resonance imaging (MRI) necessary to exclude occult hip fracture? *Injury*. 2007; 38: 1204–8.

8. Smeets SJ, Vening W, Winkes MB *et al.* The patellar pubic percussion test: A simple bedside tool for suspected occult hip fractures. *International Orthopaedics*. 2018; 42: 2521–4.

9. Tiru M, Goh SH, Low BY. Use of percussion as a screening tool in the diagnosis of occult hip fractures. *Singapore Medical Journal*. 2002; 43: 467–9.

10. Haubro M, Stougaard C, Torfing T, Overgaard S. Sensitivity and specificity of CT- and MRI-scanning in evaluation of occult fracture of the proximal femur. *Injury*. 2015; 46: 1557–61.

11. Ohishi T, Ito T, Suzuki D *et al.* Occult hip and pelvic fractures and accompanying muscle injuries around the hip. *Archives of Orthopaedic and Trauma Surgery*. 2012; 132: 105–12.

12. Oka M, Monu JU. Prevalence and patterns of occult hip fractures and mimics revealed by MRI. *American Journal of Roentgenology.* 2004; 182: 283–8.
13. Lubovsky O, Liebergall M, Mattan Y *et al.* Early diagnosis of hip fractures: MRI versus CT scan. *Injury.* 2005; 36: 788–92.
14. Verbeeten KM, Hermann KL, Hasselqvist M *et al.* The advantages of MRI in the detection of occult hip fractures. *European Radiology.* 2005; 15: 165–9.
15. Kellock TT, Khurana B, Mandell JC. Diagnostic performance of CT for occult proximal femoral fractures: A systematic review and meta-analysis. *American Journal of Roentgenography.* 2019; 213: 1324–30.
16. Eggenberger E, Hildebrand G, Vang S *et al.* Use of CT vs. MRI for diagnosis of hip or pelvic fractures in elderly patients after low energy trauma. *The Iowa Orthopaedic Journal.* 2019; 39: 179–83.
17. Yun BJ, Hunink MG, Prabhakar AM *et al.* Diagnostic imaging strategies for occult hip fractures: A decision and cost-effectiveness analysis. *Academic Emergency Medicine.* 2016; 23: 1161–9.
18. Lanotte SJ, Larbi A, Michoux N *et al.* Value of CT to detect radiographically occult injuries of the proximal femur in elderly patients after low-energy trauma: Determination of non-inferiority margins of CT in comparison with MRI. *European Radiology.* 2020; 30: 1113–26.

Chapter 15 **Blunt Soft Tissue Neck Trauma**

Ali S. Raja[1] and Jesse M. Pines[2,3]

[1] Department of Emergency Medicine, Massachusetts General Hospital, Harvard Medical School, Boston, MA, USA
[2] US Acute Care Solutions, Canton, OH, USA
[3] Department of Emergency Medicine, Drexel University, Philadelphia, PA, USA

Highlights

- Blunt cerebrovascular injury is a rare but potentially severe outcome of blunt trauma.
- While no definitive evidence exists to determine which patients with blunt soft tissue neck trauma should be tested for cerebrovascular injury, we recommend advanced imaging in otherwise asymptomatic patients with blunt neck trauma who also have associated cervical spine injuries, basilar skull or severe facial injuries, or ligature mechanisms, and patients with a high suspicion of injury based on clinical judgment.
- While cerebral angiography is the criterion standard for the diagnosis of blunt cerebrovascular injury, modern CT angiography (>16 slice) has similar test characteristics and is an acceptable screening modality.

Background

Blunt neck trauma is a rare event, accounting for only 5–10% of all trauma to the neck. It occurs most commonly following motor vehicle accidents, although clothesline mechanisms and strangulation can also cause blunt injury to the aerodigestive tract and cervical vasculature. While blunt esophageal injuries are exceptionally rare (a 1988 review found only 96 cases reported since 1900),[1] airway and vascular injuries are far more common.

Evidence-Based Emergency Care: Diagnostic Testing and Clinical Decision Rules, Third Edition.
Edited by Jesse M. Pines, Fernanda Bellolio, Christopher R. Carpenter, and Ali S. Raja.
© 2023 John Wiley & Sons Ltd. Published 2023 by John Wiley & Sons Ltd.

The most common mechanism for blunt neck trauma, motor vehicle accidents, typically occurs due to impact with the steering column or dashboard. The "padded dash syndrome" primarily causes crushing of the trachea and the cricoid ring, although it can lead to esophageal compression against the cervical vertebral bodies. The next most common mechanism, clothesline injuries, is commonly the result of motorcycle, all-terrain vehicle, or snowmobile riders and unseen wire fences or tree branches. Since the force involved is applied to a smaller area, the injuries are usually more localized but also more severe. Crushed laryngeal cartilage and even cricotracheal separation can be seen with clothesline injuries. The third most common blunt neck injury is strangulation and includes several distinct mechanisms. Manual strangulation can occlude and traumatize the carotid arteries, and the blunt force involved can result in delayed laryngeal edema. Ligature strangulation results in injuries similar to clothesline mechanisms. Lastly, suicidal strangulation (i.e., hanging) typically leads to jugular venous compression and occlusion, leading to increased intracranial pressure, loss of consciousness, and eventual airway occlusion.

Blunt trauma patients *in extremis* with obvious airway compromise should be emergently intubated with a well-thought-out rescue plan in case direct or video laryngoscopy is unsuccessful. Patients with any stridor or dysphonia should undergo bronchoscopy and observation. Patients with neurologic deficits, neck hematomas, or new carotid bruits should undergo imaging of both the cervical spine and cervical vasculature. However, the evaluation of stable patients with the potential for blunt cerebrovascular injury is more controversial. Although these injuries are rare, with an incidence of approximately 1% with blunt trauma, they are associated with mortality rates between 23% and 28%.[2-4] In addition, there is commonly a delay in symptom onset; 25–50% of patients develop symptoms more than 12 hours after the traumatic event, prompting evaluation for blunt cerebrovascular injury in patients who are initially asymptomatic.[4] While the mainstay of less severe blunt cerebrovascular injury treatment, antithrombotic therapy, may be contraindicated in some patients with blunt trauma, more severe blunt cerebrovascular injuries are typically treated endovascularly or surgically, necessitating screening in patients with suspected disease.

Clinical question

Which stable patients with no apparent blunt cerebrovascular injury should undergo screening with an imaging test?
Several studies have demonstrated that blunt cerebrovascular injury can present in a delayed fashion, sometimes days after the initial injury,

making diagnosis of these injuries extremely difficult.[5,6] However, given their potentially devastating nature and the fact that treatment in this "silent period" before the onset of neurologic symptoms can improve outcomes, some authors have advocated for standardized screening protocols based on the mechanism of injury and associated injuries.[4] While there are no published clinical decision rules applicable to blunt cerebrovascular injuries, a recent meta-analysis by Franz et al.[7] evaluated studies with proposed screening criteria for blunt cerebrovascular injury to determine which mechanisms or associated findings were most associated with the diagnosis of blunt cerebrovascular injury.

The authors included 10 studies in their meta-analysis, all of which used either four-vessel digital subtraction angiography (DSA) or computed tomography (CT) angiography as the criterion standard and seven of which used routine diagnostic screening based on specified protocols. These studies included 24,435 patients and had incidences of blunt cerebrovascular injury between 0.2% and 2.7%. In the pooled analysis, no specific mechanisms of injury (including head injury, basilar skull fracture, "seatbelt sign," and facial fracture) were significantly associated with blunt cerebrovascular injury, while both cervical spine injuries and thoracic injuries were significantly associated with blunt cerebrovascular injury.

The meta-analysis was limited by the fact that some centers used specified protocols that mandated screening for blunt cerebrovascular injury, which may have biased the results, and the fact that extremely broad definitions may have led to increased weight being given to certain associated injuries ("thoracic injury," e.g., included all injuries of any severity to the thorax). While national guidelines do exist,[8,9] they do not yet include data from this recent study. However, given the limitations of the study, we would not advocate for changing practice based on its results.

Clinical question

In patients requiring screening for blunt cerebrovascular injury after blunt trauma, which imaging modality has the best test characteristics?

Four-vessel DSA has long been the criterion standard for the diagnosis of blunt cerebrovascular injury. However, Willinsky et al.[10] found a 1.3% neurologic complication rate for DSA, with 0.5% of all patients undergoing DSA having a permanent neurologic impairment. In addition, it is not rapidly available in all centers and so other imaging modalities have been studied for screening these patients. While no systematic reviews or meta-analyses exist, a number of studies have directly compared duplex ultrasound, CT angiography (CTA), and magnetic resonance imaging (MRI)/MR angiography (MRA) to DSA.

Mutze *et al.*[11] evaluated 1471 patients who were screened for blunt cerebrovascular injury using duplex ultrasound and found a sensitivity of 38.5% (confidence interval [CI] 13.9–68.4%) and a specificity of 100% (CI 99.7–100%). Sturzenegger *et al.*[12] found higher (86%) sensitivity for duplex ultrasound but noted that the sensitivity was still too low for an appropriate screening modality.

CTA is much more widely available than duplex sonography in the emergency department (ED) and has become the screening modality of choice for blunt cerebrovascular injury. However, early reports indicated that CT scanners with 1–4 slices were not sensitive enough to detect blunt cerebrovascular injury. A 2002 study by Biffl *et al.*[13] found that, in 46 symptomatic blunt trauma patients undergoing screening with both DSA and early CTA, CTA had a sensitivity of 68%, a specificity of 67%, a positive predictive value (PPV) of 65%, and a negative predictive value (NPV) of 70%. More recent reports using 16-slice CT scanners have shown more promising results, although only one study to date has directly compared 16-slice CTA to DSA. Eastman *et al.*[14] evaluated 162 patients at risk for blunt cerebrovascular injury, 146 of whom had both CTA and DSA. Test characteristics for CTA in this study were a sensitivity of 97.7%, a specificity of 100%, a PPV of 100%, and a NPV of 99.3%. In addition, a recent cost-effectiveness analysis found CTA to be a cost-effective method for screening patients for blunt cerebrovascular injury after blunt trauma.[15]

A few studies have evaluated the use of MRI or MRA in patients being screened for blunt cerebrovascular injury. While MRA is more expensive and time-consuming than CTA, MRA avoids both the risks of contrast as well as radiation. However, its test characteristics have demonstrated that, like duplex ultrasound, it is not appropriate for screening these patients. Biffl *et al.* in their 2002 study also evaluated MRA and found that it had a sensitivity of 75%, a specificity of 67%, a PPV of 43%, and a NPV of 89%.[13] These results were supported by a study by Miller *et al.* who found that MRA had a sensitivity of 50% for carotid injury and only 47% for vertebral injury.[16]

Comments

Patients with blunt neck trauma can have airway, vascular, and esophageal injuries. While esophageal injuries are extremely rare and airway injuries are typically apparent or easily evaluated by direct visualization in patients stable enough for bronchoscopy, the evaluation of blunt cerebrovascular injury is much more controversial.

While there are no large randomized trials regarding treatment for blunt cerebrovascular injury, the mainstay of therapy involves anticoagulation even in asymptomatic patients, based on small prospective and database studies.[15–18] Given both the potential for delayed symptoms, as well as the fact that earlier treatment during the asymptomatic period may improve outcomes, we recommend using CTA for asymptomatic patients thought to be at risk for blunt cerebrovascular injury. The meta-analysis by Franz et al. found that the presence of any cervical spine injury or any thoracic injury was significantly associated with blunt cerebrovascular injury.[7] However, the study has several limitations. Instead, we recommend imaging otherwise asymptomatic patients with blunt neck trauma who have associated cervical spine injuries, basilar skull or severe facial injuries, or ligature mechanisms with CTA to evaluate for blunt cerebrovascular injury, as well as patients with a high suspicion of injury based on clinical judgment.

References

1. Beal SL, Pottmeyer EW, Spisso JM. Esophageal perforation following external blunt trauma. *Journal of Trauma*. 1988; 28(10): 1425–32.
2. Biffl WL, Moore EE, Ryu RK et al. The unrecognized epidemic of blunt carotid arterial injuries: Early diagnosis improves neurologic outcome. *Annals of Surgery*. 1998; 228(4): 462–70.
3. Fabian TC, Patton JH Jr, Croce MA et al. Blunt carotid injury: Importance of early diagnosis and anticoagulant therapy. *Annals of Surgery*. 1996; 223(5): 513–22; discussion 522–5.
4. Berne JD, Norwood SH, McAuley CE et al. The high morbidity of blunt cerebrovascular injury in an unscreened population: More evidence of the need for mandatory screening protocols. *Journal of the American College of Surgeons*. 2001; 192(3): 314–21.
5. Fakhry SM, Jaques PF, Proctor HJ. Cervical vessel injury after blunt trauma. *Journal of Vascular Surgery*. 1988; 8(4): 501–8.
6. Batnitzky S, Price HI, Holden RW, Franken EA Jr. Cervical internal carotid artery injuries due to blunt trauma. *American Journal of Neuroradiology*. 1983; 4(3): 292–5.
7. Franz RW, Willette PA, Wood MJ, Wright ML, Hartman JF. A systematic review and meta-analysis of diagnostic screening criteria for blunt cerebrovascular injuries. *Journal of the American College of Surgeons*. 2012; 214(3): 313–27.
8. Biffl WL, Cothren CC, Moore EE et al. Western Trauma Association critical decisions in trauma: Screening for and treatment of blunt cerebrovascular injuries. *Journal of Trauma*. 2009; 67(6): 1150–3.
9. Bromberg WJ, Collier BC, Diebel LN et al. Blunt cerebrovascular injury practice management guidelines: The Eastern Association for the Surgery of Trauma. *Journal of Trauma*. 2010; 68(2): 471–7.

10. Willinsky RA, Taylor SM, TerBrugge K *et al.* Neurologic complications of cerebral angiography: Prospective analysis of 2,899 procedures and review of the literature. *Radiology.* 2003; 227(2): 522–8.
11. Mutze S, Rademacher G, Matthes G, Hosten N, Stengel D. Blunt cerebrovascular injury in patients with blunt multiple trauma: Diagnostic accuracy of duplex Doppler US and early CT angiography. *Radiology.* 2005; 237(3): 884–92.
12. Sturzenegger M, Mattle HP, Rivoir A, Rihs F, Schmid C. Ultrasound findings in spontaneous extracranial vertebral artery dissection. *Stroke.* 1993; 24(12): 1910–21.
13. Biffl WL, Ray CE Jr, Moore EE *et al.* Noninvasive diagnosis of blunt cerebrovascular injuries: A preliminary report. *Journal of Trauma.* 2002; 53(5): 850–6.
14. Eastman AL, Chason DP, Perez CL, McAnulty AL, Minei JP. Computed tomographic angiography for the diagnosis of blunt cervical vascular injury: is it ready for primetime? *The Journal of Trauma.* 2006; 60(5): 925–9.
15. Kaye D, Brasel KJ, Neideen T, Weigelt JA. Screening for blunt cerebrovascular injuries is cost-effective. *Journal of Trauma.* 2011; 70(5): 1051–6; discussion 1056–7.
16. Miller PR, Fabian TC, Croce MA *et al.* Prospective screening for blunt cerebrovascular injuries. *Annals of Surgery.* 2002; 236(3): 386–95.
17. Biffl WL, Ray CE Jr, Moore EE *et al.* Treatment-related outcomes from blunt cerebrovascular injuries: Importance of routine follow-up arteriography. *Annals of Surgery.* 2002; 235(5): 699–706; discussion 706–7.
18. Cothren CC, Moore EE, Biffl WL *et al.* Anticoagulation is the gold standard therapy for blunt carotid injuries to reduce stroke rate. *Archives of Surgery.* 2004; 139(5): 540–5; discussion 545–6.

Chapter 16 **Occult Scaphoid Fractures**

Christopher R. Carpenter[1] and Ali S. Raja[2]

[1] Department of Emergency Medicine, Washington University School of Medicine, St. Louis, MO, USA
[2] Department of Emergency Medicine, Massachusetts General Hospital, Harvard Medical School, Boston, MA, USA

Highlights

- Suspicion for a scaphoid fracture should be raised based on the mechanism of injury (fall on an outstretched hand) and physical examination findings but merits a broader differential diagnosis.
- Physical exam findings concerning for scaphoid fracture include pain with longitudinal compression (axial loading) of the thumb, tenderness over the scaphoid tubercle, anatomical snuffbox tenderness, clamp sign, and pain with resisted supination.
- Initial plain radiography will not detect 10–15% of scaphoid fractures in the emergency department (ED).
- Missed scaphoid fractures are associated with poor outcomes, including nonunion, delayed union, and avascular necrosis.
- Advanced imaging (typically MRI or CT) may be considered in patients with initially nondiagnostic X-rays but suspicious physical exam findings. Those with high suspicion but no confirmatory testing should be splinted using a thumb spica splint and have specialist follow-up within 2 weeks.
- MRI is the preferred advanced imaging test for occult scaphoid fractures and may be cost-effective, but CT or bone scintigraphy may be considered in some settings based on resource availability.

Evidence-Based Emergency Care: Diagnostic Testing and Clinical Decision Rules, Third Edition.
Edited by Jesse M. Pines, Fernanda Bellolio, Christopher R. Carpenter, and Ali S. Raja.
© 2023 John Wiley & Sons Ltd. Published 2023 by John Wiley & Sons Ltd.

Background

Scaphoid fractures account for 70% of all carpal fractures presenting to the emergency department (ED). Missed scaphoid injuries represent an uncommon but expensive source of malpractice risk.[1] The most common reasons for litigated missed scaphoid fractures include failure to obtain an X-ray and inadequate return instructions.[2] In ED studies of adult patients with suspicious acute wrist injuries, the prevalence of a scaphoid fracture ranges from 12% to 57%.[3] The differential diagnosis of scaphoid fracture includes other fractures, ligamentous injuries, or arthritis (Box 16.1).

Suspicion of a scaphoid fracture is based largely on a patient's mechanism of injury, classically a fall on an outstretched hand. Scaphoid fractures are most common in adolescents and young adults. Various physical examination tests exist for scaphoid fracture (Figures 16.1–16.6).[3] Clinicians should maintain a high level of suspicion either when a compatible mechanism is described or if any of the associated signs are elicited on exam for patients with acute wrist trauma and pain. As the scaphoid bone has a retrograde blood supply, failure to diagnose a scaphoid fracture in the ED can increase the risk of avascular necrosis, nonunion, and delayed union, all of which can lead to varying degrees of degenerative osteoarthritis and arthrosis. Once a scaphoid fracture is diagnosed, referral to a hand surgeon and prompt immobilization of the wrist are therefore imperative. Treatment in the ED should include immobilizing the suspected injury with a thumb spica (or other similar) splint.

Box 16.1   Differential Diagnosis and Common Injuries that Mimic Scaphoid Fracture

Fractures
Intra-articular distal radius
  Styloid
  Salter-Harris III/IV
Trapezium ridge fracture

Soft Tissue
Scapholunate ligament rupture

Arthritis
Scapholunate joint
Scaphotrapezium-trapezoid joint
Thumb carpometacarpal joint

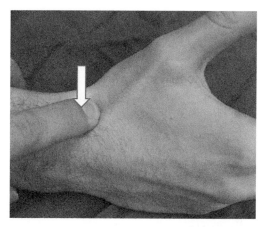

Figure 16.1 Anatomical snuffbox tenderness. Dorsal wrist tenderness in the anatomic snuffbox elicited between the extensor pollicis longus (EPL) and extensor pollicis brevis (EPB) tendons.

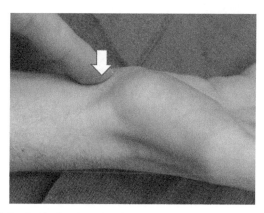

Figure 16.2 Scaphoid tubercle tenderness. Tenderness over the distal scaphoid tubercle is elicited on the palmar surface at the level of the wrist flexion crease.

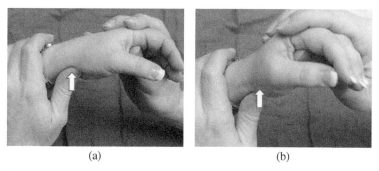

(a)   (b)

Figure 16.3 Scaphoid shift (Watson's test). Scaphoid shift test is performed with the examiner placing one thumb under the distal scaphoid tubercle distally and using the other hand to hold the patient's hand. Gentle ulnar and radial deviation makes the scaphoid tubercle identifiable as it becomes more prominent with radial deviation.

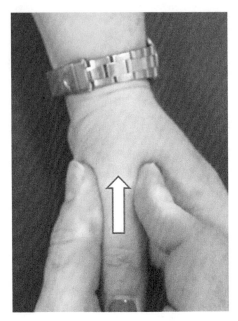

Figure 16.4 Starting in ulnar deviation, the examiner puts pressure under the distal scaphoid pushing dorsally as the wrist is radially deviated. If the scapholunate ligament is incompetent then scaphoid flexion is blocked and the proximal scaphoid subluxes over the dorsal radius rim and then reduces with a clunk as pressure is released from the volar scaphoid. A positive test must reproduce pain and result in the palpable subluxation and reduction of the scaphoid. Figure 16.3 is in ulnar deviation and this figure is in radial deviation as the maneuver is completed.

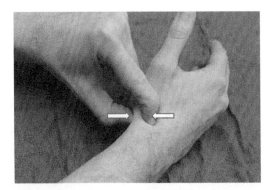

Figure 16.5 Axial load (thumb compression test). To axial load the scaphoid, the examiner grasps the patient's thumb and provides axial compression to reproduce pain over the scaphoid.

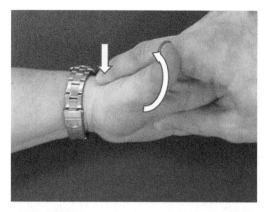

Figure 16.6 Clamp sign. The clamp sign is demonstrated when asking the patient to point to the location of pain and they will clasp the scaphoid with the opposite hand pinching between the dorsal and volar scaphoid waist.

While plain radiography is typically used as the initial imaging modality for suspected scaphoid fractures (Figure 16.7), the first ED X-ray has a positive likelihood ratio (LR+) of only 2.4 (95% confidence interval [CI] 0.84–6.6) and negative likelihood ratio (LR−) of 0.23 (95% CI 0.08–0.70).[4,5] In patients with a suspected fracture despite negative initial X-rays, follow-up X-rays (typically in 5–14 days) reveal an initially occult fracture in approximately 10–15% of cases with LR+ 4.7 (95% CI 1.6–14.4) and LR− 0.67 (95% CI 0.50–0.89). If X-ray imaging is nondiagnostic and significant clinical concern for occult scaphoid fracture persists, ultrasound, computed tomography (CT), bone scintigraphy (BS), and magnetic resonance imaging (MRI) are current advanced imaging options for patients with suspected occult scaphoid fractures.

Clinical question

Which physical exam finding is most sensitive and specific for scaphoid fractures?

The accuracy of the physical exam tests depicted in Figures 16.1–16.5 in ED settings is summarized in Table 16.1.[3] To rule in scaphoid fracture, the clamp sign and resisted supination demonstrate the highest LRs, although the CIs cross 1 for each. To rule out scaphoid fracture, the absence of snuffbox tenderness was most accurate.[3] More recent diagnostic systematic reviews in settings that include the ED and orthopedic offices provided similar ranges of physical exam accuracy.[6] One scaphoid fracture decision aid has been

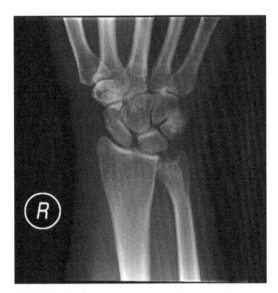

Figure 16.7 Resisted supination. Pain is demonstrable with resisted supination. The seated patient rests with the shoulder adducted with the elbow at their side flexed at 90° and the forearm in neutral rotation (thumb toward ceiling). Holding the patient's hand with the examiner's index finger over the dorsal scaphoid the patient attempts to supinate against the examiner.

derived and awaits external validation.[7] However, the rule necessitates the use of a dynamometer (a device not typically available in the ED) to assess supination strength, so it is less practical for emergency medicine. Another instrument named the "Clinical Scaphoid Score" awaits validation and relies upon anatomical snuffbox tenderness with ulnar deviation, along with pain overlying the scaphoid tubercle or with thumb axial load.[8]

Clinical question

Which diagnostic imaging modality is preferred to evaluate a clinically suspected scaphoid fracture when X-rays are nondiagnostic?

In the era before widespread access to CT or MRI, bone scan was the more readily available advanced imaging available. Historically, bone scan remains the most frequently studied advanced imaging test and may be superior to ultrasound or CT to rule out scaphoid fracture (Table 16.2).[3] Formal ultrasound is another option but is diagnostically inferior to bone scan, CT, or MRI. CT and MRI rule in scaphoid fracture with similar accuracy, but MRI is superior to rule out scaphoid fracture and provides the added advantage of

Table 16.1 Physical exam diagnostic accuracy for scaphoid fracture

Finding	Sensitivity, % (95% CI)	Specificity, % (95% CI)	Positive LR (95% CI)	Negative LR (95% CI)
Snuffbox tenderness				
Pooled estimate	96 (92–99)	39 (36–43)	1.5 (1.1–2.1)	0.15 (0.05–0.43)
Thumb compression				
Pooled estimate	82 (77–87)	58 (54–62)	2.0 (1.1–3.5)	0.24 (0.06–0.99)
Vibration pain				
Pooled estimate	67 (59–75)	57 (51–62)	1.8 (0.9–3.4)	0.56 (0.24–1.32)
Clamp sign				
Pooled estimate	73 (67–78)	92 (89–95)	8.6 (0.51–147.0)	0.40 (0.14–1.18)
Ulnar deviation pain				
Pooled estimate	77 (68–84)	42 (34–49)	1.4 (0.8–2.4)	0.53 (0.13–2.16)
Radial deviation pain				
Pooled estimate	69 (59–77)	32 (24–41)	1.0 (0.9–1.2)	0.97 (0.67–1.40)
Scaphoid tubercle				
Pooled estimate	92 (86–96)	47 (43–52)	1.7 (1.3–2.1)	0.23 (0.09–0.56)
Resisted supination				
Pooled estimate	94 (85–98)	73 (63–84)	6.1 (0.04–10.86)	0.09 (0.00–11.9)
Resisted pronation	65 (51–81)	24 (13–36)	0.9 (0.6–1.3)	1.44 (0.54–3.87)
"Clinical exam"	89 (67–99)	50 (17–66)	1.8 (0.8–2.9)	0.22 (0.80–2.90)
Swelling	61 (44–77)	52 (38–64)	1.3 (0.7–2.1)	0.76 (0.36–1.48)
Discoloration	22 (9–36)	76 (66–87)	0.9 (0.3–2.8)	1.0 (0.73–1.38)

Table 16.2 Advanced imaging diagnostic accuracy for scaphoid fracture

Imaging type (number of studies)	Sensitivity, % (95% CI)	Specificity, % (95% CI)	Positive LR (95% CI)	Negative LR (95% CI)
Bone scan (18)				
Pooled estimate	91 (87–94)	86 (83–88)	6.6 (3.9–11.1)	0.11 (0.05–0.23)
Formal ultrasound (6)				
Pooled estimate	80 (67–90)	87 (81–91)	5.6 (3.0–10.5)	0.27 (0.13–0.56)
CT (8)				
Pooled estimate	83 (75–89)	97 (94–99)	15.4 (8.8–27.0)	0.23 (0.16–0.34)
MRI (13)				
Pooled estimate	96 (92–99)	98 (96–99)	22.0 (11.9–40.1)	0.09 (0.04–0.19)

identifying ligamentous injuries commonly confused with scaphoid fracture (Box 16.1).[3] The inter-observer agreement (reliability) of CT and MRI between radiologists, hand surgeons, and ED physicians appears similar.[3]

The superiority of MRI and concerns about malpractice risk with missed scaphoid fracture have fueled recommendations to obtain MRI on all suspected scaphoid fractures in the ED if initial X-ray imaging is nondiagnostic.[2,9] Operationally, increasing MRI ordering for wrist injuries could exacerbate ED crowding, although one Irish hospital's experience with a wrist MRI protocol disputes that possibility.[10] A small diagnostic randomized controlled trial comparing ED MRI versus fracture clinic appointment 14-days later demonstrated significant reductions in downstream X-ray rates and clinic appointments with no differences in mean costs, but improved patient pain and satisfaction scores.[11] Another study also demonstrated improved identification of scaphoid fracture with a 3-month cost-savings of €174 per patient.[12]

Comments

Based upon available ED diagnostic research, the probability of a radiologically occult scaphoid fracture after initial X-rays is about 25%.[3] When patients with radial-side wrist pain and a suspicious mechanism have no appreciable scaphoid fracture on the initial ED X-ray, management options include thumb spica immobilization until specialist re-evaluation and, if appropriate, re-imaging in 10- to 14-days versus immediate ED CT or MRI.[13] Another option would be no further imaging and no immobilization, using shared decision-making to facilitate patient understanding of the risks and functional consequences if an occult scaphoid fracture is not immobilized.[14] With a 25% residual probability after initial X-ray, three individuals without an actual scaphoid fracture would require immobilization for everyone with a scaphoid fracture.[3] The risks of immobilization include difficulty performing fine hand tasks, diminished driving performance, and pain/pruritis of the splint.[15] The risk of splint-related complications requiring further management is estimated at 6.7%.[16] On the other hand, the absolute risk reduction to prevent nonunion via operative repair is estimated at 4% with minor surgical complication occurring in up to 29%.[17,18] Based upon these estimates of risk and benefit for MRI, one meta-analysis quantified a testing threshold of 0.4% below which MRI harms outweigh benefits and a treatment threshold of 80% above which MRI harms outweigh benefits.[3]

We recommend initial plain X-ray or CT, with immobilization with a thumb spica splint and follow-up for patients with pain on axial loading, tenderness over the scaphoid tubercle, anatomical snuffbox tenderness, clamp sign, or pain with resisted pronation. Also, the absence of anatomical snuffbox tenderness should prompt investigation into other potential causes of wrist pain. While CT imaging can rule in fractures, the LR– of 0.23 (95% CI 0.16–0.34) is not sufficient to confidently dissuade immobilization and should not be used to rule out scaphoid fractures. Recognizing the superior LR– and benefit of differentiating soft tissue and ligamentous injury from true bony injury as well as identification of other related wrist injuries, we recommend early outpatient MRI as the follow-up modality of choice when wrist pain persists in the weeks following ED evaluation, noting that either X-ray or bone scan is appropriate when early MRI is unavailable. Ultrasound may someday have a role in the early evaluation of wrist fractures but further studies are needed to establish benefit.

References

1. Harrison W, Newton AW, Cheung G. The litigation cost of negligent scaphoid fracture management. *European Journal of Emergency Medicine*. 2015; 22(2): 142–3.
2. Jamjoom BA, Davis TRC. Why scaphoid fractures are missed. A review of 52 medical negligence cases. *Injury*. 2019; 50(7): 1306–8.
3. Carpenter CR, Pines JM, Schuur JD, Muir M, Calfee RP, Raja AS. Adult scaphoid fracture. *Academic Emergency Medicine*. 2014; 21(2): 101–21.
4. Dias JJ, Finlay DB, Brenkel IJ, Gregg PJ. Radiographic assessment of soft tissue signs in clinically suspected scaphoid fractures: The incidence of false negative and false positive results. *Journal of Orthopaedic Trauma*. 1987; 1(3): 205–8.
5. Banerjee B, Nashi M. Abnormal scaphoid fat pad: Is it a reliable sign of fracture scaphoid. *Injury*. 1999; 30(3): 191–4.

6. Krastman P, Mathijssen NM, Bierma-Zeinstra SMA, Kraan G, Runhaar J. Diagnostic accuracy of history taking, physical examination and imaging for phalangeal, metacarpal and carpal fractures: A systematic review update. *BMC Musculoskeletal Disorders.* 2020; 21(1): 12.
7. Rhemrev SJ, Beeres FJ, van Leerdam RH, Hogervorst M, Ring D. Clinical prediction rule for suspected scaphoid fractures: A prospective cohort study. *Injury.* 2010; 41(10): 1026–30.
8. Bergh TH, Lindau T, Soldal LA *et al.* Clinical scaphoid score (CSS) to identify scaphoid fracture with MRI in patients with normal X-ray after a wrist trauma. *Emergency Medicine Journal.* 2014; 31(8): 659–64.
9. Burns MJ, Aitken SA, McRae D, Duckworth AD, Gray A. The suspected scaphoid injury: Resource implications in the absence of magnetic resonance imaging. *Scottish Medical Journal.* 2013; 58(3): 143–8.
10. Ramasubbu B, Mac Suibhne E, El-Gammal A, Sheehy N, Shields D. Utilising magnetic resonance imaging as the gold-standard in management of suspected scaphoid fractures in the emergency department setting. *Irish Medical Journal.* 2017; 110(2): 515.
11. Patel NK, Davies N, Mirza Z, Watson M. Cost and clinical effectiveness of MRI in occult scaphoid fractures: A randomised controlled trial. *Emergency Medicine Journal.* 2013; 30(3): 202–7.
12. Rua T, Malhotra B, Vijayanathan S *et al.* Clinical and cost implications of using immediate MRI in the management of patients with a suspected scaphoid fracture and negative radiographs results from the SMaRT trial. *The Bone & Joint Journal.* 2019; 101-B(8): 984–94.
13. Schramm JM, Nguyen M, Wongworawat MD, Kjellin I. Does thumb immobilization contribute to scaphoid fracture stability? *Hand (New York, NY).* 2008; 3(1): 41–3.
14. Hess EP, Grudzen CR, Thomson R, Raja AS, Carpenter CR. Shared decision-making in the emergency department: Respecting patient autonomy when seconds count. *Academic Emergency Medicine.* 2015; 22(7): 856–64.
15. Chong PY, Koehler EA, Shyr Y *et al.* Driving with an arm immobilized in a splint: A randomized higher-order crossover trial. *The Journal of Bone and Joint Surgery. American Volume.* 2010; 92(13): 2263–9.
16. Buijze GA, Mallee WH, Beeres FJ, Hanson TE, Johnson WO, Ring D. Diagnostic performance tests for suspected scaphoid fractures differ with conventional and latent class analysis. *Clinical Orthopaedics and Related Research.* 2011; 469(12): 3400–7.
17. Alshryda S, Shah A, Odak S, Al-Shryda J, Ilango B, Murali SR. Acute fractures of the scaphoid bone: Systematic review and meta-analysis. *The Surgeon.* 2012; 10(4): 218–29.
18. Vinnars B, Pietreanu M, Bodestedt A, Ekenstam F, Gerdin B. Nonoperative compared with operative treatment of acute scaphoid fractures. A randomized clinical trial. *The Journal of Bone and Joint Surgery. American Volume.* 2008; 90(6): 1176–85.

Chapter 17 **Penetrating Abdominal Trauma**

Jesse M. Pines[1,2] and Ali S. Raja[3]

[1] US Acute Care Solution, Canton, OH, USA
[2] Department of Emergency Medicine, Drexel University, Philadelphia, PA, USA
[3] Department of Emergency Medicine, Massachusetts General Hospital, Harvard Medical School, Boston, MA, USA

Highlights

- Patients with penetrating stab wounds to the abdomen and high-risk clinical signs, including unstable vital signs, evisceration, or peritonitis, should be taken for immediate laparotomy.
- In patients with penetrating thoraco-abdominal injuries, CT can miss diaphragmatic injuries, so additional testing (thoracoscopy or laparoscopy) should be considered.
- In patients with penetrating back and flank wounds, fewer than 5% will have intraperitoneal injury, and the absence of apparent injury on CT scan can rule out these injuries.
- In patients with penetrating anterior abdominal trauma, both CT and focused assessment with sonography in trauma (FAST) have imperfect sensitivity and specificity in detecting intraperitoneal injuries and should not be used as the only basis to rule out injuries. In these patients, local wound exploration (LWE), when done properly, is highly sensitive and can rule out peritoneal violation.
- Diagnostic peritoneal lavage (DPL) is not useful to rule in or rule out injuries. Because of its invasiveness and the availability of other diagnostic strategies, it should not be a part of the evaluation of stable abdominal stab wounds.

Evidence-Based Emergency Care: Diagnostic Testing and Clinical Decision Rules, Third Edition.
Edited by Jesse M. Pines, Fernanda Bellolio, Christopher R. Carpenter, and Ali S. Raja.
© 2023 John Wiley & Sons Ltd. Published 2023 by John Wiley & Sons Ltd.

Background

Over the past 150 years, there has been a major revolution in the management of penetrating abdominal injuries. Prior to the Civil War and into the latter nineteenth century, penetrating injuries were managed with observation; significant organ injuries that led to peritonitis, or other serious infections, were almost universally fatal. During World Wars I and II, early laparotomy became the treatment of choice. Laparotomy involves surgical exploration of intra-abdominal injuries and repair or removal of damaged structures. Early exploration has led to dramatic improvements in survival. However, not all patients with penetrating abdominal injuries have serious injuries. Using early laparotomy or potentially less invasive laparoscopy for all cases of penetrating abdominal trauma may be the most conservative strategy, but it is not always necessary. In certain subsets of patients with penetrating wounds, such as stab wounds, the rate of negative laparotomy can approach 70%.[1]

In the past 25 years, there has been a proliferation of availability of rapid diagnostic testing in emergency departments (EDs). In hemodynamically stable patients with abdominal stab wounds, management strategies have been developed to provide more rapid and less invasive ways to risk-stratify intra-abdominal injuries.[2] It is important to distinguish stab wounds from penetrating gunshot wounds (GSWs). Because of the high prevalence of peritoneal penetration in abdominal GSWs, most surgeons will perform immediate laparotomy in GSW cases.[3] It is also important to distinguish which patients can be managed conservatively and the importance of the physiology and anatomy of the injury. This is particularly true in high-volume trauma centers where the presence of multiple patients with severe injuries at once (i.e., multiple GSW cases) can overwhelm operating room (OR) resources. Indications for immediate surgical exploration include signs of evisceration, unstable vital signs such as hypotension and tachycardia, and clinical signs of peritonitis, all of which are evidence of significant injury to the intra-abdominal organs or vasculature.

By contrast, patients with abdominal stab wounds with otherwise stable vital signs and without peritonitis present a diagnostic challenge. Some patients will have injuries requiring immediate repair, others can be managed expectantly without invasive laparotomy. Anterior abdominal wounds can be explored with local wound exploration (LWE). In addition, contrast-enhanced computed tomography (CT) and focused assessment with sonography in trauma (FAST), and serial clinical assessment (SCA) are commonly used modalities to help risk-stratify stable patients with penetrating abdominal injuries. Historically, diagnostic peritoneal lavage (DPL) performed at the bedside in the ED has been used to risk-stratify these injuries; however, this modality is mostly of historical interest in hospitals with advanced technology. However, without access to FAST or other technology, DPL may still be a useful tool.

Clinical question

What is the sensitivity of different types of diagnostic testing and management strategies (including CT, ultrasound, LWE, DPL, and SCA) to detect important injuries in stable patients with penetrating abdominal stab wounds?
Because management strategies can vary by body site, it is important to divide injuries into three separate regions, the anterior abdomen, the thoraco-abdomen, and the flank and back region.

Thoraco-abdominal injuries

Thoraco-abdominal stab wounds can damage structures in the chest and abdomen, including the diaphragm (Figure 17.1). Diaphragmatic injuries due to stab wounds frequently do not result in specific signs and

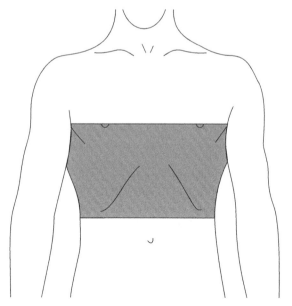

Figure 17.1 The thoraco-abdominal region for penetrating injuries.

symptoms, requiring diagnostic testing. Diaphragmatic injuries can sometimes go unnoticed during an initial hospitalization and can cause delayed sequelae. Using radiography to diagnose these injuries alone can be a problem because even small injuries can go undetected using advanced radiography. In a case series at the University of Maryland Shock Trauma Center, 50 patients had CT findings of potential diaphragmatic injuries and only 40% were termed as "specific," including contiguous organ injury and/or herniation of abdominal fat through a diaphragmatic defect.[4] In that study, patients' nonspecific findings included wound tracts extending to the diaphragm, thickening of the diaphragm from blood or edema, and an apparent diaphragmatic defect. About one-third (31%) had surgical evaluations of the diaphragm; of those, 71% had confirmed diaphragmatic injuries. Importantly, there were two cases where the CT demonstrated a diaphragmatic injury that was not identified on surgical evaluation.

Historically, another helpful modality for detecting diaphragmatic wounds was DPL. A red blood cell (RBC) threshold of $5000\,RBCs/mm^3$ is positive for diaphragmatic injury after instillation of 1 L of normal saline because peritoneal aspirate cell counts above $5000\,RBCs/mm^3$ are thought to likely not be caused by the procedure.[5] More recent data have studied other ways to assess the diaphragm, including thoracoscopy and laparoscopy. In 28 patients with penetrating thoraco-abdominal trauma, nine had diaphragmatic injuries on thoracoscopy, and eight of those nine had concomitant intra-abdominal injuries on laparotomy.[6] In another series of 110 patients with left lower chest penetrating trauma, 24% had diaphragmatic injuries on laparoscopy.[7] A more recent study confirmed these findings in 34 patients with penetrating thoraco-abdominal trauma – eight (24%) had diaphragmatic injuries.

Recently, a management strategy has been proposed for stable patients with penetrating thoraco-abdominal injuries; however, the strategy has not been formally studied. The authors suggested that an initial upright chest X-ray and FAST should be performed on stable patients with penetrating thoraco-abdominal trauma.[2] If the FAST is positive, laparoscopy or laparotomy should be performed. In the case of a hemo- or pneumothorax with a negative FAST, thoracoscopy is performed because it will result in no additional invasive treatment–tube thoracostomy will already be required. In the case of diaphragmatic injury on thoracostomy, a laparoscopy or laparotomy should be performed. If both X-ray and FAST are negative, then a DPL should be performed, and if positive (by the threshold of $5000/mm^3$), then laparoscopy or laparotomy would be the next step.

Back and flank injuries

Penetrating injuries to the back and the flank (Figure 17.2) have a lower likelihood of intraperitoneal injury than thoraco-abdominal or anterior abdominal injuries. However, these injuries can be challenging because of the difficulty in assessing injuries with FAST, which detects intraperitoneal blood only and does not adequately evaluate the retroperitoneum. Two studies have evaluated the use of CT scanning in penetrating flank injuries.[8,9] One study investigated 88 stable patients; of those, 78 received a DPL before CT scan.[8] A total of 9/88 (10%) had high-risk CT scans, and two had significant injuries identified on laparotomy. Of the 79 patients with non-high-risk scans, 77 were observed without complication, and no high-risk lesions were found in the two patients with non-high-risk scans and positive DPLs. The authors concluded that the negative predictive value of a non-high-risk scan was close to 100%.

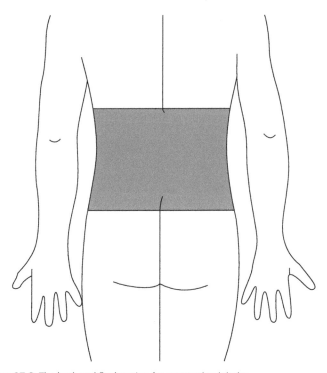

Figure 17.2 The back and flank region for penetrating injuries.

Anterior abdominal injuries

There is currently a debate over how best to manage stable patients with penetrating anterior abdominal injuries without obvious signs of peritonitis, evisceration, or hemodynamic instability (Figure 17.3). A study was conducted that observed the management of these injuries across 11 medical centers in the Western Trauma Association (WTA) Multicenter Clinical Trials Group.[10] Over a 2-year period, 359 patients were enrolled, of whom 77% did not have an immediate indication for laparotomy. Of those 278 patients, 61 (22%) required a therapeutic laparotomy (the main study outcome). There were several management strategies employed, including CT, FAST, LWE, DLP, and SCA. The sensitivities and specificities of each of these modalities are summarized in Table 17.1, where the criterion standard was a therapeutic laparotomy.

These data were notably limited by spectrum and incorporation bias (Chapter 6) and the fact that these are observational data; however, this was

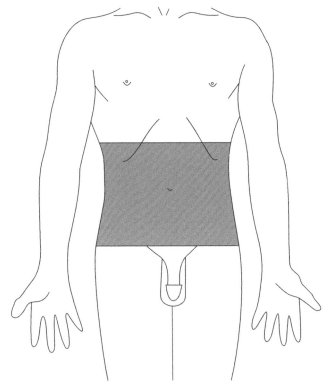

Figure 17.3 The anterior abdominal region for penetrating injuries.

Table 17.1 Test characteristics of various diagnostic modalities in detecting serious intra-abdominal injuries in stable patients with penetrating abdominal trauma

Test	N	Prevalence	Sensitivity, %	Specificity, %	Positive predictive value, %	Negative predictive value, %
Computed tomography	145	35 (24%)	77	73	47	91
Focused assessment with sonography in trauma (FAST)	132	29 (22%)	21	94	50	81
Local wound exploration	125	25 (20%)	100	54	35	100
Diagnostic peritoneal lavage	45	11 (24%)	82	88	69	94
Serial clinical examinations	26	2 (8%)	100	96	67	100

Source: Data from [10].

the largest study on the topic to date. The study is also limited by nonuniform follow-up of patients. In addition, determining if someone needs a laparotomy is not accurately assessed in analyzing whether the surgeon provided a therapeutic intervention because in many cases, some of these injuries may have been managed nonoperatively.

The authors also calculated the proportion of patients with negative test results who underwent a therapeutic laparotomy as an additional value of the test. This could be calculated for tests that were not 100% sensitive. For CT the rate was 7%, for DPL it was 6%, and for FAST it was higher at 19%.

A Cochrane review investigated the sensitivity and specificity of FAST to detect either intraperitoneal or pericardial fluid.[11] This was different from the WTA study because the outcome was therapeutic laparotomy. The authors found in eight observational studies (*n* = 565 patients) that the prevalence of an abnormal FAST exam after penetrating trauma was low (24–56%). FAST is highly specific (94–100%) but demonstrated low sensitivity (28–100%). The Cochrane review authors concluded that a positive FAST should prompt immediate laparotomy, but a negative FAST requires additional testing.

Comment

Patients with abdominal stab wounds and high-risk signs or symptoms (instability, evisceration, and peritonitis) should be taken to the OR immediately. In stable patients, several diagnostic strategies can be undertaken, depending upon the site of the injury. In thoraco-abdominal injuries, advanced radiography is not sensitive. Therefore, even in cases where the initial chest X-ray and FAST are normal, patients should still receive a diagnostic thoracoscopy or laparotomy because of the possibility for occult diaphragmatic injuries. In flank and back penetrating trauma, patients have a low prevalence of intra-abdominal injury that can be ruled out if stable with a negative CT.

In penetrating anterior abdominal stab wounds, FAST is a useful test to rule in significant injuries, but not to rule out injuries. In the WTA study, it was performed in almost half of the cases; however, it affected the management in only 5% of cases. In addition, a positive FAST was associated with either a nontherapeutic laparotomy or no laparotomy performed in 28% of the cases. However, a negative FAST can also be deceiving in that 19% of patients with negative FASTs went on to have a therapeutic laparotomy. Therefore, in the case of stable penetrating trauma to the abdomen, FAST should not be used to exclude important injuries.

Similar to FAST, CT is poorly sensitive and specific in predicting the need for therapeutic laparotomy. CT often identifies patients with injuries of questionable significance since 24% of patients with positive CT findings ultimately have a negative laparotomy. In addition, a negative CT scan can be falsely reassuring. Therefore, CT should not be the only determinant of laparotomy in stable anterior abdominal stab injuries.

LWE was performed in about half of the WTA patients. The primary value of LWE is to assess if the stabbing object violated the peritoneal cavity. Positive LWEs should not be the only indicator for laparotomy because more than half (57%) of the laparotomies performed were nontherapeutic. These studies used a variety of definitions of a positive LWE across the sites in the WTA (some defining it as violation of the anterior fascia – which is not necessarily intraperitoneal – while others defined it as violation of the posterior fascia). However, given the high sensitivity and negative predictive value of LWE, it may be suggested that negative LWE patients can be discharged home if explored properly by a surgeon. Patients with a positive LWE may be admitted and observed with serial exams.

Data on DPL demonstrated low sensitivity and specificity, which are dependent upon the cutoff for DPL positivity. In most centers, the cutoff for a positive DPL is >100,000 RBC/mm^3, >500 WBC/mm^3, or elevated alkaline phosphatase and bilirubin in the effluent in addition to grossly positive blood, succus, bile, or food. Reducing the cutoffs for these numbers would increase sensitivity but result in greater false positives. The WTA authors calculated that reducing the DPL cutoff to 10,000 RBC/mm^3 would result in two additional nontherapeutic laparotomies for every therapeutic laparotomy. Given the shortcomings of DPL and the reduction in the volume of training in these procedures that can cause iatrogenic injury, it has been suggested that DPL be removed from management pathways in stable patients with anterior abdominal stab wounds.

References

1. Shaftan GW. Indications for operation in abdominal trauma. *American Journal of Surgery*. 1960; 99: 657–64.
2. Biffl WL, Moore EE. Management guidelines for penetrating abdominal trauma. *Current Opinion in Critical Care*. 2010; 16: 609–17.
3. Moore EE, Moore JB, Van Duzer-Moore S, Thompson JS. Mandatory laparotomy for gunshot wounds penetrating the abdomen. *American Journal of Surgery*. 1980; 140: 847–51.
4. Shanmuganathan K, Mirvis SE, Chiu WC *et al*. Penetrating torso trauma: Triplecontrast helical CT in peritoneal violation and organ injury: A prospective study in 200 patients. *Radiology*. 2004; 231: 775–84.
5. Moore EE, Marx JA. Penetrating abdominal wounds: Rationale for exploratory laparotomy. *Journal of the American Medical Association*. 1985; 253: 2705–8.
6. Uribe RA, Pachon CE, Frame SB *et al*. A prospective evaluation of thoracoscopy for the diagnosis of penetrating thoracoabdominal trauma. *Journal of Trauma*. 1994; 37: 650–4.
7. Murray JA, Demetriades D, Asensio JA *et al*. Occult injuries to the diaphragm: Prospective evaluation of laparoscopy in penetrating injuries to the left lower chest. *Journal of the American College of Surgeons*. 1998; 187: 626–30.
8. Himmelman RG, Martin M, Gilkey S, Barrett JA. Triple-contrast CT scans in penetrating back and flank trauma. *Journal of Trauma*. 1991; 31: 852–6.
9. Boyle EM Jr, Maier RV, Salazar JD *et al*. Diagnosis of injuries after stab wounds to the back and flank. *Journal of Trauma*. 1997; 42: 260–5.
10. Biffl WL, Kaups KL, Cothren CC *et al*. Management of patients with anterior abdominal stab wounds: A Western Trauma Association Multicenter Trial. *Journal of Trauma*. 2009; 66: 1294–301.
11. Quinn AC, Sinert R. What is the utility of the focused assessment with sonography in trauma (FAST) exam in penetrating torso trauma? *Injury*. 2011; 42: 482–7.

Chapter 18 Penetrating Trauma to the Extremities and Vascular Injuries

Christopher R. Carpenter[1] and Ali S. Raja[2]

[1]Department of Emergency Medicine, Washington University School of Medicine, St. Louis, MO, USA
[2]Department of Emergency Medicine, Massachusetts General Hospital, Harvard Medical School, Boston, MA, USA

Highlights

- Definitions of "hard" and "soft" signs of vascular injury differ across organizations.
- Hard signs of vascular injury accurately rule in arterial injury and affected patients should proceed directly to the operating room.
- Soft signs should not be used to rule in or rule out vascular injury.
- Ankle–brachial index (ABI) can be used to rule in arterial injury but should not be used in isolation to rule out arterial injury.
- The absence of "hard signs" in conjunction with ABI > 0.9 accurately rules out arterial injury.
- Multidetector CT angiography (CTA) accurately rules in or rules out arterial injury and is associated with less complications than traditional angiography.

Background

Firearms account for over half of penetrating injuries to the extremities in the United States.[1] In contrast, blunt mechanisms and penetrating knife wounds are more common in Europe and Asia for extremity vascular trauma.[2,3] Penetrating vascular injuries across the United States were associated with 3.8% mortality rate and 1.3% of patients had amputations.[4] Missed vascular injuries delay time to definitive operative or nonoperative management, but occult injuries are

Evidence-Based Emergency Care: Diagnostic Testing and Clinical Decision Rules, Third Edition.
Edited by Jesse M. Pines, Fernanda Bellolio, Christopher R. Carpenter, and Ali S. Raja.
© 2023 John Wiley & Sons Ltd. Published 2023 by John Wiley & Sons Ltd.

Table 18.1 Differing definitions of hard and soft signs between organizations

Guideline	Hard sign	Soft sign
EAST	Bruit	History of arterial bleeding
	Expanding hematoma	Neurologic deficit
	Pulsatile bleeding	Nonexpanding hematoma
	Pulse deficit	Wound proximity to artery
	Thrill	
WTA	Bruit	History of arterial bleeding
	Expanding hematoma	Neurologic deficit
	External bleeding	Small nonpulsatile hematoma
	Pain	Wound proximity to artery
	Pallor	
	Paralysis	
	Paresthesia	
	Pulselessness	
	Thrill	

common. In fact, trauma guidelines sometimes differ in providing diagnostic evaluation recommendations. For example, the Eastern Association for the Surgery of Trauma (EAST) practice management guideline[5] and Western Trauma Association (WTA) position papers[6,7] provide slightly different definitions of "hard" and "soft" signs (Table 18.1).[8] The presence of hard signs indicates the need for immediate exploration in the operating room, but vascular injuries can be present in the absence of hard signs. Specifically, the presence of peripheral pulses cannot exclude arterial injury.[9]

Trauma care of extremity vascular injuries has evolved over the last 60 years. Rather than resulting in amputations, the majority of extremity vascular injuries can now be repaired. As operative repair has improved, the role of the diagnostic evaluation has also evolved. In addition to evaluating hard and soft signs, the ankle–brachial index (ABI) is used to identify patients at risk for vascular injury.[9] Since traditional angiography is invasive and carries risks that outweigh its benefits in routine use, noninvasive diagnostic techniques have emerged as accurate alternatives to angiography or surgical exploration. CT angiography (CTA) has replaced Doppler ultrasonography as the imaging modality of choice to identify the presence or absence of an extremity vascular injury.[9] Many centers have developed diagnostic algorithms that utilize all these diagnostic modalities to avoid invasive angiography and surgical exploration while still maximizing limb salvage and patient outcomes. For this chapter, we reviewed studies of civilian penetrating extremity trauma, as military injuries typically involve much higher energy trauma than typical civilian injuries caused by knives and handguns.

Table 18.2 Diagnostic characteristics of hard signs

Author	N	Prevalence (%)	Sensitivity (%)	Specificity (%)	LR+	LR−
Schwartz et al.[11]	469	16	49	83	3	0.6
Gonzalez (1999)	489	10	92	95	19	0.08
Inaba et al.[12]	212	16	60	100	210	0.4

Note: LR+ = positive likelihood ratio; and LR− = negative likelihood ratio.
Source: Data from [7–11,13].

Clinical question

What clinical signs and symptoms reliably predict a penetrating vascular injury?
For emergency medicine, the physical examination remains the mainstay of the evaluation of penetrating extremity wounds, so as not to indiscriminately obtain vascular imaging on every patient with the accompanying risks of medical radiation exposure and healthcare costs.[10] Soft signs should not be used to rule in or rule out the possibility of penetrating vascular injury, as they do not add diagnostic value. Although the definitions of hard signs varied between studies, and individual study designs were at risk for spectrum bias, incorporation bias, and differential verification bias, one emergency department-based diagnostic meta-analysis summarizes the accuracy of hard signs (Table 18.2).[8,13] Notably, high heterogeneity in pooled estimates of LR+ (I^2 = 96.5%) and LR− (I^2 = 92.6%) precluded meta-analysis. This heterogeneity probably reflects between-study differences in defining and evaluating hard signs. For example, Schwartz et al. included neurologic deficit as a hard sign but Gonzalez labeled that a soft sign.[11,14] Bruit represented a hard sign for Gonzalez and Inaba, but a soft sign by Schwartz.[11,12,14] None of these studies reported intra- or inter-rater reliability of these physical exam findings, so their reproducibility remains unknown.

Clinical question

Can ABI be used to rule out penetrating vascular injury?
The ABI is a test to compare arterial pressures and is used for both acute and chronic vascular evaluation. The ABI is the ratio between systolic blood pressures measured distal to a penetrating lower extremity injury and the systolic blood pressure measured on an uninjured and nondiseased upper extremity. In contrast, the arterial pressure index (API) is the ratio between systolic blood pressures measured distal to a penetrating injury in one extremity and measured at the same location on the contralateral uninjured extremity. The

Table 18.3 Diagnostic characteristics of the ankle–brachial index (ABI)

Author	N	Prevalence (%)	Sensitivity (%)	Specificity (%)	LR+	LR–
Anderson et al.[15]	23	26	67	100	23	0.37
Schwartz et al.[11]	469	16	47	85	3	0.63
Inabe et al.[12]	200	8	56	95	12	0.46
Pooled	**692**	**14**	**49.5**	**I^2=89%**	**I^2=82%**	**0.59**

Note: LR+ = positive likelihood ratio; and LR– = negative likelihood ratio.
Source: Data from [8].

ABI and API are valid for injuries distal to the "shoulder" and "groin." These are inexact terms, so the more proximal the injury, the less valid the use of these indices becomes. Generally, pressures are obtained using a Doppler vascular probe and a blood pressure cuff. The injured limb's pressure is divided by the noninjured limb's pressure, and the resulting proportion is the ABI or API. One emergency department-based diagnostic meta-analysis summarizes the accuracy of the ABI (Table 18.3).[8]

This diagnostic systematic review actually identified five ABI studies, but only reports meta-analysis results for three of them.[11,12,15] Nassoura et al. was excluded as a statistical outlier with LR+ 409, probably because that study only included patients with injuries proximal to an artery and without other signs.[16] Gagne et al.[17] was excluded because they reported 25 penetrating extremity cases without any vascular injuries identified, so ABI likelihood ratios could not be computed.[17] The summary accuracy described in Table 18.3 uses ABI < 0.9 as the threshold of abnormal. Inaba et al. and Schwartz et al. attempted to follow-up patients who did not have criterion standard testing with follow-up intervals ranging from 3 days to 18 months; however, 63% were lost to follow-up, so partial verification bias is likely.[11–13] The results indicate that an abnormal ABI accurately rules in a vascular injury, but a normal ABI alone does not exclude a vascular injury. Most studies used Doppler ultrasound when assessing ABI. None of these studies reported ABI intra-rater or inter-rater reliability.

The diagnostic systematic review next identified two studies with similar populations of "no hard or soft signs" and then pooled the results of these findings with ABI (Table 18.4).[8,11,12] Based on these two studies, the combination of a normal physical exam (no hard or soft signs) with a normal ABI accurately rules out vascular injury (LR– 0.01 with 95% confidence interval [CI] 0.0–0.1, I^2 = 0%).

Table 18.4 Diagnostic characteristics of the hard or soft signs in combination with ABI

Author	N	Prevalence (%)	Sensitivity (%)	Specificity (%)	LR+	LR−
Schwartz et al.[11]	469	16	100	85	3	0.01
Inabe et al.[12]	212	16	100	95	12	0.02
Pooled	**681**	**16**	**100**	$I^2=98\%$	$I^2=98\%$	**0.01**

Note: LR+ = positive likelihood ratio; and LR− = negative likelihood ratio.
Source: Data from [8].

Table 18.5 Diagnostic characteristics of computed tomography angiography (CTA)

Author	N	Prevalence (%)	Sensitivity (%)	Specificity (%)	LR+	LR−
4 Slice CTA						
Soto et al.[18]	43	44	89	100	46	0.08
Soto et al.[19]	137	45	95	99	72	0.05
Joshi et al[21]	23	57	100	100	21	0.04
Inaba et al.[20]	82	28	100	100	68	0.02
Rieger et al.[21]	99	65	98	83	6	0.02
Iezzi et al.[22]	47	57	96	90	10	0.04
Hogan et al.[23]	32	34	100	95	14	0.04
Pooled	**463**		**97**	**95**	**16**	**0.04**
			$I^2=0\%$	$I^2=66\%$	$I^2=49\%$	$I^2=0\%$
16–64 Slice CTA						
Seamon et al.[24]	21	52	100	100	23	0.05
Foster et al.[25]	262	16	100	99	87	0.01
Inaba et al.[12]	66	29	100	100	88	0.02
Pooled	**328**		**100**	**99**	**72**	**0.02**
			$I^2=0\%$	$I^2=0\%$	$I^2=0\%$	$I^2=0\%$

Note: CTA = computed tomography angiography; I^2 = index of inconsistency;
LR+ = positive likelihood ratio; and LR− = negative likelihood ratio.
Source: Data from [26].

Clinical question

Can CTA rule out vascular injury?

One surgical meta-analysis re-evaluated the accuracy and reliability of CTA for the diagnosis of peripheral arterial injury and is summarized in Table 18.5.[26] These 11 studies have similar attributes.[12,18–25,27] First, most were small studies performed at a single center. Second, most studies evaluated CTA in patients of intermediate risk who had no hard signs and at least one soft sign. Third, they generally excluded the 2–10% of CTAs that were inde-terminate. Finally, the choice of criterion standard varied, both between studies and within certain studies. Many studies used a composite criterion standard of surgical findings, other imaging, and follow-up, increasing the risk of incorporation bias.[13] Most studies allowed CTA to serve as its own criterion standard, thereby significantly inflating both sensitivity and speci-ficity. Four of the studies also reported inter-observer agreement between radiologists with kappa results ranging from 0.89 to 1.0.[18,19,21,22] Based on these results, CTA is an accurate and reliable imaging test to rule in or rule out vascular injury to an extremity after penetrating trauma, although with less heterogeneity with 16–64 slice computed tomography (CT) imaging.

Comments

There are several reasonable approaches to the diagnosis of major-vessel injuries following penetrating extremity injury. The American Association for the Surgery of Trauma-World Society of Emergency Surgery discour-ages additional imaging if ABI > 0.9 and encourages CTA as first-line imag-ing for penetrating extremity injuries in adults and children who are hemodynamically stable without active bleeding when arterial injury is suspected.[9] Invasive catheter angiography is indicated if CTA is unavailable or equivocal, or when required by surgical services for interventional decision-making. Every emergency department should create a standard protocol in collaboration with their trauma and vascular surgeons. We present one well-designed algorithm in Figure 18.1.

Since CTA exposes patients to the risks of contrast and medical radiation exposure, understanding the probability of vascular injury after physical exam is important. Using the Bayesian logic described in Chapter 3, a diag-nostic meta-analysis depicted the posttest probability of vascular injury with ultrasound, ABI, or a combination of hard signs and ABI (Figure 18.2).[8] These authors then used an approach described by Pauker and Kassirer[8,28] to estimate a test–treatment threshold for CTA imaging based upon CTA sensi-tivity 96.2% and specificity 99.2%, risk of vascular surgery 10%, lifetime risk of medical radiation 0.05%, and benefit of surgical repair 95% (estimating that 5% will resolve without operative intervention). Their test–treatment estimates resulted in a test threshold of 0.14%, meaning that if the posttest probability is above 0.14%, continued testing with CTA is justified (Figure 18.3). Continuing to test below that threshold potentially harms more patients than testing benefits.

The physical exam remains critically important in the evaluation of these injuries. Although their definition varies across studies and surgical

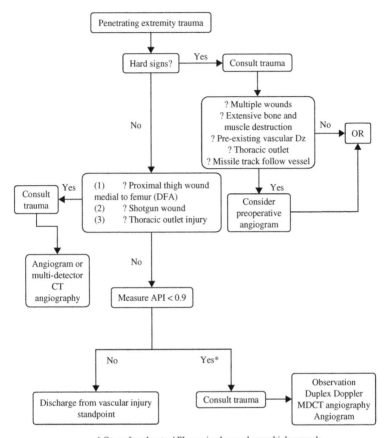

* Or confounders to API: proximal wound or multiple wounds

Figure 18.1 Management algorithm for evaluation of vascular injury due to penetrating extremity trauma. Note: Dz = disease; DFA = deep femoral artery; CT = computed tomography; US = ultrasound; API = arterial pressure indices; and MDCT angiography = multidetector computed tomography angiography. (Reproduced from [1]/With permission from Elsevier.)

societies, hard signs of vessel injury can accurately rule in vascular injury and are often an indication for operative repair. The posttest probability with a hard sign is too high for any diagnostic test to rule out injury, and the risk of delay with angiogram is greater than the benefit of preventing unnecessary operations. In a select group of cases with hard signs, an angiogram may be useful preoperatively to guide operative management, but the decision to activate surgical resources should not be predicated on the angiogram's results. Factors that necessitate surgical intervention include multiple sites of

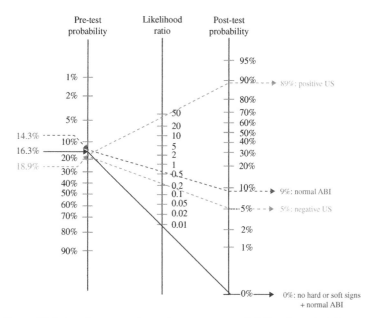

Figure 18.2 Bayesian approach to estimate posttest probability of vascular injury. (Data from [8].)

$$\text{Testing threshold} = [(P_{pos/nd}) \times (R_{rx}) + R_t] \div [(P_{pos/nd} \times R_{rx}) + (P_{pos/d} \times B_{rx})] = 0.14\%$$

$$\text{Treatment threshold} = [(P_{neg/nd}) \times (R_{rx}) - R_t] \div [(P_{neg/nd} \times R_{rx}) + (P_{neg/d} \times B_{rx})] = 72.95\%$$

$P_{pos/nd}$ = probability of a positive result in patients without disease = 1–specificity = 1–0.992 = 0.008

$P_{neg/nd}$ = probability of a negative result in patients without disease = specificity = 0.992

R_{rx} = risk of treatment in patients without disease = 0.10

R_t = risk of diagnostic test = 0.0005

$P_{pos/d}$ = probability of a positive result in patients with disease = sensitivity = 0.962

$P_{neg/d}$ = probability of a negative result in patients with disease = 1–sensitivity = 0.038

B_{rx} = benefit of treatment in patients with disease = 0.95

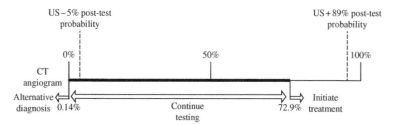

Figure 18.3 Testing and treatment threshold of CTA for penetrating extremity vascular injury. (Data from [8].)

injury, such as a shotgun wound; preexisting vascular disease in the injured extremity; missile track parallel to a vessel; extensive bone and muscle injury mimicking arterial injury; and thoracic outlet injury. Hard signs in the presence of high-risk features are an indication for an intraoperative angiogram to assess the extent and location of the injury.

References

1. Manthey DE, Nicks BA. Penetrating trauma to the extremity. *The Journal of Emergency Medicine.* 2008; 34: 187–93.
2. Pöyhönen R, Suominen V, Uurto I, Salenius J. Non-iatrogenic civilian vascular trauma in a well-defined geographical region in Finland. *European Journal of Trauma and Emergency Surgery.* 2015; 41: 545–9.
3. Gopinathan NR, Santhanam SS, Saibaba B, Dhillon MS. Epidemiology of lower limb musculoskeletal trauma with associated vascular injuries in a tertiary care institute in India. *Indian Journal of Orthopaedics.* 2017; 51: 199–204.
4. Tan TW, Joglar FL, Hamburg NM *et al.* Limb outcome and mortality in lower and upper extremity arterial injury: A comparison using the National Trauma Data Bank. *Vascular and Endovascular Surgery.* 2011; 45: 592–7.
5. Fox N, Rajani RR, Bokhari F *et al.* Evaluation and management of penetrating lower extremity arterial trauma: An Eastern Association for the Surgery of Trauma practice management guideline. *Journal of Trauma and Acute Care Surgery.* 2012; 73: S315–20.
6. Feliciano DV, Moore FA, Moore EE *et al.* Evaluation and management of peripheral vascular injury. Part 1. Western Trauma Association/critical decisions in trauma. *The Journal of Trauma.* 2011; 70: 1551–6.
7. Feliciano DV, Moore EE, West MA *et al.* Western Trauma Association critical decisions in trauma: Evaluation and management of peripheral vascular injury, part II. *Journal of Trauma and Acute Care Surgery.* 2013; 75: 391–7.
8. deSouza IS, Benabbas R, McKee S *et al.* Accuracy of physical examination, ankle-brachial index, and ultrasonography in the diagnosis of arterial injury in patients with penetrating extremity trauma: A systematic review and meta-analysis. *Academic Emergency Medicine.* 2017; 24: 994–1017.
9. Kobayashi L, Coimbra R, Goes AMO *et al.* American Association for the Surgery of Trauma-World Society of Emergency Surgery guidelines on diagnosis and management of peripheral vascular injuries. *Journal of Trauma and Acute Care Surgery.* 2020; 89: 1183–96.
10. Carpenter CR, Raja AS, Brown MD. Overtesting and the downstream consequences of overtreatment: Implications of "preventing overdiagnosis" for emergency medicine. *Academic Emergency Medicine.* 2015; 22: 1484–92.
11. Schwartz MR, Weaver FA, Bauer M, Siegel A, Yellin AE. Refining the indications for arteriography in penetrating extremity trauma: A prospective analysis. *Journal of Vascular Surgery.* 1993; 17: 116–22.

12. Inaba K, Branco BC, Reddy S et al. Prospective evaluation of multidetector computed tomography for extremity vascular trauma. *The Journal of Trauma.* 2011; 70: 808–15.

13. Kohn MA, Carpenter CR, Newman TB. Understanding the direction of bias in studies of diagnostic test accuracy. *Academic Emergency Medicine.* 2013; 20: 1194–206.

14. Gonzalez RP, Falimirski ME. The utility of physical examination in proximity penetrating extremity trauma. *The American Surgeon.* 1999; 65: 784–9.

15. Anderson RJ, Hobson RW, Lee BC et al. Reduced dependency on arteriography for penetrating extremity trauma: Influence of wound location and noninvasive vascular studies. *The Journal of Trauma.* 1990; 30: 1059–63.

16. Nassoura ZE, Ivatury RR, Simon RJ, Jabbour N, Vinzons A, Stahl W. A reassessment of Doppler pressure indices in the detection of arterial lesions in proximity penetrating injuries of extremities: A prospective study. *The American Journal of Emergency Medicine.* 1996; 14: 151–6.

17. Gagne PJ, Cone JB, McFarland D et al. Proximity penetrating extremity trauma: The role of duplex ultrasound in the detection of occult venous injuries. *The Journal of Trauma.* 1995; 39: 1157–63.

18. Soto JA, Munera F, Cardoso N, Guarin O, Medina S. Diagnostic performance of helical CT angiography in trauma to large arteries of the extremities. *Journal of Computer Assisted Tomography.* 1999; 23: 188–96.

19. Soto JA, Munera F, Morales C et al. Focal arterial injuries of the proximal extremities: Helical CT arteriography as the initial method of diagnosis. *Radiology.* 2001; 218: 188–94.

20. Inaba K, Potzman J, Munera F et al. Multi-slice CT angiography for arterial evaluation in the injured lower extremity. *The Journal of Trauma.* 2006; 60: 502–6.

21. Rieger M, Mallouhi A, Tauscher T, Lutz M, Jaschke WR. Traumatic arterial injuries of the extremities: Initial evaluation with MDCT angiography. *AJR. American Journal of Roentgenology.* 2006; 186: 656–64.

22. Iezzi R, Cotroneo AR, Pascali D, Merlino B, Storto ML. Multi-slice CT (MSCT) angiography for assessment of traumatic lesions of lower limbs peripheral arteries. *Emergency Radiology.* 2007; 14: 389–94.

23. Hogan AR, Lineen EB, Perez EA, Neville HL, Thompson WR, Sola JE. Value of computed tomographic angiography in neck and extremity pediatric vascular trauma. *Journal of Pediatric Surgery.* 2009; 44: 1236–41.

24. Seamon MJ, Smoger D, Torres DM et al. A prospective validation of a current practice: The detection of extremity vascular injury with CT angiography. *The Journal of Trauma.* 2009; 67: 238–43.

25. Foster BR, Anderson SW, Uyeda JW, Brooks JG, Soto JA. Integration of 64-detector lower extremity CT angiography into whole-body trauma imaging: Feasibility and early experience. *Radiology.* 2011; 261: 787–95.

26. Jens S, Kerstens MK, Legemate DA, Reekers JA, Bipat S, Koelemay MJW. Diagnostic performance of computed tomography angiography in peripheral arterial injury due to trauma: A systematic review and meta-analysis. *European Journal of Vascular and Endovascular Surgery.* 2013; 46: 329–37.

27. Joshi A, Nimbkar V, Merchant S, Mhashelkar Y, Talekar K. The role of CT angiography in the evaluation of peripheral vascularture using MSCT - our initial experience. *Indian Journal of Radiology and Imaging*. 2004; 14: 309–15.

28. Pauker SG, Kassirer JP. The threshold approach to clinical decision making. *The New England Journal of Medicine*. 1980; 302: 1109–17.

SECTION 3
Cardiology

Chapter 19 **Heart Failure**

Ian T. Ferguson and Christopher R. Carpenter

Department of Emergency Medicine, Washington University School of Medicine, St. Louis, MO, USA

Highlights

- The prevalence of heart failure is increasing: nearly 1 in 33 people will be diagnosed by 2030.
- No elements of history alone significantly increase diagnostic accuracy, but on physical examination, the presence of a S3 heart sound increases the likelihood of heart failure.
- BNP or NT-proBNP < 100 pg/mL or BNP > 1500 significantly decrease or increase the probability of heart failure in undifferentiated dyspnea.
- Multiple CXR findings increase the probability of heart failure, but 20% of heart failure patients present with a normal or nondiagnostic CXR.
- Lung ultrasound and echocardiography can significantly increase or decrease the probability of heart failure.

Background

Heart failure is a widespread disease that accounts for more than one million hospitalizations annually in the United States, and nearly half a million new cases arise each year. Heart failure is a syndrome diagnosed by clinical signs and symptoms demonstrating a reduction in cardiac function. Severity is typically stratified by functional status using the New York Heart Association (NYHA) classification system, and by echocardiography measurements of left ventricular ejection fraction, which is either preserved, mid-range, or reduced.[1] Heart failure is both a highly prevalent and highly morbid condition, affecting 6.2 million people in the United States alone: a number

---

Evidence-Based Emergency Care: Diagnostic Testing and Clinical Decision Rules, Third Edition.
Edited by Jesse M. Pines, Fernanda Bellolio, Christopher R. Carpenter, and Ali S. Raja.
© 2023 John Wiley & Sons Ltd. Published 2023 by John Wiley & Sons Ltd.

estimated to grow to eight million by 2030, representing nearly 1 in 33 people.[2] Prompt diagnosis and management from the emergency department (ED) is an important benchmark in the care of heart failure patients, as 80% of all hospitalizations due to heart failure are through the ED and inpatient mortality ranges from anywhere from 4% up to 25%. However, the diagnosis is not always straightforward. A study utilizing a national database found the most common specified diagnoses associated with dyspnea in ED patients (aside from the grouped diagnosis of "other and unspecified lower respiratory disease") were asthma (12.9%), chronic obstructive pulmonary disease (COPD, 11.9%), acute heart failure (8%), and pneumonia (7.1%), followed by injury (1.9%), arrhythmia (1.4%), acute coronary syndrome (0.9%), and pulmonary embolism (0.5%).[3]

The undifferentiated dyspneic patient requires careful consideration by the ED clinician, as dyspnea has a nearly two-fold odds of increased in-hospital mortality.[4] Differentiating between these diagnoses can be difficult when faced with limited information in the ED: the clinician must utilize the history, physical exam, and diagnostic tests – including natriuretic peptides, chest X-ray (CXR), and bedside ultrasound – when available in order to most accurately diagnose acute heart failure in the ED. This review will focus on the utility of the history and physical exam, natriuretic peptides, chest radiography, and lung ultrasound in the diagnosis of acute heart failure in the ED.

Clinical question

Can history, physical exam, and/or decision aids accurately and reliably distinguish congestive heart failure (CHF) from other causes of acute dyspnea in ED patients?

Two diagnostic systematic reviews quantified the role of physical examination in the diagnosis of heart failure at the time. Wang *et al.*[5] identified 815 citations from 1966 to 2005, including 22 studies in the final analysis. Martindale *et al.*[6] focused on ED-based studies and included 57 studies from 52 unique cohorts, totaling 17,893 patients. One difficulty in evaluating the diagnostic accuracy for CHF is the lack of an objective and universally accepted criterion standard; however, the most agreed-upon standard is the adjudication of the diagnosis by independent reviewers after retrospective evaluation of clinical data. Both systematic reviews only included studies with a criterion standard based on retrospective adjudication by independent reviewers.

The physical exam in acute heart failure assesses volume and perfusion in order to categorize the patient into one of four clinical profiles (Figure 19.1).[7,8]

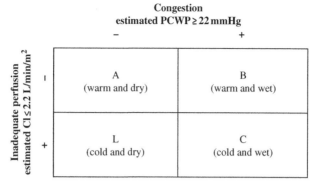

Figure 19.1 Assessing hemodynamic profiles in patients with heart failure.

Volume status can be appreciated by clinical findings such as jugular venous distension (JVD), hepatojugular reflux (HJR), orthopnea, rales, and ascites. In a sub-analysis of the Evaluation Study of Congestive Heart Failure and Pulmonary Artery Catheterization Effectiveness (ESCAPE) trial on patients with pulmonary artery catheter measurements, only JVP ≥ 12 remained associated with elevated pulmonary capillary wedge pressure (PCWP) in a multivariate analysis (odds ratio [OR] 3.3, 95% confidence interval [CI] 1.8–6.1).[9] There are fewer signs and symptoms of poor perfusion, with the two most prominent being low pulse pressure and cool extremities. Only a global assessment by the treating clinician of a "cold profile" was significantly associated with a cardiac index ≤2.2l/min/m² (OR 2.97, 95% CI 1.24–7.13).[9] Similarly in Wang et al., the "overall clinical impression" was found to be moderately specific (86%) but insensitive (61%). Summary likelihood ratios (LRs) for the initial treating physician's overall clinical impression of the diagnosis of heart failure were LR+ 4.4 (CI 1.8–10) and LR– 0.45 (CI 0.28–0.73).[5]

Thirty-one studies on history and physical examination were included in the analysis by Martindale et al. Of the variables identified in the history and physical examination, the presence of an S3 was most likely to rule in the diagnosis (LR+ 4.0, range 1.6–13) and the presence of fever was most likely to rule out the diagnosis (LR– 0.4). Electrocardiogram (ECG) findings were not helpful in ruling in or ruling out the diagnosis of CHF. Summary LRs are included in Table 19.1. Existing acute heart failure clinical decision rules were designed to estimate the risk of adverse outcome to guide admission or discharge decisions, not to rule in or rule out the diagnosis of CHF.[10]

Table 19.1 Summary of diagnostic accuracy of findings on history and physical examination, chest X-ray, and electrocardiogram (ECG)

Finding	Sensitivity, % (95% CI)	Specificity, % (95% CI)	LR+ (95% CI)	LR– (95% CI)
History				
Atrial fibrillation	30 (27–33)	85 (83–88)	2.1 (1.6–2.9)	0.82 (0.71–0.93)
Chronic renal insufficiency	32 (29–35)	91 (90–93)	3.4 (2.7–4.5)	0.75 (0.71–0.80)
Heart failure	56 (54–57)	80 (79–81)	2.7 (2.0–3.7)	0.58 (0.49–0.68)
Myocardial infarction	32 (30–34)	87 (86–88)	2.1 (1.8–2.5)	0.82 (0.76–0.89)
No history of COPD	79 (77–80)	34 (33–36)	1.2 (1.1–1.4)	0.70 (0.6–0.8)
Symptoms				
Paroxysmal nocturnal dyspnea	46 (44–49)	74 (72–76)	1.6 (1.2–2.1)	0.79 (0.71–0.88)
Orthopnea	52 (50–54)	71 (69–72)	1.9 (1.4–2.5)	0.74 (0.64–0.85)
Dyspnea at rest	55 (51–58)	50 (47–53)	1.1 (0.9–1.4)	0.88 (0.74–1.0)
Absence of cough	82 (80–84)	26 (24–28)	1.1 (1.0–1.3)	0.60 (0.5–0.8)
Physical examination				
Third heart sound	13 (12–14)	98 (97–98)	4.0 (2.7–5.9)	0.91 (0.88–0.95)
Hepatojugular reflux	14 (12–17)	93 (91–95)	2.2 (1.3–3.7)	0.91 (0.88–0.94)
Jugular vein distension	37 (36–39)	87 (86–88)	2.8 (1.7–4.5)	0.91 (0.88–0.95)
Rales	62 (61–64)	68 (67–69)	1.8 (1.5–2.1)	0.60 (0.51–0.69)
Any murmur	28 (26–30)	83 (82–85)	1.9 (0.9–3.9)	0.93 (0.79–1.1)
Leg edema	52 (51–53)	75 (74–76)	1.9 (1.6–2.3)	0.68 (0.61–0.75)
Wheezing	22 (21–24)	64 (63–65)	0.6 (0.5–0.8)	1.2 (1.1–1.3)
No fever	92 (91–94)	21 (19–23)	1.1 (1.0–1.3)	0.4 (0.3–0.6)
Chest X-ray				
Alveolar edema	6 (5–7)	99 (98–99)	5.3 (3.3–8.5)	0.95 (0.94–0.97)
Cardiomegaly	75 (73–76)	62 (59–64)	2.3 (1.6–3.4)	0.43 (0.36–0.51)
Interstitial edema	31 (28–34)	95 (94–96)	6.4 (3.4–12.2)	0.73 (0.68–0.78)
Kerley B-lines	9.2 (6.5–12.5)	99 (97–100)	6.5 (2.6–16.2)	0.88 (0.69–1.1)
Pleural effusion	16 (14–19)	93 (90–95)	2.4 (1.6–3.6)	0.89 (0.80–0.99)
Pulmonary edema	57 (55–59)	89 (88–90)	4.8 (3.6–6.4)	0.48 (0.39–0.58)
ECG				
Atrial fibrillation	20 (18–23)	90 (88–92)	2.2 (1.4–3.5)	0.88 (0.85–0.91)
Ischemic changes	34 (30–38)	84 (81–87)	2.9 (1.2–7.1)	0.78 (0.73–0.84)
Normal sinus rhythm	55 (51–60)	18 (15–21)	0.7 (0.5–0.9)	2.9 (1.3–6.6)
T-wave inversion	10 (7–13)	96 (92–98)	2.4 (1.2–4.8)	0.94 (0.90–0.98)
ST-depression	5.6 (4–8)	96 (94–98)	2.0 (1.0–3.8)	0.97 (0.95–1.0)
ST-elevation	5.2 (2–11)	92 (84–97)	0.6 (0.2–1.7)	1.0 (0.96–1.1)

Source: Data from [6].

Table 19.2 BNP levels for ED patients with acute dyspnea

BNP value (pg/mL)	Interval likelihood ratio (95% CI)	NT-proBNP value (pg/mL)	Interval likelihood ratio (95% CI)
0–100	0.14 (0.12–0.18)	0–100	0.09 (0.05–0.17)
100–200	0.29 (0.23–0.38)	100–300	0.23 (0.16–0.33)
200–300	0.89 (0.67–1.17)	300–600	0.28 (0.20–0.39)
300–400	1.34 (0.98–1.83)	600–900	0.63 (0.46–0.87)
400–500	2.05 (1.47–2.84)	900–1500	0.84 (0.67–1.06)
500–600	3.50 (2.30–5.35)	1500–3000	1.49 (1.19–1.86)
600–800	4.13 (3.01–5.68)	3000–5000	2.36 (1.81–3.08)
800–1000	5.00 (3.21–7.89)	5000–10,000	2.48 (1.91–3.21)
1000–1500	7.12 (4.53–11.18)	10,000–15,000	2.84 (1.90–4.23)
1500–2500	8.33 (4.60–15.12)	15,000–30,000	2.93 (1.95–4.39)
2500–5000	8.91 (4.09–19.43)	30,000–200,000	3.30 (2.05–5.31)

Source: Data from [6].

Clinical question

Do B-type natriuretic peptide (BNP) or N-terminal proB-type natriuretic peptide (NT-proBNP) accurately distinguish CHF from other causes of acute dyspnea in ED patients?
BNP and NT-proBNP are neurohormones secreted by cardiac ventricles under conditions of increased ventricular volumes and pressures. A diagnostic meta-analysis that included 41 studies, including 20 that evaluated BNP and 14 that evaluated NT-proBNP and seven that evaluated both is summarized in Table 19.2 with interval LRs (see Chapter 3).[6] BNP and NT-proBNP below 100 pg/mL are sufficient to rule out heart failure (interval LR when <100). Unfortunately, levels this low are not common among patients with common symptom mimics like COPD.

Clinical question

Does CXR accurately differentiate heart failure from other causes of acute dyspnea?
CXR findings that raise concern for heart failure include pulmonary edema, cardiomegaly, and pleural effusion (Figure 19.2). Other conditions have similar CXR findings. Martindale *et al.*[6] summarized 18 studies that evaluated CXR findings (Table 19.3). Notably no interobserver agreement measurements were included in any of the included studies. Interstitial edema (LR+ 6.4) and Kerley B-lines (LR+ 6.5) most accurately increased the probability of heart failure. The absence of any of these findings does not significantly decrease the probability of heart failure.

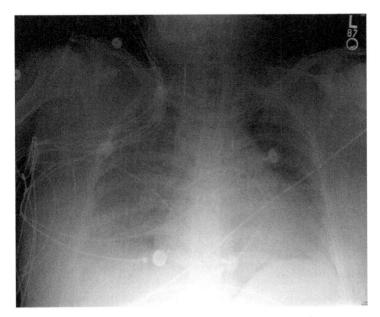

Figure 19.2 Interstitial edema seen on the chest X-ray of a patient with decompensated heart failure.

Table 19.3 Summary of diagnostic accuracy of chest X-ray findings

Finding	Sensitivity, % (95% CI)	Specificity, % (95% CI)	LR+ (95% CI)	LR– (95% CI)
Chest X-ray				
Alveolar edema	6 (5–7)	99 (98–99)	5.3 (3.3–8.5)	0.95 (0.94–0.97)
Cardiomegaly	75 (73–76)	62 (59–64)	2.3 (1.6–3.4)	0.43 (0.36–0.51)
Interstitial edema	31 (28–34)	95 (94–96)	6.4 (3.4–12.2)	0.73 (0.68–0.78)
Kerley B-lines	9.2 (6.5–12.5)	99 (97–100)	6.5 (2.6–16.2)	0.88 (0.69–1.1)
Pleural effusion	16 (14–19)	93 (90–95)	2.4 (1.6–3.6)	0.89 (0.80–0.99)
Pulmonary edema	57 (55–59)	89 (88–90)	4.8 (3.6–6.4)	0.48 (0.39–0.58)

Source: Data from [6].

Clinical question

Does point-of-care ultrasound differentiate heart failure from other causes of acute dyspnea?

Table 19.4 Summary of diagnostic accuracy of POCUS-lung and bedside echocardiography

Finding	Sensitivity, % (95% CI)	Specificity, % (95% CI)	LR+ (95% CI)	LR− (95% CI)
POCUS-lung				
Positive B-lines	85 (83–88)	93 (91–94)	7.4 (4.2–12.8)	0.16 (0.05–0.51)
Pleural effusion	64 (50–75)	72 (61–81)	2.0 (1.4–2.8)	0.49 (0.22–1.1)
Bedside echocardiography				
Increased LV end-diastolic dimension	80 (66–90)	69 (51–83)	2.5 (1.5–4.2)	0.30 (0.16–0.54)
Restrictive mitral pattern	82 (69–91)	90 (81–96)	8.3 (4.0–16.9)	0.21 (0.12–0.36)
Pulmonary edema	81 (73–87)	81 (73–86)	4.1 (2.4–7.2)	0.24 (0.17–0.35)

Source: Data from [6].

Point of care ultrasound (POCUS) for the diagnosis of CHF in the ED includes echocardiography and lung (POCUS-lung). Martingdale et al.[6] summarized eight studies in which the emergency provider was the clinician performing and interpreting POCUS-lung at bedside (Table 19.4). At least three B-lines in two lung zones bilaterally defined a "positive" POCUS-lung for heart failure. This finding had a higher LR+ point estimate (7.4, 95% CI 4.2–12.8) than any finding on radiography, history, or physical examination. The absence of B-lines was also helpful in ruling out the diagnosis (LR− 0.16, 95% CI 0.05–0.51). The authors also quantified the accuracy of bedside echocardiography based on four studies.[6] Visual estimation of reduced ejection fraction (EF) has an LR+ of 4.1 (95% 2.4–7.2) based on three studies. Restrictive mitral inflow using Doppler analysis defined as an E/A ratio >2 or E/A between 1 and 2 and deceleration time <130 msec had an LR+ of 8.3 (95% CI 4–16.9).

A more recent systematic review and meta-analysis synthesized six studies focused on directly comparing POCUS-lung US and chest radiography.[11] Five of these studies used retrospective expert review as the criterion standard, while the sixth used a combination of echocardiography, BNP, and CXR. CXR had LR+ of 7.36 (95% CI, 2.70–20.07) and LR− of 0.30 (95% CI 0.26–0.35). POCUS-lung had LR+ of 8.63 (95% CI, 6.93–10.74) and LR− of 0.14 (95% CI 0.06–0.29). The difference in LR between POCUS-lung and CXR may be larger than reported given the lack of blinding in evaluating CXR and incorporating CXR into the reference standard in one study. This incorporation bias would falsely elevate the reported sensitivity and specificity of CXR in that study (Chapter 6).[12]

Comment

The diagnosis of heart failure in adult patients presenting to the ED with undifferentiated dyspnea remains challenging and current emergency medicine clinical practice guidelines are outdated.[13] These challenges should probably not be surprising because heart failure represents a range of pathologies that include systolic and diastolic dysfunction in addition to valvular heart disease, pulmonary hypertension, and end-stage renal disease-related hypervolemia. In addition, ED patients at higher risk for heart failure often present with co-morbidities that may not have been previously documented including COPD and venous thromboembolism. In addition, access to previous echocardiography results is sometimes limited and multidisciplinary research or clinical practice guidelines are lacking.[14,15]

Specific elements of the history, physical examination, CXR, and POCUS-lung are valuable in evaluating patients with suspected heart failure. In addition to the initial clinician's clinical judgment, patient histories of heart failure and myocardial infarction are both useful for increasing the probability of heart failure when present. On physical exam, the presence of a third heart sound (ventricular filling gallop) significantly increases the probability of heart failure. The absence of any common history (exertional dyspnea, orthopnea) or exam findings (edema, rales) does not significantly decrease the probability of heart failure as the etiology of undifferentiated dyspnea. Notably absent are reliability studies quantifying intra- or inter-clinician agreement on the presence or absence of these subjective physical exam findings. Future researchers might quantify the accuracy of an ED walk test for the diagnosis of heart failure in undifferentiated dyspnea.[16]

The presence of pulmonary edema and/or Kerley B-lines on CXR significantly increases the probability of heart failure, but their absence does not decrease that probability significantly. Indeed, 20% of heart failure patients will present to the ED with a normal CXR.[17] ECG findings are unhelpful to rule in or to rule out heart failure but are essential to identify acute coronary syndrome as an etiology of undifferentiated dyspnea.[18]

BNP or NT-proBNP levels less than 100 pg/mL or BNP levels greater than 1500 pg/mL can significantly decrease or increase the probability of heart failure. However, BNP can also be elevated secondary to acute cardiac syndrome or pulmonary embolism and in the chronic setting, these might include pulmonary hypertension and systemic conditions of volume overload (as in the case of end-stage renal disease necessitating hemodialysis). Therefore, an elevated BNP should be interpreted with these other conditions in mind. In addition, multiple randomized controlled trials suggest that awareness of BNP in ED patients with suspected heart failure does not improve measurable operational or patient-centered outcomes.[19] BNP levels may be more helpful in the dyspneic patient in whom there is not a high suspicion of heart failure, since an elevated level may prompt consideration of the diagnosis in a patient otherwise thought to have another pulmonary disease (e.g., asthma or COPD).

Appropriate ED assessment of the acutely dyspneic patient using physical exam, CXR, and BNP/NT-proBNP level can allow clinicians to tailor appropriate therapies for suspected heart failure. While a number of decision rules allow risk stratification of patients with heart failure, they were designed to prognosticate outcomes after the diagnosis of heart failure has been made and not as diagnostic aids.[9,10]

References

1. Ponikowski P, Voors AA, Anker SD *et al.* 2016 ESC guidelines for the diagnosis and treatment of acute and chronic heart failure: The Task Force for the diagnosis and treatment of acute and chronic heart failure of the European Society of Cardiology (ESC). Developed with the special contribution of the Heart Failure Association (HFA) of the ESC. *European Journal of Heart Failure.* 2016; 18(8): 891–975.

2. Hollenberg SM, Warner Stevenson L, Ahmad T *et al.* 2019 ACC expert consensus decision pathway on risk assessment, management, and clinical trajectory of patients hospitalized with heart failure: A report of the American College of Cardiology Solution Set Oversight Committee. *Journal of the American College of Cardiology.* 2019; 74(15): 1966–2011.

3. Hale ZE, Singhal A, Hsia RY. Causes of shortness of breath in the acute patient: A national study. *Academic Emergency Medicine.* 2018; 25(11): 1227–34.

4. Safwenberg U, Terent A, Lind L. The emergency department presenting complaint as predictor of in-hospital fatality. *European Journal of Emergency Medicine.* 2007; 14(6): 324–31.

5. Wang CS, FitzGerald JM, Schulzer M, Mak E, Ayas NT. Does this dyspneic patient in the emergency department have congestive heart failure? *JAMA.* 2005; 294(15): 1944–56.

6. Martindale JL, Wakai A, Collins SP *et al.* Diagnosing acute heart failure in the emergency department: A systematic review and meta-analysis. *Academic Emergency Medicine.* 2016; 23(3): 223–42.

7. Nohria A, Tsang SW, Fang JC *et al.* Clinical assessment identifies hemodynamic profiles that predict outcomes in patients admitted with heart failure. *Journal of the American College of Cardiology.* 2003; 41(10): 1797–804.

8. Thibodeau JT, Drazner MH. The role of the clinical examination in patients with heart failure. *JACC. Heart Failure.* 2018; 6(7): 543–51.

9. Drazner MH, Hellkamp AS, Leier CV *et al.* Value of clinician assessment of hemodynamics in advanced heart failure: The ESCAPE trial. *Circulation. Heart Failure.* 2008; 1(3): 170–7.

10. Stiell IG, Perry JJ, Clement CM *et al*. Prospective and explicit clinical validation of the Ottawa heart failure risk scale, with and without use of quantitative NT-proBNP. *Academic Emergency Medicine*. 2017; 24(3): 316–27.
11. Maw AM, Hassanin A, Ho PM *et al*. Diagnostic accuracy of point-of-care lung ultrasonography and chest radiography in adults with symptoms suggestive of acute decompensated heart failure: A systematic review and meta-analysis. *JAMA Network Open*. 2019; 2(3): e190703.
12. Kohn MA, Carpenter CR, Newman TB. Understanding the direction of bias in studies of diagnostic test accuracy. *Academic Emergency Medicine*. 2013; 20(11): 1194–206.
13. Silvers SM, Howell JM, Kosowsky JM, Rokos IC, Jagoda AS. Clinical policy: Critical issues in the evaluation and management of adult patients presenting to the emergency department with acute heart failure syndromes. *Annals of Emergency Medicine*. 2007; 49(5): 627–69.
14. Collins SP, Levy PD, Fermann GJ *et al*. What's next for acute heart failure research. *Academic Emergency Medicine*. 2018; 25(1): 85–93.
15. Wallace PJ. What's next for acute heart failure research: A call for multidisciplinary collaborations. *Academic Emergency Medicine*. 2018; 25(8): 969–70.
16. Pan AM, Stiell IG, Clement CM, Acheson J, Aaron SD. Feasibility of a structured 3-minute walk test as a clinical decision tool for patients presenting to the emergency department with acute dyspnoea. *Emergency Medicine Journal*. 2009; 26(4): 278–82.
17. Collins SP, Lindsell CJ, Storrow AB, Abraham WT. Prevalence of negative chest radiography results in the emergency department patient with decompensated heart failure. *Annals of Emergency Medicine*. 2006; 47(1): 13–8.
18. Kohn MA, Steinhart B. Broadcasting not properly: Using B-type natriuretic peptide interval likelihood ratios and the results of other emergency department tests to diagnose acute heart failure in dyspneic patients. *Academic Emergency Medicine*. 2016; 23(3): 347–50.
19. Carpenter CR, Keim SM, Worster A, Rosen P, Beem. Brain natriuretic peptide in the evaluation of emergency department dyspnea: Is there a role? *The Journal of Emergency Medicine*. 2012; 42(2): 197–205.

Chapter 20 **Syncope**

Lucas Oliveira Junqueira e Silva[1,2] and Fernanda Bellolio[1]

[1] Department of Emergency Medicine, Mayo Clinic, Rochester, MN, USA
[2] Department of Emergency Medicine, Hospital de Clínicas de Porto Alegre, Porto Alegre, Brazil

Highlights

- Most patients with syncope are well appearing in the ED, and only a small proportion will have a life-threatening precipitant.
- Several clinical decision rules have been developed to differentiate patients who can safely be discharged from the ED.
- The Canadian Syncope Risk Score has been externally validated and has shown promising results.
- Cardiac biomarkers, especially high-sensitive troponin and NT-proBNP, have a prognostic role in patients presenting with syncope and might be a potential additional tool for emergency physicians.
- Head CT in patients presenting with syncope has a very low diagnostic yield and clinical decision rules need to be developed in order to decrease unnecessary imaging in this population.

Background

Syncope is a transient loss of consciousness associated with a return to preexisting neurological function. It accounts for up to 2% of all emergency department (ED) visits. Syncope is a symptom and has a wide variety of causes, ranging from benign to life threatening. The evaluation of patients with "unstable" syncope where there is a clear etiology (e.g., ongoing chest pain, gastrointestinal bleeding, or cardiac rhythm disturbances) can typically be focused on correcting or treating the underlying cause. The evaluation of

Evidence-Based Emergency Care: Diagnostic Testing and Clinical Decision Rules, Third Edition.
Edited by Jesse M. Pines, Fernanda Bellolio, Christopher R. Carpenter, and Ali S. Raja.
© 2023 John Wiley & Sons Ltd. Published 2023 by John Wiley & Sons Ltd.

syncope that is "stable" poses a greater diagnostic conundrum to the emergency physician because in approximately half of these cases, the cause for syncope is unclear, even after a thorough ED evaluation.[1-3] Even in stable patients with syncope, there are several potentially lethal causes including cardiac arrhythmias, myocardial infarction, ruptured ectopic pregnancy, subarachnoid hemorrhage, and pulmonary embolism. The clinical presentation can sometimes be confused with other conditions where there is a loss of consciousness like seizures (see Chapter 49), vertigo, dizziness, coma, or shock, and can be the result of trauma, alcohol intoxication, or other toxic substances.

As a result of the diagnostic uncertainty and the multiple potentially serious etiologies of syncope, patients are frequently admitted to the hospital for further evaluation, monitoring, and additional testing. As an inpatient, patients may receive further diagnostic testing such as echocardiogram, electroencephalogram, cardiac monitoring, and cardiac stress testing.[4] The yield of hospitalizations in this population with diagnostic uncertainty, however, has been questioned.[5] Specific treatments, such as pacemakers or defibrillators, can be used if a cardiac arrhythmia is determined as the cause for syncope (see Chapter 22), or changes in medication that impact blood pressure, heart rate, or underlying rhythm disturbances may be made to reduce the risk of syncope in the future. Over the last decade, numerous studies have been performed to identify lower-risk syncope patients who may be safe for discharge after ED evaluation, as well as to identify those at higher risk for short-term major adverse events.

Clinical question

Can elements of the history, physical exam, and basic workup risk stratify adult patients who present with syncope to the ED?

A review[6] in the JAMA Rational Exam Series has identified key elements from the ED evaluation that both increase and decrease the probability of cardiac syncope (Table 20.1). Gibson *et al.*[7] conducted a systematic review on predictors of short-term outcomes (30 days) after syncope, and among 17 studies, the following predictors were found to have the highest yield, (i) *clinical findings*: elevated blood urea nitrogen (BUN) (positive likelihood ratio [LR+] 2.86), history of congestive heart failure (CHF) (LR+ 2.65), initial low blood pressure (LR+ 2.62), history of arrhythmia (LR+ 2.32), abnormal troponin (LR+ 2.49); (ii) *symptoms:* dyspnea (LR+ 2.29); and (iii) *physical exam findings:* hypotension (LR+ 2.62), altered respiratory rate (LR+ 2.26).

Toarta *et al.*[8] investigated the emergency physician's syncope diagnosis and its association with 30-day serious outcome after ED disposition. In a large

Table 20.1 Elements of history, physical exam, and basic workup and their ability to increase or decrease the probability of cardiac syncope

Increased probability of cardiac syncope	Decreased probability of cardiac syncope
Age at first episode ≥35 (LR+ 3.3)	Age < 35 (LR+ 0.13)
History of atrial fibrillation or flutter (LR+ 7.3)	Warm place (LR+ 0.17)
Severe structural heart disease (LR+ 3.3–4.8)	Pain or medical procedure (LR+ 0.12)
Dyspnea (LR+ 3.5)	After using the toilet (LR+ 0.05)
Chest pain prior to syncope (LR+ 3.4–3.8)	Headache prior to syncope (LR+ 0.17)
Witnessed cyanosis during syncope (LR+ 6.2)	Feeling cold prior to syncope (LR+ 0.16)
Elevated cardiac troponin (LR+ 2.3–5.4)	Mood change or prodromal preoccupation with details prior to syncope (LR+ 0.09)
Elevated BNP (LR+ 1.8–47)	Normal cardiac troponin (LR+ 0.15–0.39) Normal BNP (LR+ 0.16–0.20)

Source: Data from [6].

prospective cohort of 5010 patients of whom 177 (3.5%) had serious short-term outcomes, the ED diagnostic category assigned by the emergency physician strongly correlated with the probability of 30-day serious outcome. There were no reported deaths in the vasovagal syncope group, and patients in this group had the lowest serious outcome rates. Patients with a clear history of vasovagal syncope as identified by an emergency physician had a very good prognosis in this study.

A 2010 systematic review[9] identified nine different clinical decision rules (CDRs) for adults presenting with syncope to the ED. Among all of these instruments, only two rules were externally validated at that time (The San Francisco Syncope Rule [SFSR] and the Osservatorio Epidemiologico sulla Sincope nel Lazio [OESIL] risk score). The SFSR focused on predicting 7 and 30-day outcomes, while the OESIL looked at 1-year endpoints. An expert consortium developed standardized reporting guidelines for ED syncope stratification research in 2012,[10] and it was determined that ED-based risk stratification tools should identify serious outcomes occurring at the ED visit or within 7–30 days after discharge. For this reason, in this chapter, we will consider only those CDRs that have their outcomes defined in accordance with this timeframe. This includes the following CDRs in various stages of derivation and validation: the SFSR, the Boston syncope criteria, the Risk stratification of syncope in the ED (ROSE) rule, the Short-Term Prognosis of

Syncope (STePS), the Syncope Risk Score, the Canadian Syncope Risk Score (CSRS), and the FAINT score.

San Francisco Syncope Rule (SFSR)

In 2004, Quinn et al. derived[11] and, 2 years later, validated, the SFSR. The authors used outcomes at 7 days as the standard by which to assess whether a patient with syncope requires hospital admission. The outcomes included mortality, myocardial infarction, arrhythmia, pulmonary embolism, stroke, subarachnoid hemorrhage, significant hemorrhage, or return to the ED. In the derivation study, the authors followed 684 patients with syncope or near syncope who were evaluated in the ED. Of the 684, there were 79 (11.5%) serious outcomes. They performed a kappa analysis (test of interrater agreement) and only used variables with good agreement (0.5–1.0) for the decision rule. The rule, which required the absence of all the risk factors listed in Table 20.2, was 96% (confidence interval [CI] 92–100%) sensitive and 62% (CI 58–66%) specific for identifying serious outcomes at 7 days (Table 20.3). If the rule had been applied to the derivation cohort, it could have safely decreased admission rates for syncope by 10%.

The initial validation of the SFSR conducted by the same group included 791 consecutive ED visits for syncope, with 53 (6.7%) serious reported outcomes within 30 days. The authors found that the rule was 98% sensitive (CI 89–100%) and 56% specific (CI 52–60%). Some limitations of the study included that it was conducted at only one hospital. Because they used a composite outcome that included multiple serious outcomes, the study was not powered to detect any outcome (such as pulmonary embolism) individually. The authors advocated that the rule should be used as a risk stratification instrument rather than as an admission guideline, citing the fact that there are many reasons for admission to the hospital.

Saccilotto et al.[13] conducted a systematic review and found 11 validation studies from five different countries (Australia, Canada, Italy, the United Kingdom, and the United States) looking at the performance of the SFSR. For nine studies including all patients presenting with syncope to the ED, the

Table 20.2 San Francisco Syncope Rule

• Abnormal electrocardiogram (ECG) • Complaint of shortness of breath • Hematocrit less than 30% • Triage systolic blood pressure of less than 90 mmHg • History of congestive heart failure	**Interpretation:** the presence of at least one of these variables identified the patient as high risk (SFSR positive)

Table 20.3 Performance of San Francisco Syncope Rule (SFSR) in derivation and validation studies

Rule	N	Sensitivity	Specificity	NPV	PPV	LR–	LR+
Quinn et al. (the United States)[11] – 7-day serious outcomes*							
SFSR	684	76/79, 96.2%	375/605, 61.9%	99.2%	24.8%	0.06	2.53
Quinn et al. (the United States)[12] – 30-day serious outcomes							
SFSR	713	52/53, 98%	370/660, 56%	99.7%	15%	0.03	2.23
Serrano et al. (meta-analysis, 10 studies)[9]							
SFSR	5468	86%	49%	NR	NR	0.28	1.74
Saccilotto et al. (meta-analysis, 12 studies)[13]							
SFSR	5316	87%	53%	97%	19%	NR	NR
Tan et al. (Singapore)[14] – 7-day serious outcomes							
SFSR	1194	130/138, 94.2%	536/1056, 50.8%	98.5%	20%	0.1	1.9
Costantino et al. (individual data meta-analysis, three studies)[15] – 10-day serious outcome							
SFSR	2348	76%	53%	NR	NR	0.45	1.61
Costantino et al. (individual data meta-analysis, three studies)[15] – 30-day serious outcome							
SFSR	2348	74%	61%	NR	NR	0.43	1.89

* *Serious outcomes* were defined as death, myocardial infarction, arrhythmia, pulmonary embolism, stroke, subarachnoid hemorrhage, significant hemorrhage, or any condition causing or likely to cause a return ED visit, and hospitalization for a related event.
NR = not reported by the systematic review and numbers unavailable for calculations; NPV = negative predictive value; PPV = positive predictive value; LR = likelihood ratio.

pooled sensitivity and specificity were 85% (CI 76–92%) and 51% (CI 39–64%), respectively. When looking at the five studies that included a subgroup analysis on patients without a cause for syncope identified in the ED, the pooled sensitivity and specificity were 88% (CI 70–96%) and 54% (CI 44–63%), respectively. The authors reported substantial between-study heterogeneity that resulted in a 95% prediction interval for sensitivity of 55–98%. In patients with all high-risk factors absent, the probability of a serious outcome was 5% or lower, and it was 2% or lower when the rule was used for patients where no cause of syncope was identified after initial ED evaluation.

When looking individually across the different validation studies of SFSR,[13] sensitivity levels ranged from as low as 52% to as high as 100%. However, it is important to note that none of the validation studies applied the SFSR as originally outlined in the derivation study, which may explain its variable performance across different settings.

In 2013, the SFSR was prospectively validated in two Asian EDs.[14] A total of 1194 patients (age $\geq$ 12) presenting with syncope or near syncope to the ED were included for analysis, of whom 138 (11.6%) had a serious outcome at 7 days. Sensitivity was 94.2% (CI 89–97%) and specificity was 50.8% (CI 47.7–53.8%). However, when excluding events that happened in the ED, sensitivity went down to 93.6% (CI 82.8–97.8%). In this cohort, there were nine adverse events in eight patients who were not identified by the rule as high-risk. Emergency physician's judgment, independent of the rule, correctly identified all 138 patients and admitted them to the hospital.

In a 2014 individual data meta-analysis,[15] Costantino *et al.* compared the SFSR with clinical judgment to predict 10- and 30-day serious outcomes. SFSR had a sensitivity of 76% for 10-day outcomes and 74% for 30-day outcomes, with a specificity of 53% for 10-day outcomes and 61% for 30-day outcomes. Independent clinical judgment of the emergency physician, however, had a much better performance (sensitivity of 95% and specificity of 55% for 10-day outcomes; sensitivity of 94% and specificity of 50% for 30-day outcomes).

In 2018, a large prospective cohort study[16] included 1490 patients (age $\geq$ 40) presenting with syncope to 13 different EDs in eight countries (Switzerland, Spain, Germany, Italy, Poland, New Zealand, Australia, and the United States), and compared nine risk stratification scores with early clinical judgment in regards to the ability of predicting death, major cardiac adverse events (MACE), and the diagnosis of cardiac syncope. When looking at the accuracy of analyzed scores for the prediction of MACE at 30 days, the SFSR had the lowest area under the curve (AUC) when compared to other tools. Its ability to predict death and MACE at 2-year follow-up included sensitivities of 84% (death) and 85.7% (MACE). Again, emergency physician judgment outperformed all risk scores when predicting cardiac syncope (AUC 0.87). The authors published an analysis from the same cohort[17] evaluating the prognostic accuracy of cardiac biomarkers (B-type natriuretic peptide [BNP] and troponin) when compared to different risk scores. The SFSR had significantly inferior prognostic accuracy for MACE (AUC 0.64) when compared to biomarkers such as BNP, N-terminal proB-type natriuretic peptide (NT-proBNP), high-sensitivity troponin I (hs-cTnI), and high-sensitivity troponin T (hs-cTnT) (AUCs 0.75–0.79).

Boston syncope criteria

In 2007, Grossman *et al.*[18] derived the Boston syncope criteria. They conducted a prospective observational study that included patients 18 and older with syncope from a single, academic hospital. The primary outcome was a critical intervention or adverse outcome that occurred during the ED stay or subsequent hospitalization, or within 30 days after the initial visit. Critical interventions were the placement of a pacemaker or implantable cardiac defibrillator, coronary intervention, surgery, blood transfusion, cardiopulmonary resuscitation (CPR), alterations in antiarrhythmic therapy, endoscopy with intervention, or intervention for carotid stenosis. Adverse outcomes were death, pulmonary embolism, stroke, severe infection or sepsis, ventricular dysrhythmia, atrial dysrhythmia, intracranial hemorrhage, myocardial infarction, cardiac arrest, or life-threatening sequelae of syncope (e.g., rhabdomyolysis or long-bone or cervical spine fractures). The Boston syncope criteria are described in Table 20.4.

Among 362 patients enrolled with syncope, there was complete follow-up in 81% at 30 days. A total of 68 patients (23% of 293) had either a critical intervention or adverse outcome. The derived rule identified 66 of 68 patients with a sensitivity of 97% (95% CI 93–100%) and a specificity of 62% (95% CI 56–69%). Notably, the rule was not derived using standard decision rule methods such as recursive partitioning (see Chapter 4). Instead, according to

Table 20.4 Boston syncope criteria

• Signs and symptoms of acute coronary syndrome (e.g., chest pain, ischemic ECG, or other significant arrhythmia)	**Interpretation:** the presence of at least one of these variables identified the patient as high risk (Boston positive)
• Worrisome cardiac history (e.g., history of coronary disease, heart failure, or significant arrhythmia)	
• Family history of sudden death in first-degree relative	
• Valvular heart disease (murmur noted in history or on ED examination)	
• Signs of cardiac conduction disease	
• Volume depletion (gastrointestinal bleeding, hematocrit <30, and dehydration not corrected in the ED)	
• Persistence (>15 min) of abnormal vital signs in the ED without the need of concurrent interventions such as oxygen, pressors, and temporary pacemakers	
• Primary central nervous system event (stroke or subarachnoid hemorrhage)	

the authors, the Boston syncope criteria were developed using previous work such as the SFSR, clinical guidelines, and clinical judgment.

In the same ED, the authors conducted a before–after study to assess the effectiveness of implementing the Boston syncope criteria.[19] They conducted an in-service training on the rule and implemented it as a clinical guideline that encouraged emergency physicians to make admission decisions based on the criteria. In the "before" phase, 69% of patients with syncope were admitted (which was the original cohort for the derivation), while in the "after" phase, 58% were admitted (an 11% reduction in admission rate). In the 160 patients admitted in the "after" phase, 64 (40%) had adverse events during hospitalization, compared to none in the discharged group. When follow-up was conducted at 30 days, six additional patients (4%) had adverse outcomes, all of whom were admitted initially. The authors concluded that a real-time application of the Boston syncope criteria had a sensitivity of 100% (CI 94–100%) and a specificity of 57% (CI 50–63%). In a prospective cohort study by du Fay de Lavallaz et al.,[16] for the prediction of death and MACE at 2 years of follow-up, the rule had a sensitivity of 100% and 99.7%, respectively. However, the performance for short-term outcomes was not explicitly reported by the authors.

Short-Term Prognosis of Syncope (STePS)

In 2008, Costantino et al.[20] conducted a prospective cohort study at four different EDs in Italy. A total of 676 patients presenting with syncope to the ED were included, of which 41 (6.1%) experienced severe outcomes (death, the need for major therapeutic procedures, and readmission to hospital) within 10 days after presentation. Through logistic regression and stepwise backward technique, they identified four variables significantly associated with severe short-term outcomes (10-day follow-up): abnormal electrocardiogram (ECG) at presentation (adjusted odds ratio [aOR] 6.9), concomitant trauma (aOR 2.9), absence of previous symptoms (aOR 2.4), and male gender (aOR 2.2). Although they have identified the variables in this derivation study, the authors did not proceed to create a CDR, and the performance of these variables together as a tool on predicting short-term outcomes was not described.

Syncope risk score

In 2009, Sun et al.[21] performed a retrospective cohort study to identify predictors of 30-day serious events after syncope in older adults (age ≥ 60) presenting with syncope or near syncope to the ED. Serious events were defined as 30-day endpoints such as death, arrhythmias, myocardial infarction, a new diagnosis of structural heart disease thought to be related to

Table 20.5 Syncope risk score

Age > 90 years (+1 point)	Interpretation:
Male sex (+1 point)	−1, 0: low risk (2.5% risk in 30 days)
History of arrhythmia (+1 point)	1, 2: intermediate risk (6.3%)
Triage systolic blood pressure > 160 (+1 point)	3–6: high risk (20%)
Abnormal ECG (+1 point)	
Abnormal troponin I (+1 point)	
Near-syncope (−1 point)	

syncope, pulmonary embolism, aortic dissection, stroke/transient ischemic attack, subarachnoid or nontraumatic cerebral hemorrhage, and significant hemorrhage or anemia requiring blood transfusion. Cardiac interventions were also considered as serious events. In this cohort of 2584 older adults, 173 (7%) had a serious event within 30 days after their initial ED evaluation. Through the development of a multivariable logistic regression model, they identified six variables associated with increased risk and one variable associated with decreased risk (Table 20.5). This risk score is yet to be externally validated.

Risk stratification of syncope in the ED (ROSE)

In 2010, a group from the United Kingdom aimed to derive and validate a CDR for syncope, called the ROSE.[22] They conducted the study in a single center and used a split derivation and validation cohort, both consisting of 550 patients. The authors defined their outcome as all-cause death, or serious outcomes (acute myocardial infarction, life-threatening arrhythmia, decision to implant a pacemaker or cardiac defibrillator, pulmonary embolism, stroke, intracranial hemorrhage, subarachnoid hemorrhage, hemorrhage requiring a blood transfusion of ≥2 units, acute surgical procedure, or endoscopic intervention). In the derivation cohort, 1-month serious outcome or all-cause death happened in 40 (7.3%) patients. Predictors included an elevated BNP (odds ratio [OR] 7.3), fecal occult blood (OR 13.2), a low hemoglobin (OR 6.7), an oxygen saturation ≤94% (OR 3.0), and a Q-wave on the presenting ECG (OR 2.8). In the validation cohort, 1-month serious outcome or all-cause death occurred in 39 (7.1%) patients. The ROSE rule that was derived is listed in Table 20.6.

In the validation cohort,[22] the ROSE rule had a sensitivity of 87% and a specificity of 66%. The negative predictive value of the rule was 99%. The authors noted that an elevated BNP alone was the major predictor of serious cardiovascular outcomes (i.e., it predicted 36% of the events) and deaths (i.e., 89% of the deaths).

Table 20.6 The ROSE rule

Bradycardia (heart rate ≤ 50 beats per minutes in the ED) or prehospital BNP level ≥ 300 pg/mL **R**ectal exam showing fecal occult blood **A**nemia – hemoglobin (90 g/dL) **C**hest pain associated with syncope **E**CG showing a Q wave (not in lead III) **S**aturation of oxygen ≤ 94% on room air	**Interpretation:** the presence of at least one of these variables identified the patient as high risk (ROSE positive)

In an external validation study including 356 adult patients (age ≥ 18) in Iran, there were 26 (7.3%) serious outcomes.[23] Bozorgi et al. found a sensitivity of only 46% (12/26) and a specificity of 95%.

One large prospective multicenter cohort study[17] to risk stratify syncope and compare CDRs reported that cardiac biomarkers were significantly higher in cardiac syncope versus other causes of syncope. The prognostic accuracy of these laboratory markers for MACE was moderate-to-good (AUC 0.75–0.79); superior to ROSE, OESIL, and SFSR, and inferior to the CSRS.

Canadian Syncope Risk Score (CSRS)

In 2016, a group from Canada derived the CSRS through a prospective cohort study including 4030 adults (age ≥ 16) presenting within 24 hours of syncope to six different EDs.[24] Within the 30-day follow-up period, there were 147 (3.6%) serious adverse events after disposition from the ED. Serious adverse events were defined as any serious condition related to syncope within 30 days after disposition from the ED and included: death, arrhythmia, myocardial infarction, serious structural heart disease, aortic dissection, pulmonary embolism, severe pulmonary hypertension, severe hemorrhage, subarachnoid hemorrhage, any other serious condition causing syncope, and procedural interventions for the treatment of syncope. The derived rule is illustrated in Table 20.7 and included variables related to clinical evaluation, investigations, and diagnosis in the ED. The sensitivity and specificity for a threshold of −2 were 99.2% and 25.4%, respectively. For a threshold of −1, the sensitivity and specificity were 97.7% and 45.1%, respectively. The same authors derived a similar tool[25] to predict 30-day arrhythmia after ED disposition in 5010 patients. The outcome included a composite of death (due to arrhythmia or unknown cause), arrhythmia, and procedural interventions to treat arrhythmias within 30 days of ED disposition. At 30-day follow-up, 106 (2.1%) suffered study outcomes. The model included eight variables as depicted in Table 20.8. The sensitivity was 97.1% for a threshold score of 0.

Table 20.7 Canadian Syncope Risk Score (CSRS) – outcome of all 30-day serious adverse events

Clinical evaluation	Interpretation:
Predisposition to vasovagal symptoms (–1 point)	–3, –2: very low risk (0.4–0.7% risk in 30 days)
History of heart disease (+1 point)	–1, 0: low risk (1.2–1.9%)
Any systolic pressure <90 or >180mmHg (+2 points)	+1–3: medium risk (3.1–8.1%)
Investigations	+4, 5: high risk (12.9–19.7%)
Elevated troponin (>99th percentile) (+2 points)	+6–11: very high risk (28.9–83.6%)
Abnormal QRS axis (< –30 or >100) (+1 point)	**Performance:**
QRS duration>130ms (+1 point)	
Corrected QT interval>480ms (+2 points)	–2 points or higher threshold:
Diagnosis in the emergency department	Sensitivity 99.2% (CI 95.9–100%)
Vasovagal syncope (–2 points)	Specificity 25.4% (CI 23.9–26.8%)
Cardiac syncope (+2 points)	
Total score: –3–+11	

Source: Data from [24].

Table 20.8 Canadian Syncope Arrhythmia Risk Score (CSARS) – outcome of 30-day arrhythmia

Clinical evaluation	Interpretation:
Predisposition to vasovagal symptoms (–1 point)	–2–0: very low risk (0.2–0.9% risk in 30 days)
History of heart disease (+1 point)	+1: low risk (1.9%)
Any systolic pressure <90 or >180mmHg (+1 point)	+2, 3: medium risk (3.8–7.5%)
Investigations	+4, 5: high risk (14.3–25.4%)
Elevated troponin (>99th percentile) (+ 1 point)	+6–8: very high risk (41.1–74.5%)
QRS duration>130ms (+2 points)	**Performance:**
Corrected QT interval>480ms (+1 point)	
Diagnosis in the emergency department	0 points or higher
Vasovagal syncope (–1 point)	Sensitivity 97.1% (CI 91.6–99.4%)
Cardiac syncope (+2 points)	Specificity 53.4% (CI 52–54.9%)
Total score: –2–+8	

Source: Data from [25].

Most recently, the CSRS rule has been externally validated in a prospective multicenter cohort study conducted at nine EDs across Canada.[26] Among 3819 patients analyzed, 139 (3.6%) experienced 30-day serious outcomes after ED disposition. The accuracy of the CSRS remained high with an AUC of 0.91 (CI 0.88–0.93), similar to the derivation phase (AUC 0.87). The very low-risk category had 0.3% rate of serious events, the low-risk category 0.7%, and the very high-risk category had 51.3% rate of serious events. For a threshold of −1, the sensitivity was 97.8%.

The authors and collaborators went one step further and developed a clinical decision aid[27] based on CSRS risk estimates to be used in patients with syncope in the ED whenever shared decision-making is appropriate (Chapter 59). The implementation of this tool is yet to be evaluated in regards to decreasing admission rates and improving patient-centered outcomes.

In a large prospective multicenter cohort study performed by the BASEL investigators from eight different countries including 1913 patients,[16] the CSRS outperformed all cardiac biomarkers and other risk stratification scores in regards to the prediction of MACE at 2-year follow-up (AUC 0.88). The raw numbers to calculate sensitivity and specificity, however, were not reported by authors.

FAINT score

Probst et al.[28] derived and internally validated the FAINT score, a geriatric-specific syncope risk stratification tool, in 11 different EDs in the United States (Table 20.9) A total of 3177 older adults (age ≥ 60) presenting with unexplained syncope or near syncope to the ED were included, of which 181 (5.7%) experienced the primary outcome. Primary outcome was defined as 30-day all-cause death and serious cardiac outcome (significant cardiac arrhythmia, myocardial infarction, new diagnosis of significant structural

Table 20.9 FAINT score

History of heart **F**ailure (+1 point)	Interpretation:
History of cardiac **A**rrhythmia (+1 point)	0: low risk (0.9% risk in 30 days)
Initial abnormal ECG result (+1 point)	≥1: high risk (6.9%)
Elevated pro-B**N**P (+2 points)	**Performance:**
Elevated high-sensitivity **T**roponin (+1 point)	Threshold of ≥1 point:
Total score: 0–6 points	Sensitivity 97% (CI 93–99%)
	Specificity 22% (CI 21–24%)
	PPV: 7% (CI 6–8%)
	NPV: 99% (98–100%)

Source: Data from [28].

heart disease, or cardiac intervention). The FAINT score was derived as shown in Table 20.9. The tool was developed to identify patients at low risk and primarily rule out serious cardiac outcomes, which may allow emergency physicians to avoid unnecessary hospital admissions of geriatric patients. When they compared the FAINT score with unstructured physician judgment, the score had higher AUC (0.70 versus 0.63). This score is yet to be externally validated.

Clinical question

Can cardiac biomarkers identify patients with syncope who are at high risk for short-term serious outcomes?

Thiruganasambandamoorthy et al.[29] included 11 studies with low to moderate risk of bias in a systematic review published in 2015 to evaluate the ability of cardiac biomarkers to predict MACE. Pooled test characteristics of contemporary troponin, natriuretic peptide, and high-sensitivity troponin are illustrated in Table 20.10.

In a large prospective multicenter study with a median patient age of 71 years,[17] the BASEL group found that the prognostic accuracy of BNP, NT-proBNP, hs-cTnI, and hs-cTnT for death and MACE was moderate-to-good (AUCs 0.74–0.78 for death; AUCs 0.75–0.76 for MACE). All biomarkers performed similarly in the short-term 30-day follow-up, and were superior to the clinical prediction rules ROSE, OESIL, and SFSR, but inferior to the CSRS. In the short-term outcomes, however, troponins performed better for ischemic MACE, whereas BNPs performed better for arrhythmic MACE. When the diagnostic accuracy of biomarkers was evaluated for the diagnosis of cardiac syncope, it also had moderate-to-good performance (all AUCs 0.77–0.78).

Table 20.10 Pooled test characteristics of cardiac biomarkers to predict MACE

Sensitivity (CI)	Specificity (CI)	LR+	LR−
Contemporary troponin (4 studies, 2693 patients)			
29% (24–34%)	88% (86–89%)	2.31	0.81
Natriuretic peptide (4 studies, 1353 patients)			
77% (69–85%)	73% (70–76%)	2.87	0.31
High-sensitivity troponin (3 studies, 819 patients)			
74% (65–83%)	65% (62–69%)	2.15	0.39

Source: Data from [29].

In a planned secondary analysis of the FAINT score,[30] hs-cTnT and NT-proBNP measurements were independently predictive of 30-day serious events. When using a cut point of 5, the hs-cTnT had a sensitivity of 93.4% and specificity of 21.1%. For a cut point of 125, the NT-proBNP had a sensitivity of 89.3% and specificity of 35%. A refinement of the score was performed and these biomarkers were added to the final score.[28]

Clinical question

Is there an optimal time period for monitoring patients with syncope in the ED?
The CSRS investigators evaluated the time to occurrence of serious arrhythmias relative to time of ED arrival based on the CSRS risk category.[31] A total of 5581 patients were included in this analysis and 417 (7.5%) experienced serious outcomes, of which 207 (3.7%) were arrhythmias. One-half of the arrhythmias were identified within 2 hours of ED arrival in low-risk patients, and within 6 hours in medium- and high-risk patients. The residual risk of arrhythmic outcomes beyond 2 hours of observation was found to be very low (0.2%) in low-risk CSRS patients. However, patients classified as medium or high-risk by CSRS had a residual risk of 4.4% for arrhythmic events after 6 hours of observation. The vast majority of the arrhythmic serious outcomes occurred within 15 days of the index visit among the non-low-risk patients. The authors suggested a 2-hour monitoring for patients classified as low risk, and 6 hours for medium- and high-risk patients, followed by selective admission or 15-day outpatient monitoring.

The Syncope Monitoring and Natriuretic peptides in the Emergency department (SyMoNE) study was a prospective multicenter investigation conducted in six Italian EDs to assess the role of ECG monitoring in the ED management of patients with syncope.[32] A total of 242 non-low-risk patients without an obvious etiology of syncope after ED evaluation received ECG monitoring in the ED and were analyzed. Low-risk patients were defined at the discretion of emergency physicians and those who were discharged without ECG monitoring (e.g., those with clear vasovagal etiology). Thirty-two (13.2%) patients had positive monitoring in the ED, while 210 (86.7%) had a negative test. Among those who were positive, there were 19 (59.3%) 30-day adverse events, and among those who were negative, there were 20 (9.5%) adverse events. The performance of ECG monitoring in the ED to predict both 7-day and 30-day adverse events is depicted in Table 20.11. The diagnostic accuracy of ECG monitoring in the ED in non-low-risk patients

Table 20.11 Performance of ECG monitoring in the ED to predict 7-day and 30-day adverse events

	N	Sensitivity (CI)	Specificity (CI)
7-day adverse events			
Overall	242	55% (36–74%)	93% (89–96%)
<6 hours	242	7% (1–23%)	98% (95–99%)
6–12 hours	198	29% (13–51%)	95% (90–98%)
>12 hours	88	89% (65–99%)	78% (67–87%)
30-day adverse events			
Overall	242	49% (32–65%)	94% (90–97%)
<6 hours	242	8% (2–21%)	98% (96–100%)
6–12 hours	198	24% (11–42%)	95% (91–98%)
>12 hours	88	86% (65–97%)	82% (70–90%)

Source: Data from [32].

was poor, and the authors suggested the use of prolonged (>12 hours) monitoring as a safe alternative.

Clinical question

What is the diagnostic yield of head computerized tomography (CT) in patients presenting with syncope to the ED?

Viau et al.[33] performed a systematic review in which they included 17 studies with 3361 syncope patients. A total of 1821 (54.2%) patients underwent head CT, of whom 53 patients (2.9%) had serious intracranial conditions identified. In the meta-analytic pooled estimates of eight ED-based studies with 1669 patients, 54.4% received a head CT with a 3.8% diagnostic yield (positive for serious intracranial conditions). Since the rates of imaging in this population seem to be very high with a low diagnostic yield, future studies should address how to identify patients with syncope who require an imaging in the ED.

Comment

The current decision rules available for syncope in the ED do provide good risk stratification schemes to identify patients at low risk for serious outcomes in the short term. That is, clinicians can look at the factors that were significant across the different rules (many of which were the same) and make their own decisions regarding the risk of a serious diagnosis. Most recently, the CSRS has been developed and externally validated, showing adequate ability to identify individuals at very low and low risk of subsequent 30-day clinically important outcomes. Importantly, this tool includes the physician diagnostic impression, which may facilitate its use by emergency physicians. The validation of this tool, however, occurred in academic centers and its performance in nonacademic settings is yet to be studied. Also, an impact analysis to evaluate whether the use of this rule improves patient outcomes is needed before its widespread implementation in clinical practice. As for cardiac biomarkers specifically, they seem to have an important short-term prognostic role in this population and should be considered for inclusion into the decision-making of these patients.

Can clinical judgment be better than CDRs?

CDRs use objective variables, with higher reproducibility, like troponin test, or history of heart failure. An individual patient meta-analysis comparing syncope risk stratification tools with clinical judgment showed that prediction tools did not have better sensitivity, specificity, or prognostic yield compared with clinical judgment, in predicting short-term serious outcomes after syncope.[15] Schriger et al.[34] described that physician judgment was infrequently reported or compared to the performance of a CDR, and when reported, the decision aid rarely outperformed physician judgment. A systematic review of studies comparing diagnostic CDRs with clinical judgment found that CDRs are rarely superior to clinical judgment, and there is a trade-off between the proportion classified as not having disease and the proportion of missed diagnoses when one or the other is used for decision-making.[35]

There are several explanations to how and why clinical judgment can outperform CDRs. When we are evaluating an individual patient, we have more information than what was included in the rule; for example, a syncope patient with family history of sudden death. Another explanation is that a CDR is made with the information of the average population included, and the tails of the distribution are beyond the standard deviations, toward the edges of a distribution curve (Figure 20.1). Population distributions with "broad tails" are more likely to outperform clinical judgment. In conclusion, CDRs are tools to inform your decision, but should not be followed blindly. Use your judgment.

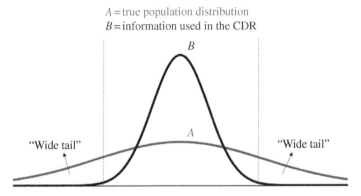

A = true population distribution
B = information used in the CDR

B

"Wide tail"

A

"Wide tail"

Figure 20.1 Information used for CDRs versus true population distribution.

References

1. Martin GJ, Adams SL, Martin HG, Mathews J, Zull D, Scanlon PJ. Prospective evaluation of syncope. *Annals of Emergency Medicine.* 1984; 13(7): 499–504.
2. Kapoor WN, Hanusa BH. Is syncope a risk factor for poor outcomes? Comparison of patients with and without syncope. *The American Journal of Medicine.* 1996; 100(6): 646–55.
3. Sarasin FP, Pruvot E, Louis-Simonet M *et al.* Stepwise evaluation of syncope: A prospective population-based controlled study. *International Journal of Cardiology.* 2008; 127(1): 103–11.
4. Strickberger SA, Benson W, Biaggioni I *et al.* AHA/ACCF scientific statement on the evaluation of syncope: From the American Heart Association Councils on Clinical Cardiology, Cardiovascular Nursing, Cardiovascular Disease in the Young, and Stroke, and the Quality of Care and Outcomes Research Interdisciplinary Working Group; and the American College of Cardiology Foundation: In collaboration with the Heart Rhythm Society: Endorsed by the American Autonomic Society. *Circulation.* 2006; 113(2): 316–27.
5. Probst MA, Su E, Weiss RE *et al.* Clinical benefit of hospitalization for older adults with unexplained syncope: A propensity-matched analysis. *Annals of Emergency Medicine.* 2019; 74(2): 260–9.
6. Albassam OT, Redelmeier RJ, Shadowitz S, Husain AM, Simel D, Etchells EE. Did this patient have cardiac syncope?: The rational clinical examination systematic review. *JAMA - Journal of the American Medical Association.* 2019; 321(24): 2448–57.
7. Gibson TA, Weiss RE, Sun BC. Predictors of short-term outcomes after syncope: A systematic review and meta-analysis. *The Western Journal of Emergency Medicine.* 2018; 19(3): 517–23.
8. Toarta C, Mukarram M, Arcot K *et al.* Syncope prognosis based on emergency department diagnosis: A prospective cohort study. *Academic Emergency Medicine.* 2018; 25(4): 388–96.

9. Serrano LA, Hess EP, Bellolio MF *et al.* Accuracy and quality of clinical decision rules for syncope in the emergency department: A systematic review and meta-analysis. *Annals of Emergency Medicine.* 2010; 56(4): 362–73.e1.

10. Sun BC, Thiruganasambandamoorthy V, Dela Cruz J. Standardized reporting guidelines for emergency department syncope risk-stratification research. *Academic Emergency Medicine.* 2012; 19(6): 694–702.

11. Quinn JV, Stiell IG, McDermott DA, Sellers KL, Kohn MA, Wells GA. Derivation of the San Francisco Syncope Rule to predict patients with short-term serious outcomes. *Annals of Emergency Medicine.* 2004; 43(2): 224–32.

12. Quinn J, McDermott D, Stiell I, Kohn M, Wells G. Prospective validation of the San Francisco Syncope Rule to predict patients with serious outcomes. *Annals of Emergency Medicine.* 2006; 47(5): 448–54.

13. Saccilotto RT, Nickel CH, Bucher HC, Steyerberg EW, Bingisser R, Koller MT. San Francisco Syncope Rule to predict short-term serious outcomes: A systematic review. *CMAJ.* 2011; 183(15): E1116–26.

14. Tan C, Sim TB, Thng SY. Validation of the San Francisco syncope rule in two hospital emergency departments in an Asian population. *Academic Emergency Medicine.* 2013; 20(5): 487–97.

15. Costantino G, Casazza G, Reed M *et al.* Syncope risk stratification tools vs clinical judgment: An individual patient data meta-analysis. *The American Journal of Medicine.* 2014; 127(11): 1126.e13–25.

16. du Fay de Lavallaz J, Badertscher P, Nestelberger T *et al.* Prospective validation of prognostic and diagnostic syncope scores in the emergency department. *International Journal of Cardiology.* 2018; 269: 114–21.

17. Du Fay De Lavallaz J, Badertscher P, Nestelberger T *et al.* B-type natriuretic peptides and cardiac troponins for diagnosis and risk-stratification of syncope. *Circulation.* 2019; 139(21): 2403–18.

18. Grossman SA, Fischer C, Lipsitz LA *et al.* Predicting adverse outcomes in syncope. *The Journal of Emergency Medicine.* 2007; 33(3): 233–9.

19. Grossman SA, Bar J, Fischer C *et al.* Reducing admissions utilizing the Boston syncope criteria. *The Journal of Emergency Medicine.* 2012; 42(3): 345–52.

20. Costantino G, Perego F, Dipaola F *et al.* Short- and long-term prognosis of syncope, risk factors, and role of hospital admission. Results from the STePS (short-term prognosis of syncope) study. *Journal of the American College of Cardiology.* 2008; 51(3): 276–83.

21. Sun BC, Derose SF, Liang LJ *et al.* Predictors of 30-day serious events in older patients with syncope. *Annals of Emergency Medicine.* 2009; 54(6): 769–78.e5.

22. Reed MJ, Newby DE, Coull AJ, Prescott RJ, Jacques KG, Gray AJ. The ROSE (risk stratification of syncope in the emergency department) study. *Journal of the American College of Cardiology.* 2010; 55(8): 713–21.

23. Bozorgi A, Hosseini K, Jalali A, Tajdini M. A new feasible syncope risk score appropriate for emergency department: A prospective cohort study. *Critical Pathways in Cardiology.* 2018; 17(3): 151–4.

24. Thiruganasambandamoorthy V, Kwong K, Wells GA *et al.* Development of the Canadian Syncope Risk Score to predict serious adverse events after emergency department assessment of syncope. *CMAJ.* 2016; 188(12): E289–98.

25. Thiruganasambandamoorthy V, Stiell IG, Sivilotti MLA *et al.* Predicting short-term risk of arrhythmia among patients with syncope: The Canadian syncope arrhythmia risk score. *Academic Emergency Medicine.* 2017; 24(11): 1315–26.

26. Thiruganasambandamoorthy V, Sivilotti MLA, Le Sage N *et al.* Multicenter emergency department validation of the Canadian syncope risk score. *JAMA Internal Medicine.* 2020; 180(5): 737–44.

27. Probst MA, Hess EP, Breslin M *et al.* Development of a patient decision aid for syncope in the emergency department: The SynDA tool. *Academic Emergency Medicine.* 2018; 25(4): 425–33.

28. Probst MA, Gibson T, Weiss RE *et al.* Risk stratification of older adults who present to the emergency department with syncope: The FAINT score. *Annals of Emergency Medicine.* 2020; 75(2): 147–58.

29. Thiruganasambandamoorthy V, Ramaekers R, Rahman MO *et al.* Prognostic value of cardiac biomarkers in the risk stratification of syncope: A systematic review. *Internal and Emergency Medicine.* 2015; 10(8): 1003–14.

30. Clark CL, Gibson TA, Weiss RE *et al.* Do high-sensitivity troponin and natriuretic peptide predict death or serious cardiac outcomes after syncope? *Academic Emergency Medicine.* 2019; 26(5): 528–38.

31. Thiruganasambandamoorthy V, Rowe BH, Sivilotti MLA *et al.* Duration of electrocardiographic monitoring of emergency department patients with syncope. *Circulation.* 2019; 139(11): 1396–406.

32. Solbiati M, Dipaola F, Villa P *et al.* Predictive accuracy of electrocardiographic monitoring of patients with syncope in the emergency department: The SyMoNE multicenter study. *Academic Emergency Medicine.* 2020; 27(1): 15–23.

33. Viau JA, Chaudry H, Hannigan A, Boutet M, Mukarram M, Thiruganasambandamoorthy V. The yield of computed tomography of the head among patients presenting with syncope: A systematic review. *Academic Emergency Medicine.* 2019; 26(5): 479–90.

34. Schriger DL, Elder JW, Cooper RJ. Structured clinical decision aids are seldom compared with subjective physician judgment, and are seldom superior. *Annals of Emergency Medicine.* 2017; 70(3): 338–44.e3.

35. Sanders S, Doust J, Glasziou P. A systematic review of studies comparing diagnostic clinical prediction rules with clinical judgment. *PLoS One.* 2015; 10(6): e0128233.

Chapter 21 **Chest Pain**

Christopher R. Carpenter[1] and Ali S. Raja[2]

[1]Department of Emergency Medicine, Washington University School of Medicine, St. Louis, MO, USA
[2]Department of Emergency Medicine, Massachusetts General Hospital, Harvard Medical School, Boston, MA, USA

Highlights

- Atraumatic chest pain has a broad differential diagnosis ranging from acute coronary syndrome (ACS) to pericarditis, pericardial effusion, pneumothorax, and pulmonary embolism.
- Multiple emergency medicine clinical practice guidelines exist for the diagnostic approach to acute chest pain and do not recommend routine stress testing or admission for low-risk patients.
- Pericardial tamponade more commonly presents with dyspnea than chest pain.
- Pulsus paradoxus is the most accurate physical exam finding for pericardial tamponade.
- Point-of-care ultrasound can be diagnostic for pericardial effusion, but confirming tamponade may require quantifying the duration of right atrial collapse.
- The HEART Score and HEART Pathway are becoming the most commonly used risk stratification instruments for ACS prediction of major adverse cardiac event risk.
- High-sensitivity troponin predominates in Europe and is increasingly prevalent in North America with equivocal impact on emergency department (ED) operational flow.

Evidence-Based Emergency Care: Diagnostic Testing and Clinical Decision Rules, Third Edition. Edited by Jesse M. Pines, Fernanda Bellolio, Christopher R. Carpenter, and Ali S. Raja.
© 2023 John Wiley & Sons Ltd. Published 2023 by John Wiley & Sons Ltd.

- Computed tomography (CT) coronary angiography is superior to stress echocardiography or myocardial scintigraphy for the assessment of obstructive coronary artery disease in emergency department settings.
- Safely disseminating guideline recommendations, risk assessment scores, and cardiac imaging decisions across dissimilar emergency departments will require patient-shared decision-making and implementation science approaches.

Background

Chest pain accounted for 4.7% of emergency department (ED) visits in 2017, and is the second most common presenting complaint after abdominal pain at an estimated cost of $10 billion annually in the United States.[1,2] ED physicians prioritize the identification of potentially life-threatening etiologies of chest pain, including acute coronary syndrome (ACS), aortic dissection, pneumothorax, and pericardial effusion, in addition to lesser immediate threats like pericarditis, pneumonia, and gastroesophageal reflux disease. This chapter will focus on the diagnostic approaches for pericardial effusion, pericarditis, and ACS.

The first step in the ED evaluation and management of patients who present with chest pain or other symptoms concerning for ACS is a 12-lead electrocardiogram (ECG). While findings on the initial ECG may be diagnostic or suggestive of ACS, the initial ECG can also be normal or nondiagnostic, underscoring the need for additional monitoring and testing of patients with suspected ACS. Evaluation of the initial ECG in patients with suspected ACS should focus on the presence of ST-segment elevations, new left bundle branch blocks, or new dynamic ST changes, all indicative of acute myocardial infarction (AMI). In patients with known left bundle branch blocks or paced rhythm, the Sgarbossa criteria (ST-segment elevation of 1 mm or more concordant with the QRS complex; ST-segment depression of 1 mm or more in lead V1, V2, or V3; and ST-segment elevation of 5 mm or more discordant with the QRS complex) can still be used to diagnose ACS.[3] A modification of Sgarbossa criteria that replaces the ST-segment elevation of 5 mm or more with the ratio of ST-segment elevation divided by S-segment depth (ST/S) less than −0.25 may improve overall accuracy for ST-segment elevation myocardial infarction (STEMI).[4] More recently, additional modification of the Sgarbossa criteria called the BARCELONA algorithm further improves sensitivity without significantly reducing specificity. The BARCELONA algorithm is "positive" for ACS with ST deviation ≥ 1 mm concordant with QRS polarity in *any* lead, or ST deviation ≥1 mm discordant with the QRS in leads in which the largest deflection of the R or S wave ≤ 6 mm.[5] However, while the standard ECG is the single best test to identify patients with AMI upon their presentation to the ED, it has relatively low sensitivity.[6] In patients with AMI, ST segments may be elevated in only 50% of initial ECGs.[7] In addition, most left bundle branch block is not ACS and ST-elevation can be observed with myopericarditis, early repolarization, hyperkalemia, Takotsubo cardiomyopathy, and left ventricular hypertrophy or ventricular aneurysm, among other causes.[8,9] Due to these limitations, distinguishing AMI and unstable angina from other noncardiac chest pain in patients at risk for ACS typically involves serial ECGs and/or serial serum biomarkers of myocardial injury, also with diagnostic imaging [provocative stress tests or computed tomography (CT) imaging] or cardiac catheterization.[10,11]

Clinical questions relevant to the assessment of a patient with acute undifferentiated chest pain involve the test characteristics of history and physical examination findings, cardiac biomarkers, point-of-care ultrasound, and cardiac CT imaging.

Clinical question

Can emergency medicine physicians accurately and reliably distinguish pericardial effusion and pericarditis from acute coronary syndrome?

The pericardial sac consists of the outermost parietal pericardium and the inner visceral pericardium and usually contains less than 30 mL of fluid. The pericardium is compliant so large amounts of fluid can accumulate slowly without compromising cardiac function, but rapid accumulation of pericardial fluid over minutes to hours may exceed pericardial compliance. The incidence of pericardial effusion or tamponade among ED patients with acute chest pain has not been described, but one small single-center prospective study of dyspnea patients reported an incidence of 14%.[12] In one case series of Spanish patients with moderate or large pericardial effusion, the most common causative diagnoses were pericarditis (20%), malignancy (13%), myocardial infarction (8%), end-stage renal disease (6%), congestive heart failure (5%), collagen vascular disease (5%), and tuberculosis or bacterial infection (4%).[13] Hypotension is uncommon in subacute pericardial effusion, whereas pericardial tamponade is typically associated with cardiogenic shock. Assessing for the presence or absence of pericardial tamponade is not a clinical diagnosis because both sensitivity and specificity are suboptimal for findings such as tachycardia, jugular venous distension, diminished heart sounds, and pulsus paradoxus.[14] Even in tamponade, 27% of patients may present with paradoxical hypertension.[15]

One diagnostic accuracy systematic review in 2007 synthesized the diagnostic accuracy of history, physical exam, chest X-ray, and ECG for the diagnosis of tamponade.[14] For most findings, only sensitivity was reported. The exception was pulsus paradoxus which was evaluated in a single study of 65 pericardial tamponade and 101 control patients with positive likelihood ratio 5.9 (95% CI 2.4–14) and negative likelihood ratio 0.03 (95% CI 0–0.21) for pulsus paradoxus >12 mm Hg.[16] Seven different studies found lower sensitivity for pulsus paradoxus, ranging between 56% and 86%.[14] Pulsus paradoxus is not a paradox.[17] Instead, this finding is an exaggeration of the normal inspiratory decrease in blood pressure. Pulsus paradoxus can be evaluated by auscultation of Korotkoff sounds during slow release of a blood pressure cuff. Pulsus paradoxus can be masked by the presence of hypotension, aortic regurgitation, atrial septal defects, or right ventricular hypertrophy.[6]

The most common presenting symptom in pericardial tamponade is dyspnea, which is found in 87% of cases. The next most common symptom is fever (25%) then chest pain (20%).[18] The sensitivity of other physical examination findings for the diagnosis of tamponade are summarized in Table 21.1. The most sensitive ECG finding for tamponade is low voltage with a pooled sensitivity of 42% (95% CI 32–53).[14] The sensitivity of electrical alternans ranges from 16% to 21%.[19,20] The sensitivity of cardiomegaly on chest X-ray ranges from 68% to 100% for the diagnosis of tamponade.[14]

Point-of-care bedside ultrasound is the diagnostic test of choice to identify pericardial effusion and features of tamponade. The subcostal window is the recommended window because that positions the most dependent portion of pericardium adjacent to the probe. A common error is confusing epicardial fatty tissue with an effusion, which can be avoided by noting the heterogeneous sonographic texture of fat compared with fluid, as well as the failure of fat

Table 21.1 Sensitivity of physical examination for the diagnosis of tamponade

Sign	Number of studies	Sensitivity %
Tachycardia	4	65–87
Hypotension	4	14–35
Hypertension (>140 mm)	1	33
Tachypnea	1	80
Diminished heart sounds	3	24–34
Elevated jugular venous pressure	4	53–88
Peripheral edema	2	21–28
Pericardial rub	2	19–29
Hepatomegaly	2	28–55

Source: Data from [14].

to track around the heart.[21] Right atrial collapse is a sensitive marker of tamponade but is not specific.[17] One sonographic approach to distinguish clinically inconsequential right atrial collapse associated with pericardial effusion from right atrial collapse due to tamponade is to quantify the duration of collapse during the cardiac cycle. Right atrial collapse exceeding one-third of the cardiac cycle increases accuracy from 87% (using dichotomous collapse or no collapse) to 97%.[22] Quantifying the duration of right atrial collapse can be accomplished using M-mode.[23]

Pericarditis, or inflammation of the layers surrounding the heart, usually affects young and middle-aged individuals, is idiopathic in 90% of cases, and is diagnosed in approximately 5% of North American ED chest pain patients.[24,25] Pericarditis may be attributable to infection (usually viral), autoimmune, neoplastic, or medications, but is most commonly associated with metabolic (uremia, myxedema) or traumatic causes when an etiology can be identified.[25] Classically, the presenting complaint is chest pain described as "sharp" and pleuritic with exacerbation while lying flat and improvement leaning forward. Other features that may distinguish pericarditis from ACS include more prolonged duration of pain in pericarditis and radiation of pain to the trapezius ridge.[26] ECG classically demonstrates diffuse ST-segment (J-point) elevation with PR segment depression in leads other than V1 and aVR. Another finding is a down-sloping ECG baseline and is called Spodick's sign. In one retrospective review, Spodick's sign was noted in 29% of acute pericarditis patients but also in 5% of STEMI patients. The ECG findings that most strongly distinguished pericarditis from STEMI were more profound ST-depression in lead III than in lead II as well as the absence of PR-depression (both favoring STEMI).[27] Unfortunately, inter-rater agreement for Spodick's sign (kappa 0.4–0.5) and PR-depression (kappa 0.5) is suboptimal.[27]

Clinical question

Can the HEART score accurately and reliably distinguish low- and high-risk chest pain patients?

To appreciate the potential value of the HEART score and other chest pain decision-aids in ED settings, understanding the limitations of isolated findings from the history and physical exam for the accurate diagnosis of ACS is essential. A large meta-analysis by Panju *et al.* reviewed examination findings of patients with suspected AMI and was subsequently updated in 2008.[6] Fourteen studies met their inclusion criteria, most of which used the World Health Organization definition of AMI as the criterion standard, which includes evolving changes on serial ECGs, a rise in serial biomarkers, and

Table 21.2 History and physical examination characteristics associated with either a greater or lesser risk of acute myocardial infarction

Clinical feature	Positive likelihood ratio (LR+) (CI)	Negative likelihood ratio (LR–) (CI)
Chest or center arm pain*	2.7	—
Chest pain radiation to:		
Right shoulder	2.2 (1.4–3.4)	—
Right arm	7.3 (3.9–14)	—
Left arm	2.2 (1.6–3.1)	—
Both left and right arms	9.7 (4.6–20)	—
Chest pain most important symptom*	2.0	—
History of myocardial infarction**	1.5–3.0	—
Nausea or vomiting	1.9 (1.7–2.3)	—
Diaphoresis	2.0 (1.9–2.2)	—
Third heart sound on auscultation	3.2 (1.6–6.5)	—
Hypotension***	3.1 (1.8–5.2)	—
Pulmonary crackles on auscultation	2.1 (1.4–3.1)	—
Pleuritic chest pain	—	0.2 (0.2–0.3)
Sharp or stabbing chest pain	—	0.3 (0.2–0.5)
Positional chest pain	—	0.3 (0.2–0.4)
Chest pain reproducible by palpation*	*—	0.2–0.4

*Data not available to calculate confidence intervals.
**Reported as a range due to heterogeneity of the pooled studies.
***Defined as systolic blood pressure ≤80 mm Hg.
Source: Data from [6].

either chest pain with an abnormal ECG or other symptoms with evolving changes on serial ECGs. The analysis of the pooled data in the meta-analysis (Table 21.2) demonstrates a number of historical and physical exam characteristics that increase and decrease the likelihood of AMI. For the sake of clarity, the authors chose to only report LRs that were either greater than 2.0 or less than 0.5.

Numerous decision aids have emerged over the last 40 years to risk stratify ACS among ED chest pain patients. Since the Second Edition of this textbook was published, the History/ECG/Age/Risk factors/Troponin (HEART) score (Figure 21.1) and HEART Pathway (Figure 21.2) have emerged as the most frequently researched and emergency medicine guideline-endorsed chest pain decision aid.[10,11] The American College of Emergency Physicians (ACEP) 2018 Clinical Policy on suspected non-ST-elevation ACSs gave a Level B recommendation to use HEART score ≤ 3 as a predictor of very low 30-day major adverse cardiac events. In contrast, that same Clinical Policy

The HEART score for chest pain patients in the ED		
History	• Highly suspicious • Moderately suspicious • Slightly or non-suspicious	• 2 points • 1 point • 0 points
ECG	• Significant ST-depression • Nonspecific repolarization • Normal	• 2 points • 1 point • 0 points
Age	• ≥ 65 years • > 45 – < 65 years • ≤ 45 years	• 2 points • 1 point • 0 points
Risk Factors	• ≥ 3 Risk factors or history of CAD • 1 or 2 Risk factors • No risk factors	• 2 points • 1 point • 0 points
Troponin	• ≥ 3 × Normal limit • > 1 – < 3 × Normal limit • ≤ Normal limit	• 2 points • 1 point • 0 points
Risk factors: DM, current or recent (<one month) smoker, HTN, HLP, family history of CAD, & obesity		

Figure 21.1 The HEART score. REBEL EM. Used with permission.

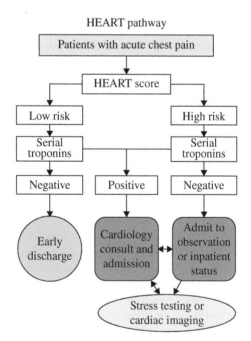

Figure 21.2 The HEART pathway. REBEL EM. Used with permission.

provided a lower Level C recommendation for the use of the thrombolysis in myocardial infarction (TIMI) score for the same purpose.[10] The ACEP Clinical Policy notes that the derivation and validation of the HEART Score in ED settings as opposed to the inpatient settings used in the older TIMI score are a strength of the HEART score. The Society for Academic Emergency Medicine (SAEM) Guidelines for Reasonable and Appropriate Care in the Emergency Department (GRACE) published recommendations for the management of recurrent low-risk chest pain and defined "low-risk" primarily by HEART score <4.[11] The SAEM GRACE rationale for selecting the HEART score and HEART Pathway (as opposed to alternative chest pain scores) included the volume of supporting ED-based research demonstrating the consistent accuracy of this approach in conjunction with associated decreased rates of hospitalization, death, and myocardial infarction when implemented into practice, which attains international standards for acceptable clinical practice.[28,29]

The HEART and TIMI scores have been compared head-to-head. In one Dutch study that included 2440 chest pain patients from 10 hospitals, HEART score ≤ 3 demonstrated 30-day major adverse cardiac event (MACE) rates of 1.7% compared with a 2.7% rate for TIMI ≤1.[30] Another study in China also demonstrated superiority of HEART compared with TIMI and two other scores as a predictor of 30-day MACE.[31]

The HEART Score was evaluated in 25 studies between 2010 and 2017, including over 25,000 patients with a pooled negative likelihood ratio for HEART ≤3 of 0.09 (95% CI 0.06–0.15) to predict short-term MACE. Despite the various study settings, use of regular versus high-sensitivity troponin, or timeline until follow-up, the HEART Score consistently demonstrated high sensitivity and clinically useful negative likelihood ratio.[32] A more recent meta-analysis of 30 studies including over 44,000 patients demonstrated an optimal HEART cutoff ≥ 4 based on hierarchical summary receiver operating characteristic curves and no impact of HEART Score accuracy when ECG interpretation was conducted by Cardiology or ED physician.[33] One reliability study quantified the interrater reliability of HEART Score ≤ 3 with kappa 0.68 (95% CI 0.60–0.77) with the history and ECG components demonstrating lower kappa than the risk factors and troponin assessment.[34] The most frequent HEART scoring error by clinicians is the failure to assign two points for history of atherosclerosis, which accounts for half of the mistakes applying the "risk factor" component of the HEART Score.[35] To quantify the clinical impact of introducing the HEART Score into ED operations, a Dutch stepped-wedge cluster randomized trial introduced the decision aid sequentially into nine hospitals and noted no statistically significant differences in early discharge rates, readmissions, ED revisits, or outpatient visits.

The authors attributed the ineffectiveness to physician hesitation to avoid admissions for low-risk HEART patients.[36]

The HEART Pathway was evaluated in a single-center randomized controlled trial comparing use of the pathway to usual care. The HEART Pathway demonstrated similar 1-year MACE rates (9.9% in HEART Pathway, 11.3% in usual care), but the HEART Pathway demonstrated a nonsignificant trend toward increased cardiac-related hospitalizations (15% versus 11%) and ED returns (21% versus 16%).[37] A subsequent prepost study introducing the HEART Pathway across three EDs demonstrated decreased admission rates, increased identification of index AMIs, and very low rates of death or myocardial infarction for low-risk patients.[28] A longitudinal follow-up of discharged low-risk HEART Pathway patients showed that 31% of patients were identified as low-risk during the index ED evaluation and 1-year hospitalization rates decreased by 7% using the pathway without increasing mortality rates.[38] Stress testing of low-risk HEART Pathway patients has also demonstrated futility with 1% diagnostic yield (abnormal stress testing followed by cardiac catheterization demonstrating coronary artery disease).[39] Perceived barriers and facilitators to successfully introducing the HEART Pathway have been identified using Implementation Science. Facilitators include the overall strength of evidence supporting the HEART Pathway capacity to reduce the length of stay, unnecessary testing, and associated iatrogenic complications. Barriers include time and resource burdens, electronic medical record challenges, as well as sustained communication and engagement with key stakeholders.[40]

Clinical question

Does high-sensitivity troponin accuracy aid in efficiency of emergency department evaluation for chest pain?

Both the ACEP Clinical Policy on non-ST-elevation ACS and the SAEM GRACE guideline on recurrent chest pain in low-risk patients advocate for a role in high-sensitivity troponin testing. The ACEP Clinical Policy provides two Level C recommendations:

1. A single high-sensitivity troponin result below the level of detection on arrival to the ED, or negative serial high-sensitivity troponin result at 0 and 2 hours, is predictive of a low rate of MACE.

2. In adult patients with suspected acute Non-ST elevation ACS who are determined to be low risk based on validated accelerated discharge pathways that include a nonischemic ECG result and negative serial high-sensitivity troponin testing results both at presentation and at 2 hours can predict a low rate of 30-day MACE, allowing for discharge from the ED.[10]

Similarly, the GRACE guideline provides a GRADE-based conditional guideline based on low-level evidence that "In adult patients with recurrent, low-risk chest pain for greater than 3 hours duration, we suggested a single, high-sensitivity troponin below a validated threshold to reasonably exclude ACS within 30 days."[11,41] Unfortunately, the American Heart Association and the European Society of Cardiology currently diverge in their recommendations for a single troponin with the former recommending serial troponin and the latter providing scenarios for a single troponin, which likely reflects the delay to adopt high-sensitivity troponin in the United States relative to Europe.[42] The GRACE guidelines are based entirely on indirect evidence across eight studies using high-sensitivity troponin.[43–50] While including these eight studies and one additional study that used conventional troponin, the 30-day MACE rate for low-risk chest pain patients was 0.5% (72/15,715 patients).[11]

Neither the ACEP Clinical Policy nor the SAEM GRACE guideline provides recommendations about the efficiency of high-sensitivity troponin. Multiple recent controlled studies raise doubts about whether high sensitivity troponin improves ED efficiency for the large-scale evaluation of chest pain. Shah *et al.* reported a stepped-wedge cluster-randomized controlled trial of over 48,000 chest pain patients evaluated with a high sensitivity assay with reclassification of 17% who were not identified by conventional troponin. As a consequence of this reclassification, cardiac catheterization rates increased 7% without any difference in percutaneous coronary intervention rates or 1-year MACE outcomes.[51] A three-center prepost analysis comparing high sensitivity to conventional troponin decreased ED length of stay for suspected ACS patients without increasing ED returns or cardiology consultations.[52] However, a subsequent randomized controlled trial across eight United Kingdom hospitals comparing a single high-sensitivity troponin with usual care did not significantly improve time-to-discharge rates or increase 30-day MACE rates, indicating that system-level factors influence operational metrics in addition to the cardiac enzyme assay.[53] One cost-effectiveness analysis reported an incremental cost-effectiveness ratio of $108,552 per adverse clinical outcome avoided through the use of high sensitivity troponin, which is reduced to $49,030 per adverse clinical outcome if limited to cases below the normal troponin threshold.[54]

Clinical question

Does CT coronary angiography accurately distinguish significant coronary artery disease from other causes of acute chest pain?

CT coronary angiography (cCTA) is increasingly available as a viable alternative to alternative imaging tests like stress echocardiography or myocardial

Table 21.3 Predictive values of cCTA for coronary artery disease in stable chest pain stratified by pretest probability from individualized patient data meta-analysis

	Pretest probability of CAD (%)			
	7	15	50	67
Including nondiagnostic cCTA				
PPV (95% CI)	51 (43–58)	56 (49–62)	75 (71–80)	83 (78–86)
NPV (95% CI)	98 (96–99)	97 (95–98)	91 (88–93)	85 (80–89)
Excluding nondiagnostic cCTA				
PPV (95% CI)	68 (61–75)	72 (65–78)	85 (80–88)	89 (85–92)
NPV (95% CI)	98 (97–99)	98 (96–99)	94 (92–96)	91 (88–94)

Source: Data from [55].

scintigraphy. While the ACEP Clinical Policy Level B recommendation is to not routinely use cCTA prior to discharge in low-risk patients in whom AMI has been ruled out, the SAEM GRACE guideline for recurrent low-risk chest pain recommends that, after a cCTA within 2 years that demonstrated no coronary stenosis, no further diagnostic testing after a single high-sensitivity troponin is required.[10,11] An individual patient data meta-analysis including 5332 patients from 65 prospective diagnostic accuracy studies for obstructive coronary artery disease (CAD) in stable chest pain patients reported sensitivity 95% (95% CI 93–97) and specificity 79% (95% CI 75–83) with area under the receiver operating characteristic curve improving from 0.897 (95 CI 0.889–0.906) to 0.949 (95% CI 0.943–0.954) when indeterminant studies were excluded. As discussed in Chapter 4, the positive and negative predictive values are generally unhelpful without the context of pretest disease probability, so these authors also provided predictive values stratified by pretest probability (Table 21.3).[55]

A meta-analysis of 10 randomized controlled trials including 6285 patients comparing cCTA with routine care for the evaluation of acute chest pain with follow-up ranging 1–19 months found no significant differences in all-cause mortality, MI, or MACE rates, but higher rates of downstream cardiac catheterization and revascularization.[56] Although ED-based cCTA is associated with higher initial costs ($4490 versus $2513–$4144) and revascularization rates (5.2% versus 2.6–3.7%) compared with routine care, cCTA is cost-effective over a lifetime at $49,428 per quality-adjusted life year.[57]

Comment

Chest pain and missed ACS remains a significant source of closed malpractice claims with legal teams recommending thorough diagnostic evaluations and liberal consultation with cardiology.[58] Not surprisingly, medicolegal concerns are associated with increased chest pain admission rates and observation units do not reduce admission rates.[59,60] Many ED physicians target a posttest probability of <1% as the objective, and often equate the probability of ACS with the likelihood of short-term MACE despite the reality that the outcomes of death or myocardial infarction are uncommon (i.e., likelihood ACS ≠ likelihood MACE).[61] Aspiring for a 0% ACS miss rate comes with the price of potential over-testing, over-diagnosis, and over-treatment.[62] For example, cCTA will inevitably identify pulmonary and upper abdominal findings that would otherwise remain unknown to patients and never cause symptoms or early demise. Even in the best situation where these incidentalomas are nonexistent and the long-term risks of medical radiation are negated, most (perhaps 85%) of cCTA patients will not benefit as a result of cCTA imaging from a cardiovascular status because the probability of over-treatment exists in that revascularization for abnormal coronary findings occur that does not improve patient outcomes or reduce MACE rates.[63]

Fortunately, ED-specific guidelines now exist for the evaluation of chest pain.[10,11] Although the recommendations are conditional and generally based upon very weak and often indirect evidence, these guidelines provide a peer-reviewed foundation of current state knowledge to inform bedside decision-making. SAEM's GRACE guidelines for recurrent low-risk chest pain (summarized in Figure 21.3) highlight the futility of routinely repeating stress testing or hospital admissions, while providing a warranty for prior cardiac angiography findings within the last five years. However, for patients presenting with concern about symptoms, simply explaining the very unlikely probability of an ACS diagnosis or MACE outcome may be inadequate to alleviate concerns. The GRACE guidelines also illustrate the oft-neglected opportunity to screen for depression or anxiety and provide appropriate referrals when indicated.[11]

Clinician gestalt alone is often inadequate to rule in or rule out ACS.[64] As previously discussed, the HEART Score and HEART Pathway are recommended by both the ACEP Clinical Policy and the SAEM GRACE guideline.[10,11] However, successfully incorporating these scoring systems into clinical care is a challenge. Using the Consolidated Framework for Implementation Research, lessons learned from introducing the HEART Pathway across four academic medical centers include engagement of clinical and financial stakeholders, as well as efficient integration with electronic medical records. Key stakeholders include patients and their advocates, nursing, cardiology, radiology, hospitalists, primary care, and laboratory medicine.[40]

Recommendations

1 In adult patients with recurrent, low-risk chest pain, for greater than 3 hours duration we suggest a single, high-sensitivity troponin below a validated threshold to reasonably exclude ACS within 30 days. [Conditional, For] [Low level of evidence]

2 In adult patients with recurrent, low-risk chest pain, and a normal stress test within the previous 12 months, we do not recommend repeat routine stress testing as a means to decrease rates of MACE at 30 days. [Conditional, Against] [Low level of evidence]

3 In adult patients with recurrent, low-risk chest pain, there is insufficient evidence to recommend admission to the hospital versus admission to the observation unit versus discharge home in relation to ACS outcomes within 30 days. [No evidence, Either]

4 In adult patients with recurrent, low-risk chest pain and non-obstructive [<50% stenosis] CAD on prior angiography within 5 years, we suggest referral for expedited outpatient testing as warranted rather than admission for inpatient evaluation. [Conditional, For] [Low level of evidence]

5 In adult patients with recurrent, low-risk chest pain and no occlusive CAD [0% stenosis] on prior angiography within 5 years, we recommend referral for expedited outpatient testing as warranted rather than admission for inpatient evaluation. [Conditional, For] [Low level of evidence]

6 In adult patients with recurrent, low-risk chest pain and prior CCTA within the past two years with no coronary stenosis, we suggest no further diagnostic testing other than a single, high-sensitivity troponin below a validated threshold to exclude ACS within that two-year time frame. [Conditional, For] [Moderate level of evidence]

7 In adult patients with recurrent, low-risk chest pain, we suggest the use of depression and anxiety screening tools as these might have an affect on healthcare use and return EC visits. [Conditional, Either] [Very low level of evidence]

8 In adult patients with recurrent, low-risk chest pain, we suggest referral for anxiety or depression management, as this might have an impact on healthcare use and return ED visits. [Conditional, Either] [Low level of evidence]

Figure 21.3 Synopsis of SAEM GRACE guideline recommendations for recurrent low-risk chest pain in the ED.

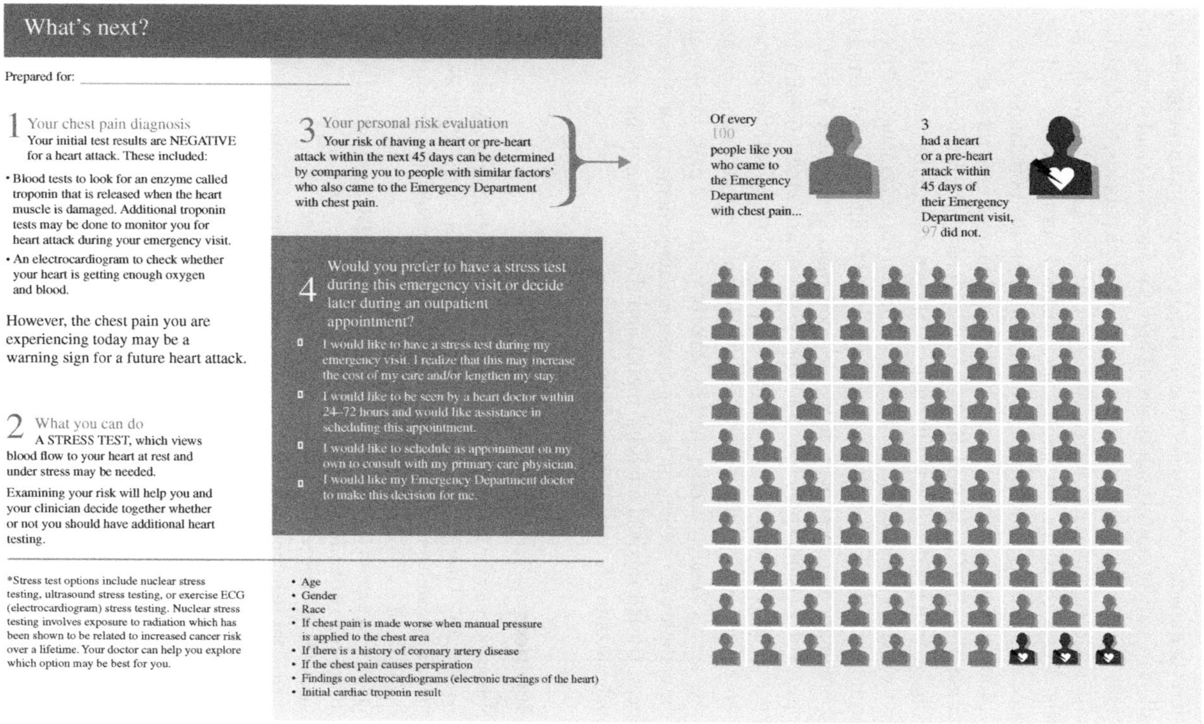

What's next?

Prepared for: _____

1 Your chest pain diagnosis

Your initial test results are NEGATIVE for a heart attack. These included:

• Blood tests to look for an enzyme called troponin that is released when the heart muscle is damaged. Additional troponin tests may be done to monitor you for heart attack during your emergency visit.

• An electrocardiogram to check whether your heart is getting enough oxygen and blood.

However, the chest pain you are experiencing today may be a warning sign for a future heart attack.

2 What you can do

A STRESS TEST, which views blood flow to your heart at rest and under stress may be needed.

Examining your risk will help you and your clinician decide together whether or not you should have additional heart testing.

*Stress test options include nuclear stress testing, ultrasound stress testing, or exercise ECG (electrocardiogram) stress testing. Nuclear stress testing involves exposure to radiation which has been shown to be related to increased cancer risk over a lifetime. Your doctor can help you explore which option may be best for you.

3 Your personal risk evaluation

Your risk of having a heart or pre-heart attack within the next 45 days can be determined by comparing you to people with similar factors' who also came to the Emergency Department with chest pain.

4 Would you prefer to have a stress test during this emergency visit or decide later during an outpatient appointment?

☐ I would like to have a stress test during my emergency visit. I realize that this may increase the cost of my care and/or lengthen my stay.

☐ I would like to be seen by a heart doctor within 24–72 hours and would like assistance in scheduling this appointment.

☐ I would like to schedule an appointment on my own to consult with my primary care physician.

☐ I would like my Emergency Department doctor to make this decision for me.

• Age
• Gender
• Race
• If chest pain is made worse when manual pressure is applied to the chest area
• If there is a history of coronary artery disease
• If the chest pain causes perspiration
• Findings on electrocardiogram (electronic tracings of the heart)
• Initial cardiac troponin result

Of every 100 people like you who came to the Emergency Department with chest pain...

3 had a heart or a pre-heart attack within 45 days of their Emergency Department visit, 97 did not.

Figure 21.4 Chest pain decision aid.

Engaging patients and their surrogates in these decisions are a pragmatic approach to balance a patient's long-term health with physician's short-term malpractice angst.[65,66] Shared decision-making provides another opportunity to alleviate patient concerns in choosing between diagnostic and therapeutic options.[67] When employed in ED settings for low-risk patients, the chest pain decision aid (Figure 21.4) increased patient ACS self-risk knowledge and safely decreased admission rates.[68] Since limited health literacy and age-related cognitive dysfunction are prevalent in some ED populations, shared decision-making instruments must be designed to overcome these communication obstacles.[69-71] Indeed, limited health literacy patients are less likely to engage with the decision aid in Figure 21.4 even though the instrument is effective across vulnerable patient groups.[72,73] In an era of personalized medicine, future researchers exploring the barriers and facilitators for meaningful and pragmatic ED chest pain shared decision-making will need acceptable measures of decisional preferences and priorities, as well as situational appropriateness and evaluations of operational impact.[74] Concurrently, implementation experts and guideline developers will need to understand optimal change agents to safely accelerate the uptake of valid chest pain decision aids in the complex ED setting, including decisional antecedents (prior ED experiences, trusted medical advisors' input) and the objective quality of decisional outcomes.[75]

References

1. National Center for Health Statistics. National Hospital Ambulatory Medical Care Survey: 2017 Emergency Department Summary Tables. 2017. https://www.cdc.gov/nchs/data/nhamcs/web_tables/2017_ed_web_tables-508.pdf. Accessed May 19, 2021.
2. Yau AA, Nguyendo LT, Lockett LL, Michaud E. The HEART pathway and hospital cost savings. *Critical Pathways in Cardiology*. 2017; 16: 126–8.
3. Tabas JA, Rodriguez RM, Seligman HK, Goldschlager NF. Electrocardiographic criteria for detecting acute myocardial infarction in patients with left bundle branch block: A meta-analysis. *Annals of Emergency Medicine*. 2008; 52: 329–36.
4. Smith SW, Dodd KW, Henry TD, Dvorak DM, Pearce LA. Diagnosis of ST-elevation myocardial infarction in the presence of left bundle branch block with the ST-elevation to S-wave ratio in a modified Sgarbossa rule. *Annals of Emergency Medicine*. 2012; 60: 766–76.
5. Di Marco A, Rodriguez M, Cinca J *et al.* New electrocardiographic algorithm for the diagnosis of acute myocardial infarction in patients with left bundle branch block. *Journal of the American Heart Association*. 2020; 9: e015573.
6. Panju AA, Hemmelgarn BA, Guyatt GH, Simel DL. The rational clinical examination. Is this patient having a myocardial infarction? *JAMA*. 1998; 280: 1256–63.

7. Gibler WB, Young GP, Hedges JR *et al*. Acute myocardial infarction in chest pain patients with nondiagnostic ECGs: Serial CK-MB sampling in the emergency department. The Emergency Medicine Cardiac Research Group. *Annals of Emergency Medicine*. 1992; 21: 504–12.

8. Nestelberger T, Cullen L, Lindahl B *et al*. Diagnosis of acute myocardial infarction in the presence of left bundle branch block. *Heart*. 2019; 105: 1559–67.

9. Wang K, Asinger RW, Marriott HJL. ST-segment elevation in conditions other than acute myocardial infarction. *The New England Journal of Medicine*. 2003; 349: 2128–35.

10. Tomaszewski CA, Nestler D, Shah KH, Sudhir A, Brown MD. Clinical policy: Critical issues in the evaluation and management of emergency department patients with suspected non-ST-elevation acute coronary syndromes. *Annals of Emergency Medicine*. 2018; 72: e65–e106.

11. Musey PI, Bellolio F, Upadhye S *et al*. Guidelines for reasonable and appropriate care in the emergency department (GRACE): Recurrent low-risk chest pain in the emergency department. *Academic Emergency Medicine*. 2021; 28: 718–44.

12. Blaivas M. Incidence of pericardial effusion in patients presenting to the emergency department with unexplained dyspnea. *Academic Emergency Medicine*. 2001; 8: 1143–6.

13. Sagristà-Sauleda J, Mercé J, Permanyer-Miralda G, Soler-Soler J. Clinical clues to the causes of large pericardial effusions. *The American Journal of Medicine*. 2000; 109: 95–101.

14. Roy CL, Minor MA, Brookhart MA, Choudhry NK. Does this patient with a pericardial effusion have cardiac tamponade? *JAMA*. 2007; 297: 1810–8.

15. Argulian E, Herzog E, Halpern DG, Messerli FH. Paradoxical hypertension with cardiac tamponade. *The American Journal of Cardiology*. 2012; 110: 1066–9.

16. Curtiss EI, Reddy PS, Uretsky BF, Cecchetti AA. Pulsus paradoxus: Definition and relation to the severity of cardiac tamponade. *American Heart Journal*. 1988; 115: 391–8.

17. Argulian E, Messerli F. Misconceptions and facts about pericardial effusion and tamponade. *The American Journal of Medicine*. 2013; 126: 858–61.

18. Cooper JP, Oliver RM, Currie P, Walker JM, Swanton RH. How do the clinical findings in patients with pericardial effusions influence the success of aspiration? *British Heart Journal*. 1995; 73: 351–4.

19. Guberman BA, Fowler NO, Engel PJ, Gueron M, Allen JM. Cardiac tamponade in medical patients. *Circulation*. 1981; 64: 633–40.

20. Levine MJ, Lorell BH, Diver DJ, Come PC. Implications of echocardiographically assisted diagnosis of pericardial tamponade in contemporary medical patients: Detection before hemodynamic embarrassment. *Journal of the American College of Cardiology*. 1991; 17: 59–65.

21. Hall MK, Coffey EC, Herbst M *et al*. The "5Es" of emergency physician-performed focused cardiac ultrasound: A protocol for rapid identification of effusion, ejection, equality, exit, and entrance. *Academic Emergency Medicine*. 2015; 22: 583–93.

22. Gillam LD, Guyer DE, Gibson TC, King ME, Marshall JE, Weyman AE. Hydrodynamic compression of the right atrium: A new echocardiographic sign of cardiac tamponade. *Circulation*. 1983; 63: 294–301.
23. Argulian E, Ramirez R. Understanding right atrial collapse: Timing is everything. *Annals of Emergency Medicine*. 2019; 73: 397–9.
24. LeWinter MW. Clinical practice. Acute pericarditis. *The New England Journal of Medicine*. 2014; 371: 2410–6.
25. Imazio M, Gaita F, LeWinter M. Evaluation and treatment of pericarditis: A systematic review. *JAMA*. 2015; 314: 1498–506.
26. Spodick DH. Acute pericarditis: Current concepts and practice. *JAMA*. 2003; 289: 1150–3.
27. Witting MD, Hu KM, Westreich AA, Tewelde S, Farzad A, Mattu A. Evaluation of spodick's sign and other electrocardiographic findings as indicators of STEMI and pericarditis. *The Journal of Emergency Medicine*. 2020; 58: 562–9.
28. Mahler SA, Lenoir KM, Wells BJ et al. Safely identifying emergency department patients with acute chest pain for early discharge. *Circulation*. 2018; 138: 2456–68.
29. Than M, Herbert M, Flaws D et al. What is an acceptable risk of major adverse cardiac event in chest pain patients soon after discharge from the Emergency Department?: A clinical survey. *International Journal of Cardiology*. 2013; 166: 752–4.
30. Backus BE, Six AJ, Kelder JC et al. A prospective validation of the HEART score for chest pain patients at the emergency department. *International Journal of Cardiology*. 2013; 168: 2153–8.
31. Chen XH, Jiang HL, Li YM et al. Prognostic values of 4 risk scores in Chinese patients with chest pain: Prospective 2-centre cohort study. *Medicine*. 2016; 95: e4778.
32. Laureano-Phillips J, Robinson RD, Aryal S et al. HEART score risk stratification of low-risk chest pain patients in the emergency department: A systematic review and meta-analysis. *Annals of Emergency Medicine*. 2019; 74: 187–203.
33. Fernando SM, Tran A, Cheng W et al. Prognostic accuracy of the HEART score for prediction of major adverse cardiac events in patients presenting with chest pain: A systematic review and meta-analysis. *Academic Emergency Medicine*. 2019; 26: 140–51.
34. Gershon CA, Yagapen AN, Lin A, Yanez D, Sun BC. Inter-rater reliability of the HEART score. *Academic Emergency Medicine*. 2019; 26: 552–5.
35. Ras M, Reitsma JB, Hoes AW, Six AJ, Poldervaart JM. Secondary analysis of frequency, circumstances and consequences of calculation errors of the HEART (history, ECG, age, risk factors and troponin) score at the emergency departments of nine hospitals in the Netherlands. *BMJ Open*. 2017; 7: e017259.
36. Poldervaart JM, Reitsma JB, Backus BE et al. Effect of using the HEART score in patients with chest pain in the emergency department: A stepped-wedge, cluster randomized trial. *Annals of Internal Medicine*. 2017; 166: 689–97.
37. Stopyra JP, Riley RF, Hiestand BC et al. The HEART pathway randomized controlled trial one-year outcomes. *Academic Emergency Medicine*. 2019; 26: 41–50.

38. Stopyra JP, Snavely AC, Lenoir KM *et al*. HEART pathway implementation safely reduces hospitalizations at one year in patients with acute chest pain. *Annals of Emergency Medicine*. 2020; 76: 555–65.

39. Ashburn NP, Smith ZP, Hunter KJ *et al*. The disutility of stress testing in low-risk HEART Pathway patients. *The American Journal of Emergency Medicine*. 2020; 45: 227–32.

40. Gesell SB, Golden SL, Limkakeng AT *et al*. Implementation of the HEART pathway: Using the consolidated framework for implementation research. *Critical Pathways in Cardiology*. 2018; 17: 191–200.

41. Carpenter CR, Bellolio F, Upadhye S, Kline JA. Navigating uncertainty with GRACE: Society for academic emergency medicine's guidelines for reasonable and appropriate care in the emergency department. *Academic Emergency Medicine*. 2021; 28: 821–5.

42. Rodriguez F, Mahaffey KW. Management of patients with NSTE-ACS: A comparison of the recent AHA/ACC and ESC guidelines. *Journal of the American College of Cardiology*. 2016; 68: 313–21.

43. Bandstein N, Ljung R, Johansson M, Holzmann MJ. Undetectable high-sensitivity cardiac troponin T level in the emergency department and risk of myocardial infarction. *Journal of the American College of Cardiology*. 2014; 63: 2569–78.

44. Cullen L, Mueller C, Parsonage WA *et al*. Validation of high-sensitivity troponin I in a 2-hour diagnostic strategy to assess 30-day outcomes in emergency department patients with possible acute coronary syndrome. *Journal of the American College of Cardiology*. 2013; 62: 1242–9.

45. Kavsak PA, Neumann JT, Cullen L *et al*. Clinical chemistry score versus high-sensitivity cardiac troponin I and T tests alone to identify patients at low or high risk for myocardial infarction or death at presentation to the emergency department. *CMAJ*. 2018; 190: E974–E84.

46. McCord J, Cabrera R, Lindahl B *et al*. Prognostic utility of a modified HEART score in chest pain patients in the emergency department. *Circulation. Cardiovascular Quality and Outcomes*. 2017; 10: e003101.

47. Mokhtari A, Lindahl B, Schiopu A *et al*. A 0-hour/1-hour protocol for safe, early discharge of chest pain patients. *Academic Emergency Medicine*. 2017; 24: 983–92.

48. Sandoval Y, Nowak R, deFilippi CR *et al*. Myocardial infarction risk stratification with a single measurement of high-sensitivity troponin I. *Journal of the American College of Cardiology*. 2019; 74: 271–82.

49. Tan JWC, Tan HJG, Sahlen AO *et al*. Performance of cardiac troponins within the HEART score in predicting major adverse cardiac events at the emergency department. *The American Journal of Emergency Medicine*. 2020; 38: 1560–7.

50. Wang G, Zheng W, Wu S *et al*. Comparison of usual care and the HEART score for effectively and safely discharging patients with low-risk chest pain in the emergency department: Would the score always help? *Clinical Cardiology*. 2020; 43: 371–8.

51. Shah ASV, Anand A, Strachan FE *et al*. High-sensitivity troponin in the evaluation of patients with suspected acute coronary syndrome: A stepped-wedge, cluster-randomised controlled trial. *Lancet*. 2018; 392: 919–28.

52. Crowder KR, Jones TD, Lang ES *et al.* The impact of high-sensitivity troponin implementation on hospital operations and patient outcomes in 3 tertiary care centers. *The American Journal of Emergency Medicine.* 2015; 33: 1790–4.
53. Carlton EW, Ingram J, Taylor H *et al.* Limit of detection of troponin discharge strategy versus usual care: Randomised controlled trial. *Heart.* 2020; 106: 1586–94.
54. Kaambwa B, Ratcliffe J, Horsfall M *et al.* Cost effectiveness of high-sensitivity troponin compared to conventional troponin among patients presenting with undifferentiated chest pain: A trial based analysis. *International Journal of Cardiology.* 2017; 238: 144–50.
55. Haase R, Schlattmann P, Gueret P *et al.* Diagnosis of obstructive coronary artery disease using computed tomography angiography in patients with stable chest pain depending on clinical probability and in clinically important subgroups: Meta-analysis of individual patient data. *BMJ Open.* 2019; 365: l1945.
56. Gongora CA, Bavishi C, Uretsky S, Argulian E. Acute chest pain evaluation using coronary computed tomography angiography compared with standard of care: A meta-analysis of randomised clinical trials. *Heart.* 2018; 104: 215–21.
57. Goehler A, Mayrhofer T, Pursnani A *et al.* Long-term health outcomes and cost-effectiveness of coronary CT angiography in patients with suspicion for acute coronary syndrome. *Journal of Cardiovascular Computed Tomography.* 2020; 14: 44–54.
58. Wu KH, Yen YL, Wu CH, Hwang CY, Cheng SY. Learning from an analysis of closed malpractice litigation involving myocardial infarction. *Journal of Forensic and Legal Medicine.* 2017; 48: 41–5.
59. Brooker JA, Hastings JW, Major-Monfried H *et al.* The association between medicolegal and professional concerns and chest pain admission rates. *Academic Emergency Medicine.* 2015; 22: 883–6.
60. Pines JM, Isserman JA, Szyld D, Dean AJ, McCusker CM, Hollander JE. The effect of physician risk tolerance and the presence of an observation unit on decision making for ED patients with chest pain. *The American Journal of Emergency Medicine.* 2010; 28: 771–9.
61. Schriger DL, Menchine M, Wiechmann W, Carmelli G. Emergency physician risk estimates and admission decisions for chest pain: A web-based scenario study. *Annals of Emergency Medicine.* 2018; 72: 511–22.
62. Carpenter CR, Raja AS, Brown MD. Overtesting and the downstream consequences of overtreatment: Implications of "Preventing Overdiagnosis" for emergency medicine. *Academic Emergency Medicine.* 2015; 22: 1484–92.
63. Tsarpalis K. Coronary computed tomographic angiography and potential for overtreatment. *JAMA Internal Medicine.* 2018; 178: 435–6.
64. Oliver G, Reynard C, Morris N, Body R. Can emergency physician gestalt "Rule In" or "Rule Out" acute coronary syndrome: Validation in a multicenter prospective diagnostic cohort study. *Academic Emergency Medicine.* 2019; 27: 24–30.
65. Probst MA, Kanzaria HK, Frosch DL *et al.* Perceived appropriateness of shared decision-making in the emergency department: A survey study. *Academic Emergency Medicine.* 2016; 23: 375–81.

66. Weinstock MD, Mattu A, Hess EP. How do we balance the long-term health of a patient with the short-term risk to the physician? *The Journal of Emergency Medicine*. 2017; 53: 583–5.
67. Hess EP, Grudzen CR, Thomson R, Raja AS, Carpenter CR. Shared decision-making in the emergency department: Respecting patient autonomy when seconds count. *Academic Emergency Medicine*. 2015; 22: 856–64.
68. Hess EP, Hollander JE, Schaffer JT *et al*. Shared decision making in patients with low risk chest pain: Prospective randomized pragmatic trial. *BMJ*. 2016; 355: i6165.
69. Carpenter CR, Kaphingst KA, Goodman MS, Lin MJ, Melson AT, Griffey RT. Feasibility and diagnostic accuracy of brief health literacy and numeracy screening instruments in an urban emergency department. *Academic Emergency Medicine*. 2014; 21: 137–46.
70. Griffey RT, McNaughton CD, McCarthy DM *et al*. Shared decision making in the emergency department among patients with limited health literacy: Beyond slower and louder. *Academic Emergency Medicine*. 2016; 23: 1403–9.
71. Hogan TM, Richmond NL, Carpenter CR *et al*. Shared decision making to improve the emergency care of older adults: A research agenda. *Academic Emergency Medicine*. 2016; 23: 1386–93.
72. Probst MA, Tschatscher CF, Lohse CM, Bellolio MF, Hess EP. Factors associated with patient involvement in emergency care decisions: A secondary analysis of the chest pain choice multicenter randomized trial. *Academic Emergency Medicine*. 2018; 25: 1107–17.
73. Rising KL, Hollander JE, Schaffer JT *et al*. Effectiveness of a decision aid in potentially vulnerable patients: A secondary analysis of the chest pain choice multicenter randomized trial. *Medical Decision Making*. 2018; 38: 69–78.
74. Sepucha KR, Breslin M, Graffeo C, Carpenter CR, Hess EP. State of the science: Tools and measurement for shared decision making. *Academic Emergency Medicine*. 2016; 23: 1325–31.
75. Kanzaria HK, Booker-Vaughns J, Itakura K *et al*. Dissemination and implementation of shared decision making into clinical practice: A research agenda. *Academic Emergency Medicine*. 2016; 23: 1368–79.

Chapter 22 **Palpitations**

Marc A. Probst[1] and Christopher R. Carpenter[2]

[1] Department of Emergency Medicine, Columbia University Irving Medical Center, New York, NY, USA
[2] Department of Emergency Medicine, Washington University School of Medicine, St. Louis, MO, USA

Highlights

- Relatively little research has been published on palpitations in the emergency care setting. Thus, clinical management regarding diagnostic and prognosis is extrapolated from the primary care setting.
- History and physical exam do not accurately identify clinically significant dysrhythmias as the etiology of palpitations, so emergency clinicians rely on clinical gestalt and electrocardiographic testing to aid in diagnosis, as opposed to clinical risk scores or patient decision aids.
- Attributing anxiety and other psychiatric conditions as the etiology of palpitations could delay diagnostic testing, and should be a diagnosis of exclusion.
- Emerging ambulatory cardiac monitors may provide alternative post-ED monitoring to identify preventable or potentially dangerous precipitants of palpitations.

Background

Palpitations are the subjectively unpleasant awareness of heartbeats. In this chapter, we will review palpitations without syncope since syncope is discussed in this chapter. Between 2001 and 2010 palpitations represented approximately 0.58% of emergency department (ED) visits in the United States.[1] Most individuals with cardiac dysrhythmias do not report

---

Evidence-Based Emergency Care: Diagnostic Testing and Clinical Decision Rules, Third Edition.
Edited by Jesse M. Pines, Fernanda Bellolio, Christopher R. Carpenter, and Ali S. Raja.

palpitations, and approximately 40% of patients with palpitations who present for evaluation are found to have a dysrhythmia.[1,2] The 1-year mortality rate for individuals evaluated for palpitations is 1.6%.[2]

The differential diagnosis for palpitations is broad (Table 22.1).[3] Some elements of the history may provide clues as to the etiology of palpitations, allowing focused additional diagnostic testing to be obtained. Patients who present with new-onset palpitations at a younger age are likely to have developed paroxysmal supraventricular tachycardia (PSVT). In older adults, atrial fibrillation and ventricular tachycardia (VT) are more often associated with structural heart disease.[4] The onset of symptoms with exercise or stress (due to catecholamine surges) can imply VT or sinus tachycardia,[5] while symptoms that occur during periods of increased vagal tone or while sleeping can be associated with atrial fibrillation or prolonged QT syndrome (an inherited abnormality of myocardial repolarization).[6] Medications associated with prolonged QT and subsequent Torsades de Pointes include antiarrhythmics, antimicrobials, antihistamines, psychotropics, diuretics, protease inhibitors, and gastrointestinal motility agents.[7,8] Young adults consumers of energy drinks high in caffeine are more likely to report palpitations than nonconsumers.[9,10] Inappropriate sinus tachycardia is characterized by atypical increases in sinus rates and occurs most frequently in young women during minimal exertion or with emotional stress, possibly due to a hypersensitivity to beta-adrenergic stimulation.[11]

Table 22.1 Differential diagnosis of palpitations

Dysrhythmia
  Supraventricular
    Atrial fibrillation or atrial flutter
    AV node re-entry
    Premature atrial complex
  Ventricular
    Ventricular tachycardia
    Premature ventricular complex
Sinus tachycardia
  Hyperthyroidism
  Hypovolemia
  Stimulants (e.g., caffeine, nicotine, cocaine, or amphetamines.)
  Hypoglycemia
  Pheochromocytoma
  Medications (e.g., sympathomimetic agents, vasodilators, anticholinergic drugs, or withdrawal from beta blockers.)
Anxiety or panic disorder

Source: Data from [3].

Although anxiety and panic disorders can be associated with palpitations, these psychiatric conditions must remain diagnoses of exclusion in the ED. One investigation of 107 consecutive PSVT patients found that 67% fulfilled DSM (*Diagnostic and Statistical Manual of Mental Disorders*) criteria for panic disorder and that true dysrhythmias were misdiagnosed for a median of 3.3 years.[12] About half of patients referred for Holter monitoring will have at least one anxiety or depressive disorder if tested using DSM criteria.[13] At 6 months, 84% of palpitation patients have recurrent palpitations with significantly higher rates of psychosocial morbidity and physician visits.[14] A 10-item screening instrument derived in primary care settings to distinguish patients whose palpitations are more likely to result from panic disorder and in whom monitoring might be avoided awaits validation in ED settings.[15] The panic disorder modules of the Patient Health Questionnaire and Psychiatric Diagnostic Screening Questionnaire are weak predictors of panic attacks or panic disorder among ED adults with chest pain or palpitations.[16]

Multiple diagnostic tests are used in an attempt to identify the etiology of palpitations and distinguish clinically significant sources. The initial test-of-choice is generally a standard 12-lead electrocardiogram (ECG) (Table 22.2). If electrical or structural abnormalities are identified on the ECG, additional cardiac evaluation may be warranted. A Holter monitor simultaneously records two or three electrocardiographic leads and may record continuously (loop recorders) or be triggered at the time of symptoms (event recorders). Stored events on the Holter monitor can be transmitted through a telephone for physician review. Electrophysiological studies are more invasive tests of cardiac conduction that require a cardiology lab. Exercise treadmill testing or other types of provocative cardiac testing (also known as stress testing) may

Table 22.2 Electrocardiographic clues to palpitation etiology

ECG finding	Possible etiology
Complete heart block	PVC, VT
LVH (Q$_i$, aVL, V4–V6)	Hypertrophic cardiomyopathy with VT
P-mitrale	Atrial fibrillation
Premature ventricular complexes	PVC, VT
Prolonged QT interval	VT
Q-waves	PVC, VT
Short PR interval, delta waves	WPW syndrome, other re-entrant tachycardia

Q$_i$ = Q-wave in lead I; PVC = premature ventricular contraction; VT = ventricular tachycardia; LVH = left ventricular hypertrophy; WPW = Wolff–Parkinson–White.
Source: Data from [17].

be useful if palpitations are precipitated by exercise or thought to be associated with myocardial ischemia.[18] Echocardiography is indicated to evaluate suspected structural heart disease that may be associated with palpitations; however, identifying structural heart disease does not establish a causal relationship with palpitations.

Clinical question

Can history, physical exam, and/or clinical risk scores accurately and reliably distinguish clinically significant dysrhythmia from other causes of palpitations?

Six studies have evaluated the diagnostic accuracy of history for significant dysrhythmias.[3] The only useful clinical finding is the sensation of rapid pounding in the neck, which has a positive likelihood ratio (LR+) of 177 (CI 25–1251) and a negative likelihood ratio (LR–) of 0.07 (CI 0.03–0.19) for AV nodal re-entry (Table 22.3).[19]

None of these studies were conducted in ED settings. Summerton *et al.* evaluated 139 adult patients with new-onset palpitations from 36 primary care practices in the United Kingdom over 9 months using an event recorder as the criterion standard.[20] Hoefman *et al.* evaluated 127 consecutive patients with palpitations and lightheadedness from 41 general practice clinics in the Netherlands using a continuous event recorder as the criterion standard.[21] Barsky *et al.* studied two cohorts of 131 and 145 patients who had been evaluated for palpitations using a 24-hour Holter monitor and DSM criteria as the criterion standard for dysrhythmia and psychiatric disorder, respectively.[13,22] Gürsoy *et al.* assessed 244 patients referred for electrophysiology to assess AV nodal reentry tachycardia.[19] Sakhuja *et al.* evaluated 239 patients referred for electrophysiology studies, cardiac ablation, or cardioversion using a combination of the electrophysiology studies, Holter monitoring, telemetry, and ECG for the criterion standard.[23]

Clinical question

Can additional testing (ECG, Holter monitoring, electrophysiology lab) accurately distinguish clinically significant dysrhythmia from other causes of palpitations?

The 12-lead ECG is the initial test of choice for palpitations, but in primary care, this is possible for only one-third of patients.[20,24] If an ECG is performed while palpitations are being reported, 48% have a rhythm abnormality, including 19% with a clinically relevant dysrhythmia.[24] The diagnostic yield

Table 22.3 Diagnostic accuracy of signs and symptoms to identify clinically significant dysrhythmia in palpitations

	Positive likelihood ratio (LR+)	Negative likelihood ratio (LR−)
History		
Family history of palpitations	1.07	0.98
Panic disorder	1.0	1.0
Any psychiatric disorder	0.67	1.12
Description		
Continuous	0.93	1.20
Duration > 5 minutes	0.79	1.23
Duration > 1 minute	1.17	0.63
Heart rate > 100 bpm	1.08	0.86
Regular	1.38	0.55
Precipitants		
Alcohol	1.94	0.90
Breathing	0.52	1.20
Caffeine	2.06	0.89
Exercise	0.78	1.07
Holiday	0.79	1.04
Lying in bed	1.02	0.97
Resting	1.02	0.97
Sleeping	2.44	0.63
Weekend	0.72	1.08
Working	1.54	0.86
Associated symptoms		
Chest pain	0.92	1.02
Dizziness	1.34	0.67
Dyspnea	0.27	1.12
Neck fullness	0.85	1.04
Neck pounding	177	0.07
Presyncope	1.04	0.95
Vasovagal	1.72	0.63
Visible neck pulsations	2.68	0.87

Source: Data from [3].

of ECG in the ED evaluation of palpitations has not been described, nor has the diagnostic yield of laboratory testing.

One systematic review evaluated six diagnostic devices for the evaluation of palpitations.[25]
1. Holter monitor: Records an ECG continuously for up to 72 hours with palpitations linked to the electrical rhythm via a patient diary.
2. External event recorders without a loop: Patient-activated ECG transmitted via telephone to a receiving center for interpretation.

3. Event recorders with looping memory (continuous event recorders [CERs]): Continuous one-lead recording with pre- and post-event electrical rhythm saved when patients activate the device.

4. Auto-triggered event monitors with looping memory (Auto-CER): Automatically recognizes prespecified brady- or tachy-dysrhythmias via continuous monitoring. Transmit ECG data to a monitor at the patient's home when triggered by prespecified criteria or patient activation. If appropriate, the rhythm is then transmitted to a monitoring center for interpretation and therapeutic intervention.

5. Implantable auto-triggered loop recorder (ILR): Same capability as number 4 above without the requirement of external electrodes. Generally reserved for longer periods of monitoring (12–24 months).

6. Pacemakers and cardiac defibrillators: Can be programmed to detect, store, and send rhythm data to remote receiving facilities.

Twenty-eight studies have evaluated these diagnostic instruments, including 12 simple descriptive studies.[25] Since the descriptive studies suffer from numerous diagnostic biases described in Chapter 6 (e.g., the criterion standard is the reference device [incorporation bias], or an unequal distribution of patients with preexisting structural heart disease or device-guided interventions [spectrum bias]),[26] the comparative studies assessing the diagnostic performance for one device against another are more informative. These comparative trials demonstrate the following:

- CER versus Holter: CER was superior at establishing a diagnosis with a range of 21–62% definitive diagnoses (versus 30% maximum for Holter) in six studies. CER was also superior at excluding a significant dysrhythmia (34% excluded by CER versus 2% for Holter).[27-30]

- CER versus ECG: Within 30 days, the CER was diagnostic in 37% versus 10% with only the initial ECG.[31]

- CER versus routine primary care physician gestalt: At 6 months, relevant dysrhythmias were diagnosed in 22% of CER versus 7% of patients using gestalt alone, while primary care physicians had no explanation for symptoms in 17% of CER and 38% of gestalt patients. CER did not alter referral rates or ancillary diagnostic testing, but cardiology referrals in the CER group may have been more productive since a cardiac problem was identified in 92% (versus 57% of gestalt patients) of referrals.[32]

- Auto-CER versus External event recorders without a loop: Both modes established a diagnosis in >80% of patients, although Auto-CER found an additional 11–17% of relevant diagnoses.[33-35]

- Auto-ILR versus patient-triggered ILR: A dysrhythmia occurred with symptoms in 16% of patient-triggered ILR. Auto-ILR had an 83% inappropriate activation rate, and no relevant dysrhythmias were detected by auto-ILR that were not detected by patient-triggered ILR.[36]

- ILR versus conventional strategy (24-hour Holter, 4-week CER, or electrophysiology testing if the first two strategies were nondiagnostic): At 1 year, a dysrhythmia diagnosis was obtained in 21% via the conventional strategy and 73% with the ILR.[37]

The cost-effectiveness of outpatient CER has been reported as $98 per new diagnosis at 1 week, rising to $5832 per new diagnosis at 3 weeks.[38] The optimal duration of External event recorders without a loop is 2 weeks during which 75% of all diagnoses are established, including 83% of all clinically relevant diagnoses.[39] Investigators continue to evaluate smartphone and other emerging monitoring technologies as alternatives to Holter devices. One study enrolling patients across three academic EDs evaluated the efficacy of Zio®Patch, an adhesive patch applied at the time of discharge, which the patient then removes and mails back after a symptomatic episode or within 2-weeks. This device detected dysrhythmia in 48% of patients in a median time of 1.5 days for an overall diagnostic yield of 63%.[40] In another open-label, randomized controlled trial of ED patients presenting with palpitations in the United Kingdom, a smartphone-based event recorder increased the detection of symptomatic rhythms at 90-days to 55.6% from 9.5% in controls. More importantly, the mean time to detection decreased from 43 to 9.5 days.[41] A scoping review on mobile self-monitoring ECG devices reported in high-risk adults palpitations could coincide with atrial fibrillation. The use of these devices can be beneficial in decreasing patient's anxiety and lowering morbidity and mortality at a low cost.[42] A systematic review of 14 studies without meta-analysis because of the large heterogeneity among the included studies, reported that smartphone-based ECG devices allow for better documentation of dysrhythmias compared to standard care and increase patient empowerment and engagement on their health care. Concern was raised for possible overdiagnosis of dysrhythmias without clinical significance.[43] Establishing smartphone-based monitoring protocol from the ED requires both institutional funding and coordination with local cardiology and primary care teams but provides a theoretically more convenient and contemporary approach to post-ED dysrhythmia detection.[44]

Comment

History and physical exam are not accurate enough to distinguish clinically significant dysrhythmias from benign etiologies in patients with palpitations. A 12-lead ECG is regularly performed in the ED and may reveal relevant information, but is not always diagnostic. Selection biases imply that existing research is not representative of ED patients presenting with palpitations. During an ED visit, clinicians monitor for the presence of malignant dysrhythmia and associated symptoms when determining disposition and referrals.[45] While awaiting the derivation and validation of clinical risk scores to identify low- or high-risk ED palpitation patients, many clinicians use unstructured clinical gestalt and shared decision-making to determine disposition and testing strategies.[45,46] Figure 22.1 provides one ED protocol to begin standardizing the diagnostic approach for palpitations based upon the available evidence. High-risk patients may require additional testing even if history, physical exam, and ECG do not delineate a clear etiology for palpitations.

High-risk patients are defined as follows:[17]

1. Abnormal heart structure including scar formation from myocardial infarction, dilated cardiomyopathy, clinically significant valvular regurgitation or stenosis, or hypertrophic cardiomyopathy
2. Family history of dysrhythmia, syncope, cardiomyopathy, long-QT syndrome, or sudden death.

Optimally, an ECG should be obtained while palpitations are being reported. Since the ECG and the initial evaluation of patients presenting to the ED for evaluation of palpitations will usually be nondiagnostic, emergency providers will have to decide upon the role of ancillary outpatient testing in conjunction with primary care physicians. Several general considerations can aid effective decision-making. The frequency of palpitations is the first factor, as daily symptoms indicate a role for Holter monitoring, while weekly symptoms make an event recorder more

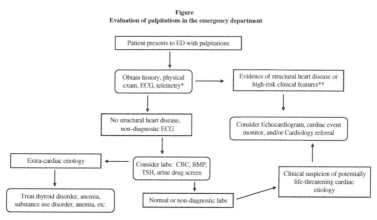

Figure
Evaluation of palpitations in the emergency department

Patient presents to ED with palpitations

Obtain history, physical exam, ECG, telemetry* → Evidence of structural heart disease or high-risk clinical features**

No structural heart disease, non-diagnostic ECG

Consider Echocardiogram, cardiac event monitor, and/or Cardiology referral

Extra-cardiac etiology ← Consider labs: CBC, BMP, TSH, urine drug screen

Clinical suspicion of potentially life-threatening cardiac etiology

Treat thyroid disorder, anemia, substance use disorder, anemia, etc.

Normal or non-diagnostic labs

* If palpitations occur while on telemetry, obtain rhythm strip and 12-lead ECG to formulate differential diagnosis and diagnostic/therapeutic decision-making.
** High-risk = known structural heart disease or family history of dysrhythmia, sudden death, prolonged QT syndrome, or cardiomyopathy.

Figure 22.1 Evaluation of palpitations in the emergency department. ECG = electrocardiogram; CBC = complete blood count; BMP = basic metabolic panel; TSH = thyroid stimulating hormone.

appropriate. Another factor is patient awareness of his or her symptoms. If patients are unaware of palpitation-inducing dysrhythmias (paroxysmal atrial fibrillation) or are unable to trigger a device (due to comorbidities or age), then an auto-triggered device is more appropriate. However, patient-triggered devices have been shown to be superior in the detection of clinically significant dysrhythmias.

Future ED-based studies are needed to assess the prevalence, incidence, and short-term sequelae of palpitations without syncope. In addition, the diagnostic and prognostic properties, including the accuracy and reliability of the history, physical exam, labs, and ECG, need to be evaluated in ED patients while defining the appropriate risk strata for whom outpatient ambulatory cardiac monitoring is most beneficial.

References

1. Probst MA, Mower MR, Kanzaria HK, Hoffman JR, Buch EF, Sun BC. Analysis of emergency department visits for palpitations (from the National Hospital Ambulatory Medical Care Survey). *The American Journal of Cardiology.* 2014; 113: 1685–90.

2. Weber BE, Kapoor WN. Evaluation and outcomes of patients with palpitations. *The American Journal of Medicine.* 1996; 100: 138–48.

3. Thavendiranathan P, Bagai A, Khoo C, Dorian P, Choudhry NK. Does this patient with palpitations have a cardiac arrhythmia? *JAMA.* 2009; 302: 2135–43.

4. Porter MJ, Morton JB, Denman R et al. Influence of age and gender on the mechanism of supraventricular tachycardia. *Heart Rhythm.* 2004; 1: 393–6.

5. Lampert R, Joska T, Burg MM, Batsford WP, McPherson CA, Jain D. Emotional and physical precipitants of ventricular arrhythmia. *Circulation.* 2002; 106: 1800–5.

6. Hansson A, Madsen-Härdig B, Olsson SB. Arrhythmia-provoking factors and symptoms at the onset of paroxysmal atrial fibrillation: A study based on interviews with 100 patients seeking hospital assistance. *BMC Cardiovascular Disorders.* 2004; 4: 13.

7. De Ponti F, Poluzzi E, Cavalli A, Recanatini M, Montanaro N. Safety of non-antiarrhythmic drugs that prolong the QT interval or induce torsade de pointes: An overview. *Drug Safety.* 2002; 25: 263–86.

8. Roden DM. Drug-induced prolongation of the QT interval. *The New England Journal of Medicine.* 2004; 350: 1013–22.

9. Nordt SP, Vilke GM, Clark RF et al. Energy drink use and adverse effects among emergency department patients. *Journal of Community Health.* 2012; 37: 976–81.

10. Busuttil M, Willoughby S. A survey of energy drink consumption among young patients presenting to the emergency department with the symptom of palpitations. *International Journal of Cardiology.* 2016; 204: 55–6.

11. Morillo CA, Klein GJ, Thakur RK, Li H, Zardini M, Yee R. Mechanism of 'inappropriate' sinus tachycardia. Role of sympathovagal balance. *Circulation.* 1994; 90: 873–7.

12. Lessmeier TJ, Gamperling D, Johnson-Liddon V *et al.* Unrecognized paroxysmal supraventricular tachycardia. Potential for misdiagnosis as panic disorder. *Archives of Internal Medicine.* 1997; 157: 537–43.

13. Barsky AJ, Cleary PD, Coeytaux RR, Ruskin JN. Psychiatric disorders in medical outpatients complaining of palpitations. *Journal of General Internal Medicine.* 1994; 9: 306–13.

14. Barsky AJ, Cleary PD, Coeytaux RR, Ruskin JN. The clinical course of palpitations in medical outpatients. *Archives of Internal Medicine.* 1995; 155: 1782–8.

15. Barsky AJ, Ahern DK, Delamater BA, Clancy SA, Bailey ED. Differential diagnosis of palpitations. Preliminary development of a screening instrument. *Archives of Family Medicine.* 1997; 6: 241–5.

16. Sung SC, Ma J, Earnest A, Rush AJ, Lim LEC, Ong MEH. Screening for panic-related anxiety in emergency department patients with cardiopulmonary complaints: A comparison of two self-report instruments. *Psychiatry Research.* 2018; 263: 7–14.

17. Zimetbaum P, Josephson ME. Evaluation of patients with palpitations. *The New England Journal of Medicine.* 1998; 338: 1369–73.

18. Abbott AV. Diagnostic approach to palpitations. *American Family Physician.* 2005; 71: 743–50.

19. Gürsoy S, Steurer G, Brugada J, Andries E, Brugada P. Brief report: The hemodynamic mechanism of pounding in the neck in atrioventricular nodal reentrant tachycardia. *The New England Journal of Medicine.* 1992; 327: 772–4.

20. Summerton N, Mann S, Rigby A, Petkar S, Dhawan J. New-onset palpitations in general practice: Assessing the discriminant value of items within the clinical history. *Family Practice.* 2001; 18: 383–92.

21. Hoefman E, Boer KR, van Weert HCPM, Reitsma JB, Koster RW, Bindels PJE. Predictive value of history taking and physical examination in diagnosing arrhythmias in general practice. *Family Practice.* 2007; 24: 636–41.

22. Barsky AJ, Cleary PD, Sarnie MK, Ruskin JN. Panic disorder, palpitations, and the awareness of cardiac activity. *The Journal of Nervous and Mental Disease.* 1994; 182: 63–70.

23. Sakhuja R, Smith LM, Tseng ZH *et al.* Test characteristics of neck fullness and witnessed neck pulsations in the diagnosis of typical AV nodal reentrant tachycardia. *Clinical Cardiology.* 2009; 32: E13–8.

24. Zwieting PJ, Knottnerus JA, Rinkens PE, Kleijne MA, Gorgels AP. Arrhythmias in general practice: Diagnostic value of patient characteristics, medical history and symptoms. *Family Practice.* 1998; 15: 343–53.

25. Hoefman E, Bindels PJE, van Weert HCPM. Efficacy of diagnostic tools for detecting cardiac arrhythmias: Systematic literature search. *Netherlands Heart Journal.* 2010; 18: 543–51.

26. Kohn MA, Carpenter CR, Newman TB. Understanding the direction of bias in studies of diagnostic test accuracy. *Academic Emergency Medicine*. 2013; 20: 1194–206.
27. Grodman RS, Capone RJ, Most AS. Arrhythmia surveillance by transtelephonic monitoring: Comparison with Holter monitoring in symptomatic ambulatory patients. *American Heart Journal*. 1979; 98: 459–64.
28. Kus T, Nadeau R, Costi P, Molin F, Primeau R. Comparison of the diagnostic yield of Holter versus transtelephonic monitoring. *The Canadian Journal of Cardiology*. 1995; 11: 891–4.
29. Kinlay S, Leitch JW, Neil A, Chapman BL, Hardy DB, Fletcher PJ. Cardiac event recorders yield more diagnoses and are more cost-effective than 48-hour Holter monitoring in patients with palpitations. A controlled clinical trial. *Annals of Internal Medicine*. 1996; 124: 16–20.
30. Scalvini S, Zanelli E, Martinelli G, Baratti D, Giordano A, Glisenti F. Cardiac event recording yields more diagnoses than 24-hour Holter monitoring in patients with palpitations. *Journal of Telemedicine and Telecare*. 2005; 11: 14–6.
31. Wu J, Kessler DK, Chakko S, Kessler KM. A cost-effectiveness strategy for transtelephonic arrhythmia monitoring. *The American Journal of Cardiology*. 1995; 75: 184–5.
32. Hoefman E, van Weert HCPM, Reitsma JB, Koster RW, Bindels PJE. Diagnostic yield of patient-activated loop recorders for detecting heart rhythm abnormalities in general practice: A randomised clinical trial. *Family Practice*. 2005; 22: 478–84.
33. Balmelli N, Naegeli B, Bertel O. Diagnostic yield of automatic and patient-triggered ambulatory cardiac event recording in the evaluation of patients with palpitations, dizziness, or syncope. *Clinical Cardiology*. 2003; 26: 173–6.
34. Martinez T, Sztajzel J. Utility of event loop recorders for the management of arrhythmias in young ambulatory patients. *International Journal of Cardiology*. 2004; 97: 495–8.
35. Reiffel JA, Schwarzberg R, Murry M. Comparison of autotriggered memory loop recorders versus standard loop recorders versus 24-hour Holter monitors for arrhythmia detection. *The American Journal of Cardiology*. 2005; 95: 1055–9.
36. Ng E, Stafford PJ, Ng GA. Arrhythmia detection by patient and auto-activation in implantable loop recorders. *Journal of Interventional Cardiac Electrophysiology*. 2004; 10: 147–52.
37. Giada F, Gulizia M, Francese M *et al*. Recurrent unexplained palpitations (RUP) study comparison of implantable loop recorder versus conventional diagnostic strategy. *Journal of the American College of Cardiology*. 2007; 49: 1951–6.
38. Zimetbaum P, Kim KY, Josephson ME, Goldberger AL, Cohen DJ. Diagnostic yield and optimal duration of continuous-loop event monitoring for the diagnosis of palpitations. A cost-effectiveness analysis. *Annals of Internal Medicine*. 1998; 128: 890–5.
39. Hoefman E, van Weert HCPM, Boer KR, Reitsma JB, Koster RW, Bindels PJE. Optimal duration of event recording for diagnosis of arrhythmias in patients with palpitations and light-headedness in the general practice. *Family Practice*. 2006; 24: 11–3.

40. Schreiber D, Sattar A, Drigalla D. Ambulatory cardiac monitoring for discharged emergency department patients with possible cardiac arrhythmias. *The Western Journal of Emergency Medicine*. 2014; 15: 194–8.
41. Reed MJ, Grubb NR, Lang CC *et al.* Multi-centre randomised controlled trial of a smartphone-based event recorder alongside standard care versus standard care for patients presenting to the emergency department with palpitations and pre-syncope: The IPED (Investigation of Palpitations in the ED) study. *EClinicalMedicine*. 2019; 8: 37–46.
42. Marston HR, Hadley R, Banks D, MDCM D. Mobile self-monitoring ECG devices to diagnose arrhythmia that coincide with palpitations: A scoping review. *Healthcare (Basel)*. 2019; 7: 96.
43. Biersteker TE, Schalij MJ, Treskes RW. Impact of mobile health devices for the detection of atrial fibrillation: Systematic review. *JMIR mHealth and uHealth*. 2021; 9: e26161.
44. Reed MJ, Muir A, Cullen J *et al.* Establishing a smartphone ambulatory ECG service for patients presenting to the emergency department with pre-syncope and palpitations. *Medicina*. 2021; 57: 147.
45. Probst MA, Kanzaria HK, Hoffman JR *et al.* Emergency physicians' perceptions and decision-making processes regarding patients presenting with palpitations. *The Journal of Emergency Medicine*. 2015; 49: 236–43.
46. Hess EP, Grudzen CR, Thomson R, Raja AS, Carpenter CR. Shared decision-making in the emergency department: Respecting patient autonomy when seconds count. *Academic Emergency Medicine*. 2015; 22: 856–64.

SECTION 4
Infectious Disease

Chapter 23 **Bacterial Meningitis in Children**

Jana L. Anderson and Fernanda Bellolio

Department of Emergency Medicine, Mayo Clinic, Rochester, MN, USA

Highlights

- All infants less than 28 days with fever should undergo a lumbar puncture to rule out bacterial meningitis.
- Infants less than 60 days with a febrile urinary tract infection should undergo a lumbar puncture to evaluate for meningitis because up to 40% of children with meningitis have an abnormal urinalysis.
- Immunization status is important when assessing the risk of bacterial meningitis.
- The Bacterial Meningitis Score can identify bacterial versus viral meningitis in children older than 2 months.
- Both the Step-by-Step and PECARN febrile infant rules risk stratify older infants to avoid unnecessary lumbar puncture.

Background

The epidemiology of acute bacterial meningitis has changed drastically since the introduction of routine vaccination with the *Haemophilus influenzae* type B (Hib) in and the polyvalent conjugated pneumococcal vaccine.[1] The incidence of invasive Hib infection among young children (<5 years of age) has decreased by 99%, from 46 to 100 cases per 100,000 children to <1 case per 100,000 children.[2] Hib vaccination is a 3 to 4 immunization series that occurs at 2, 4, possibly 6 (depending on the type of vaccine used), and a booster at 12 to 15 months.[3] Similarly, the current 13-valent pneumococcal

---

Evidence-Based Emergency Care: Diagnostic Testing and Clinical Decision Rules, Third Edition.
Edited by Jesse M. Pines, Fernanda Bellolio, Christopher R. Carpenter, and Ali S. Raja.
© 2023 John Wiley & Sons Ltd. Published 2023 by John Wiley & Sons Ltd.

conjugated vaccine is administered at 2, 4, 6, and 12 to 15 months. When the 7-valent pneumococcal vaccination was introduced in 2000, the rate of pneumococcal meningitis decreased by 66% from 7.7 per 100,000 to 2.6 per 100,000 in children less than 2 years of age. A decline of 51.5% was seen in older children 2 to 4 years of age.[4] Meningococcal disease has two peaks of increased incidence, the highest is still in young children less than 4 years at 0.69 per 100,000 persons, and then in the teenage years, 15 to 19 years, at 0.29 per 100,000 persons.[5] Currently, there is a two-dose schedule of the meningococcal vaccine that is to be given at 11 to 12 years and then a booster at 16 years.[3]

Vaccination has created four distinct populations of children at different risks of acute bacterial meningitis: neonates less than <1 month, infants 1–2 months, unvaccinated or under-vaccinated children, and vaccinated children. However, small areas of unimmunized and under-immunized children remain and may continue to serve as potential reservoirs for disease. Despite vaccination, there will always be a child with an underlying immunodeficiency or infection from a strain not covered in current vaccines.

Preterm and infants less than 28 days of age are at the highest risk for bacterial meningitis at 0.25 to 0.32 per 1000 live births.[6] This is likely due to their immature immune system and intrapartum bacterial exposures. Group B Streptococcus (GBS) continues to be a leading pathogen in neonates despite widespread intrapartum surveillance and treatment, accounting for 40% of disease.[7] Late-onset (6 to 90 days) and very late onset (>90 days) GBS diseases have the highest rates and mortality in preterm neonates.[8] Most mothers carried GBS in the rectovaginal flora and 6% of mothers had mastitis at the time of the late-onset GBS diagnosis. Intrapartum antibiotics have been associated with delayed presentation of symptoms and milder GBS disease.[8] Next to GBS, E. coli and other Gram-negative bacteria have emerged as the second leading pathogen, attributing to 30% of meningitis infections. Listeria continues to be a lingering pathogen that still is considered in this age group (Table 23.1).

Table 23.1 Most common pathogens of bacterial meningitis by age

Age	Pathogens
Newborns	Group B Streptococcus (GBS), S. pneumoniae, L. monocytogenes, E. coli
≥1 month and <3 months	GBS, Gram-negative bacilli, S. pneumoniae, N. meningitidis
≥3 months and <3 years	S. pneumoniae, N. meningitidis, GBS, Gram-negative bacilli, H. influenzae type b (Hib)
≥3 years-teen	S. pneumoniae, N. meningitidis

Clinical question

Can history or physical exam accurately and reliably distinguish meningitis from other diagnoses?

History and physical exam are not sufficient to rule out bacterial meningitis in children, particularly those younger than 2 months of age. The classic presentation of fever, headache, and neck pain, and stiffness is rare and usually late in the illness. Absence of fever does not rule out meningitis.[9] In a large multicenter study of children older than 29 days with culture-proven meningitis, 7% did not have preceding fever, and only 40% had meningismus.[10] In children younger than 4 years, only 5% had headache, and among older children aged 5 to 17 years, 71% had headache.[11] Of children with meningitis, only 16% presented critically ill; either obtundent, requiring intubation, or pressors. A total of 10% had a seizure at or prior to presentation and 4% had purpura.[10] Neonates may present with subtle signs and symptoms; fever only, hypothermia, irritability, poor feeding, vomiting, and apnea. Practitioners must remain vigilant even in this era of vaccination and have a low threshold to perform a lumbar puncture to evaluate for bacterial meningitis.

Neonatal fever is the classic situation where an infant would be evaluated for meningitis. In the infant less than 1 month of age that presents to the emergency department (ED) for fever, a meta-analysis found the estimated risk for meningitis was 1.3% (CI 0.8–2.0%).[12] Neonates that are not well-appearing or have a history of prematurity are at extremely high risk and warrant a full sepsis evaluation including ruling out meningitis, whether fever is present or not, when presenting with concerning symptoms.

Clinical question

Are clinical decision rules useful in ruling out bacterial meningitis at the time of clinical presentation in children?

The Bacterial Meningitis Score (BMS) was developed to help discern bacterial from aseptic meningitis in the setting cerebrospinal fluid (CSF) pleocytosis (white blood cell count ≥ 10 cells/μL) in children older than 29 days of age. The tool was originally developed in 2007 and then refined with further exclusion criteria added in 2012. The BMS has a sensitivity for bacterial meningitis of 99.3% (CI 98.7–99.7%) and a negative predictive value of 98.3% (CI 96.6–99.3%).[13,14] The score utilizes CSF Gram stain, CSF absolute neutrophil count (ANC) ≥1000 cells/μL, CSF protein ≥ 80 mg/dL, peripheral blood ANC ≥ 10,000 cells/μL, and seizure at presentation (Table 23.2). In the original study, there were 3295 patients with CSF pleocytosis, 3.7% had bacterial

Table 23.2 Bacterial meningitis score for children ≥ 2 months of age

Low-risk features include the following:
- Negative CSF Gram stain
- CSF ANC < 1000 cells/μL
- CSF protein < 80 mg/dL
- Peripheral blood ANC < 10,000 cells/μL
- No seizure at or prior to initial presentation

CSF = cerebrospinal fluid; ANC = absolute neutrophil count.
Source: Data from [13, 14].

meningitis and the remainder had aseptic meningitis. There were 1714 children who were categorized as low risk by the BMS (as a score of 0). Of those, 2 had bacterial meningitis, and both were younger than 2 months old. In the meta-analysis used for the refinement of the rule, 8 validation studies and 5312 patients were included. The prevalence of meningitis was 23%, and the score missed 9 patients with bacterial meningitis: 3 patients were < 2 months old and 3 had petechiae or purpura. The 6 patients who were older than 2 months all had *N. meningitidis*. BMS ≥1 predicted bacterial meningitis with sensitivity of 99.3%, specificity 62.1%, and negative predictive value of 99.6%. The authors concluded that the BMS is an accurate clinical decision rule that imparts a very low risk of bacterial meningitis in patients who fulfill the criteria (Table 23.2) but should not be used in children younger than 2 month of age, those ill appearing, those that received antibiotics prior to the presentations, have petechiae or purpura, immunocompromised, have ventriculoperitoneal shunt or recent neurosurgery.[13,14]

In an external validation of the BMS, 166 children were included, 20 of whom had bacterial meningitis. The sensitivity of the decision rule was 100% (95% CI 84–100%), and the specificity was 66% (95% CI 57–73%). The authors concluded that using the rule would make it possible to avoid two-thirds of antibiotic treatments and hospitalization in children with acute meningitis.[15]

The BMS was further refined into the Meningitest criteria that includes procalcitonin values in children aged 29 days and older (Table 23.3).[16] In a secondary analysis of retrospective multicenter hospital-based cohort studies of 6 pediatric EDs and intensive care units (ICU)s, 198 children (including 96 with bacterial meningitis) were included. Procalcitonin had an area under the receiver operating characteristic curve of 0.98 (95% CI 0.95–0.99). Using a 0.5-ng/mL threshold, the sensitivity was 99% (95% CI 97–100%) and specificity 83% (95% CI 76–90%) for distinguishing between bacterial and aseptic meningitis.[17] In a different study, the BMS and Meningitest both showed 100% sensitivity (95% CI 96–100%), with BMS having higher specificity (52% [95% CI 42–62%] versus 36% [95% CI 27–46%]). The authors

Table 23.3 Meningitis criteria for children older than 29 days of age

Antibiotic treatment and hospitalization are indicated in children
with meningitis and at least one of the following criteria:
- Seizure
- "Toxic" appearance (irritability, lethargy, or poor capillary refill)
- Purpura
- Positive CSF Gram stain
- Procalcitonin ≥ 0.5 ng/mL
- CSF protein ≥ 50 mg/dL

CSF = cerebrospinal fluid.

concluded that use of the BMS could safely avoid more unnecessary antibiotic treatments for children compared to the Meningitest.[18]

Recently, two methods to risk stratifying infants with fever and at low risk for serious bacterial infections (and therefore applicable to meningitis) have been published. One, the European study called the Step-by-Step (SbS) and the North American study performed by the Pediatric Emergency Care Applied Research Network (PECARN).[19,20] These studies are sequential in their approach and utilize procalcitonin and ANC to risk stratify infants that are at low risk for serious bacterial infections and may forego a lumbar puncture. The SbS guideline classifies neonates less than 21 days as high risk and therefore would require a lumbar puncture. Infants 21 to 28 days have been found to have prevalence of bacterial infections similar to older children,[21] nonetheless, the SbS guideline misclassified 4 of 7 invasive bacterial infections in infants aged 22 to 28 days (none of which were meningitis). Therefore, caution is warranted in the 21 to 28 day old with fever. The PECARN febrile infant rule does not require a lumbar puncture to establish risk level for invasive bacterial infections. PECARN uses urinalysis, ANC, and procalcitonin in infants less than 60 days of age, with a negative predictive value of 99.6% (CI 98.4–99.9%) for serious bacterial infection. Even with the high negative predictive value found in the PECARN study, many practitioners are still reticent not to perform a lumbar puncture in the less than 28 day and particularly the 21-day old infant with fever until further studies validate these findings. Given the pathogen of neonatal bacteremia, the coverage for meningitis follows suit with ampicillin, cefotaxime, and gentamicin. In the neonate, methicillin-resistant *Staphylococcus aureus* and *S. pneumoniae* are uncommon; however, if suspected, vancomycin should be added.

For the febrile infant aged 29 to 60 days, which presents to the ED and who appear nontoxic, the rate of meningitis was found to be 0.2% (CI 0.1–0.4%).[22] As the infant ages, *GBS* becomes less prominent as a pathogen and *E. coli* and other Gram-negative become the leading bacterial cause. In a recent study of

Table 23.4 Meningitis Score for Emergencies (MSE) for children older than 30 days of age

Laboratory value	Points
Serum procalcitonin >1.20 ng/mL	3 points
Serum CRP >40 mg/L	1 point
CSF ANC >1000/mcL	1 point
CSF protein >80 mg/dL	2 points

infants less than 3 months of age with meningitis diagnosed in the ED: 93% had fever, 63% were ill-appearing, 31% had a white blood cell (WBC) count >15,000 × 10⁹/L, 40% had an abnormal urinalysis and 15% had an abnormal chest X-ray.[23] In infants 3 to 89 days of age with bacteremia or meningitis, a WBC count less than 5000 × 10⁹/L had a seven times higher likelihood of having meningitis over bacteremia.[24] Overall, WBC counts have poor sensitivity in detecting invasive bacterial infections in children.[25] In Infants greater than 28 days and all older children with suspected meningitis treatment with vancomycin and ceftriaxone to cover for penicillin-resistant *S. pneumoniae and N. meningitidis* is warranted.

In 2020, the meningitis score for emergencies (MSE) was published. The MSE includes laboratory and CSF results (Table 23.4). The derivation included children between 29 days and 14 years old with meningitis admitted to 25 Spanish EDs. A retrospective cohort was used for derivation and a prospective cohort for validation at the same centers. A total of 1009 children, including 92 with bacterial meningitis were included. The prediction rule was developed using multivariable logistic regression analysis. A score MSE ≥ 1 predicted bacterial meningitis with a sensitivity of 100% (CI 95.0–100%), specificity of 83.2% (CI 80.6–85.5%), and a negative predictive value of 100% (CI 99.4–100%). In this study, BMS ≥1 had a sensitivity of 96.7%, specificity of 51.3%, and negative predictive value (NPV) of 99.4%. However, the study included infants as young as 30 days old and the BMS is not intended for use in children younger than 2 months.[26]

Comment

Bacterial meningitis has significantly decreased since the introduction of current immunization programs in children. History and physical exam are not sufficient to rule out bacterial meningitis in children, particularly among children younger than 2 months of age. WBC count has poor sensitivity in detecting invasive bacterial infections in children, and absence of fever does not rule out meningitis.

The SbS and PECARN studies are tools for risk stratifying infants with fever and at low risk for serious bacterial infection and might forego lumbar puncture. However, these scores use procalcitonin, which might not be readily available in all EDs. Lumbar puncture is still recommended for all febrile infants younger than 21–28 days.

References

1. Brouwer MC, van de Beek D. Epidemiology of community-acquired bacterial meningitis. *Current Opinion in Infectious Diseases*. 2018; 31: 78–84.
2. Lowther SA, Shinoda N, Juni BA et al. Haemophilus influenzae type b infection, vaccination, and H. influenzae carriage in children in Minnesota, 2008–2009. *Epidemiology and Infection*. 2012; 140: 566–74.
3. Centers for Disease Control and Prevention. Vaccines schedule. https://www.cdc.gov/vaccines/schedules/hcp/imz/child-adolescent.html. Accessed October 16, 2021.
4. Tsai CJ, Griffin MR, Nuorti JP, Grijalva CG. Changing epidemiology of pneumococcal meningitis after the introduction of pneumococcal conjugate vaccine in the United States. *Clinical Infectious Diseases*. 2008; 46: 1664–72.
5. Centers for Disease Control and Prevention. Bacterial Meningitis. https://www.cdc.gov/meningitis/bacterial.html. Accessed October 16, 2021.
6. Heath PT, Okike IO, Oeser C. Neonatal meningitis: Can we do better? *Advances in Experimental Medicine and Biology*. 2011; 719: 11–24.
7. Stoll BJ. Early-onset neonatal sepsis: A continuing problem in need of novel prevention strategies. *Pediatrics*. 2016; 138: e20163038.
8. Berardi A, Rossi C, Lugli L et al. Group B streptococcus late-onset disease: 2003–2010. *Pediatrics*. 2013; 131: e361–8.
9. Curtis S, Stobart K, Vandermeer B, Simel DL, Klassen T. Clinical features suggestive of meningitis in children: A systematic review of prospective data. *Pediatrics*. 2010; 126: 952–60.
10. Nigrovic LE, Kuppermann N, Malley R. Bacterial meningitis study group of the pediatric emergency medicine collaborative research committee of the american academy of P. Children with bacterial meningitis presenting to the emergency department during the pneumococcal conjugate vaccine era. *Academic Emergency Medicine*. 2008; 15: 522–8.
11. Johansson Kostenniemi U, Norman D, Borgstrom M, Silfverdal SA. The clinical presentation of acute bacterial meningitis varies with age, sex and duration of illness. *Acta Paediatrica*. 2015; 104: 1117–24.
12. Biondi EA, Lee B, Ralston SL et al. Prevalence of bacteremia and bacterial meningitis in febrile neonates and infants in the second month of life: A systematic review and meta-analysis. *JAMA Network Open*. 2019; 2: e190874.
13. Nigrovic LE, Kuppermann N, Macias CG et al. Clinical prediction rule for identifying children with cerebrospinal fluid pleocytosis at very low risk of bacterial meningitis. *JAMA*. 2007; 297: 52–60.

14. Nigrovic LE, Malley R, Kuppermann N. Meta-analysis of bacterial meningitis score validation studies. *Archives of Disease in Childhood.* 2012; 97: 799–805.
15. Dubos F, Lamotte B, Bibi-Triki F *et al.* Clinical decision rules to distinguish between bacterial and aseptic meningitis. *Archives of Disease in Childhood.* 2006; 91: 647–50.
16. Dubos F, Moulin F, Gajdos V *et al.* Serum procalcitonin and other biologic markers to distinguish between bacterial and aseptic meningitis. *The Journal of Pediatrics.* 2006; 149: 72–6.
17. Dubos F, Korczowski B, Aygun DA *et al.* Serum procalcitonin level and other biological markers to distinguish between bacterial and aseptic meningitis in children: A European multicenter case cohort study. *Archives of Pediatrics & Adolescent Medicine.* 2008; 162: 1157–63.
18. Dubos F, Korczowski B, Aygun DA *et al.* Distinguishing between bacterial and aseptic meningitis in children: European comparison of two clinical decision rules. *Archives of Disease in Childhood.* 2010; 95: 963–7.
19. Gomez B, Mintegi S, Bressan S *et al.* Validation of the "Step-by-Step" approach in the management of young febrile infants. *Pediatrics.* 2016; 138: e20154381.
20. Kuppermann N, Dayan PS, Levine DA *et al.* A clinical prediction rule to identify febrile infants 60 days and younger at low risk for serious bacterial infections. *JAMA Pediatrics.* 2019; 173: 342–51.
21. Schwartz S, Raveh D, Toker O, Segal G, Godovitch N, Schlesinger Y. A week-by-week analysis of the low-risk criteria for serious bacterial infection in febrile neonates. *Archives of Disease in Childhood.* 2009; 94: 287–92.
22. Powell EC, Mahajan PV, Roosevelt G *et al.* Epidemiology of bacteremia in febrile infants aged 60 days and younger. *Annals of Emergency Medicine.* 2018; 71: 211–6.
23. Greenhow TL, Hung YY, Herz AM, Losada E, Pantell RH. The changing epidemiology of serious bacterial infections in young infants. *The Pediatric Infectious Disease Journal.* 2014; 33: 595–9.
24. Bonsu BK, Harper MB. A low peripheral blood white blood cell count in infants younger than 90 days increases the odds of acute bacterial meningitis relative to bacteremia. *Academic Emergency Medicine.* 2004; 11: 1297–301.
25. Cruz AT, Mahajan P, Bonsu BK *et al.* Accuracy of complete blood cell counts to identify febrile infants 60 days or younger with invasive bacterial infections. *JAMA Pediatrics.* 2017; 171: e172927.
26. Mintegi S, Garcia S, Martin MJ *et al.* Clinical prediction rule for distinguishing bacterial from aseptic meningitis. *Pediatrics.* 2020; 146: e20201126.

Chapter 24 **Serious Bacterial Infections in Children Aged 0 to 60/90 Days**

Jana L. Anderson and Fernanda Bellolio

Department of Emergency Medicine, Mayo Clinic, Rochester, MN, USA

Highlights

- Febrile infants 28 days of age and younger are at a significant risk for serious bacterial infections and warrant a full sepsis evaluation.
- Both the Step-by-Step and PECARN febrile infant protocols use sequential analysis to determine if an infant 28 days and older are at high risk and in need of a full sepsis evaluation.
- The American Academy of Pediatrics Clinical Practice Guideline recommends the use of inflammatory markers to determine which febrile infants need lumbar puncture, IV antibiotics, or admission.
- Concurrent viral infections decrease but do not negate the need for serious bacterial infection evaluation.

Background

There is great variation in the management of febrile infants.[1] The current estimates for serious bacterial infections (SBIs) including urinary tract infection (UTI), bacteremia, and meningitis in well-appearing febrile infants less than 28 days are UTI 10.0%, bacteremia 3.1% (CI 2.3–4.1%), and meningitis 1.3% (CI 0.8–2.0%).[2,3] For older infants, 29 to 60 days of age, the rate of SBI is UTI 7.3 to 8.2%, bacteremia 1.1% (CI 0.8–1.6%), and meningitis 0.2% (CI 0.1–0.4%).[2,3] The febrile infant evaluation paradigm has shifted given two large multicenter studies, the Step by Step (SbS) and the Pediatric Emergency

---

Evidence-Based Emergency Care: Diagnostic Testing and Clinical Decision Rules, Third Edition.
Edited by Jesse M. Pines, Fernanda Bellolio, Christopher R. Carpenter, and Ali S. Raja.
© 2023 John Wiley & Sons Ltd. Published 2023 by John Wiley & Sons Ltd.

Care Applied Research Network (PECARN) febrile infant rules.[3,4] The American Academy of Pediatrics (AAP) published in 2021 a Clinical Practice Guideline (CPG) combining data from four large datasets (including PECARN), and reported the following aggregated rates of bacteremia: 8 to 21 day old – 4% bacteremia, 22 to 28 day old – 2.9% bacteremia, and 29 to 56 days – 2% bacteremia.[5]

SbS (Figure 24.1) and the PECARN febrile infant rules (Figure 24.2), both use a sequential approach to febrile infants less than 60–90 days of age to determine if the infant is at increased risk for SBI and therefore a full sepsis evaluation, antibiotics and admission are warranted. The CPG from the AAP recommends the use of inflammatory markers (CRP and procalcitonin

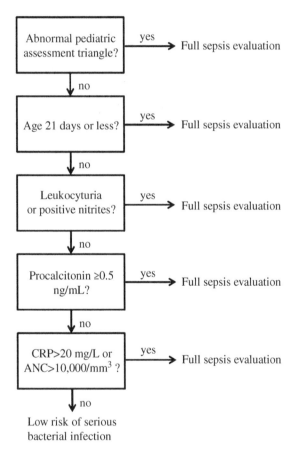

Figure 24.1 Step-by-Step febrile infant protocol. (Data from [4].)

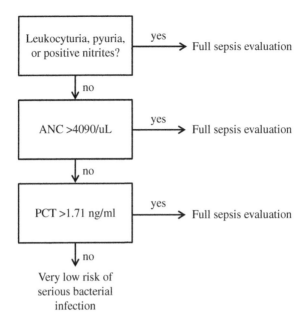

Figure 24.2 PECARN febrile infant protocol. (Data from [3].)

[PCT]) in older infant (≥22 days of age) to decide if a lumbar puncture (LP), antibiotics, or admission are necessary.[5] Previous rules like Rochester, Philadelphia, and Boston criteria,[6,7] were developed before the introduction of polyvalent conjugate pneumococcal and *Haemophilus influenzae type B* (Hib) vaccines, improved food safety for *Listeria monocytogenes,* and routine maternal group B strep testing.

Clinical question

How do newer clinical decision rules compare to previous ones? Are clinical decision rules useful in ruling out serious bacterial infection in children?

SbS, PECARN, and the AAP CPG define fever as a rectal temperature of ≥38.0 °C (100.4 °F) similar to the traditional Rochester and Boston Criteria, and lower than the Philadelphia protocol of 38.2 °C.[6,7] Overall, all protocols apply to "well-appearing" infants; while SbS protocol specifically utilizes the Pediatric Assessment Triangle (PAT) to determine ill appearance, the PECARN protocol utilized the Yale Observation Score (YOS) in the study. The AAP CPG uses the term "well-appearing" but also recognizes that there are likely three categories: ill, intermediate, and well-appearing. All the febrile infant literature recommends that appearance alone should not be utilized to determine if a full sepsis evaluation is *not* needed particularly in the younger infant.[8,9]

The SbS protocol was developed for infants less than 90 days and then classifies all infants less than 21 days as high risk. The PECARN and the AAP CPG protocols apply to all febrile infants less than 60 days of age. Both SbS and PECARN protocols use a positive urine early in the sequence to classify the infant as high risk for SBI and therefore warrant a full sepsis evaluation. The AAP CPG was developed for the 8- to 60-day-old infant and emphasizes testing for invasive bacterial infections (IBI, including bacteremia and meningitis) among those 21 days and younger.

Previous rules for febrile neonates defined an UTI as >10 WBCs/hpf (white blood counts/high power field) or >10 WBC/µL on enhanced urinalysis to define an abnormal urine.[7] With improved urinalysis technique, practice has evolved to using the presence of leukocyte esterase or nitrites, and/or >5 WBC/hpf to define an abnormal urinalysis.[10] AAP CPG defines the urinalysis as "positive" as the presence of any leukocyte esterase on dipstick, >5 WBC/hpf in centrifuged urine, or >10 WBCs/mm^3 in uncentrifuged urine on microscopic urinalysis.

Both SbS and the AAP CPG utilize PCT at different thresholds than PECARN. PECARN used recursive partitioning to determine a cut-off level, which was determined to be a PCT >1.71 ng/mL. SbS and the AAP CPG used a lower threshold at $\geq$0.5 ng/mL. To utilize PCT, fever should be present for at least 2 hours and preferably 4 to 6 hours to reflect the body's inflammatory response. Both the SbS and PECARN protocols utilize the ANC (absolute neutrophil count) to replace bands, neutrophils, and total WBC counts of the traditional protocols.[6,7,11] The threshold determined by the PECARN febrile infant rules is ANC > 4090/µL to define high risk. The SbS protocol utilizes an ANC > 10,000/mm^3 (one microliter is equivalent to one cubic millimeter) to define intermediate risk. In addition, the SbS protocol uses either elevated ANC or CRP >20 mg/L to define intermediate risk.

The sequence of the SbS algorithm to detect infants at increased risk for IBI defined as bacteremia or meningitis is (i) abnormal PAT (the three areas of assessment are: appearance, work of breathing, and circulation to skin); (ii) age $\leq$ 21 days; (iii) leukocyturia (>5 WBC/HPF) or positive leukocyte esterase or nitrites; and (iv) PCT $\geq$ 0.5 ng/mL. If any of these first four parameters are positive, the infant is classified as high-risk, with an incidence of IBI of 8.1%, and a full sepsis evaluation is recommended. The fifth and final step of the SbS protocol is CRP >20 mg/L or ANC > 10,000/mm^3, if either of those parameters are elevated, the child is identified as intermediate risk. With intermediate risk, the rate of IBI was found to be 3.4% and full sepsis evaluation is still recommended. If none of those characteristics are present the sensitivity of the SbS protocol was found to be 92% (CI 84.3–96.0%) and a negative predictive value (NPV) of 99.3% (CI 98.5–99.7%) for IBI.[4] Of note, 4 of 7 infants that were misclassified as low-risk by SbS were between 21 and 28 days of age (all with bacteremia). Subsequently, the authors caution against the protocols used on the less than 28-day-old infant. In addition, 3 of the 7 infants not identified by the protocol presented within 1 hour of fever which is likely too early for the inflammatory markers to elevate.

The PECARN febrile infant rules were developed utilizing recursive partitioning to find thresholds that would identify infants with SBI. The rules were then applied in a validation study of 913 febrile infants. The first branch point in the rule is an abnormal urinalysis (leukocyturia >5 WBC/hpf or positive leukocyte esterase or nitrites), then progresses to ANC >4090/μL, and then PCT >1.71 ng/mL. If any of these markers are positive a full sepsis evaluation is recommended. Factors that were examined but were not found to be significant were: age < 28 days, temperature degree, duration of fever, YOS, clinician suspicion, or total WBC count. The sensitivity of the prediction rule in the validation phase was found to be 97.7% (CI 91.3–99.6%) and a NPV of 99.6% (CI 98.4–99.9%). Of note, there were three infants misclassified that had SBI, one infant with bacteremia, and then two who had a normal urinalysis but subsequently had significant growth on urine culture. The one infant that was misclassified with bacteremia was 30 days of age with a negative urinalysis, ANC of 2700, PCT of 0.14 ng/mL, and negative LP. The infant was admitted and had an *Enterobacter cloacae* infection.

The AAP CPG provides recommendations on who may need a LP, parenteral antibiotics, and admission to the hospital. Their guidelines are informed by systematic reviews conducted by an Evidence-Based Practice Center. The guideline specifically separates infants: <21 days, 22 to 28 days, and 29 to 60 days.[5] This is due to the differing rates of bacteremia by the ages. The guideline emphasizes the use of the term IBI that includes bacteremia and meningitis, versus SBI that includes UTI, bacteremia, and meningitis, since UTI is very prevalent and distinct from IBI. In addition, not having a full sepsis evaluation in all infants in a study makes the denominator for bacteremia and meningitis difficult to interpret and introduces biases. Table 24.1 presents a comparison of different clinical scores to predict SBI in infants.

Clinical question

Among febrile infants with UTI, which need a lumbar puncture?
In febrile infants with a UTI, the next question is what the prevalence of concurrent bacteremia and meningitis is. Specifically, if UTI is identified, is

Table 24.1 Comparison of different clinical scores to predict serious bacterial infection in infants

	AAP CPG (2021)	PECARN (2019)	Step by Step (2016)	Rochester (1994)	Philadelphia (1992)	Boston (1992)
Age (days)	<60	<60	21–90	<60	29–56	28–89
Temp (C)	≥38.0	≥38.0	≥38.0	≥38.0	≥38.2	≥38.0
Assessment	Well appearance		Pediatric assessment triangle	Well appearance	Well appearance	Well appearance
Urine	<5 WBC/hpf, LE or nitrites	<5 WBC/hpf, LE or nitrites	<5 WBC/hpf, LE or nitrites	<10 WBC/hpf	<10 WBC/hpf, (−) gram stain	<10 WBC/hpf
WBC				b/n 5,000 to 15,000	<15,000	<20,000
Bands				<1,500	I:T ratio <0.2	
ANC	<4,090/µL		<10,000/mm^3			
Procalcitonin	<0.5 ng/mL	<1.71 ng/mL	<0.5 ng/mL			
CRP	<20 mg/L		<20 mg/L			
Chest X-ray					Negative CXR if symptoms	Negative CXR if symptoms
CSF	Obtain LP depending on age and inflammatory markers (IM)	n/a	n/a	n/a	Yes, <8 WBCs/µL, (−) gram stain	Yes, <10 WBC/µL
Sensitivity		98.8%	92.0%	81.6%	98.0%	
NPV		99.8%	99.3%	98.3%	99.7%	
Other	Applies only to well-appearing >37 wks; Variable pathways by age; <21 d (full workup), 22–28 d (LP if IM are abnormal; infant should be admitted for observation), 29–60 d (no need for LP if all IM are normal)	Not critically ill, No antibiotics within 48 h; No prematurity ≤36 wks; No pre-existing conditions, No soft tissue infections	Previously healthy	>37 wks, No antibiotics, Previously healthy	Nonfocal examination, Normal vital signs	Normal vital signs, No immunizations within 48 h, No antibiotics within 48 h, No dehydration

C = celsius; LE = leukocyte esterase; WBC = white blood cell count; ANC = absolute neutrophil count; I:T = immature to total ratio; CRP = C reactive protein; CSF = cerebrospinal fluid; NPV = negative predictive value; wks = weeks; h = hours; hpf = high power field; IM = inflammatory markers.

it still necessary to perform a LP? Tzimenatos *et al.* reported a secondary analysis of a cohort of febrile infants ≤60 days old at 26 emergency departments in the PECARN. Among the 4147 infants included, 289 (7.0%) had UTIs with colony counts ≥50,000 CFUs/mL, including 27 (9.3%) with bacteremia. A positive urinalysis was very sensitive in children (94%, CI 91–97%) for a UTI. Sensitivity was higher for those with bacteremia (sensitivity 100% [CI 87–100%] for those with bacteremia and 94% [CI 90–96%] for those without bacteremia). Specificity was 91% (CI 90–91%).[10] The rate of meningitis in a febrile <28 day old with a UTI is similar to infants without an UTI at 1.2%, which underscores the importance of LP in this population despite a positive urinalysis. By comparison, the rate of meningitis in the febrile 28 to 60-day-old infant with an UTI is very low and is estimated at 0%, but the 95% confidence intervals are between zero and 1.25%.

According to the AAP CPG, an 8 to 21-day-old with a UTI should have a full sepsis evaluation and hospitalization given the relatively high rate of bacteremia (9.3%) and meningitis (1.2%). A 22 to 28-day-old infant with a positive urinalysis would have inflammatory markers sent. If the CRP is >20 mg/L, PCT > 0.5 ng/mL, or if the infant's temperature > 38.5 °C, LP is recommended. If inflammatory markers are negative a LP may be considered. If LP is not performed parenteral antibiotics and hospitalization are recommended. If the LP is performed and negative, parenteral antibiotics should be administered, and the infant can be observed at home with follow-up within 24 hours or hospitalized. It should be emphasized that administering parenteral antibiotics without a LP in less than 28-day-old infant makes the decision for the duration of antibiotics difficult to determine. In the older infant, 29 to 60 days with a UTI, if inflammatory markers are positive or temperature >38.5, a LP may be performed. In this situation, parental antibiotics and observation at home can be performed. If inflammatory markers are negative in the 29 to 60-day old with a UTI, LP is not recommended and oral antibiotics can be administered.[5]

Clinical question

How does a positive viral test affect the chances of serious bacterial infection in children?

A 2004 study evaluated febrile infants less than 60 days old with viral infection.[12] When respiratory syncytial virus (RSV) was present, the prevalence of UTI was found to decrease from 12.5% to 7.0%, bacteremia from 2.3% to 1.1%. There were not enough cases of meningitis to reach statistical significance in the study.[12] A similar reduction in SBIs was found with influenza-positive infants. Since the initial RSV/influenza viral testing studies, viral panels have expanded to include many more viruses.

Mahajan *et al.* evaluated the prevalence of SBIs between virus-positive and virus-negative infants <60 days of age in the PECARN network. Among the febrile infants with viral testing performed, 1200 were positive for viral infection, and 44 of the 1200 had SBI (3.7%, CI 2.7–4.9%). Of the 1745 virus-negative infants, 222 had SBIs (12.7%, CI 11.2–14.4%). Rates of specific SBIs in the virus-positive group versus the virus-negative group were: UTIs (33 of 1200 [2.8%; CI 1.9–3.8%] versus 186 of 1745 [10.7%; CI 9.2–12.2%]) and bacteremia (9 of 1199 [0.8%; CI 0.3–1.4%] versus 50 of 1743 [2.9%; CI 2.1–3.8%]). The rate of bacterial meningitis was lower in the virus-positive group (0.4%) than in the virus-negative group (0.8%); the difference was not statistically significant. Negative viral status (aOR, 3.2; CI 2.3–4.6), was significantly associated with SBI in multivariable analysis.

In febrile infants, <28 days of age with a documented viral infection, the rate of UTI was found to decrease from 13.3% (CI 10.9–16.1%) to 2.6% (CI 1.3–4.8%), bacteremia decreased from 4.4 % (CI 3.0–6.1%) to 1.1% (CI 0.3–2.7%) and meningitis decreased from 1.7% (CI 0.9–2.9%) to 0.8% (CI 0.2–2.3%).[13] For the febrile infant >28 to 60 days, well appearing with fever with a documented virus, the rate of UTI decreased from 8.8% (CI 7.2–10.7%) to 2.8% (CI 1.8–4.2%), bacteremia decreased from 1.8% (CI 1.1–2.9%) to 0.6% (CI 0.2–1.4%), and meningitis was unchanged at 0.2%.[13] The rate of meningitis in the virus-positive infant is lower, but is not zero and should still be considered in the differential.

Comment

Due to their high risk of invasive bacterial infection, the care of the febrile infant <21 day old has not changed and they require a full sepsis workup including blood cultures, urinalysis, and LP. The care for the well-appearing febrile infant 22 days and older has changed with the availability of inflammatory markers (CRP and PCT) allowing for risk stratification in determining those infants that warrant a full sepsis evaluation versus those who do not need to undergo LP.

Per AAP guidelines, testing of the well-appearing 22 to 28-day old can exclude LP in some situations and with normal inflammatory marker (PCT of <0.5 ng/mL, CRP of <20 mg/L, normal ANC, and temperature <38.5 °C). After 29 days of age, the well-appearing febrile infant should undergo urinalysis, urine culture, blood culture, and inflammatory markers. They can forego LP if inflammatory markers are negative.

Both PECARN and SbS emphasize urine as a branch point for further testing, with those having a UTI being at higher risk of bacteremia and meningitis. The febrile 29 to 60-day-old infant with negative inflammatory markers and negative urinalysis, can forego LP and be observed closely at home. Among well-appearing children aged 29 days and older with a confirmed UTI, the rate of meningitis is extremely low, and LP can be avoided. Among well-appearing children 29–60 days with a confirmed viral infection, urinalysis is still indicated. The rate of bacteremia and meningitis is less than 1%.

SbS and PECARN have high NPV, meaning that if all the variables included in the score are negative, can be used to rule out SBI. The NPVs are 99.3% and 99.6%, most missed cases were in infants younger than 28 days of age.

Current guidelines apply to well-appearing infants and assessing the infant to determine that they are "well" is dependent on experience level and exposure to infants. It is important to remember that the appearance alone should not be utilized to determine if a full sepsis evaluation is needed. Also, a positive urinalysis classifies the infant as high risk of SBI, and the rate of meningitis in a febrile <28 day old with a UTI is similar to infants without an UTI. The next phase of febrile infant evaluation will be examining RNA biosignatures to more accurately identify high-risk febrile infants.[13-16] Clinical judgment and balance of testing with the risk of missing a SBI should be considered. Involving the parents in shared decision-making is important to balance different risk tolerances. Even with evidence-based guidelines, there will still be variability in who is high risk and warrants a full sepsis evaluation.

References

1. Rogers AJ, Kuppermann N, Anders J et al. Practice variation in the evaluation and disposition of febrile infants </=60 days of age. *The Journal of Emergency Medicine.* 2019; 56(6): 583–91.
2. Powell EC, Mahajan PV, Roosevelt G et al. Epidemiology of bacteremia in febrile infants aged 60 days and younger. *Annals of Emergency Medicine.* 2018; 71(2): 211–6.
3. Kuppermann N, Dayan PS, Levine DA et al. A clinical prediction rule to identify febrile infants 60 days and younger at low risk for serious bacterial infections. *JAMA Pediatrics.* 2019; 173(4): 342–51.
4. Gomez B, Mintegi S, Bressan S et al. Validation of the "Step-by-Step" approach in the management of young febrile infants. *Pediatrics.* 2016; 138(2): e20154381.
5. Pantell RH, Roberts KB, Adams WG et al. Evaluation and management of well-appearing febrile infants 8 to 60 days old. *Pediatrics.* 2021; 148(2): e2021052228.
6. Jaskiewicz JA, McCarthy CA, Richardson AC et al. Febrile infants at low risk for serious bacterial infection–an appraisal of the Rochester criteria and implications for management. Febrile Infant Collaborative Study Group. *Pediatrics.* 1994; 94(3): 390–6.

7. Baskin MN, O'Rourke EJ, Fleisher GR. Outpatient treatment of febrile infants 28 to 89 days of age with intramuscular administration of ceftriaxone. *The Journal of Pediatrics.* 1992; 120(1): 22–7.

8. Baker MD, Avner JR, Bell LM. Failure of infant observation scales in detecting serious illness in febrile, 4- to 8-week-old infants. *Pediatrics.* 1990; 85(6): 1040–3.

9. Nigrovic LE, Mahajan PV, Blumberg SM et al. The yale observation scale score and the risk of serious bacterial infections in febrile infants. *Pediatrics.* 2017; 140(1): e20170695.

10. Tzimenatos L, Mahajan P, Dayan PS et al. Accuracy of the urinalysis for urinary tract infections in febrile infants 60 days and younger. *Pediatrics.* 2018; 141(2): e20173068.

11. Baker MD, Bell LM, Avner JR. Outpatient management without antibiotics of fever in selected infants. *The New England Journal of Medicine.* 1993; 329(20): 1437–41.

12. Levine DA, Platt SL, Dayan PS et al. Risk of serious bacterial infection in young febrile infants with respiratory syncytial virus infections. *Pediatrics.* 2004; 113(6): 1728–34.

13. Mahajan P, Browne LR, Levine DA et al. Risk of bacterial coinfections in febrile infants 60 days old and younger with documented viral infections. *The Journal of Pediatrics.* 2018; 203: 86–91 e82.

14. Mahajan P, Kuppermann N, Mejias A et al. Association of RNA biosignatures with bacterial infections in febrile infants aged 60 days or younger. *Journal of the American Medical Association.* 2016; 316(8): 846–57.

15. Mahajan P, Kuppermann N, Suarez N et al. RNA transcriptional biosignature analysis for identifying febrile infants with serious bacterial infections in the emergency department: A feasibility study. *Pediatric Emergency Care.* 2015; 31(1): 1–5.

16. Mahajan P, Ramilo O, Kuppermann N. The future possibilities of diagnostic testing for the evaluation of febrile infants. *JAMA Pediatrics.* 2013; 167(10): 888–98.

Chapter 25 **Necrotizing Soft Tissue Infection**

Lucas Oliveira Junqueira e Silva[1,2] and Fernanda Bellolio[2]

[1] Department of Emergency Medicine, Hospital de Clínicas de Porto Alegre, Porto Alegre, Brazil
[2] Department of Emergency Medicine, Mayo Clinic, Rochester, MN, USA

Highlights

- Necrotizing soft tissue infection is a rare but potentially lethal condition that requires early recognition and aggressive surgical treatment.
- Physical examination findings and the Laboratory Risk Indicator for Necrotizing Fasciitis (LRINEC) criteria have high specificity but insufficient sensitivity. Therefore, the LRINEC should not be used to rule out necrotizing soft tissue infections.
- CT has the most robust evidence and the highest sensitivity to diagnose necrotizing infections. CT findings concerning for necrotizing infection include the presence of fascial edema, fascial enhancement, or fascial gas.
- Point-of-care ultrasound has appropriate positive likelihood ratio to significantly increase posttest probabilities and expedite the diagnosis when performed by experienced sonographers. A negative ultrasound, however, is not enough to rule out a necrotizing soft tissue infection.
- Imaging should not delay surgical consultation when there is a high clinical suspicion for necrotizing soft tissue infection.

Evidence-Based Emergency Care: Diagnostic Testing and Clinical Decision Rules, Third Edition.
Edited by Jesse M. Pines, Fernanda Bellolio, Christopher R. Carpenter, and Ali S. Raja.
© 2023 John Wiley & Sons Ltd. Published 2023 by John Wiley & Sons Ltd.

Background

Necrotizing soft tissue infection (NSTI), commonly referred as "necrotizing fasciitis," is a rapidly progressive infection involving the fascia and subcutaneous tissue. It most commonly affects the extremities. Differentiating necrotizing infection from other skin and soft tissue infections (Figure 25.1) is important in the emergency department (ED). While NSTI is a rare disease, it results in considerable morbidity and mortality. Mortality is estimated at 20% to 30%. NSTI is a surgically treated disease, and early recognition and debridement of necrotic fascia and other involved areas are major determinants of overall outcome (Figure 25.2). A delay in debridement has been associated with poor survival.

Early on, NSTI can be difficult to distinguish from other forms of soft tissue infections, such as cellulitis and abscess. Computed tomography (CT), magnetic resonance imaging (MRI), and ultrasound have been used in distinguishing necrotizing fasciitis from other clinical entities.

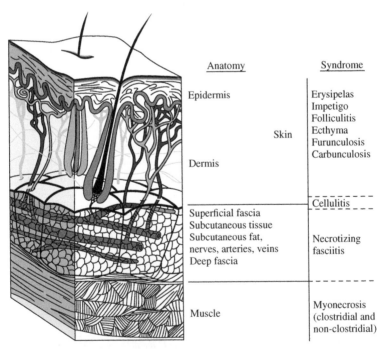

Figure 25.1 Schematic of the different layers of the skin and the corresponding infections associated with each layer.,

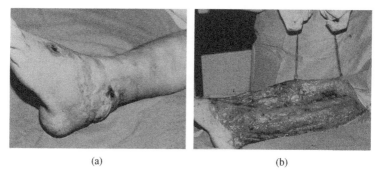

(a)   (b)

Figure 25.2 (a) A suspected case of necrotizing fasciitis. Left foot shown with oozing wound, dusky skin, and bullae formation. (b) Surgical exploration resulted in extensive debridement. (Hall *et al.* [1], Reproduced with permission from McGraw-Hill Education.)

Clinical question

Can physical examination be helpful in distinguishing necrotizing soft tissue infection from nonnecrotizing soft tissue infections?

Several clinical manifestations are classically described in patients with NSTI, including erythema (without sharp margins), edema that extends beyond the visible erythema, severe pain ("out of proportion"), fever, crepitus, and skin bullae, necrosis or ecchymosis. Some of these findings are often described as "pathognomonic," which would mean a very high positive predictive value for the diagnosis of NSTI.

However, a diagnostic test accuracy systematic review and meta-analysis found limited evidence for the use of physical examination findings, especially regarding their ability to rule out the diagnosis of NSTI.[2] The authors calculated summary estimates for three examination findings: fever, hemorrhagic bullae, and hypotension (Table 25.1). While the pooled positive likelihood ratio was high for hemorrhagic bullae (LR+ 5.97, CI 2.89–12.32) and hypotension (LR+ 9.20, CI 3.87–21.86), these two findings, when absent, had limited ability to change posttest probabilities (pooled negative likelihood ratios of 0.78 and 0.81, respectively). These data illustrate that their absence should not be individually used to rule out the presence of NSTI. The authors also provided a Bayesian-based clinical reasoning exercise in their discussion, where they reported that a patient with a pretest probability of NSTI of 50% without fever, hemorrhagic bullae, or hypotension, still remains with a posttest probability of 41.3%, 43.9%, and 44.7%, respectively.

Table 25.1 Physical examination findings to differentiate necrotizing soft tissue infections from other nonnecrotizing skin and soft-tissue infections

	No. of studies (No. of patients)	Pooled sensitivity (95% CI)	Pooled specificity (95% CI)	Pooled positive likelihood ratio (95% CI)	Pooled negative likelihood ratio (95% CI)
Fever	4 (647)	46.0% (38.9–53.2%)	77.0% (59.7–88.1%)	1.98 (1.12–3.51)	0.70 (0.59–0.84)
Hemorrhagic bullae	5 (951)	25.2% (12.8–43.7%)	95.8% (87.3–98.7%)	5.97 (2.89–12.32)	0.78 (0.66–0.93)
Hypotension	6 (1014)	21.0 (9.4–40.4%)	97.7% (91.4–99.4%)	9.20 (3.87–21.86)	0.81 (0.68–0.96)

Source: Data from [2].

Physical examination findings may be used to increase the posttest probabilities to levels where no further diagnostic procedures are needed. In other words, these findings may aid clinicians to cross through the threshold for requesting surgical evaluation. For example, a patient with a pretest probability of NSTI of 20% presenting with hypotension (LR+ 9.20) remains with a posttest probability of 70%. This relatively high posttest probability should lead to immediate surgical consultation. On the other hand, if hypotension was absent, the remaining posttest probability would be at 17%, almost not changed from the initial 20%.

Clinical question

Can laboratory tests be reliably used in the ED in distinguishing necrotizing soft tissue infection from other nonnecrotizing soft tissue infections?
The Laboratory Risk Indicator for Necrotizing Fasciitis (LRINEC) investigators developed a scoring system to differentiate necrotizing fasciitis from other skin and soft tissue infections.[3] They derived the LRINEC scoring system in a retrospective cohort of 314 patients and validated it in 140 patients in two teaching hospitals in Singapore. They included 140 patients who had necrotizing fasciitis and 309 patients with severe cellulitis or abscesses. They found that WBC, hemoglobin, sodium, glucose, creatinine, and C-reactive protein were associated with a diagnosis of necrotizing fasciitis. They constructed the LRINEC score through conversion of the independent predictors of necrotizing fasciitis into an integer scoring system. This scoring system is detailed in Table 25.2.

Table 25.2 The LRINEC score to differentiate necrotizing fasciitis from severe cellulitis

Variable, units	Value	Score	Interpretation
C-reactive protein, mg/L	<150	0	The score ranges from 0 to
C-reactive protein, mg/L	≥150	4	13, where a score of ≥ 6 is
WBC (per mm³)	<15	0	considered "positive"
WBC (per mm³)	15–25	1	(probability of necrotizing
WBC (per mm³)	>25	2	fasciitis 50–75%)
Hemoglobin, g/dL	>13.5	0	
Hemoglobin, g/dL	11–13.5	1	
Hemoglobin, g/dL	<11	2	
Sodium, mmol/L	≥135	0	
Sodium, mmol/L	<135	2	
Creatinine, mg/dL	≤1.6	0	
Creatinine, mg/dL	>1.6	2	
Glucose, mg/dL	≤180	0	
Glucose, mg/dL	<180	1	

WBC = white blood cell.

Using a cutoff of 6 points or higher, there was a positive predictive value of 92% and a negative predictive value of 96%. The authors did not report sensitivities and specificities in their results section. The area under the receiver operator characteristic (ROC) curve was 0.98 in the derivation set and 0.976 in the validation cohort, showing a high degree of accuracy in differentiating necrotizing fasciitis from cellulitis or abscess.

In 2009, a single-center retrospective study was published from Australia that aimed to externally validate the LRINEC.[2] The authors calculated the performance of a LRINEC score of ≥6 compared with the findings of a surgical biopsy. In 28 patients who were identified with an admission diagnosis of necrotizing fasciitis, 10 had biopsy-proven necrotizing fasciitis. In this small group of patients using a score ≥6, the LRINEC score had a sensitivity of 80%, a specificity of 67%, a positive predictive value of 57%, and a negative predictive value of 86% in distinguishing the patients with proven necrotizing fasciitis from those with other severe soft tissue infections. The authors concluded that at this cutoff level, the LRINEC score would have only minimal effect on posttest probability for having necrotizing fasciitis.

In another 2010 study in France, a LRINEC ≥ 6 was retrospectively applied to risk-stratify patients for the diagnosis of necrotizing fasciitis.[4] Three criteria were used: time from initiation of antibiotics to regression of erythema, duration of fever, and occurrence of complications (abscess, surgery, septic shock, necrotizing fasciitis, death, and transfer to intensive care). There were several potential predictor variables, including a

LRINEC score ≥ 6 at admission. In 50 patients, the authors reported that the complication rate was higher for patients with a LRINEC score ≥ 6 (54%) than for patients with a score <6 (12%, P = 0.008). However, a LRINEC score ≥ 6 did not appear to be related to an increased duration of erythema or fever.

Most recently, Fernando *et al.* evaluated the diagnostic accuracy of the LRINEC score in a meta-analysis of 14 studies (4339 patients) that used a threshold of ≥ 6 and 9 studies (1905 patients) that used a threshold of ≥ 8.[2] This is the same systematic review that provided diagnostic accuracy estimates for physical examination findings described earlier in this chapter. The diagnosis of NSTI was defined as the presence of classic operative findings (presence of grayish necrotic fascia, lack of resistance to normally adherent muscular fascia to blunt dissection, lack of bleeding of the fascia during dissection, or the presence of foul-smelling "dishwater" pus), histopathologic tissue examination, or death from suspected NSTI. The pooled sensitivities found for these two score thresholds were low and the negative likelihood ratios insufficient to significantly reduce posttest probabilities in patients with moderate pretest probabilities. The authors provided an example where a patient with a pretest probability of 50% but a LRINEC < 6 (likelihood ratio of 0.38) still retains a 27.3% risk of NSTI. The pooled diagnostic accuracy estimates of the two different score thresholds are illustrated in Table 25.3.

The authors of the systematic review have also identified important source of biases that are common to diagnostic studies. This included the lack of information about whether the diagnostic test (namely LRINEC score) was interpreted by individuals who were blinded to the final diagnosis of NSTI, and the use of case-control study designs, which may introduce significant spectrum bias (see Chapter 6).

Table 25.3 Diagnostic accuracy of two different score thresholds for the LRINEC score

Score threshold	No. of studies (No. of patients)	Pooled sensitivity (95% CI)	Pooled specificity (95% CI)	Pooled positive likelihood ratio (95% CI)	Pooled negative likelihood ratio (95% CI)
LRINEC ≥ 6	14 (4339)	68.2% (51.4–81.3%)	84.8% (75.8–90.9%)	4.49 (2.74–7.35)	0.38 (0.24–0.60)
LRINEC ≥ 8	9 (1905)	40.8% (28.6–54.2%)	94.9% (89.4–97.6%)	7.94 (3.44–18.32)	0.62 (0.50–0.78)

Source: Data from [2].

The limited ability of this score to rule out necrotizing fasciitis has also been shown in a recent prospective observational study of ED patients.[5] Hsiao *et al.* analyzed a total of 825 patients with severe cellulitis and 106 with necrotizing fasciitis in the extremities. With the cutoff score ≥ 6, the sensitivity was only 43% (CI 34–53%) for the presence of necrotizing fasciitis, and with the cutoff score ≥ 8, the sensitivity was even lower at 27% (CI 19–37%).

Emergency physicians need to recognize the limited sensitivity of the LRINEC score. While a score of ≥ 6 or ≥ 8 may have appropriate ability to rule in the diagnosis of NSTI (relatively high specificities and positive likelihood ratios), the sensitivities are low and the score should not be used to rule out the diagnosis due to the unacceptable risk of missing this deadly condition. Also, this score requires the use of six laboratory measurements and its execution should not delay surgical consultation in scenarios of moderate to high pretest probabilities.

Clinical question

What is the accuracy of CT, plain radiography, ultrasound, and MRI for the diagnosis of necrotizing soft tissue infections?

Computed tomography and plain radiographs

In a similar approach that evaluated the diagnostic accuracy of physical examination and the LRINEC score, the systematic review by Fernando *et al.* evaluated the performance of different imaging.[2] In a meta-analysis, the authors evaluated plain radiography from 4 studies (478 patients), and CT from 7 studies (787 patients). The visualization of soft tissue gas on plain radiography was associated with a pooled sensitivity of 48.9% (CI 24.9–73.4%) for the diagnosis of NSTI, while the visualization of fascial gas on CT had a sensitivity of 88.5% (CI 55.5–97.9%) and the composite findings of fascial enhancement, fascial edema, or fascial gas on CT had a sensitivity of 94.3% (CI 81.2–98.5%). Table 25.4 illustrates the summary estimates for the performance of plain radiography and CT.

When the need of immediate surgical intervention is not clinically obvious, CT is better than plain radiography on ruling out a diagnosis of NSTI. In another Bayesian-based clinical reasoning exercise provided by the authors of the systematic review, in a patient with an equivocal pretest probability of 50%, the presence of fascial gas in the CT increases the probability to 93%, while the absence of fascial enhancement, edema or gas decreases the probability to less than 7%.

Table 25.4 Diagnostic accuracy of plain radiography and CT for the diagnosis of necrotizing soft tissue infection

Imaging	No of studies (No of patients)	Pooled sensitivity (95% CI)	Pooled specificity (95% CI)	Pooled positive likelihood ratio (95% CI)	Pooled negative likelihood ratio (95% CI)
Plain radiography	4 (478)	48.9% (24.9–73.4%)	94.0% (63.8–99.3%)	8.17 (1.61–41.47)	0.54 (0.36–0.82)
Computed tomography (fascial gas only)	7 (787)	88.5% (55.5–97.9%)	93.3% (80.8–97.9%)	13.27 (4.24–41.50)	0.12 (0.03–0.62)
Computed tomography (fascial edema or fascial enhancement or fascial gas)	6 (700)	94.3% (81.2–98.5%)	76.6% (21.3–97.5%)	4.04 (0.62–26.47)	0.07 (0.02–0.24)

Source: Data from [2].

Ultrasound

Point-of-care ultrasound (POCUS) is commonly used as a diagnostic tool by emergency physicians. Its utility has been recently supported by a diagnostic test accuracy systematic review and meta-analysis for differentiating abscesses from cellulitis in the ED.[6] However, the evidence for the use of POCUS for the diagnosis of NSTI is less established.

Yen et al. prospectively studied 62 patients with clinically suspected necrotizing fasciitis presenting to an ED in Taiwan. All patients underwent POCUS using a linear-array transducer. The diagnosis of necrotizing fasciitis was based on the criterion of a diffuse thickening of the subcutaneous tissue, accompanied by a layer of fluid accumulation more than 4 mm in depth along the deep fascial layer when compared with the contralateral position on the corresponding normal limb. A total of 17 (27.4%) patients were eventually diagnosed with necrotizing fasciitis (pathological findings for patients who underwent fasciotomy or biopsy results for patients who were managed nonoperatively). The estimated sensitivity and specificity were 88.2% (95% CI 63.6–98.5%) and 93.3% (95% CI 81.7–98.6%), respectively. It is important to note that all scans were obtained by only one clinician, which raises concerns about the applicability and reproducibility of the protocol, as ultrasound is operator-dependent.

Most recently, another study from Taiwan evaluated the diagnostic accuracy of POCUS to diagnose necrotizing fasciitis.[7] Lin et al. analyzed a convenience sample of 95 patients with suspected necrotizing fasciitis. A total of 48 (50.5%) patients were diagnosed with necrotizing fasciitis based on pathological findings. Using the definition of necrotizing fasciitis in the POCUS as fluid accumulation in the deep fascial layer ≥ 2 mm in depth, the authors reported a sensitivity of 75.0% and a specificity of 70.2%, positive likelihood ratio of 2.51 and negative likelihood ratio of 0.35. When the authors used a similar cutoff from the previous study by Yen *et al.* (4 mm), the sensitivity was only 42.3% and the specificity 93.6%, positive likelihood ratio of 6.60, and negative likelihood ratio of 0.62. Based on these two limited studies, POCUS may have a role in rapidly rule in necrotizing fasciitis in the ED, but it cannot be used to rule out the diagnosis. More studies exploring the different ultrasonographic findings and their diagnostic accuracy are needed.

Magnetic resonance imaging (MRI)

As for MRI in the diagnosis of NSTI, there is yet limited evidence to support its use, and MRI has limited availability in most EDs.

A case-control study[8] of 30 patients (7 with necrotizing fasciitis and 23 with nonnecrotizing fasciitis) found that certain MRI findings were more common in patients with necrotizing fasciitis, and the authors suggested that the use of MRI may be useful for the differential diagnosis. The MRI findings are potentially useful and suggested by the authors included: thick (≥3 mm) abnormal signal intensity on fat-suppressed T2-weighted images, low signal intensity in the deep fascia on fat-suppressed T2-weighted images, a focal or diffuse nonenhancing portion in the area of abnormal signal intensity in the deep fascia, extensive involvement of the deep fascia, and involvement of 3 or more compartments in one extremity.

A study[9] in South Korea derived and externally validated a score that integrates the LRINEC score with specific MRI findings to predict necrotizing fasciitis. This was done using an observational study of 144 subjects (96 patients in the derivation cohort, and 48 patients in the validation cohort) who underwent surgery for necrotizing fasciitis or cellulitis. The final model consisted of three variables: thickening of the deep fascia ≥ 3 mm (MRI finding), multicompartmental involvement (MRI finding), and LRINEC score. The authors used the coefficients of the variables from the final model to derive a score ranging from 0 to 17 with increasing scores representing increasing probabilities of necrotizing fasciitis. The model had an area under the curve (AUC) of 0.862 in the derivation cohort, as compared to an AUC of 0.814 using the LRINEC score alone. The AUC of the model was 0.933 in the validation cohort. The new scoring system with a cutoff of ≥ 5.5 had a sensitivity of 77% in the derivation cohort, while in the validation cohort the sensitivity was 96%. The LRINEC score alone with a cutoff ≥ 6 had sensitivity of 57% and 70% in the derivation and validation cohorts, respectively. Although with promising findings in regards to the differentiation of necrotizing versus non-NSTI, the study had important limitations in regards to potential selection and referral bias as the authors included only patients who underwent MRI including fat-suppressed T2-weighted images and those who underwent surgical intervention in tertiary referral centers.

More recently, another observational study[10] in South Korea evaluated the diagnostic accuracy of MRI by comparing 34 patients with necrotizing fasciitis and 15 with severe cellulitis. The authors developed an MRI-based algorithm using classification and regression tree analysis, including the presence and absence of T2 hyperintensity of intermuscular deep fascia (step one), and diffuse T2 hyperintensity of deep peripheral fascia (step two). Of the 49 patients who underwent MRI, the sensitivity and specificity of the algorithm to differentiate necrotizing fasciitis from severe cellulitis were 94% (CI 80–99%) and 60% (CI 32–84%), respectively. These estimates of diagnostic accuracy for this MRI-based diagnostic algorithm are similar to the ones found with the use of CT imaging. Importantly, when the authors analyzed the diagnostic accuracy of the algorithm in the subset of patients with low LRINEC scores (≤5), the sensitivity was 88% and specificity was 69%. This subset of patients is likely the group where clinical dilemma is most important and imaging is an important diagnostic aid. On the other hand, patients with higher risks should probably get immediate surgical intervention and MRI is neither feasible nor advisable due to the importance of timely treatment. We do not know the diagnostic accuracy of CT in this subset of "low-risk" patients (aka low LRINEC scores), and future research is needed to compare the diagnostic yield of MRI with CT in this subgroup. It is possible that the diagnostic yield of MRI is better in this subset of patients because of its ability to detect subtle and initial findings of NSTI.

Comment

Certain physical examination findings such as the presence of hypotension and hemorrhagic bullae, as well as the LRINEC score, are specific and helpful in ruling in NSTI. Yet, the sensitivity of both physical exam findings and the LRINEC score is low and should not be used to definitively rule out necrotizing fasciitis.

CT findings of fascial edema, fascial enhancement, or fascial gas are sensitive and specific to help identify low-risk patients and rule out NSTI. Plain radiography has very low sensitivity and a negative X-ray is insufficient to rule out the diagnosis. MRI and ultrasound are promising but yet to be further investigated. In the hands of experienced sonographers, point-of-care ultrasound has appropriate positive likelihood ratio to significantly increase posttest probabilities and expedite the diagnosis. A negative ultrasound, however, is not enough to rule out NSTI and further imaging (e.g., CT) may be necessary. New scoring algorithms integrating MRI and laboratory findings have been developed and although promising to differentiate necrotizing from non-NSTIs, MRI is not currently widely available in EDs.

Based on the current evidence, a reasonable diagnostic pathway seems to start with POCUS (if readily available) for suspected cases and if positive, proceed with immediate surgical consultation. If the ultrasound is negative, CT should be the exam of choice to rule in or rule out the diagnosis of NSTI. Imaging should not delay surgical consultation when there is a high clinical suspicion for necrotizing fasciitis.

References

1. Hall JB, Schmidt GA, Wood L. *Principles of critical care*. 3rd ed. New York: McGraw-Hill Companies; 2005.

2. Fernando SM, Tran A, Cheng W *et al*. Necrotizing soft tissue infection: Diagnostic accuracy of physical examination, imaging, and LRINEC score: A systematic review and meta-analysis. *Annals of Surgery*. 2019; 269(1): 58–65.

3. Wong CH, Khin LW, Heng KS, Tan KC, Low CO. The LRINEC (Laboratory Risk Indicator for Necrotizing Fasciitis) score: A tool for distinguishing necrotizing fasciitis from other soft tissue infections. *Critical Care Medicine*. 2004; 32(7): 1535–41.

4. Corbin V, Vidal M, Beytout J *et al*. Valeur pronostique du score Laboratory Risk Indicator for Necrotizing Fasciitis (LRINEC) dans les dermohypodermites infectieuses: Étude prospective au CHU de Clermont-Ferrand. *Annales de Dermatologie et de Vénéréologie*. 2010; 137(1): 5–11.

5. Hsiao CT, Chang CP, Huang TY, Chen YC, Fann WC. Prospective validation of the laboratory risk indicator for necrotizing fasciitis (LRINEC) score for necrotizing fasciitis of the extremities. *PLoS One*. 2020; 15(1): e0227748.

6. Gottlieb M, Avila J, Chottiner M, Peksa GD. Point-of-care ultrasonography for the diagnosis of skin and soft tissue abscesses: A systematic review and meta-analysis. *Annals of Emergency Medicine*. 2020; 76(1): 67–77.

7. Lin CN, Hsiao CT, Chang CP *et al*. The relationship between fluid accumulation in ultrasonography and the diagnosis and prognosis of patients with necrotizing fasciitis. *Ultrasound in Medicine and Biology*. 2019; 45(7): 1545–50.

8. Kim KT, Kim YJ, Lee JW *et al*. Can necrotizing infectious fasciitis be differentiated from nonnecrotizing infectious fasciitis with MR imaging? *Radiology*. 2011; 259(3): 816–24.

9. Yoon MA, Chung HW, Yeo Y *et al.* Distinguishing necrotizing from non-necrotizing fasciitis: A new predictive scoring integrating MRI in the LRINEC score. *European Radiology.* 2019; 29(7): 3414–23.

10. Kim M-C, Kim S, Cho EB *et al.* Utility of magnetic resonance imaging for differentiating necrotizing fasciitis from severe cellulitis: A magnetic resonance indicator for necrotizing fasciitis (MRINEC) algorithm. *Journal of Clinical Medicine.* 2020; 9(9): 3040.

Chapter 26 **Infective Endocarditis**

W. Mason Bonner and Jonathan Sheele

Department of Emergency Medicine, Mayo Clinic, Jacksonville, FL, USA

Highlights

- Endocarditis requires a high clinical suspicion for diagnosis and confirmation usually cannot be made in the emergency department (ED).
- The modified Duke criteria allow for effective risk stratification in suspected patients.
- Groups at high risk for endocarditis include patients abusing intravenous drugs, patients with abnormal valvular anatomy, prosthetic valves, and indwelling catheters.
- Transesophageal echocardiography (TEE) is highly sensitive and specific for the diagnosis of endocarditis and is superior to transthoracic echocardiography (TTE).
- *Staphylococcus aureus* is the most common pathogen, followed by *Streptococcus* species, and these account for roughly 80% of infections.

Background

Infective endocarditis is a bacterial infection of the endothelial lining of the heart which begins as an infection of cardiac valve leaflets and can evolve to include other portions of the heart and vasculature. These vegetations can cause devastating illness when they form abscesses or embolize to extracardiac sites. In industrialized countries, the incidence is ~3–9 cases per 100,000 population with a male to female predilection of roughly 2:1. Classically, endocarditis has been associated with intravenous drug abuse and patients with underlying cardiac valvular pathology (rheumatic heart

Evidence-Based Emergency Care: Diagnostic Testing and Clinical Decision Rules, Third Edition.
Edited by Jesse M. Pines, Fernanda Bellolio, Christopher R. Carpenter, and Ali S. Raja.
© 2023 John Wiley & Sons Ltd. Published 2023 by John Wiley & Sons Ltd.

disease, congenital cyanotic valvular disease). Mortality associated with endocarditis is high with some estimates approaching 18%.[1] Healthcare-associated illness is increasingly recognized as a cause and accounts for roughly one-fourth to one-third of cases. Patients with prosthetic valves, indwelling catheters, and intracardiac devices represent a growing percentage of endocarditis cases.

The most common complications of endocarditis include heart failure, stroke, nonstroke embolization, and intracardiac abscess. The mitral and aortic valves are more commonly affected and account for >70% of cases. Left-sided endocarditis overall tends to carry a worse prognosis than right-sided disease. The most common presenting symptom is fever which is present in up to 80% of cases. Relapsing fever >5 days without a clear source increases the possibility of endocarditis. Other presenting findings include new murmur (48%), worsening known murmur (20%), hematuria (26%), and splenomegaly (11%).[1] More uncommon but well-known cutaneous and mucous membrane manifestations of disease such as splinter hemorrhages, Janeway's lesions (Figure 26.1), and Roth spots occur in fewer than 10% of patients. Other presentations can include sepsis, meningitis, new heart failure, and symptoms of embolization such as pulmonary embolus (PE), stroke, peripheral arterial occlusion, hepatic abscess, and renal failure.[3]

The most common pathogen causing endocarditis is *Staphylococcus* and this is followed by *Streptococcus*.[4] Together they account for 80% of cases of infectious endocarditis. Gram-negative bacteria are less frequently implicated, and total around 5% of cases and can involve *Haemophilus, Aggregatibacter, Cardiobacterium, Eikenella,* and *Kingella,* referred to as

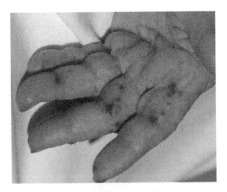

Figure 26.1 Janeway's lesions from bacterial endocarditis. (Fitzpatrick *et al.* [2], Reproduced with permission from McGraw-Hill Education.)

HACEK.[5] Fungal infections represent 1–2% of cases. Emergency providers must maintain a high index of suspicion for endocarditis because most cases are not confirmed in the emergency department.

Clinical question

What is the most accurate method to diagnose suspected infective endocarditis in the ED?

Diagnosis of endocarditis in the ED relies primarily upon effective patient risk stratification and the most validated tool is the modified Duke criteria.[6] The Duke criteria have a sensitivity and specificity approaching 80% and have a strong negative predictive value.[7] Initially proposed in 1994 by Durack *et al.*, the Duke criteria aided clinicians in their approach to the diagnosis of endocarditis.[8] The Duke criteria stratify the probability of endocarditis into three categories: definite, possible, and rejected. These categories utilize a combination of major and minor criteria to define the likelihood of infectious endocarditis. The Major Duke criteria include positive echocardiography and positive blood cultures. Minor Duke criteria consist of fever, predisposition, secondary vascular phenomena, and suggestive but nondiagnostic echocardiogram. A list of these criteria can be found in Table 26.1.

Additional revisions of the Duke criteria have been suggested, and propose removal of the minor criterion *echocardiogram consistent with infective endocarditis*. Other proposals for new minor criteria include splenomegaly, and C-reactive protein (CRP) of >100 mg/L.[9]

In diagnosing endocarditis laboratory testing, while helpful, is often nonspecific. The CBC reveals anemia or leukocytosis in about 50% of patients. Inflammatory markers such as erythrocyte sedimentation rate (ESR) and CRP are abnormal in 2/3 of cases. Procalcitonin can be important for its negative predictive value. The urinalysis may reveal microscopic hematuria.

At initial evaluation, imaging options for infectious endocarditis can be limited. Transesophageal echocardiography (TEE) has a sensitivity >90% and has excellent ability to appraise both native and prosthetic valves. It can also identify smaller vegetations and abscesses with greater diagnostic accuracy than transthoracic echocardiography (TTE). In some instances, TTE despite its inferiority to TEE can be an acceptable initial imaging study as it has the advantages of being more readily available and not requiring sedation (Figure 26.2). It should be noted that TEE may ultimately be required when TTE results are nondiagnostic, or suspicion for endocarditis remains high.

Table 26.1 The modified Duke criteria for infective endocarditis[9]

Infective endocarditis
Definite pathologic criteria
- Presence of microorganisms demonstrated by culture of a vegetation, vegetative embolus, or in an intracardiac abscess
- Histologic evidence of endocarditis on pathologic examination proving presence of a vegetation or intracardiac abscess

Definite clinical criteria
- 2 major criteria, 1 major and 3 minor criteria, or 5 minor criteria

Possible clinical criteria
- 1 major criterion and 1 minor criterion, or 3 minor criteria

Rejected clinical criteria
- Firm alternative diagnosis, no pathologic evidence of infective endocarditis at surgery or autopsy, resolution of symptoms after antibiotic therapy of 4 days or less, or does not meet criteria for possible endocarditis as described

Major criteria
Positive blood culture with agent known to cause infectious endocarditis from two separate blood cultures
- *Streptococcus viridans, Streptococcus bovis*, HACEK group; or *Staphylococcus aureus* or community-acquired enterococci
- Minimum of two positive blood cultures drawn more than 12 hours apart; or
- Persistently positive blood culture, with recovery of a microorganism known to cause infective endocarditis
- Single positive blood culture for Coxiella brunette or antiphase I IgG antibody titer >1:800
- All or 3, or majority of 4 or more separate blood cultures, with first and last drawn at least 1 hour apart

Evidence of endocardial involvement on echocardiogram
- Oscillating intracardiac mass, on valve or supporting structures, or in the path of regurgitant jets, or on implanted material, in the absence of an alternative anatomic explanation; or
- Abscess
- New partial dehiscence of a prosthetic valve
- New valvular regurgitation (increase or change in preexisting murmur not sufficient)

Minor criteria
- Predisposition: predisposing heart condition or intravenous drug use
- Fever ≥38.0 °C (100.4 °F)
- Vascular phenomena: major arterial emboli, septic pulmonary infarcts, mycotic aneurysm, intracranial hemorrhage, conjunctival hemorrhages, Janeway's lesions
- Immunologic phenomenon: glomerulonephritis, Osler's nodes, Roth's spots, rheumatoid factor
- Echocardiogram consistent with infective endocarditis but not meeting major criteria above
- Microbiological evidence: positive blood culture but not meeting major criteria

Abbreviations: HACEK = grouping of Gram-negative bacilli; *Haemophilus* species, *Aggretiabacter, Cardiobacterium, Eikenella,* and *Kingella* species.

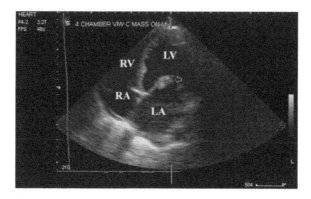

Figure 26.2 Apical four-chamber view demonstrating a large mitral valve vegetation (*arrow*). Abbreviations: RA = right atrium; LA = left atrium; LV = left ventricle; and RV = right ventricle. (Courtesy of Anthony J. Dean.)

Comment

Infectious endocarditis remains largely a clinical diagnosis for the emergency clinician. The modified Duke criteria can be used when there is high clinical suspicion,[10] but it may not be possible to satisfy the Duke criteria in the ED. TEE continues to be the most sensitive imaging modality available, though resource limitations often make the study impractical in most EDs. Arguably, blood cultures are the single most important laboratory test that can be ordered when endocarditis is suspected. Cultures serve to identify causative organisms and their sensitivity report can guide antibiotic therapy. Ideally, a set of 2–3 cultures should be obtained from different anatomic sites, with the third set drawn 1 hour after the first 2 are collected. Other tests such as the CBC will be abnormal with leukocytosis or anemia being present in 50% of cases. Additionally, ESR and CRP are abnormal in 2/3 of cases. Procalcitonin can serve as an adjunct to the diagnostic workup and can be useful for its negative predictive value; however, it has poor specificity for endocarditis.

Given the high mortality, variability of presentation, and severity of complications, the diagnosis of endocarditis requires vigilance and a low threshold for consideration. Unfortunately, the definitive diagnosis of endocarditis requires tissue biopsy, or a combination of echocardiography and blood cultures, the results of which are typically unavailable during the ED encounter. Clinical suspicion of endocarditis combined with knowledge of subtle exam findings and risk factors are essential for making the diagnosis.

References

1. Murdoch DR, Corey GR, Hoen B *et al.* Clinical presentation, and outcome of infective endocarditis in the 21st century: The international collaboration on endocarditis prospective cohort study. *Archives of Internal Medicine*. 2009; 169(5): 463–73.

2. Fitzpatrick T, Johnson RA, Wolff K, Suurmond D. *Color Atlas and synopsis of clinical dermatology*. New York: McGraw-Hill Companies; 2001.

3. Crawford D. Clinical presentation of infective endocarditis. *Cardiology Clinics*. 2003; 21: 159–66.

4. Selton-Suty C, Célard M, Le Moing V *et al.* Preeminence of *Staphylococcus aureus* in infective endocarditis: A 1 year population-based survey. *Clinical Infectious Diseases*. 2012; 54(9): 1230–9.

5. Fernández Guerrero ML, González López JJ, Goyenechea A, Fraile J, de Górgolas M *et al.* Endocarditis caused by *Staphylococcus aureus*: A reappraisal of the epidemiologic, clinical, and pathologic manifestations with analysis of factors determining outcome. *Medicine (Baltimore)*. 2009; 88(1): 1–22.

6. Hoen D. Infective endocarditis. *New England Journal of Medicine*. 2013; 368: 1425–33.

7. Topan A, Carstina D, Slavcovici A *et al.* Assessment of the Duke criteria for the diagnosis of infective endocarditis after twenty-years. An analysis of 241 cases. *Cluju Medical*. 2015; 88(3): 321–6.

8. Durack DT, Lukes AS, Bright DK. New criteria for diagnosis of infective endocarditis: Utilization of specific echocardiographic findings. Duke Endocarditis Service. *American Journal of Medicine*. 1994; 96(3): 200–9.

9. Li JS, Sexton DJ, Mick N *et al.* Proposed modifications to the Duke criteria for the diagnosis of infective endocarditis. *Clinical Infectious Diseases*. 2000; 3(4): 633–8.

10. Dodds GA III, Sexton DJ, Durack DT *et al.* Negative predictive value of the Duke criteria for infective endocarditis. *The American Journal of Cardiology*. 1996; 77: 403–7.

Chapter 27 **Pharyngitis**

Jesse M. Pines[1,2] and Christopher R. Carpenter[3]

[1] US Acute Care Solutions, Canton, OH, USA
[2] Department of Emergency Medicine, Drexel University, Philadelphia, PA, USA
[3] Department of Emergency Medicine, Washington University School of Medicine, St. Louis, MO, USA

> **Highlights**
>
> - Differentiating bacterial pharyngitis, specifically GAS (Group A Streptococci) infection from other causes of sore throat is a challenge.
> - The Centor criteria with the McIssac classification and the FeverPAIN criteria predict the probability of GAS infection based on clinical criteria.
> - While complications from GAS are relatively rare, in a large cohort study, many adult patients with low Centor and FeverPAIN scores had GAS-related complications. This suggest that patients with intermediate scores on Centor and FeverPAIN may benefit from confirmatory rapid strep testing/cultures, or potentially delaying antibiotics before starting therapy to balance the avoid overtreatment of viral infections with the potential for GAS-related complications.
> - There is an emerging discussion in the medical literature and guidelines as to whether antibiotics are beneficial in GAS because of the very high number needed to treat to prevent complications.

Background

The complaint of sore throat is common in emergency medicine, as well as in ambulatory settings such as doctor's offices and clinics. In 2017, there were more than 1.186 million visits to US emergency departments (EDs) for acute

---

Evidence-Based Emergency Care: Diagnostic Testing and Clinical Decision Rules, Third Edition.
Edited by Jesse M. Pines, Fernanda Bellolio, Christopher R. Carpenter, and Ali S. Raja.

pharyngitis, according to the National Hospital Ambulatory Medical Care Survey.[1] The most common bacterial cause for sore throat is Group A Streptococci (GAS). The value of using antibiotics has been debated for GAS because it usually resolves spontaneously without complications. However, antibiotics are currently recommended for patients in cases where there is a high likelihood of, or culture-confirmed, streptococcal infection in the throat.[2]

Antibiotics for sore throat should prevent complications, reduce symptoms, and prevent transmission of the disease. A recent Cochrane review found that at 3 days, antibiotics reduced symptoms of sore throat, headache, and fever, as well as complications following GAS pharyngitis include suppurative (acute otitis media and acute sinusitis) and nonsuppurative complications (acute glomerulonephritis and acute rheumatic fever).[3] Notably, the same Cochrane review highlights that most streptococcal pharyngitis studies occurred in the 1950s and with the shifting epidemiology of disease in high-income countries (where absolute rates of complications are lower) the NNTB (number needed to treat for benefit) will rise above a rate at which it might be regarded as worthwhile to treat. In low-income countries where the absolute rate may be much higher, the lower NNTB will mean antibiotics are more likely to be effective. A study in the UK reported that the overall incidence of suppurative complications in a large cohort to be low, on the order of 1.4% in an ambulatory population.[4] In adults without a previous history of rheumatic heart disease the number needed to treat to prevent one case of rheumatic heart disease is 3 million.[5] This literature suggests that the general paradigm for detecting and treatment GAS pharyngitis with antibiotics may need to be reconsidered.

Nonetheless, physicians routinely treat sore throat with antibiotics. Clinical gestalt is inadequate to rule in or rule out GAS pharyngitis, and no standardized diagnostic testing guideline exist for which ED patients with sore throat require antibiotics. Although rapid antigen detection and molecular tests exist, their cost-effectiveness remains undefined.[6] However, clinical decision rules such as the Centor criteria (Table 27.1) and FeverPAIN (Table 27.2) can help in risk-stratifying patients who require testing. According to the American Academy of Family Practice, the statement, "Use of clinical decision rules for diagnosing GABHS pharyngitis improves quality of care while reducing unwarranted treatment and overall cost" was given an evidence grade A.[9] The American College of Emergency Physicians and other groups within the specialty of emergency medicine have not released specific guidelines on pharyngitis.

Table 27.1 Centor score (modified McIssac) for strep pharyngitis

Patient age	3–14 yrs	+1
	15–44 yrs	0
	≥45 yrs	–1
Exudate or swelling on the tonsils	Yes	+1
	No	0
Tender/swollen anterior cervical lymph nodes	Yes	+1
	No	0
Temperature > 38 °C (100.4 °F)	Yes	+1
	No	0
Cough	Absent	+1
	Present	0

Centor score	Probability of GAS pharyngitis	Recommendation
0	1–2.5%	No further testing or antibiotics
1	5–10%	No further testing or antibiotics
2	11–17%	Optional rapid strep testing and/or culture
3	28–35%	Consider rapid strep testing and/or culture
≥4	51–53%	Consider rapid strep testing and/or culture. Empirical antibiotics may be appropriate

Source: Adapted from reference [7].

Clinical question

Which physical examination findings significantly alter the likelihood of a positive GAS culture in patients with sore throat?

A diagnostic systematic review compiled data and calculated likelihood ratios (likelihood ratio [LR]+ and LR−) for clinical findings and the chance of a positive GAS culture.[10] All data are reported here with either the 95% CI or the ranges provided by the studies. The most predictive elements included pharyngeal exudates LR+ 2.1 (CI 1.4–3.1), LR− 0.90 (CI 0.75–1.1); tonsillar swelling or enlargement LR+ 1.8 (CI 1.5–2.3), LR− 0.63 (CI 0.56–0.72);

Table 27.2 The FeverPAIN score for strep pharyngitis

Fever in the past 24 h	Yes	+1
	No	0
Absence of cough or coryza	Yes	+1
	No	0
Symptom onset ≤3 days	Yes	+1
	No	0
Purulent tonsils	Yes	+1
	No	0
Severe tonsil inflammation	Yes	+1
	No	0

FeverPAIN score	Probability of GAS pharyngitis	Recommendation
0	13–18%	No antibiotics
1	13–18%	No antibiotics
2	30–35%	Delayed antibiotic to be considered or rapid strep testing
3	39–48%	Delayed antibiotic to be considered or rapid strep testing
4	62–65%	Consider antibiotics if symptoms are severe, rapid strep testing, or short delayed prescribing

Source: Adapted from reference [8].

tender anterior cervical nodes LR+ 1.2–1.9, LR– 0.60 (CI 0.49–0.71); tonsillar exudates LR+ 3.4 (1.8–6.0), LR– 0.72 (0.60–0.88); no cough LR+ 1.1–1.7, LR– 0.53–0.89; and strep exposure within the previous 2 weeks, LR+ 1.9 (1.3–2.8), LR– 0.92 (0.86–0.99). Notably, no single clinical finding showed a sufficient accuracy to discriminate through its presence or absence between GAS-positive and GAS-negative patients with sore throat.

More recently, Paul Little and colleagues published a series of studies on sore throat, specifically examining the impact of the Centor criteria, as well as the FeverPAIN criteria on the incidence of suppurative complications in sore throat in an adult primary care population in the UK.[4,11] In more than 14,000 adults with symptoms of sore throat for less than 2 weeks, there were two independent predictors of complications, specifically severe tonsillar inflammation which was noted in 13% of the sample (odds ratio 1.92) and severe earache which was in 5% of the population (odds ratio 3.02). However, 70% of the complications occurred when neither finding was present. When the Centor criteria and FeverPAIN were applied, there were higher rates of complications with higher scores for both clinical decision rules. However, the predictive values were relatively poor and the majority of the complications in the study occurred in patients with low scores (i.e., Centor score ≤2 and FeverPAIN ≤2).

Clinical question

What are the clinical prediction rules for GAS pharyngitis, and how can they guide therapy for ED patients with sore throat?

The Centor criteria (Table 27.1) is a prediction rule based on selected signs and symptoms in patients with pharyngitis and can identify patients at low risk for GAS pharyngitis.[10] The Centor criteria include (i) history of fever, (ii) anterior cervical adenopathy, (iii) tonsillar exudates, and (iv) absence of cough. Using a positive culture for GAS as a criterion standard, in the initial derivation study of the Centor criteria, probabilities assigned to each score include: a 56% probability of positive culture in patients with four criteria, a 32% probability with three criteria, a 15% probability with two, 6.5% with one, and 2.5% with zero.[12] Since the probability of a strep infection is higher in children than adults, McIssac *et al.* suggested an age-based revision to the Centor criteria.[13] In the McIssac revision to the Centor criteria, patients who are <5 years old receive an additional point, whereas if they are >45 years old they have a point subtracted.[7] Using the McIssac modification, the risk of streptococcal infection is listed in Table 27.1.

FeverPAIN (Table 27.2) is another clinical prediction tool that has been developed to be used in both adults and children age 3 or older. FeverPAIN uses five clinical criteria including (i) fever in past 24 hours, (ii) absence of cough or coryza, (iii) symptom onset ≤3 days, (iv) purulent tonsils, and (v) severe tonsil inflammation to identify patients at low risk for GAS pharyngitis.[8] A score of 0 or 1 is associated with a 13–18% rate of GAS isolation. This is notably close to the background carriage rate for GAS in asymptomatic individuals. For 0 or 1, no antibiotics are recommended. For a score of 2, the rate of GAS increases to 30–35%, for 3 it is 39–48%. For scores of 2 or 3, the authors recommend a delayed antibiotic strategy, where antibiotics are prescribed but delayed (only to be started in 3–5 days if symptoms were either worsening or unremitting symptoms). For a score of 4 or more, the rate of isolation of GAS is 62–65%, where antibiotics are recommended for severe symptoms or a short, delayed prescribing approach (i.e., waiting 48 hours to assess if symptoms improve).

To determine the effect of clinical scoring, delayed antibiotics, and antigen tests used according to a clinical score, a pragmatic, randomized trial approach was used.[8] Outcomes were symptom severity 2–4 days after consultation, duration of symptoms, and the use of antibiotics. Symptom severity was lowest in the clinical score group (−0.33) equivalent to one in three rating sore throat a slight versus moderate problem, and also demonstrated a similar reduction in the antigen testing group (−0.30). Symptoms that were rated either moderately bad or worse also resolved significantly faster in the clinical score group (hazard ratio 1.3), but not the antigen testing group (1.11). Antibiotic use was lower in both the clinical score group (29%) and in the antigen testing group (27%), compared to the delayed antibiotics group (46%). The study did not find any significant differences in complications or patients who required additional consultation. The authors concluded that targeted use of antibiotics with clinical scoring improves both reported symptoms as well as lowers antibiotic use; however, the clinical scoring system had similar benefits as the antigen testing approach.

Comment

A few signs and symptoms can increase or reduce the likelihood of patients with sore throat having positive throat cultures for GAS. Yet, in an era of increasing antimicrobial resistance and a philosophy of emergency medicine stewardship, the philosophical relevance of whether the individual does or does not have GAS is germane. For strategies that favor treatment, the Centor criteria with the McIssac modification as well as the FeverPAIN score have been validated in both adults and children for use in predicting the probability of GAS pharyngitis.[8,13] Using these criteria may be helpful implementation strategies to guide guideline-adherent testing and antimicrobial treatment decisions in the ED.[14,15]

There is, however, considerable controversy over how these rules should be applied in clinical practice. The concern is the overtreatment of acute pharyngitis with antibiotics. A review of 17 international guidelines in 2014 on the treatment of GAS found that nine were more pro-treatment, five favored no treatment, and two had special considerations.[2]

Specifically, the guidelines from the European Society for Clinical Microbiology and Infectious Diseases (ESCMID) recommends that antibiotics should avoided in patients with Centor 0–2, and that modest benefits of antibiotics that are observed in Centor 3–4 have to be weighed against antibiotic side effects, the effects of antibiotics on microbiota, as well as antibiotic resistance and costs of care.[16] By contrast, the Infectious Disease Society of America (IDSA) recommends antibiotic treatment for all adults and children with GAS pharyngitis, and the American Academy of Pediatrics (AAP) recommends antibiotics for children with pharyngitis that is confirmed to be caused by GAS.[2,17]

Broadly the literature to date demonstrates that compared to no antibiotics, antibiotic use in confirmed or suspected GAS pharyngitis can reduce both the nonsuppurative as well as the suppurative complications.[8,16,18,19] In the Little *et al.* study, suppurative complications in GAS were rare in adults, yet most of the complications occurred in patients with low Centor and FeverPAIN scores.[8] Based on these findings, taking a more liberal approach to confirmatory testing and/or delayed antibiotics would be recommended in adults. In addition, there is a suggestion that antibiotics improves symptoms in adults.[15]

By comparison, the literature is more limited in children. It is a clinical balancing act of overtreatment (which may result in inappropriate use of antibiotics for cases that are not GAS) versus undertreatment, which may result in missed cases and potentially lead to complications such as longer times to clinical improvement and higher rates of both suppurative and nonsuppurative complications of GAS.[4,20] Yet given that the prevalence of GAS is higher among children as compared to adults, a more liberal approach to testing also makes good sense in children.

References

1. National Hospital Ambulatory Medical Care Survey: 2017 Emergency Department Summary Tables. Available at: https://www.cdc.gov/nchs/data/nhamcs/web_tables/2017_ed_web_tables-508.pdf.
2. Shulman ST, Bisno AL, Clegg HW *et al.* Clinical practice guideline for the diagnosis and management of group A streptococcal pharyngitis: 2012 update by the Infectious Diseases Society of America. *Clinical Infectious Diseases.* 2012; 55(10): 1279–82.
3. Spinks A, Glasziou PP, Del Mar CB. Antibiotics for sore throat (Cochrane Methodology Review). In: *The cochrane library, issue 9.* Chichester, UK: John Wiley & Sons, Ltd; 2011.
4. Little P, Stuart B, Hobbs FD *et al.* DESCARTE investigators. Antibiotic prescription strategies for acute sore throat: a prospective observational cohort study. *The Lancet Infectious Diseases.* 2014; 14: 213–9.
5. Luo R, Sickler J, Vahidnia F, Lee YC, Frogner B, Thompson M. Diagnosis and Management of Group a Streptococcal Pharyngitis in the United States, 2011–2015. *BMC Infectious Diseases.* 2019; 19(1): 193.
6. Fraser H, Gallacher D, Achana F *et al.* Rapid antigen detection and molecular tests for group A streptococcal infections for acute sore throat: Systematic reviews and economic evaluation. *Health Technology Assessment.* 2020; 24(31): 1–232.

7. McIsaac WJ, Kellner JD, Aufricht P, Vanjaka A, Low DE. Empirical validation of guidelines for the management of pharyngitis in children and adults. *Journal of the American Medical Association.* 2004; 291: 1587–95.
8. Little P, Hobbs FD, Moore M et al. PRISM investigators. Clinical score and rapid antigen detection test to guide antibiotic use for sore throats: Randomised controlled trial of PRISM (primary care streptococcal management). *BMJ.* 2013; 347: f5806.
9. Choby BA. Diagnosis and treatment of streptococcal pharyngitis. *American Family Physician.* 2009; 79: 383–90.
10. Ebell MH, Smith MA, Barry HC et al. The rational clinical examination: Does this patient have strep throat? *Journal of the American Medical Association.* 2000; 284: 2912–8.
11. Little P, Stuart B, Hobbs FD et al. DESCARTE investigators. Predictors of suppurative complications for acute sore throat in primary care: Prospective clinical cohort study. *BMJ.* 2013; 347: f6867.
12. Centor R, Witherspoon J, Dalton H, Brody C, Link K. The diagnosis of strep throat in adults in the emergency room. *Medical Decision Making.* 1981; 1(3): 239–46.
13. McIsaac WJ, Goel V, To T et al. The validity of a sore throat score in family practice. *Canadian Medical Association Journal.* 2000; 168: 811–5.
14. Meeker D, Knight TK, Friedberg MW et al. Nudging guideline-concordant antibiotic prescribing: A randomized clinical trial. *JAMA Internal Medicine.* 2014; 174(3): 425–31. doi: 10.1001/jamainternmed.2013.14191.
15. Yadav K, Meeker D, Mistry RD et al. A multifaceted intervention improves prescribing for acute respiratory infection for adults and children in emergency department and urgent care settings. *Academic Emergency Medicine.* 2019; 26(7): 719–31. doi: 10.1111/acem.13690.
16. ESCMID Sore Throat Guideline Group, Pelucchi C, Grigoryan L et al. Guideline for the management of acute sore throat. *Clinical Microbiology and Infection.* 2012; 18(Suppl 1): 1–28.
17. Van Brusselen D, Vlieghe E, Schelstraete P et al. Streptococcal pharyngitis in children: To treat or not to treat? *European Journal of Pediatrics.* 2014; 173(10): 1275–83.
18. Hersh AL, Jackson MA, Hicks LA. American academy of pediatrics committee on infectious diseases. Principles of judicious antibiotic prescribing for upper respiratory tract infections in pediatrics. *Pediatrics.* 2013; 132(6): 1146–54.
19. Kenealy T. Sore throat. *BMJ Clinical Evidence.* 2011; 2011: 1509.
20. Centor R, Allison JJ, Cohen SJ. Pharyngitis management: Defining the controversy. *Journal of General Internal Medicine.* 2007; 22: 127–30.

Chapter 28 **Rhinosinusitis**

W. Mason Bonner and Jonathan Sheele

Department of Emergency Medicine, Mayo Clinic, Jacksonville, FL, USA

Highlights

- The majority of rhinosinusitis cases are viral in etiology and the course of illness is typically self-limited.
- Watchful waiting without the use of antibiotic therapy is recommended for the first 7–10 days.
- The most reliable findings suggesting bacterial sinusitis include cacosmia, tooth pain, a biphasic course of illness or "double sickening," and the overall clinical impression.
- Imaging is not recommended upon initial evaluation unless invasive disease or severe complications are suspected.

Background

Rhinosinusitis is an inflammatory process of the mucosal lining of nasal cavity and paranasal sinuses. The natural pathogenesis involves inflammation of sinus mucous membranes which disrupts mucociliary function, resulting in sinus obstruction. It is typically caused by viruses, bacterial infections, noninfectious allergies, and fungi.[1] It can be subdivided by chronicity with an acute phase lasting <4 weeks, subacute 4–12 weeks, chronic >12 weeks, and recurrent disease defined as >4 episodes in a given year.[2] Rhinosinusitis is one of the most common complaints in primary care and emergency medicine affecting ~1 in 7 adults, or about 31 million people per year. Rhinosinusitis is a common diagnosis, often leading to an antibiotic prescription in the United States.[3] The overwhelming majorities of cases of rhinosinusitis are viral, and account

---

Evidence-Based Emergency Care: Diagnostic Testing and Clinical Decision Rules, Third Edition.
Edited by Jesse M. Pines, Fernanda Bellolio, Christopher R. Carpenter, and Ali S. Raja.
© 2023 John Wiley & Sons Ltd. Published 2023 by John Wiley & Sons Ltd.

for > 90% of acute infections. The most common viruses include rhinoviruses, adenoviruses, coronaviruses, influenza viruses, and parainfluenza viruses.[4] Bacterial infections are much less common. The most common bacteria include *Streptococcus pneumoniae, Haemophilus influenzae, Moraxella catarrhalis, and Staphylococcus aureus*.[5] Clinical adjuncts such as blood work and imaging are not routinely advised on initial presentation and add little to the diagnostic work up.[6] Differentiating viral from bacterial rhinosinusitis can be difficult, and the treatment decision continues to be made on clinical grounds.

Clinical question

Which clinical features are associated with acute bacterial rhinosinusitis in ambulatory ED patients?

A diagnosis of viral versus bacterial acute rhinosinusitis is typically made clinically. Rhinosinusitis is present when there is inflammation of the nose/paranasal sinuses with a combination of purulent nasal discharge, nasal obstruction, and/or facial pain or fullness.[1] Additional complaints are variable, and can include maxillary dental pain, headache, postnasal drip, cough (particularly in children), fever, sore throat, and halitosis. Unfortunately, there are no validated clinical decision rules to guide the diagnosis, and laboratory studies and imaging do not have sufficient specificity to justify routine usage. Clinicians should rely upon a combination of signs and symptoms to make the diagnosis.

A key to distinguishing viral from bacterial illness is symptom course and duration. Most viral sinusitis will be self-limited, last <10 days, and have clinical improvement over time. Duration of illness >10 days or worsening of symptoms generally indicate bacterial illness.[7] Often there is a pattern of symptom improvement followed by a worsening of the symptoms and this biphasic pattern of illness or "double sickening" can be a reliable indicator of bacterial infection.[7,8] This is hypothesized to occur secondary to bacterial overgrowth in the setting of damaged sinonasal mucosa from an initial viral insult.

The physical exam is also important for diagnosing rhinosinusitis, identifying complications, and excluding alternative diagnoses. A 2019 meta-analysis found that rhinosinusitis can be ruled in based on both purulent secretions in the middle meatus (LR+ 3.2), as well as the overall clinical impression (LR+ 3.0).[9] Conversely, rhinosinusitis can be ruled out using the overall clinical impression (LR− 0.48), normal transillumination (LR− 0.55), and the absence of: a preceding respiratory tract infection (LR− 0.48), any nasal discharge (LR− 0.49), or purulent nasal discharge (LR− 0.54). The distinction between rhinosinusitis and bacterial rhinosinusitis can be made by a fetid breath odor (cacosmia (LR+ 4.3, LR− 0.86)), tooth pain (LR+ 2.0, LR− 0.77), and the overall clinical impression (LR+ 3.8, LR− 0.34).[9]

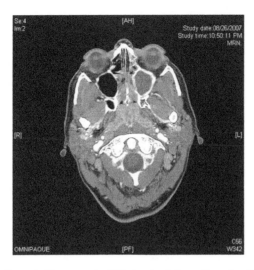

Figure 28.1 Computed tomography (CT) showing left maxillary sinusitis.

Sinus imaging including noncontrast maxillofacial CT (Figure 28.1), and Waters view X-rays are not clinically indicated for uncomplicated acute rhinosinusitis.[6] This is primarily due to the lack of specificity in abnormal imaging. Pathologic findings such as mucous membrane inflammation, opacified sinuses, and air fluid levels, fail to effectively differentiate viral from bacterial disease. Some studies have also demonstrated these findings in asymptomatic patients and those with allergic rhinitis.[10]

Complications of acute bacterial rhinosinusitis are uncommon. Imaging is indicated in cases of suspected invasive disease or in the presence of concurrent neurologic deficits, ophthalmologic abnormalities, or soft tissue concerns (i.e., orbital/preseptal cellulitis) findings. Sinus culture or other microbiologic evaluation is only indicated in cases of a suspected complicated bacterial rhinosinusitis. Sinus puncture, if indicated, is not generally performed in the Emergency Department and should be performed by a specialist.

Comment

Acute bacterial rhinosinusitis is a common complaint in primary and emergency care. The diagnosis of rhinosinusitis is clinical, and it can be difficult to distinguish viral from bacterial causes. More than 90% of rhinosinusitis cases are viral, so watchful waiting is the recommended course of treatment. Antibiotics should not be routinely prescribed until at least 7–10 days from symptom onset.[6,11] Therefore, a watchful strategy is recommended for the first 10 days in the absence of high risk features for bacterial rhinosinusitis.[7]

Common symptoms suggesting bacterial etiology include a biphasic course of illness "double sickening," cacosmia, tooth pain, and the overall clinical impression. Patients without access to appropriate follow up may be prescribed a "safety net" antibiotic prescription along with instructions directing when the

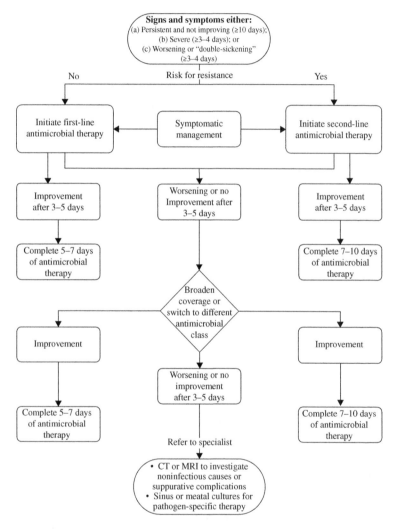

Figure 28.2 Treatment and imaging recommendations for the management of patients with acute bacterial rhinosinusitis. (Adapted from [6].)

prescription should be filled and used. Imaging is not routinely recommended and should be reserved only for cases refractory to maximal medical therapy, if complications are present, or if invasive disease is suspected. If disease is severe or recurrent patients should be referred for otorhinolaryngogologist evaluation. The Infectious Diseases Society of America published an algorithm for treatment and imaging recommendations in patients with acute bacterial rhinosinusitis, which we have adapted in Figure 28.2.[6]

References

1. Fokkens WJ, Lund VJ, Mullol J et al. EPOS 2012: European position paper on rhinosinusitis and nasal polyps 2012. A summary for otorhinolaryngologists. *Rhinology*. 2012; 50(1): 1–12.
2. Wyler B, Mallon WK. Sinusitis update. *Emergency Medicine Clinics of North America*. 2019; 37(1): 41–54.
3. Lowery JL, Alexander B, Nair R, Heintz BH, Livorsi DJ. Evaluation of antibiotic prescribing in emergency departments and urgent care centers across the Veterans' Health Administration. *Infection Control and Hospital Epidemiology*. 2021; 42(6): 694–701.
4. Jaume F, Valls-Mateus M, Mullol J. Common cold and acute rhinosinusitis: Up-to-date management in 2020. *Current Allergy and Asthma Reports*. 2020; 20(7): 28.
5. Virtanen J, Hokkinen L, Karjalainen M et al. in vitro detection of common rhinosinusitis bacteria by the eNose utilising differential mobility spectrometry. *European Archives of Oto-Rhino-Laryngology*. 2018; 275(9): 2273–9.
6. Chow AW, Benninger MS, Brook I et al. IDSA clinical practice guideline for acute bacterial rhinosinusitis in children and adults. *Clinical Infectious Diseases*. 2012; 54(8): e72–112.
7. Aring AM, Chan MM. Current concepts in adult acute rhinosinusitis. *American Family Physician*. 2016; 94(2): 97–105.
8. Lindbaek M, Hjortdahl P, Johnsen UL. Use of symptoms, signs, and blood tests to diagnose acute sinus infections in primary care: Comparison with computed tomography. *Family Medicine*. 1996; 28(3): 183–8.
9. Ebell MH, McKay B, Dale A, Guilbault R, Ermias Y. Accuracy of signs and symptoms for the diagnosis of acute rhinosinusitis and acute bacterial rhinosinusitis. *The Annals of Family Medicine*. 2019; 17(2): 164–72.
10. Gregurić T, Prokopakis E, Vlastos I et al. Imaging in chronic rhinosinusitis: A systematic review of MRI and CT diagnostic accuracy and reliability in severity staging. *Journal of Neuroradiology*. 2021; 48(4): 277–81.
11. Lin MP, Nguyen T, Probst MA, Richardson LD, Schuur JD. Emergency physician knowledge, attitudes, and behavior regarding ACEP's choosing wisely recommendations: A survey study. *Academic Emergency Medicine*. 2017; 24(6): 668–75.

Chapter 29 **Pneumonia**

John Bedolla[1] and Jesse M. Pines[2,3]

[1] Department of Surgery and Perioperative Care, Dell Medical School, University of Texas, Austin, TX, USA
[2] US Acute Care Solutions, Canton, OH, USA
[3] Department of Emergency Medicine, Drexel University, Philadelphia, PA, USA

Highlights

- The presence or absence of several elements of the history, physical examination, and laboratory testing can raise or lower the likelihood of a radiographic diagnosis of pneumonia.
- The chest radiograph has a 10% false-negative rate and does not exclude pneumonia if the pretest probability for pneumonia is moderate or high.
- The Pneumonia Severity Index accurately determines which patients are at low risk for 30-day mortality.
- The CURB-65 rule accurately stratifies patients at high risk for 30-day mortality.
- Procalcitonin is a promising tool for predicting which patients with pneumonia may benefit from antibiotics; however, additional studies are needed to justify widespread use.
- There is significant overlap in the radiologic and clinical appearance of COVID-19 and bacterial pneumonia.
- Risk stratification tools can improve clinical decision-making and help identify a group of patients who can be safely managed as outpatients.
- Chest CT and lung ultrasound are promising tools to help diagnose pneumonia in the ED.

Evidence-Based Emergency Care: Diagnostic Testing and Clinical Decision Rules, Third Edition.
Edited by Jesse M. Pines, Fernanda Bellolio, Christopher R. Carpenter, and Ali S. Raja.

Background

Community-acquired pneumonia (CAP) is an acute infection of the lung's parenchyma accompanied by symptoms of acute illness (Figure 29.1). There are several challenges in the ED evaluation of patients with CAP. The chest radiograph has a false-negative rate of 7–10%. Therefore, by itself, a negative chest X-ray does not entirely rule out pneumonia. The history and physical exam, as well as serum testing, inform a structured and unstructured estimation of pretest probability for CAP. Illness severity in diagnosed CAP often guides decisions about admission, further diagnostic testing in the ED, and the choice of antibiotics. There are diagnostic scoring systems for estimating the pretest probability of CAP, and scoring systems for estimating the severity of illness, expressed as mortality.[1,2]

The prevalence of CAP in unselected patients presenting with cough and fever is 5–10%. Beginning with this prevalence, a pretest probability for CAP can be estimated using a structured or unstructured approach. An unstructured approach means the clinician simply adds of positives and negatives to arrive at a general sense or high or low probability of pneumonia. A more structured approach, as advocated by Diehr and Heckerling, involves using the 6–7 of the most salient clinical and laboratory elements to establish a more continuous range of pretest probabilities, ranging from less than 1% to greater than 50%. The pretest probability along with the chest radiograph interpretation and the negative predictive value (NPV) or positive predictive value to arrive at posttest probability for CAP. When considering CAP in the setting of a viral respiratory pandemic, it is essential to know that some viral disease, such as severe acute respiratory syndrome (SARS), middle east

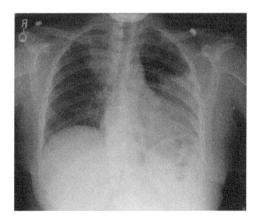

Figure 29.1 Left lower lobe pneumonia.

respiratory syndrome (MERS), coronavirus 2019 (COVID-19), and Hantavirus, can present dense lobular findings typical of bacterial pneumonia, and multifocal infiltrates usually associated with pneumonia.[3-5]

One of the most widely used severity scoring systems is the pneumonia severity index (PSI) which was developed by Fine *et al.*[6] Table 29.1 details the elements of the PSI and its association with risk of death at 30 days. The PSI helps guide disposition by identifying patients who are at low risk for death

Table 29.1 The pneumonia severity index

Characteristic	Points assigned
Demographic factor	
Men	Age (years)
Women	Age (years)–10
Nursing home resident	+10
Coexisting illnesses	
Neoplastic disease	+30
Liver disease	+20
Congestive heart failure	+10
Cerebrovascular disease	+10
Renal disease	+10
Physical examination findings	
Altered mental status	+20
Respiratory rate $\geq$ 30 breaths/min	+20
Systolic blood pressure <90 mm Hg	+20
Temperature <35 °C (95 °F) or 40 °C (104 °F)	+15
Pulse $\geq$ 125 beats/min	+10
Laboratory and radiographic findings (if performed)	
Arterial blood pH < 7.35	+30
Blood urea nitrogen level $\geq$ 30 mg/dL	+20
Sodium level < 130 mmol/L	+20
Glucose level $\geq$ 250 mg/dL	+10
Hematocrit < 30%	+10
Partial pressure of arterial O_2 < 60 mm Hg or O_2 Sat <90%	+10
Pleural effusion	+10

Class	Points	Mortality
I	<51	0.1%
II	51–70	0.6%
III	71–90	0.9%
IV	91–130	9.5%
V	>130	26.7%

Source: Data from [6].

Table 29.2 The CURB-65 scoring system*

Confusion
Elevated blood urea nitrogen (BUN) (>7 mmol/L)
Respiratory rate (≥30/min)
Blood pressure (systolic <90 mmHg or diastolic ≤60 mmHg)
Age ≥65 years

* Each element, when positive, is assigned one point.

and therefore candidates for outpatient management. The PSI score places patients with pneumonia into tiers I, II, III, IV, and V, with a mortality of 0.1%, 0.6%, 0.9%, 9.5%, and 26.7%, respectively. Tiers I, II, and III have mortality rates sufficiently low for these patients to be treated as outpatients. The PSI has a sensitivity of 99.7% for mortality, but a low specificity at 23%, for a NPV of 99.7 and a PPV of 6. The PSI weighs patient co-morbidities and age more heavily than other scoring systems. The PSI is also relatively cumbersome and requires an arterial blood gas.[7]

The CURB-65 was developed by the British Thoracic Society. The purpose of the CURB-65 is to identify patients who are at high risk of mortality from pneumonia. The elements of the CURB-65 are detailed in Table 29.2. In the CURB-65, similar to the PSI, higher numbers of points correlated with higher 30-day mortality rates. In an international derivation and validation study, the 30-day mortality rates for the CURB-65 were 0.7% for score 0, 3.2% for score 1, 3% for score 2, 17% for score 3, 41.5% for score 4, and 57% for score 5. The authors of the CURB-65 criteria have suggested that patients who score 0 or 1 are at low risk for mortality and can be managed as outpatients, while those who have a score of 2 are at intermediate risk, and those with scores >2 have severe CAP and are at high risk and should be managed in an intensive care unit. CURB-65 has a sensitivity of 96% for mortality and a specificity of 34%, for a NPV of 99.4% and a PPV of 7%. CURB-65 has slightly lower sensitivity and specificity compared with PSI. On the other hand, it is relatively easier and more reliably performed, as it takes into account only 5 elements: mental status, blood urea nitrogen (BUN), respiratory rate, blood pressure, and age cut off of 65. It relatively underestimates the severity of asthma in young patients.[8,9]

Other scores that have been used to predict mortality are: CURB (CURB-65 minus age), CRB (CURB minus BUN), a qSOFA Score (quick Sequential Organ Failure Assessment), SIRS (systemic inflammatory response syndrome), and early warning scores such as NEWS and SEWS. CURB and CRB have not been validated in large studies and appear to have lower sensitivity and specificity than both PSI and SIRS. qSOFA, SIRS, and the warning system score, are primarily sepsis screening tools, and have proven ineffective in predicting mortality in pneumonia, since sepsis is only one of several causes of death precipitated by pneumonia.[10]

Clinical question

Which elements of the history and physical examination findings are associated with a diagnosis of pneumonia?

Metlay *et al.* addressed this question in a systematic review evaluating history and physical findings against the criterion standard of findings on chest radiography.[11] They reported likelihood ratios based on history and physical examination findings where there were two or more studies; however, an important limitation of this approach is that chest radiography is neither 100% sensitive nor specific for the diagnosis of pneumonia. These likelihood ratios are listed in Table 29.3. The most known scores for estimating pretest probability of pneumonia are the Heckerling Score and the Diehr Score, listed in Tables 29.4 and 29.5.

Table 29.3 Positive and negative likelihood ratios for history, examination, and laboratory findings in diagnosing pneumonia

Finding	Likelihood ratio positive (LR+)	Likelihood ratio negative (LR−)
Patient history		
Fever	1.7–2.1	0.6–0.7
Chills	1.3–1.7	0.7–0.9
Vital signs		
Tachypnea	1.5–3.4	0.8
Tachycardia	1.6–2.3	0.5–0.7
Hyperthermia	1.4–4.4	0.6–0.8
Chest examination		
Dullness to percussion	2.2–4.3	0.8–0.9
Decreased breath sounds	2.3–2.5	0.8–0.9
Crackles	1.6–2.7	0.6–0.9
Rhonchi	1.4–1.5	0.8–0.9
Egophony	2.0–8.6	0.8–1.0
Laboratory findings		
Leukocytosis	1.9–3.7	0.3–0.6

Note: The intervals represent ranges in published studies.
Source: Data from [2].

Table 29.4 Heckerling score

Factors
Absence of asthma
Heart rate >100
Crackles
$T > 37.8$ Celsius
Decreased breath sounds

Number of factors present	Prevalence of pneumonia (%)	Posttest probability of pneumonia if chest radiograph negative (%)
0	1.6	<1
1	4	1
2	13.5	3
3	25	10
4	60	25
5	81	50

Source: Adapted from Heckerling et al. [5].

Table 29.5 Diehr score

Clinical symptom or finding	Points
Rhinorrhea	−2
Sore throat	−1
Night sweats	1
Myalgia	1
Sputum all day	1
Respiratory rate > 25	2
Temp > 100 Fahrenheit (37.8 C)	2

Score	Likelihood ratio positive	Likelihood ratio negative	Probability of pneumonia (%)
−3	1.1	0	5
−1	2.2	0.37	12
0	4.9	0.47	21
1	8.3	0.7	30
3	11	0.9	37

Source: Adapted from Diehr et al. [4].

Clinical question

When should treatment for CAP be given even if the chest radiograph is negative?

There are approximately 4.2 million yearly cases of pneumonia in the United States with a mortality of about 1–2%.[12] The chest radiograph has a false negative rate of 10% and a false positive rate of 6%.[1] The decision to treat or not should be dependent on the calculated pretest and posttest probabilities, as well as the mortality of treated versus untreated CAP. There are no controlled studies of antibiotics versus placebo for CAP, and such a study would be unethical. The best estimate is that antibiotics confer a 10% reduced mortality in CAP.[13] The calculated number needed to treat (NNT) for a macrolide of 21 to prevent one death, and the number needed to harm (NNH) by causing one MI is 144.[14] For a pretest probability of 5%, the NPV is 99.5%. For a pretest probability of 10%, the NPV is 99%. For a pretest probability of 34%, the NPV is 95%, meaning about 5% of negative will be false negatives. At this point, the NNT expressed as 1/21 and the NPV are approximately equal. Alternately, given a 1–2% mortality for treated pneumonia versus a 10% higher predicted mortality untreated, at a pretest probability of 34% or higher, antibiotics confer at least a 1% survival benefit compared to no antibiotics.

Clinical question

Can procalcitonin be used to predict a bacterial etiology of infection and survival in pneumonia?

One study followed 185 patients who had procalcitonin levels measured within 24 hours of admission for CAP.[15] They found that higher procalcitonin levels correlated with PSI score and also predicted complications including the development of empyema, need for mechanical ventilation, septic shock, and mortality. An interesting finding of this study was that procalcitonin predicted a bacterial etiology for pneumonia in patients with low PSI scores, but these findings did not apply to those with more severe CAP.

Another large trial studied 1641 ED patients with dyspnea and measured procalcitonin levels, as well as several other biomarkers.[16] The diagnosis of pneumonia was made based on strict, validated guidelines. They found that a model that used procalcitonin was more accurate with an area under the curve of 72% than any other clinical variable for a strict diagnosis of pneumonia. They reported that combining physician estimates of the probability of pneumonia along with procalcitonin levels increased the accuracy of diagnosis to greater than 86%. They found that patients with a diagnosis of acute heart failure and an elevated procalcitonin level (>0.21 ng/mL) had a worse outcome if they were not treated with antibiotics. Patients with lower procalcitonin levels (<0.05 ng/mL) had better outcomes if they did not receive any antibiotic therapy.

However, a more recent randomized trial (2012–2015) across 12 French hospitals, randomly assigned patients to either procalcitonin-guided treatment or clinical assessment-guided treatment in patients >18 years with CAP.[17] Patients were randomly assigned to either the procalcitonin-guided or clinical assessment group, with the primary outcome being antibiotic duration. Secondary outcomes were antibiotic duration ≤5 days, clinical success, and serious adverse outcomes at 30 days. In 285 patients, half were randomized to each arm. The median age was 67 years and 40% of the cohort had a PSI class of IV or V (high risk). Adherence with the procalcitonin protocol was 76%. Overall, there were no significant differences in antibiotic duration, clinical success rates, or serious adverse outcomes.

Clinical question

Which severity adjustment tool provides the best discriminatory power in predicting survival in patients with pneumonia in the emergency department?
A recent retrospective study compared PSI to CURB and CURB-65 in 3181 ED patients.[7] Both PSI and CURB-65 were good predictors of 30-day mortality and for identifying patients at low risk for mortality. However, PSI appeared to discriminate better in identifying patients at lower risk of mortality. Using PSI, 68% were identified as low risk (class I–III) with a mortality rate of 1.4% while CURB-65 identified 61% as low risk (score of 0 or 1) with a mortality rate of 1.7%. In more severe CAP (score of 2 or higher), CURB-65 seemed to be somewhat more valuable because each score (2, 3, 4, or 5) was associated with a progressive increase in mortality while PSI only discriminated a high-risk versus a low-risk group. Another study used PSI and CURB-65 in a large group of both inpatients and outpatients with CAP in Spain.[18] They found that the CURB-65 and CRB-65 (which is a simpler version that excludes the BUN measurement) accurately predicted 30-day mortality rate, mechanical ventilation, and to some degree, hospitalization. CURB-65 also correlated with time to clinical stability and was predictive of a longer duration of intravenous antibiotics. Higher PSI numbers also predicted increased mortality, similarly to previous studies.

Clinical question

What is the role of other imaging like lung ultrasound (US) and computed tomography (CT) for CAP?
Chest radiography is the standard method to diagnose pneumonia. However, CT scan is more sensitive than chest radiography for differentiating CAP from other lung conditions. One study followed 319 patients with clinically

suspected CAP, as well as chest radiography, and who also had a chest CT scan within 4 hours.[19] The probability of CAP diagnosis as well as therapeutic plans were recorded by emergency physicians before and after CT scan result. On chest radiography, a parenchymal infiltrate was seen in 188 (59%) patients. Based on these findings, the diagnosis was definite in 45% of patients, possible in 54%, and excluded in 1%. CT demonstrated a parenchymal infiltrate in 40 (33%) of patients who did not have an infiltrate on chest radiography. In addition, CT chest changed the clinical classification in 187 (59%) patients, leading to 51% with definite CAP, and 29% with CAP excluded. As a result of the CT scan, management changes with antibiotics occurred. In 51 patients (16%) antibiotics were initiated, 29 (9%) had antibiotics discontinued, and changed hospitalization decisions to admit in 22 (7%) and discharge in 23 (7%). The authors concluded that chest CT markedly changed clinical management.

There has also been increased use of lung ultrasound to diagnose pneumonia. A meta-analysis by Ye et al. compared lung US versus chest X-ray and included 742 patients.[20] All ultrasounds were performed by emergency physicians. The gold standard for CAP was clinical diagnosis and/or CT imaging (a total of 138 patients had CT imaging, 18.6%). The authors reported a pooled sensitivity of 0.95 (CI 0.93–0.97) and a specificity of 0.90 (CI 0.86–0.94) for lung US, and a pooled sensitivity of 0.77 (CI 0.73–0.80) and a specificity of 0.91 (CI 0.87–0.94) for chest X-ray when compared to the gold standard.

A separate meta-analysis of lung US for the diagnosis of CAP by Long et al. included 12 studies (1515 subjects) and reported a pooled sensitivity of 0.88 (CI 0.86–0.90) and specificity of 0.86 (CI 0.83–0.88), LR (−) of 0.13 (CI 0.08–0.23), LR (+) 5.37 (CI 2.76–10.43), and diagnostic odds ratio (DOR) of 65.5 (CI 29.2–146.6).[21] Another meta-analysis of lung US for CAP by Llamas-Alvarez et al. including 16 studies (2359 subjects) reported an Area under the receiver operator characteristic curve (ROC) of 0.93, with a DOR of 50 (CI 21–120).[22] Finally, a meta-analysis of lung US for the emergency diagnosis of CAP, heart failure, COPD by Staub et al. included 25 studies and reported ROC for lung US of 0.948 for pneumonia, 0.914 for acute heart failure, and 0.906 for exacerbations of COPD/asthma.[23] In patients suspected to have pneumonia, consolidation had sensitivity of 0.82 (CI 0.74–0.88) and specificity of 0.94 (CI 0.85–0.98). The authors reported that the modified diffuse interstitial pattern and the B-lines had the highest sensitivity and specificity for heart failure (sensitivity 0.90, CI 0.87–0.93 and specificity of 0.93, CI 0.91–0.95, and B-lines had a sensitivity of 0.93, CI 0.72–0.98 and specificity of 0.92, CI 0.79–0.97).

Lung US is reportedly very good at detecting superficial pneumonia, however, it can miss deeper alveolar pneumonia. False-positive findings with lung US have been reportedly due to sepsis of other origin, pulmonary embolism, acute respiratory distress syndrome, pulmonary edema, and pulmonary fibrosis. Most ultrasound studies noted that diagnostic performance also varies with ultrasonographer experience.[24] The possibility of a dynamic evaluation gives ultrasound an advantage over repeated chest radiography.

Clinical question

Does the chest radiograph accurately distinguish between COVID-19 Pneumonia and CAP?

COVID-19 has typical findings of ground glass infiltrates and is not confined to a lobar pattern. However, there is significant overlap in the radiologic and clinical appearance of COVID-19 and bacterial pneumonia (see Chapter 63). When the findings are diffuse and not confined to a lobar pattern and the typical ground glass pattern is noted, it is safe to treat for COVID-19 without antibiotics in COVID-positive patients. Nasopharyngeal swab testing for COVID-19 can help distinguish between COVID-19 and CAP.[25–27] That being said, in patients with severe COVID-19 bacterial superinfection can occur due to severe damage of the lung parenchyma.

Comment

Several findings in the history, physical examination, and laboratory results are associated with a diagnosis of pneumonia on chest radiography. The presence of a single finding does not have a major impact on the overall probability of disease, reflecting the fact that combinations of findings are typically more important in predicting a radiographic diagnosis. Several studies have demonstrated that a combination of findings together are associated with considerably higher likelihood of disease.[4,28]

While procalcitonin is a promising tool for predicting which patients with pneumonia (particularly equivocal diagnoses) may benefit from empiric antibiotic therapy, a moderate-sized randomized trial did not demonstrate any changes in clinical management with antibiotics, clinical success rates, or adverse outcomes, suggesting that procalcitonin may not impact management in higher-risk CAP patients. Additional study is needed to determine the role of procalcitonin in ED patients with CAP.

PSI and CURB-65 are the two major widely studied scoring systems for severity of illness in CAP. PSI better identifies patients who are at low risk of mortality. There is a tendency with PSI, however, to underestimate severity of illness in younger patients with comorbid illness because it places heavy weight on age and comorbidities. CURB-65 seems somewhat better at identifying patients at higher risk for mortality and discriminates better among more severely ill patients. One problem with CURB-65 is that it does not account as well for comorbidities. It also may be difficult to use in older patients with other chronic conditions who are at high risk for mortality, even though they may have a lower CURB-65 score.

While both scoring systems predict 30-day survival in large populations, neither can perfectly predict which patients with CAP can be safely admitted or discharged from ED. Additionally, clinical variables, social circumstances, and adequate access to follow-up care, among other factors, must be considered in the disposition plan. A recent commentary has suggested that PSI and CURB-65 be combined, recognizing that each system has its own limitations. The authors suggested that low-risk patients (PSI classes I to III or CURB-65 scores of 0–1) could be managed at home if there are no vital sign abnormalities or significant comorbidities, as measured by both scoring systems, and if no other factors (such as social situation) necessitate hospital admission.[29]

Using chest CT and lung ultrasound are promising tools to help diagnose pneumonia in the ED. Chest CT has been shown to change clinical management in a high proportion of patients, suggesting a more central role of the use of chest CT in clinically equivocal cases. Lung ultrasound has been shown to be sensitive and specific to rule out CAP and also diagnose other causes of shortness of breath, however, may miss more central infiltrates. Finally, there is significant overlap in the radiographic appearance of COVID-19 and bacterial pneumonia. Therefore, adjunctive diagnostic testing (i.e., nasal swab for COVID-19) is recommended for definitive diagnosis.

References

1. Self WH, Courtney DM, McNaughton CD, Wunderink RG, Kline JA. High discordance of chest X-ray and computed tomography for detection of pulmonary opacities in ED patients: Implications for diagnosing pneumonia. *The American Journal of Emergency Medicine*. 2013; 31(2): 401–5.
2. Emerman CL, Dawson N, Speroff T *et al.* Comparison of physician judgment and decision aids for ordering chest radiographs for pneumonia in outpatients. *Annals of Emergency Medicine*. 1991; 20(11): 1215–9.
3. Graffelman AW, le Cessie S, Knuistingh Neven A, Wilemssen FE, Zonderland HM, van den Broek PJ. Can history and exam alone reliably predict pneumonia? *The Journal of Family Practice*. 2007; 56(6): 465–70.
4. Diehr P, Wood RW, Bushyhead J, Krueger L, Wolcott B, Tompkins RK. Prediction of pneumonia in outpatients with acute cough – a statistical approach. *Journal of Chronic Diseases*. 1984; 37(3): 215–25.
5. Heckerling PS, Tape TG, Wigton RS *et al.* Clinical prediction rule for pulmonary infiltrates. *Annals of Internal Medicine*. 1990; 113(9): 664–70.

6. Fine MJ, Auble TE, Yealy DM *et al.* A prediction rule to identify low-risk patients with community-acquired pneumonia. *The New England Journal of Medicine.* 1997; 336(4): 243–50.

7. Aujesky D, Auble TE, Yealy DM *et al.* Prospective comparison of three validated prediction rules for prognosis in community-acquired pneumonia. *The American Journal of Medicine.* 2005; 118(4): 384–92.

8. Man SY, Lee N, Ip M *et al.* Prospective comparison of three predictive rules for assessing severity of community-acquired pneumonia in Hong Kong. *Thorax.* 2007; 62(4): 348–53.

9. Buising KL, Thursky KA, Black JF *et al.* A prospective comparison of severity scores for identifying patients with severe community acquired pneumonia: Reconsidering what is meant by severe pneumonia. *Thorax.* 2006; 61(5): 419–24.

10. Barlow G, Nathwani D, Davey P. The CURB65 pneumonia severity score outperforms generic sepsis and early warning scores in predicting mortality in community-acquired pneumonia. *Thorax.* 2007; 62(3): 253–9.

11. Metlay JP, Fine MJ. Testing strategies in the initial management of patients with community-acquired pneumonia. *Annals of Internal Medicine.* 2003; 138(2): 109–18.

12. File TM Jr, Marrie TJ. Burden of community-acquired pneumonia in North American adults. *Postgraduate Medicine.* 2010; 122(2): 130–41.

13. File TM Jr, Schentag JJ. What can we learn from the time course of untreated and partially treated community-onset Streptococcus pneumoniae pneumonia? A clinical perspective on superiority and noninferiority trial designs for mild community-acquired pneumonia. *Clinical Infectious Diseases.* 2008; 1(47 Suppl 3): S157–65.

14. Mortensen EM, Halm EA, Pugh MJ *et al.* Association of azithromycin with mortality and cardiovascular events among older patients hospitalized with pneumonia. *Journal of the American Medical Association.* 2014; 311(21): 2199–208.

15. Masia M, Gutierrez F, Shum C *et al.* Usefulness of procalcitonin levels in community-acquired pneumonia according to the patients outcome research team pneumonia severity index. *Chest.* 2005; 128: 2223–9.

16. Maisel A, Neath SX, Landsberg J *et al.* Use of procalcitonin for the diagnosis of pneumonia in patients presenting with a chief complaint of dyspnoea: Results from the BACH (Biomarkers in Acute Heart Failure) trial. *European Journal of Heart Failure.* 2012; 14(3): 278–86.

17. Montassier E, Javaudin F, Moustafa F *et al.* Guideline-based clinical assessment versus procalcitonin-guided antibiotic use in pneumonia: A pragmatic randomized trial. *Annals of Emergency Medicine.* 2019; 74(4): 580–91.

18. Capelastegui A, Espana PP, Quintana JM *et al.* Validation of a predictive rule for the management of community-acquired pneumonia. *The European Respiratory Journal.* 2006; 27: 151–7.

19. Claessens YE, Debray MP, Tubach F *et al.* Early chest computed tomography scan to assist diagnosis and guide treatment decision for suspected community-acquired pneumonia. *American Journal of Respiratory and Critical Care Medicine.* 2015; 192(8): 974–82.

20. Ye X, Xiao H, Chen B, Zhang S. Accuracy of lung ultrasonography versus chest radiography for the diagnosis of adult community-acquired pneumonia: Review of the literature and meta-analysis. *PLoS One*. 2015; 10(6): e0130066.

21. Long L, Zhao HT, Zhang ZY, Wang GY, Zhao HL. Lung ultrasound for the diagnosis of pneumonia in adults: A meta-analysis. *Medicine (Baltimore)*. 2017; 96(3): e5713.

22. Llamas-Álvarez AM, Tenza-Lozano EM, Latour-Pérez J. Accuracy of lung ultrasonography in the diagnosis of pneumonia in adults: Systematic review and meta-analysis. *Chest*. 2017; 151(2): 374–82.

23. Staub LJ, Mazzali Biscaro RR, Kaszubowski E, Maurici R. Lung ultrasound for the emergency diagnosis of pneumonia, acute heart failure, and exacerbations of chronic obstructive pulmonary disease/asthma in adults: A systematic review and meta-analysis. *The Journal of Emergency Medicine*. 2019; 56(1): 53–69.

24. Tsou PY, Chen KP, Wang YH *et al*. Diagnostic accuracy of lung ultrasound performed by novice versus advanced sonographers for pneumonia in children: A systematic review and meta-analysis. *Academic Emergency Medicine*. 2019; 26(9): 1074–88.

25. Cleverley J, Piper J, Jones MM. The role of chest radiography in confirming covid-19 pneumonia. *BMJ*. 2020; 16(370): m2426.

26. Kerpel A, Apter S, Nissan N *et al*. Diagnostic and prognostic value of chest radiographs for COVID-19 at presentation. West. *The Journal of Emergency Medicine*. 2020; 21(5): 1067–75.

27. Metlay JP, Waterer GW. Treatment of community-acquired pneumonia during the coronavirus disease 2019 (COVID-19) pandemic. *Annals of Internal Medicine*. 2020; 173(4): 304–5.

28. Macfarlane J, Holmes W, Gard P *et al*. Prospective study of the incidence, aetiology and outcome of adult lower respiratory tract illness in the community. *Thorax*. 2001; 56: 109–14.

29. Niederman MS, Feldman C, Richards GA. Combining information from prognostic scoring tools for CAP: An American view on how to get the best of all worlds. *The European Respiratory Journal*. 2006; 27: 9–11.

Chapter 30 **Urinary Tract Infection**

Jonathan Sheele[1] and Ali S. Raja[2]

[1]Department of Emergency Medicine, Mayo Clinic, Jacksonville, FL, USA
[2]Department of Emergency Medicine, Massachusetts General Hospital, Harvard Medical School, Boston, MA, USA

Highlights

- Urinary tract infections (UTIs) commonly affect women and older men.
- Urine culture is the criterion standard for UTIs, but its results are not available at the time of Emergency Department care.
- Urine dipsticks are not highly sensitive indicators of positive urine cultures; however, information from the urine dipstick can be combined with clinical pretest probability to improve accuracy.

Background

Urinary tract infections (UTIs) are common complaints in emergency medicine practice, affecting both women of all ages and older men. The lifetime incidence of UTIs in women is between 50% and 60%,[1] and approximately 5% of women presenting to U.S. EDs have genitourinary complaints.[2] UTIs are relatively uncommon in young men but do affect older men and are often associated with disorders of the prostate. The most common method for diagnosing UTI in the ED is either a urine dip or laboratory urinalysis. The dipstick urine test measures leukocytes, nitrite, blood, protein, and pH, while a urinalysis quantifies cell counts such as white blood cells, red blood cells, and squamous cells. The diagnosis of UTI can be difficult in the ED because of the inconsistent relationship between the clinical symptoms, bacteriuria, and pyuria. In addition, because the criterion standard test – a clean-catch or

---

Evidence-Based Emergency Care: Diagnostic Testing and Clinical Decision Rules, Third Edition.
Edited by Jesse M. Pines, Fernanda Bellolio, Christopher R. Carpenter, and Ali S. Raja.

catheterized specimen urine culture – cannot be completed in the ED (because it can take 2–3 days to grow), and the reality that some patients cannot obtain follow-up within that timeframe to act upon the culture result, emergency physicians must often diagnose and treat UTIs without criterion standard testing. The consequence of these uncertainties is tension between emergency medicine and other specialties regarding the overdiagnosis and overtreatment of UTI.[3-5] These differences in approach have led some specialists to analyze the root cause of ED physician's propensity to misdiagnose UTI that identify factors such as time constraints, knowledge deficits, automatic testing, and malpractice fears as likely precipitants.[6]

Clinical question

Can history or physical exam accurately rule in or rule out urinary tract infection?

A 2013 diagnostic systematic review addressed this question for women and reported positive likelihood ratio (LR+s) and negative likelihood ratio (LR−s) for several symptoms and signs and combinations using data from published literature, focusing on four studies that included ED patients.[7] These are listed in Tables 30.1 and 30.2. Overall, neither history and

Table 30.1 History and symptoms predicting urinary tract infections (UTIs)

	LR+ (95% confidence interval)	LR− (95% confidence interval)
Previous UTI	1.4 (0.9–2.0)	0.9 (0.7–1.0)
Dysuria	1.0 (0.8–1.4)	1.0 (0.7–1.2)
Urgency	1.3 (0.8–2.1)	0.9 (0.8–1.1)
Frequency	2.3 (1.4–3.6)	0.2 (0.0–0.6)
Back pain	1.6 (1.0–2.4)	0.8 (0.7–1.0)
Abdominal pain	0.8 (0.5–1.1)	2.0 (0.8–5.0)
Fever	2.2 (1.0–4.6)	0.9 (0.8–1.0)
Hematuria	1.4 (0.6–3.4)	1.0 (0.9–1.0)

Source: Data from [7].

Table 30.2 Physical examination findings predicting urinary tract infections (UTIs)

	LR+ (95% confidence interval)	LR− (95% confidence interval)
Temperature > 37.2 C	1.9 (1.2–3.0)	0.8 (0.6–0.9)
Costovertebral (CVA) tenderness	1.4 (0.8–2.4)	0.9 (0.8–1.0)
Vaginal discharge	0.4 (0.2–1.0)	1.1 (1.0–1.1)

Source: Data from [7].

Table 30.3 Microscopic findings predicting urinary tract infections (UTIs)

	LR+ (95% confidence interval)	LR− (95% confidence interval)
WBC > 0	1.8 (1.3–2.5)	0.1 (0.0–0.6)
WBC > 5	2.2 (1.9–2.6)	0.3 (0.2–0.4)
WBC > 10	2.3 (1.9–2.7)	0.3 (0.2–0.4)
WBC > 15	2.1 (1.7–2.5)	0.3 (0.2–0.4)
WBC > 50	6.4 (2.4–16.6)	0.3 (0.2–0.6)
WBC > 200	9.8 (2.4–39.4)	0.5 (0.3–0.8)
RBC > 5	2.0 (1.6–2.6)	0.6 (0.5–0.6)
Organisms > 0	2.5 (2.0–3.2)	0.3 (0.2–0.4)
Organisms > 1+	2.0 (1.7–2.2)	0.3 (0.3–0.4)
Organisms > 2+	21.9 (7.0–68.6)	0.6 (0.5–0.7)
Organisms > 3+	9.0 (2.1–39.4)	0.9 (0.8–1.0)

Source: Data from [7].

symptoms nor physical examination findings demonstrated large positive or negative LRs to predict the presence of UTI.

Clinical question

Can the presence or absence of microscopic pyuria, hematuria, or bacteriuria guide urine culture ordering or antibiotic prescribing?

While criterion standard urine culture testing cannot be completed during a typical ED visit, microscopic analysis of clean-catch urinary samples can typically be obtained. The 2013 diagnostic systematic review of female UTI included three studies that contained data regarding microscopic findings and calculated LR+ and LR− for pyuria, hematuria, and bacteriuria. These results are shown in Table 30.3.

Overall, both moderate pyuria (WBC > 50/HPF) and moderate bacteriuria (Organisms >2+) were predictive of a UTI, while hematuria was not.

Clinical question

Can urine dipstick accurately rule in or rule out urinary tract infection without additional testing?

The use of urinary dipsticks allows for testing for UTIs without any laboratory analysis at all, using a point-of-care test strip to determine the presence of urinary leukocyte esterase, nitrite, and protein. The accuracy for each of these was calculated by Meister, *et al.* in their systematic review of female UTI, and LR+ and LR− are included in Table 30.4.

Based on these results, the presence of urinary nitrite is the only finding on the urinary dipstick sufficient to rule in UTI. Conversely, the absence of

Table 30.4 Urinary dipstick findings predicting urinary tract infections (UTIs)

	LR+ (95% confidence interval)	LR− (95% confidence interval)
LE > 0	1.5 (1.3–1.8)	0.2 (0.1–0.4)
LE > 1+	1.9 (1.2–2.9)	0.4 (0.2–0.8)
LE > 2+	3.6 (1.5–8.9)	0.6 (0.4–0.9)
Nitrite positive	24.6 (3.4–178.4)	0.6 (0.5–0.8)
Protein > 0	1.5 (1.1–2.1)	0.4 (0.1–0.9)
Protein > 1+	3.3 (1.3–8.3)	0.6 (0.4–0.9)
Protein > 2+	4.5 (0.5–40.7)	0.9 (0.8–1.1)
Blood > 0	2.6 (1.2–2.1)	0.2 (0.1–0.8)
Blood > 1+	2.1 (1.4–3.4)	0.3 (0.1–0.7)

LE = leukocyte esterase.
Source: Data from [7].

either leukocyte esterase or blood on a urinary dipstick has a LR− sufficient to rule out UTI.

Clinical question

Should geriatric patients with nonspecific symptoms be tested for a UTI?
While the presence of nonspecific symptoms is often used to justify the testing of older patients for various infectious processes (respiratory, gastrointestinal, urinary, etc), this practice is not evidence-based. In a 2018 single-center study evaluating 242 patients over the age of 65 years, Caterino, *et al.* found that symptoms like altered mental status, malaise, lethargy, and fever did not have sufficient LR+ or LR− to either rule in or rule out respiratory, gastrointestinal, or urinary infections.[8]

They did, however, find that a fever of 38.0 °C or higher, either before or during the ED visit, had an LR+ of 5.15–18.10 for the diagnosis of one of these infections. In contrast, the absence of fever had an LR− of 0.79–0.92 and was not sufficient to rule out infection. In another 2017 study by Caterino *et al.*, significant disagreements between guideline criteria and clinician diagnosis of UTI in older adults were noted.[5]

Comment

This chapter highlights the continued difficulty in identifying ED patients with UTIs without criterion standard testing. In the context of clinical ED practice, this review identifies a number of conclusions and observations from the literature describing the care of patients with suspected UTI. Clinical signs and symptoms alone are not particularly helpful in diagnosing UTI. The test

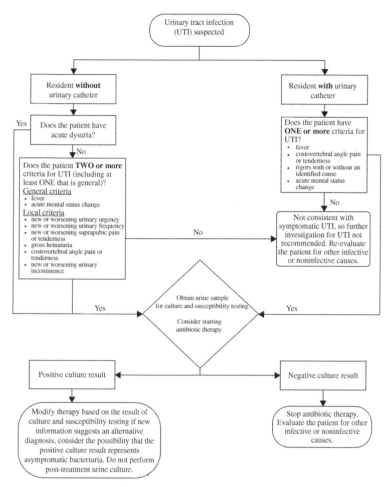

Figure 30.1 Evaluation and treatment of patients living in aged-care facilities suspected of having a UTI. (Adapted from [10].)

performance of urinary dipstick suggests that the most accurate way to define a positive UTI is the identification of the presence of urinary nitrite, while negative leukocyte esterase or blood should prompt the consideration of alternative diagnoses. Microscopic results should focus on pyuria and bacteriuria, moderate results of either of which can rule in UTI. Finally, the presence of nonspecific symptoms such as malaise and altered mental status should not, on their own, lead to UTI testing in older adults (Figure 30.1). A fever, on the other hand, should prompt consideration of an infectious process.

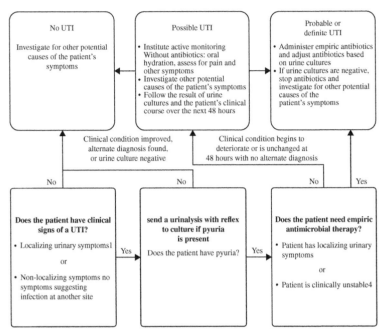

Figure 30.2 Evaluation and treatment of community-dwelling older adults suspected of having a UTI. (Adapted from [11].)

The relative nonspecific nature of most exam findings and tests for UTI, especially in older patients, has resulted in the development of algorithms for the evaluation of older patients with suspected UTI.[9] We present two such algorithms here, noting that they have not been prospectively evaluated, but represent multidisciplinary accepted strategies for the evaluation of older patients; the former is for use in patients residing in aged-care facilities, and the latter is for community-dwelling older adults (Figure 30.2).[10,11]

References

1. Medina M, Castillo-Pino E. An introduction to the epidemiology and burden of urinary tract infections. *Therapeutic Advances in Urology.* 2019;1(11):1756287219832172.
2. McCaig LF, Nawar EW. National Hospital Ambulatory Medical Care Survey: 2004 emergency department summary. *Advance Data.* 2006; 372: 1–29.
3. Caterino JM, Stephens JA, Camargo CA et al. Asymptomatic bacteriuria versus symptom underreporting in older emergency department patients with suspected urinary tract infection. *Journal of the American Geriatrics Society.* 2020; 68(11): 2696–9.

4. Finucane TE. "Urinary Tract Infection"-requiem for a heavyweight. *Journal of the American Geriatrics Society*. 2017; 65(8): 1650–5.

5. Caterino JM, Leininger R, Kline DM *et al*. Accuracy of current diagnostic criteria for acute bacterial infection in older adults in the emergency department. *Journal of the American Geriatrics Society*. 2017; 65(8): 1802–9.

6. O'Kelly K, Phelps K, Regen EL *et al*. Why are we misdiagnosing urinary tract infection in older patients? A qualitative inquiry and roadmap for staff behaviour change in the emergency department. *European Geriatric Medicine*. 2019; 10(4): 585–93.

7. Meister L, Morley EJ, Scheer D, Sinert R. History and physical examination plus laboratory testing for the diagnosis of adult female urinary tract infection. *Academic Emergency Medicine*. 2013; 20(7): 631–45.

8. Caterino JM, Kline DM, Leininger R *et al*. Nonspecific symptoms lack diagnostic accuracy for infection in older patients in the emergency department. *Journal of the American Geriatrics Society*. 2019; 67(3): 484–92.

9. Burkett E, Carpenter CR, Arendts G, Hullick C, Paterson DL, Caterino JM. Diagnosis of urinary tract infection in older persons in the emergency department: To pee or not to pee, that is the question. *Emergency Medicine Australasia*. 2019; 31(5): 856–62.

10. Australian Aged Care Quality and Safety Commission Suspected Urinary Tract Infections: User Guide to the Clinical Pathway for older people in aged care homes. From the Australian Aged Care Quality and Safety Commission. [Internet]. Available from: https://www.agedcarequality.gov.au/sites/default/files/media/guide-clinical-pathway-aged-care-homes-suspected-utis.pdf. 2022.

11. Cortes-Penfield NW, Trautner BW, Jump RLP. Urinary tract infection and asymptomatic bacteriuria in older adults. *Infectious Disease Clinics*. 2017; 31(4): 673–88.

Chapter 31 **Sepsis**

Lucas Oliveira Junqueira e Silva[1,2] and Fernanda Bellolio[2]

[1] Department of Emergency Medicine, Hospital de Clínicas de Porto Alegre, Porto Alegre, Brazil
[2] Department of Emergency Medicine, Mayo Clinic, Rochester, MN, USA

Highlights

- Sepsis is life-threatening organ dysfunction caused by a dysregulated host response to infection.
- The diagnosis of sepsis is challenging as it is largely a clinical diagnosis, and it lacks a gold standard diagnostic test.
- qSOFA has a better discriminative ability to predict in-hospital mortality than SIRS, but should not be used as a "rule out" screening tool in the emergency department given its low sensitivity across validation studies.
- Elevated serum lactate is an independent predictor of mortality in patients with sepsis, but the benefit of pursuing lactate clearance is controversial.
- Procalcitonin can help identify patients at higher risk of bacterial infection, but its sensitivity and specificity are below 80%, so it is not accurate enough to either rule in or rule out bacterial infection.

Background

Sepsis is a clinical syndrome that was initially seen as a systemic inflammatory response that is a sequela of an acute infection. Further understanding of the pathophysiology of sepsis demonstrated that it is not simply systemic inflammation that leads to pathology but also major modifications in nonimmunologic pathways.[1] Given significant changes in the understanding of the disease, the Third Annual Consensus Definitions for Sepsis and Septic Shock

---

Evidence-Based Emergency Care: Diagnostic Testing and Clinical Decision Rules, Third Edition.
Edited by Jesse M. Pines, Fernanda Bellolio, Christopher R. Carpenter, and Ali S. Raja.
© 2023 John Wiley & Sons Ltd. Published 2023 by John Wiley & Sons Ltd.

(Sepsis-3) redefined the core concepts in 2016 using a data-driven approach.[2] The systemic inflammatory response syndrome (SIRS) criteria (Table 31.1) from the definition of sepsis were removed and sepsis was defined as a *"life-threatening organ dysfunction caused by a dysregulated host response to infection."* Table 31.2 illustrates the old (based on Sepsis-1 and Sepsis-2 consensus)[3,4] and new (based on Sepsis-3 consensus)[2,5] definitions of sepsis. Recent estimates indicate that in the United States (U.S.), up to 850,000 sepsis-related emergency department (ED) visits occur annually, with an approximately 70% admission rate.[6] The burden associated with sepsis includes significant morbidity and mortality across all ages and populations. Although high-income countries have reported decreasing mortality rates,[7]

Table 31.1 Systemic inflammatory response syndrome (SIRS) criteria

SIRS is defined as the presence of two or more of the following:
- Heart rate >90 beats/min
- Respiratory rate >20 breaths/min or oxygen saturation <90% or need for >0.4 FiO_2 to maintain saturation
- Temperature >38 °C or <35.5 °C
- White blood cell count >15,000 cells/mm³ or bands >10%

Source: Data from [3].

Table 31.2 Old and new definitions of sepsis

	Sepsis-1 and Sepsis-2[3,4]	Sepsis-3[2]
Sepsis	The presence of two or more SIRS criteria associated with the presence of an infection	"Life-threatening organ dysfunction caused by a dysregulated host response to infection" Organ dysfunction is identified as an acute change in total SOFA score ε 2 consequent to the infection Outside the ICU, qSOFA ε 2 should be used as a predictor of in-hospital mortality and ICU stay
Severe sepsis	Sepsis and at least one sign of hypoperfusion or organ dysfunction	This term no longer exists
Septic shock	Sepsis and at least one sign of hypoperfusion or the requirement for a vasopressor	Septic patient with persisting hypotension requiring vasopressors to maintain MAP ε 65 mmHg and having a serum lactate level >2 mmol/L (18 mg/dL) despite adequate volume resuscitation

MAP = mean arterial pressure; qSOFA = quick SOFA; SOFA = sequential (sepsis-related) organ failure assessment.

the mortality rates in low- and middle-income countries (LMICs) are still high, ranging from 30% to 70%.[8]

In the ED, clinicians are challenged to identify sepsis early in its course and to identify patients at risk of adverse events. Early identification is required to initiate a bundle of interventions associated with improved outcomes such as early antibiotics, source control, hemodynamically-based fluid resuscitation, and vasopressors.[9] The diagnosis of sepsis is often a challenging task for the emergency physician as it is largely a clinical diagnosis and lacks a gold standard diagnostic test.

Clinical question

Can clinical scoring systems identify patients with suspected infection in the ED who are at high risk of clinical deterioration?

The Sepsis-3 Task Force recommends the use of quick sequential (sepsis-related) organ failure assessment (qSOFA, Table 31.3) in the ED to identify among patients with suspected infection as those with a higher risk of poor outcomes.[2] They suggest the use of this score rather than the old SIRS-based criteria to further investigate for organ dysfunction and initiate or escalate therapy as appropriate for the clinical syndrome of sepsis. In their proposed algorithm, any patient with suspected infection and qSOFA ε 2 should undergo evaluation for evidence of organ dysfunction and, if they have a sequential (sepsis-related) organ failure assessment (SOFA) ε 2, they are considered septic[2,10] (Tables 31.3 and 31.4).

The qSOFA was derived and internally validated through a large retrospective U.S.-based cohort study including both encounters in- and outside of the intensive care unit (ICU).[10] The primary cohort included 148,907 encounters with suspected infection of whom 6347 (4%) died in the hospital. In the population outside of the ICU (i.e., ED and wards), there were 66,617 encounters in the derivation cohort and 66,522 in the validation cohort. Patients with suspected infection were defined as those who had body fluids sampled for culture and received antibiotics. The primary outcome was

Table 31.3 Quick SOFA (qSOFA)

Patients with suspected infection who are likely to have prolonged ICU stay or to die in the hospital can be identified at the beside with the presence of two or more of the following:
- Respiratory rate ε 22/min
- Altered mental status
- Systolic blood pressure δ 100 mmHg

Source: Data from [2].

Table 31.4 Sequential (sepsis-related) organ failure assessment (SOFA)

A SOFA score of two or more reflects an overall mortality risk of approximately 10% in a general hospital population with suspected infection

- **Respiration:** PaO_2/FiO_2 ε 400 mmHg (**0 points**), <400 (**1 point**), <300 (**2 points**), <200 with respiratory support (**3 points**), <100 with respiratory support (**4 points**)
- **Coagulation:** platelets ε $150 \times 10^3/\mu L$ (**0 points**), <150 (**1 point**), <100 (**2 points**), <50 (**3 points**), <20 (**4 points**)
- **Liver:** bilirubin <1.2 mg/dL (**0 points**), 1.2–1.9 (**1 point**), 2.0–5.9 (**2 point**), 6.0–11.9 (**3 points**), >12 (**4 points**)
- **Cardiovascular:** MAP ε 70 mmHg (**0 points**), MAP <70 (**1 point**), Dopamine <5 or dobutamine (any dose) (**2 points**), dopamine 5.1–15 or epinephrine δ 0.1 or norepinephrine δ 0.1 (**3 points**), dopamine >15 or epinephrine >0.1 or norepinephrine >0.1 (**4 points**)
- **Central nervous system:** GCS 15 (**0 points**), GCS 13–14 (**1 point**), GCS 10–12 (**2 points**), GCS 6–9 (**3 points**), GCS <6 (**4 points**)
- **Renal:** creatinine <1.2 mg/dL (**0 points**), 1.2–1.9 (**1 point**), 2.0–3.4 (**2 points**), 3.5–4.9 (**3 points**), >5 (**4 points**). Urine output <500 mL/day (**3 points**), <200 (**4 points**)

Source: Data from [2].

in-hospital mortality. In the derivation cohort, the area under the curve (AUC) for in-hospital mortality of qSOFA was 0.81 (confidence interval [CI] 0.80–0.82). In the validation cohort (n = 66,552 with suspected infection of whom 1886 [3%] died), qSOFA had the same AUC of 0.81 (95% CI 0.80–0.82), which was better than SOFA (AUC 0.79) and SIRS (AUC 0.76). The same authors explored the discrimination of qSOFA to predict in-hospital mortality in external datasets including four U.S.-based cohorts and one cohort from Germany. The AUCs of qSOFA ranged from 0.71 (95% CI 0.69–0.73) in a cohort of 6508 patients with community-acquired infections to 0.78 (95% CI 0.78–0.79) in a cohort of 377,325 patients with all types of suspected infections. Although the authors stated that the failure to meet the two or more qSOFA criteria should not delay the management deemed appropriate by providers, this tool became a screening tool to "rule out" sepsis in many EDs, especially in resource-limited settings where laboratory testing is often not readily available.[11]

After the publication of Sepsis-3, several external validation studies were carried out and the evidence was comprehensively analyzed by subsequent systematic reviews and meta-analyses. Fernando et al.[12] compared the prognostic accuracy of qSOFA and SIRS for mortality in patients with suspected infection. They included 19 ED-based cohorts including 61,894 patients and found a pooled sensitivity and specificity for qSOFA ε 2 of 46.7% (95% CI 38.3–55.2%) and 81.3% (95% CI 72.8–87.5%), respectively. Among

9 ED-based cohorts with 49,640, SIRS ε 2 had a higher sensitivity although lower specificity (sensitivity 83.6% [95% CI 75.9–89.1%], specificity 30.6% [95% CI 17.7–39.5%]). It is important to note that studies have used different definitions for the primary outcome such as in-hospital mortality, 28- or 30-day mortality. However, the summary estimates did not significantly change in subgroup and sensitivity analyses. Serafim et al.[13] compared qSOFA with SIRS for the diagnosis of sepsis. They included 10 studies with a total of 229,480 patients. The sensitivity of SIRS ε 2 for diagnosis of sepsis ranged from 39.5% to 88.3%, while the sensitivity of qSOFA ε 2 ranged from 10.2% to 54.4%. Song et al.[14], compared both tools for in-hospital mortality prediction and acute organ dysfunction. They included 23 studies with a total of 146,551 patients in their quantitative analysis. In the meta-analysis, qSOFA had AUCs for in-hospital mortality and acute organ dysfunction of 0.74 (95% CI 0.70–0.78) and 0.86 (95% CI 0.83–0.89), respectively; SIRS had an AUC of 0.71 (CI 0.67–0.75) for predicting in-hospital mortality and of 0.76 (95% CI 0.73–0.80) for predicting acute organ dysfunction. The sensitivities for both outcomes were significantly higher with SIRS (Table 31.5). Jiang et al.[15] included 8 studies with 52,849 patients in their systematic review. The pooled sensitivity for predicting mortality in infected ED patients was higher with SIRS (81% [95% CI 75–86%]) than with qSOFA (42% [95% CI 31–54%]). Tan et al.[16] included 35 studies that looked at short-term mortality outcomes among 269,544 patients presenting outside of the ICU. The pooled sensitivity and specificity of qSOFA were 48% and 86%, respectively. In 2019, Liu et al.[17] performed a systematic review and analyzed 17 ED-based studies with 71,331 patients. For studies that used in-hospital mortality as the primary outcome (13 studies, 27,978 patients), sensitivity of qSOFA was 61% (95% CI 50–71) and specificity was 70% (95% CI 59–82%). For studies that used 28- or 30-day mortality outcomes (4 studies, 11,954 patients), sensitivity of qSOFA was 32% (95% CI 15–49) and specificity was 92% (95% CI 85–99).

The lower sensitivity of the qSOFA across several external validation studies raises concerns regarding potential delays in sepsis identification and treatment. Prasad et al.[18] compared SIRS with qSOFA and SOFA with regards to their time to recognition of sepsis in a large retrospective study including 16,612 patients. SIRS resulted in earlier electronic health record sepsis identification in greater than 50% of patients.

In places where laboratory testing is often not available, providers might be tempted to use qSOFA as a "rule out" screening tool. However, this approach might lead to significant consequences. In a large observational study in Brazil including 4711 patients presenting outside the ICU with sepsis from 54 different hospitals,[11] the mortality rate for patients with qSOFA δ 1 was 17.3%. The authors suggested the use of a cutoff of one or more, which

Table 31.5 Main results of systematic reviews comparing qSOFA and SIRS

Score	AUC (95% CI)	Sensitivity (95% CI)	Specificity (95% CI)
Fernando et al.[12] **(19 ED-based studies for qSOFA and 9 ED-based studies for SIRS)**			
• Outcome of mortality (in-hospital or 28- or 30-day mortality)			
qSOFA	NR	46.7%	81.3%
		(38.3–55.2%)	(72.8–87.5%)
SIRS	NR	83.6%	30.6%
		(75.9–89.1%)	(17.7–39.5%)
Serafim et al.[13] **(10 all-settings studies)**			
• Outcome of diagnosis of sepsis			
qSOFA	NR	10.2–54.4%*	97.3%**
SIRS	NR	39.5–88.3%*	84.4%**
Serafim et al.[13] **(10 all-settings studies)**			
• Outcome of mortality (in-hospital or 28- or 30-day mortality)			
qSOFA	NR	22.8–90%	27.4–91.3%
SIRS	NR	19.9–97.4%	2.3–90.2%
Song et al.[14] **(23 studies outside of the ICU)**			
• Outcome of in-hospital mortality			
qSOFA	0.74 (0.70–0.78)	51% (39–62%)	83% (75–89%)
SIRS	0.71 (0.67–0.75)	86% (79–92%)	29% (17–45%)
Song et al.[14] **(23 studies outside of the ICU)**			
• Outcome of acute organ dysfunction			
qSOFA	0.86 (0.83–0.89)	47% (28–66%)	93% (88–97%)
SIRS	0.76 (0.73–0.80)	83% (71–91%)	49% (29–69%)
Jiang et al.[15] **(8 ED-based studies)**			
• Outcome of mortality (in-hospital or 30-day mortality)			
qSOFA	0.78 (0.74–0.81)	42% (31–54%)	88% (83–92%)
SIRS	0.70 (0.65–0.73)	81% (75–86%)	41% (32–50%)
Tan et al.[16] **(35 ED-based studies)**			
• Outcome of short-term mortality (in-hospital mortality or 30-day mortality)			
qSOFA	NR	48%	86%
Liu et al.[17] **(17 ED-based studies)**			
• Outcome of mortality (in-hospital or 28- or 30-day mortality)			
qSOFA	NR	54% (43–65%)	77% (66–86%)
Liu et al.[17] **(5 ED-based studies for qSOFA and 3 ED-based studies for SIRS)**			
• Outcome of sepsis diagnosis			
qSOFA	NR	54% (50–58%)	67% (65–68%)
SIRS	NR	72% (67–77%)	71% (69–73%)

AUC = area under the curve (receiver operating characteristic); NR = not reported; qSOFA ε 2 was used as a "positive qSOFA"; SIRS ε 2 was used as a "positive SIRS."
*Pooled sensitivity was not reported and these values represent the range of sensitivities reported by the studies included.
**Only one study reported specificity.

increased the sensitivity of qSOFA from 53.9% to 84.9%. Rudd *et al.*[19] also evaluated the qSOFA in LMICs and found an 8% mortality rate among those patients with a qSOFA δ 1.

When the performance of qSOFA for predicting in-hospital mortality was compared to unstructured emergency physician judgment, the latter had similar discrimination results (AUC 0.80 [95% CI 0.70–0.89] for emergency physician judgment versus AUC 0.60 [95% CI 0.53–0.73] for qSOFA). When the clinician gestalt was added to qSOFA, it did not improve its ability to predict mortality.[20]

Although originally developed to identify any hospitalized patient at risk of clinical deterioration,[21] the National Early Warning Score (NEWS) had recently been compared to SIRS and qSOFA to assess its ability to predict in-hospital mortality and ICU admission. The NEWS, similar to the qSOFA, involves only clinical variables that do not require laboratory testing. See Table 31.6 Churpek *et al.*[22] performed a large retrospective cohort study including 30,677 patients with suspected infection from the ED and wards, of whom 1649 (5%) died in the hospital. NEWS had an AUC of 0.77 (95% CI 0.76–0.79) for predicting in-hospital mortality, while qSOFA had an AUC of 0.69 (95% CI 0.67–0.70) and SIRS had an AUC of 0.65 (95% CI 0.63–0.66). Goulden *et al.*[23] performed a retrospective cohort study in the United Kingdom including admissions from the ED in whom sepsis was suspected and treated. Among 1818 patients included, 53 (3%) were admitted to the ICU and 265 (15%) died during hospitalization. The NEWS discrimination measures (AUC 0.65 [95% CI 0.61–0.68]) outperformed the qSOFA (AUC 0.62 [95% CI 0.59–0.66]) and SIRS (AUC 0.49 [95% CI 0.45–0.52]). Usman *et al.*[24] performed a retrospective cohort study including 115,734 ED patients.

Table 31.6 National Early Warning Score (NEWS)

A high score (NEWS ≥ 7) should prompt emergency assessment by a clinical team/ critical care outreach team with critical-care competencies and/or transfer the patient to a higher level of care area

- Respiratory rate (**0 points** if 12–20 rpm; **+1** if 9–11; **+2** if 21–24; **+3** if ≤8 or ≥25)
- Oxygen saturation (**0 points** if ≥96%; **+1** if 94–94%; **+2** if 92–93%; **+3** if ≤91%)
- Any supplemental oxygen (**0 points** if No; **+2** if Yes)
- Temperature (**0 points** if 36.1–38° C; **+1** if 35.1–36 or 38.1–39; **+2** if ≥39.1; **+3** if ≤35)
- Systolic blood pressure (**0 points** if 111–219 mmHg; **+1** if 101–110; **+2** if 91–100; **+3** if <90 or ≥220)
- Heart rate (**0 points** if 51–90; **+1** if 41–50 or 91–110; **+2** if 111–130; **+3** if ≤40 or ≥131)
- AVPU Score (**A**lert: **0 points**; Altered **V**oice, **P**ain, **U**nresponsive: **+3**)

Source: Data from [21].

They compared the ability of NEWS, qSOFA, and SIRS in early identification of sepsis in the ED. NEWS was more accurate than SIRS and qSOFA for the triage detection of sepsis/septic shock, septic shock alone, and sepsis-related mortality. The AUC of NEWS for triage detection of sepsis/septic shock was 0.91, which was better than SIRS (0.88) and qSOFA (0.81). The AUC of NEWS for diagnosis of septic shock was 0.93, which was superior to SIRS (0.88) and qSOFA (0.84). Finally, for sepsis-related mortality, NEWS had an AUC of 0.95, while SIRS had 0.85 and qSOFA 0.87.

In 2011, before the release of Sepsis-3, Calle et al.[25] conducted a systematic review of severity scores in ED patients with suspected infection. Although the literature was scant at that time, they found the Mortality in Emergency Department Sepsis (MEDS) score to be promising. The MEDS score was derived by Shapiro et al.[26] in a single-center study at a tertiary, academic ED in the United States to identify risk factors for mortality in ED patients with suspected infection. All adults older than 18 years for whom a blood culture was sent were eligible. Over 1 year, 3179 patient visits were included, 2070 were randomly assigned to the derivation group, and the other 1109 were assigned to the validation group. Patient characteristics including clinical and laboratory data, demographics, and terminal illness (defined as >50% likelihood of death within 30 days) were assessed retrospectively by medical record review. The outcome was 28-day in-hospital mortality. The association of predictive variables with mortality was assessed using multivariate logistic regression. In-hospital mortality was 5.3% in the derivation group and 5.7% in the validation group. Nine variables were independently associated with mortality and are part of the MEDS score (Table 31.7). The AUC for the derivation set was 0.82, and 0.76 in the validation set. Mortality increased with higher MEDS scores in the validation group.

Table 31.7 Mortality in Emergency Department Sepsis (MEDS) score

	Points
Rapidly terminal comorbid illness	6
Age >65 years	3
Bands >5%	3
Tachypnea or hypoxemia	3
Shock	3
Platelet count <150,000 mm^3	3
Altered mental status	2
Nursing home resident	2
Lower respiratory infection	2

Source: Data from [16].

Table 31.8 Mortality in Emergency Department Sepsis (MEDS) score mortality estimate

Clinical category	MEDS score range	28-day mortality rate (%)
Very low risk	0–4	0.4–11
Low risk	5–7	3–5
Moderate risk	8–12	7–19
High risk	13–15	16–32
Very high risk	>15	39–40

Source: Data from [27].

Several studies have subsequently studied the MEDS score. A detailed evidence-based review of the MEDS score was published by Carpenter *et al.* in 2009.[27] They summarized the mortality rates associated with different MEDS scores, which are shown in Table 31.8. Carpenter *et al.* concluded that increasing MEDS scores are associated with increasing mortality and that the score is accurate and reliable, except in patients with severe sepsis, where the scale may underestimate mortality. This is an example of spectrum bias (see Chapter 6), as the MEDS score performs better in populations of undifferentiated SIRS patients than in the sicker populations eligible for early goal-directed therapy. This is not surprising, as the MEDS score was derived in a cohort of ED patients getting blood cultures and admitted to the hospital, with an in-hospital mortality of approximately 5%.

Zhang *et al.*[28] performed a comprehensive systematic review and meta-analysis in 2019 to assess the MEDS score. They included 24 studies evaluating the MEDS score involving 21,246 ED patients with suspected infection. The pooled sensitivity and specificity of MEDS for predicting mortality were 79% (95% CI 72–84%) and 74% (95% CI 68–80%), respectively. The summarized AUC was 0.83 (95% CI 0.80–0.86). The authors found significant heterogeneity across the literature. After performing a meta-regression, they showed that the time at which the MEDS score was measured, and the cutoff values used, were important sources of heterogeneity. When they separated studies with outcomes of in-hospital mortality (5 studies) vs. 28- or 30-day mortality (19 studies), MEDS had better discriminatory ability using the 28- or 30-day mortality outcome (AUC 0.85 versus 0.73).

Clinical question

Which laboratory tests are useful in risk stratifying ED patients with sepsis?
Lactic acid, procalcitonin, and central venous oxygen saturation ($ScvO_2$) have been prospectively studied as prognostic tests in sepsis. During sepsis,

lactate production exceeds the rate of lactate removal, which leads to accumulation in venous blood. Multiple studies have identified an association between elevated serum lactate levels and mortality in critically ill ED patients, including those with sepsis, burns, and traumatic injuries. Initially elevated serum lactate (e.g., >2 mmol/L) is associated with poorer prognosis regardless of the presence of hypotension and shock.[29] The mechanism behind hyperlactatemia reflects organ dysfunction and the development of anaerobic metabolism.[30]

The evidence is robust with regards to serum lactate as a good biomarker in predicting sepsis severity.[31] It can be accurately measured either in a central lab or using a point-of-care test.[32] However, whether or not we should be pursuing lactate clearance as a resuscitation goal is controversial. Some studies, in particular the Rivers study of early goal-directed therapy, have recommended the use of $ScvO_2$ as a prognostic and diagnostic tool to judge adequacy of resuscitation.[9] As $ScvO_2$ requires invasive monitoring via a central line with a special probe, or repeated analysis from central blood specimens, it is important to know if it adds value above routine lactate testing.

In a comprehensive systematic review, Vincent et al.[31] found 97 studies that evaluated the role of lactate kinetics across different populations of critically ill patients (not only sepsis). They found that a decrease in lactate levels over time was consistently associated with lower mortality rates in all subgroups of patients; however, summary estimates were not reported. In 2015, Gu et al.[33] included four randomized controlled trials (RCTs) in a meta-analysis to evaluate the effect of early lactate clearance-guided therapy in septic patients. Lactate clearance was compared with the $ScvO_2$-guided therapy, and it was associated with a reduction in mortality (relative rate [RR] 0.65 [95% CI 0.49–0.85]). The quality of evidence was deemed to be moderate. In a more recent systematic review and meta-analysis published in 2019,[34] Pan et al. included seven RCTs comparing lactate clearance-guided therapy vs. $ScvO_2$-guided therapy. In the meta-analysis, the authors report a significant reduction of in-hospital mortality with the lactate-clearance approach (RR 0.68 [95% CI 0.56–0.82], no significant heterogeneity [$I^2 = 0\%$]).

In contrast, Hernández et al.[35] conducted a multicenter RCT at 28 ICUs in five countries including 424 septic shock patients. Patients were randomized to a step-by-step resuscitation protocol aimed at either normalizing capillary refill time ($n = 212$) or normalizing or decreasing lactate levels at rates greater than 20% per 2 hours ($n = 212$), during an 8-hour intervention period. Lactate level was assessed every 2 hours, while capillary refill time was evaluated every 30 minutes until normalization and then every hour during the intervention period. There was no difference in 28-day mortality between groups (HR 0.75 [95% CI 0.55–1.02]), but peripheral perfusion-targeted resuscitation was associated with less organ dysfunction at 72 hours (mean difference of SOFA score −1 [95% CI −1.97 to −0.02]). Also, the lactate-guided strategy led to a higher volume of fluids administered, more vasopressor use, and more frequent use of epinephrine. However, this "overtreatment" did not translate into better clinical outcomes. Although this trial showed that capillary refill time-guided therapy is at least as good as lactate-guided resuscitation, the former requires significant physicians' time for frequent capillary refill checks, which may not be feasible in a busy ED.

Procalcitonin is a peptide precursor of the hormone calcitonin, which is involved with calcium homeostasis. In healthy individuals, the level of procalcitonin is below the limit of detection of clinical assays (10 pg/mL), but it rises in response to proinflammatory stimuli, for example bacterial infection. Some studies have reported that procalcitonin levels are a reliable method of diagnosing severe bacterial infection and sepsis. Two systematic reviews of procalcitonin were published in 2007. Tang et al.[36] assessed accuracy of procalcitonin for sepsis diagnosis in critically ill patients and included 18 studies. Pooled sensitivity and specificity were both 71% (95% CI 67–76%) with an AUC of 0.78 (95% CI 0.73–0.83). Jones et al.[37] evaluated the diagnostic performance of procalcitonin for the diagnosis of bacteremia in the ED population. They identified prospective studies that assessed the diagnostic accuracy of procalcitonin for bacteremia, with blood culture as the criterion standard, and included adults and children with suspected infection in the ED or at admission. They calculated unweighted summary AUC and random-effects pooled sensitivity and specificity. Seventeen studies including 2008 patients met the inclusion criteria. There was a substantial degree of inconsistency between studies. As different studies used different test thresholds, they analyzed the subgroup of studies that used a test threshold of 0.5 or 0.4 ng/mL and calculated pooled estimates for the sensitivity of 76% (95% CI 66–84%) and specificity of 70% (95% CI 60–79%). The unweighted summary AUC was 0.84 (95% CI 0.75–0.90). The authors of both systematic reviews concluded that procalcitonin cannot reliably differentiate sepsis from other noninfectious causes of SIRS in critically ill adult patients and suggested further testing in ambulatory populations.

Several recent studies have examined procalcitonin as a diagnostic test for infection in the ED. Riedel et al.[38] studied procalcitonin as a marker for the detection of bacteremia and sepsis in adults admitted to a single urban ED with symptoms of systemic infection. They enrolled 367 patients and analyzed data on the 295 patients in whom a serum sample was obtained at the same time as blood cultures, allowing analysis of procalcitonin. Procalcitonin levels were compared with blood culture results and other clinical data obtained during the ED visit – positive cultures were classified as representing real disease or contaminants according to accepted protocols. Using a predefined procalcitonin test threshold of 0.1 ng/mL led to a sensitivity of 75% and a specificity of 71% for clinically significant bacteremia. Lai et al.[39] prospectively examined 370 adult ED patients with fever and suspected bacterial infection in one urban ED. Bacterial infection was confirmed in 72% of patients; pneumonia was the most common infection (31%) followed by bacteremia (26%), urinary tract infection (27%), intra-abdominal infection (19%), skin and soft tissue infection (15%), and others (2%). The AUC for identification of bacteremia by procalcitonin was 0.76 (95% CI 0.70–0.81). Using a retrospectively derived cutoff level of 0.47 ng/mL, the sensitivity and specificity of procalcitonin for diagnosing bacteremia in patients with fever at admission to the ED were 75% and 70%, respectively. While the authors of both studies concluded that procalcitonin is useful in the diagnosis of bacterial infection in ED patients with symptoms of systemic infection, we think this oversimplifies the issue. In a recent systematic review, Hoeboer et al.[40] evaluated the diagnostic accuracy of procalcitonin for bacteremia including 58 studies. The pooled AUC was 0.79, and the optimal and most widely used procalcitonin cutoff value was 0.5 ng/mL with a corresponding sensitivity of 76% and specificity of 69%.

Liu et al.[41] performed a systematic review and meta-analysis to evaluate the diagnostic accuracy of a single procalcitonin concentration and procalcitonin nonclearance in predicting all-cause sepsis mortality. In a meta-analysis of 16 studies including 3126 patients, an elevated procalcitonin level was associated with higher mortality (RR 2.60 [95% CI 2.05–3.30]). They found, however, that initial procalcitonin measures were of limited prognostic value. The lack of clearance of procalcitonin was also found to be associated with increased mortality in nine studies (RR 3.05 [95% CI 2.35–3.95]), most in the ICU setting. The optimal cutoff and definition of nonclearance were also not well established. Wu et al.[42] performed a systematic review to compare different biomarkers to diagnose sepsis and found six studies with a total of 1822 patients evaluating procalcitonin in the ED. In their meta-analysis, they found a summarized AUC of 0.88 (95% CI 0.85–0.90) for diagnosing sepsis. When procalcitonin was compared to C-reactive protein for the diagnosis of sepsis in a different meta-analysis of nine studies, Tan et al.[43] found that procalcitonin had better discriminatory ability (AUC 0.85 [95% CI 0.82–0.88]) than C-reactive protein (AUC 0.73 [95% CI 0.69–0.77]). It is important to note that the cutoff values of both biomarkers varied significantly across studies.

As the sensitivity and specificity of procalcitonin are below 80%, it is not accurate enough to either rule in or rule out bacterial infection. It may be reasonable for clinicians to use procalcitonin to identify patients at higher risk and prioritize such patients for interventions, such as early, broad-spectrum antibiotics, but such algorithms need to be studied independently.

Comments

Identifying patients at risk from sepsis and prognosticating short-term mortality are clinically important as they can help determine who should receive early aggressive therapies, disposition to ICUs, and guidance to family and other caregivers.

Although the use of qSOFA as a bedside tool for predicting poor outcomes is recommended by the Sepsis-3 Task Force, one should not use it as a "rule out" screening tool given its low sensitivity across several external validation studies. When compared with SIRS, the qSOFA has better discrimination ability (i.e., higher AUCs). One should use clinical judgment combined with scoring systems and biomarkers rather than adopting an approach based only on one tool.

The UK-based NEWS score seems promising to be used as an early tool in the ED to predict clinical deterioration in septic patients, however further prospective validation is needed.

The MEDS score has been derived and multiply validated in ED populations and can be used to identify which ED patients being admitted with infection are at risk of in-hospital mortality. Clinicians should be aware that the MEDS may underestimate the likelihood of mortality in severely ill patients, such as those with septic shock.

Many biomarkers have been evaluated to predict severity of sepsis, organ dysfunction, and mortality. Serum lactate either calculated in a central lab or using a point-of-care test is an accurate single biomarker in predicting sepsis severity. However, lactate clearance-guided therapy remains controversial, and less invasive strategies such as peripheral perfusion-guided resuscitation seems to perform just as well with avoidance of "overtreatment." Procalcitonin has promising discriminative ability but the ideal cutoff value, as well as measurement time, are yet to be determined in the sepsis population. At this point, procalcitonin and other biomarkers do not have a clear additive benefit to serum lactate and we do not recommend their routine use in the emergent care of septic patients.

References

1. Deutschman CS, Tracey KJ. Sepsis: Current dogma and new perspectives. *Immunity*. 2014; 40(4): 463–75. doi: 10.1016/j.immuni.2014.04.001.
2. Singer M, Deutschman CS, Seymour C *et al*. The third international consensus definitions for sepsis and septic shock (sepsis-3). *JAMA: The Journal of the American Medical Associatio*. 2016; 315(8): 801–10. doi: 10.1001/jama.2016.0287.

3. Bone RC, Balk RA, Cerra FB *et al*. Definitions for sepsis and organ failure and guidelines for the use of innovative therapies in sepsis. *Chest*. 1992; 101: 1644–55. doi: 10.1378/chest.101.6.1644.

4. Levy MM, Fink MP, Marshall JC *et al*. SCCM/ESICM/ACCP/ATS/SIS International Sepsis Definitions Conference. *Critical Care Medicine*. 2001, 2003; 31: 1250–6. doi: 10.1097/01.CCM.0000050454.01978.3B.

5. Shankar-Hari M, Phillips GS, Levy ML *et al*. Developing a new definition and assessing new clinical criteria for septic shock: For the third international consensus definitions for sepsis and septic shock (sepsis-3). *JAMA: The Journal of the American Medical Association*. 2016; 315(8): 775–87. doi: 10.1001/jama.2016.0289.

6. Wang HE, Jones AR, Donnelly JP. Revised National Estimates of Emergency Department visits for sepsis in the United States. *Critical Care Medicine*. 2017; 45(9): 1443–9. doi: 10.1097/CCM.0000000000002538.

7. Fleischmann C, Scherag A, Adhikari NKJ *et al*. Assessment of global incidence and mortality of hospital-treated sepsis current estimates and limitations. *American Journal of Respiratory and Critical Care Medicine*. 2016; 193(3): 259–72. doi: 10.1164/rccm.201504-0781OC.

8. Machado FR, Azevedo LCP. Sepsis: A threat that needs a global solution. *Critical Care Medicine*. 2018; 46(3): 454–9. doi: 10.1097/CCM.0000000000002899.

9. Rivers E, Nguyen B, Havstad S *et al*. Early goal-directed therapy in the treatment of severe sepsis and septic shock. *The New England Journal of Medicine*. 2001; 345(19): 1368–77. doi: 10.1056/NEJMoa010307.

10. Seymour CW, Liu VX, Iwashyna TJ *et al*. Assessment of clinical criteria for sepsis for the third international consensus definitions for sepsis and septic shock (sepsis-3). *JAMA: The Journal of the American Medical Association*. 2016; 315(8): 762–74. doi: 10.1001/jama.2016.0288.

11. Machado FR, Cavalcanti AB, Monteiro MB *et al*. Predictive accuracy of the quick sepsis-related organ failure assessment score in Brazil: A prospective multicenter study. *American Journal of Respiratory and Critical Care Medicine*. 2020; 20: 789–98. doi: 10.1164/rccm.201905-0917OC.

12. Fernando SM, Tran A, Taljaard M *et al*. Prognostic accuracy of the quick sequential organ failure assessment for mortality in patients with suspected infection, a systematic review and meta-analysis. *Annals of Internal Medicine*. 2018; 168(4): 266–75. doi: 10.7326/M17-2820.

13. Serafim R, Gomes JA, Salluh J, Póvoa P. A comparison of the quick-SOFA and systemic inflammatory response syndrome criteria for the diagnosis of sepsis and prediction of mortality: A systematic review and meta-analysis. *Chest*. 2018; 153(3): 646–55. doi: 10.1016/j.chest.2017.12.015.

14. Song JU, Sin CK, Park HK, Shim SR, Lee J. Performance of the quick sequential (sepsis-related) organ failure assessment score as a prognostic tool in infected patients outside the intensive care unit: A systematic review and meta-analysis. *Critical Care*. 2018; 22(1): 28. doi: 10.1186/s13054-018-1952-x.

15. Jiang J, Yang J, Mei J, Jin Y, Lu Y. Head-to-head comparison of qSOFA and SIRS criteria in predicting the mortality of infected patients in the emergency department: A meta-analysis. *Scandinavian Journal of Trauma, Resuscitation and Emergency Medicine*. 2018; 26(1): 56. doi: 10.1186/s13049-018-0527-9.

16. Tan TL, Tang YJ, Ching LJ, Abdullah N, Neoh HM. Comparison of prognostic accuracy of the quick sepsis-related organ failure assessment between short- & long-term mortality in patients presenting outside of the intensive care unit – a systematic review & meta-analysis. *Scientific Reports.* 2018; 8(1): 16698. doi: 10.1038/s41598-018-35144-6.

17. Liu YC, Luo YY, Zhang X *et al.* Quick sequential organ failure assessment as a prognostic factor for infected patients outside the intensive care unit: A systematic review and meta-analysis. *Internal and Emergency Medicine.* 2019; 14(4): 603–15. doi: 10.1007/s11739-019-02036-0.

18. Prasad PA, Fang MC, Abe-Jones Y, Calfee CS, Matthay MA, Kangelaris KN. Time to recognition of sepsis in the emergency department using electronic health record data: A comparative analysis of systemic inflammatory response syndrome, sequential organ failure assessment, and quick sequential organ failure assessment. *Critical Care Medicine.* 2020; 48(2): 200–9. doi: 10.1097/CCM.0000000000004132.

19. Rudd KE, Seymour CW, Aluisio AR *et al.* Association of the quick sequential (sepsis-related) organ failure assessment (qSOFA) score with excess hospital mortality in adults with suspected infection in low- and middle-income countries. *JAMA: The Journal of the American Medical Association.* 2018; 319(21): 2202–11. doi: 10.1001/jama.2018.6229.

20. Cleek WR, Johnson NJ, Watsjold BK, Hall MK, Henning DJ. Comparing mortality prediction by quick sequential organ failure assessment with emergency physician judgment. *Shock.* 2020; 54(2): 213–7. doi: 10.1097/shk.0000000000001496.

21. Smith GB, Prytherch DR, Meredith P, Schmidt PE, Featherstone PI. The ability of the National Early Warning Score (NEWS) to discriminate patients at risk of early cardiac arrest, unanticipated intensive care unit admission, and death. *Resuscitation.* 2013; 84(4): 465–70. doi: 10.1016/j.resuscitation.2012.12.016.

22. Churpek MM, Snyder A, Han X *et al.* Quick sepsis-related organ failure assessment, systemic inflammatory response syndrome, and early warning scores for detecting clinical deterioration in infected patients outside the intensive care unit. *American Journal of Respiratory and Critical Care Medicine.* 2017; 195(7): 906–11. doi: 10.1164/rccm.201604-0854OC.

23. Goulden R, Hoyle M-C, Monis J *et al.* qSOFA, SIRS and NEWS for predicting in hospital mortality and ICU admission in emergency admissions treated as sepsis. *Emergency Medicine Journal.* 2018; 35(6): 345–9. doi: 10.1136/emermed-2017-207120.

24. Usman OA, Usman AA, Ward MA. Comparison of SIRS, qSOFA, and NEWS for the early identification of sepsis in the emergency department. *The American Journal of Emergency Medicine.* 2019; 37(8): 1490–7. doi: 10.1016/j.ajem.2018.10.058.

25. Calle P, Cerro L, Valencia J, Jaimes F. Usefulness of severity scores in patients with suspected infection in the emergency department: A systematic review. *The Journal of Emergency Medicine.* 2012; 42(4): 379–91. doi: 10.1016/j.jemermed.2011.03.033.

26. Shapiro NI, Wolfe RE, Moore RB, Smith E, Burdick E, Bates DW. Mortality in emergency department sepsis (MEDS) score: a prospectively derived and validated clinical prediction rule. *Critical Care Medicine.* 2003; 31(3): 670–5. doi: 10.1097/01.CCM.0000054867.01688.D1.

27. Carpenter CR, Keim SM, Upadhye S, Nguyen HB, Best Evidence in Emergency Medicine Investigator Group. Risk stratification of the potentially septic patient in the emergency department: The mortality in the emergency department sepsis (MEDS) score. *The Journal of Emergency Medicine*. 2009; 37(3): 319–27. doi: 10.1016/j.jemermed.2009.03.016.

28. Zhang G, Zhang K, Zheng X, Cui W, Hong Y, Zhang Z. Performance of the MEDS score in predicting mortality among emergency department patients with a suspected infection: A meta-analysis. *Emergency Medicine Journal*. 2020; 37: 232–9. doi: 10.1136/emermed-2019-208901.

29. Mikkelsen ME, Miltiades AN, Gaieski DF *et al*. Serum lactate is associated with mortality in severe sepsis independent of organ failure and shock. *Critical Care Medicine*. 2009; 37(5): 1670–7. doi: 10.1097/CCM.0b013e31819fcf68.

30. Kraut JA, Madias NE. Lactic acidosis. *The New England Journal of Medicine*. 2014; 371(24): 2309–19. doi: 10.1056/NEJMra1309483.

31. Vincent JL, e Silva AQ, Couto L, Taccone FS. The value of blood lactate kinetics in critically ill patients: A systematic review. *Critical Care*. 2016; 20(1). doi: 10.1186/S13054-016-1403-5.

32. Shapiro NI, Fisher C, Donnino M *et al*. The feasibility and accuracy of point-of-care lactate measurement in emergency department patients with suspected infection. *The Journal of Emergency Medicine*. 2010; 39(1): 89–94. doi: 10.1016/j.jemermed.2009.07.021.

33. Gu WJ, Zhang Z, Bakker J. Early lactate clearance-guided therapy in patients with sepsis: A meta-analysis with trial sequential analysis of randomized controlled trials. *Intensive Care Medicine*. 2015; 41(10): 1862–3. doi: 10.1007/s00134-015-3955-2.

34. Pan J, Peng M, Liao C, Hu X, Wang A, Li X. Relative efficacy and safety of early lactate clearance-guided therapy resuscitation in patients with sepsis: A meta-analysis. *Medicine (Baltimore)*. 2019; 98(8): e14453. doi: 10.1097/MD.0000000000014453.

35. Hernández G, Ospina-Tascón GA, Damiani LP *et al*. Effect of a resuscitation strategy targeting peripheral perfusion status vs serum lactate levels on 28-day mortality among patients with septic shock: The ANDROMEDA-SHOCK randomized clinical trial. *JAMA: The Journal of the American Medical Association*. 2019; 321: 654–64. doi: 10.1001/jama.2019.0071.

36. Tang BM, Eslick GD, Craig JC, McLean AS. Accuracy of procalcitonin for sepsis diagnosis in critically ill patients: Systematic review and meta-analysis. *The Lancet Infectious Diseases*. 2007; 7(3): 210–7. doi: 10.1016/S1473-3099(07)70052-X.

37. Jones AE, Fiechtl JF, Brown MD, Ballew JJ, Kline JA. Procalcitonin test in the diagnosis of bacteremia: A meta-analysis. *Annals of Emergency Medicine*. 2007; 50(1): 34–41. doi: 10.1016/j.annemergmed.2006.10.020.

38. Riedel S, Melendez JH, An AT, Rosenbaum JE, Zenilman JM. Procalcitonin as a marker for the detection of bacteremia and sepsis in the emergency department. *American Journal of Clinical Pathology*. 2011; 135(2): 182–9. doi: 10.1309/AJCP1MFYINQLECV2.

39. Lai CC, Tan CK, Chen SY *et al*. Diagnostic performance of procalcitonin for bacteremia in patients with bacterial infection at the emergency department. *The Journal of Infection*. 2010; 61(6): 512–5. doi: 10.1016/j.jinf.2010.10.005.

40. Hoeboer SH, van der Geest PJ, Nieboer D, Groeneveld ABJ. The diagnostic accuracy of procalcitonin for bacteraemia: A systematic review and meta-analysis. *Clinical Microbiology and Infection.* 2015; 21(5): 474–81. doi: 10.1016/j. cmi.2014.12.026.

41. Liu D, Su L, Han G, Yan P, Xie L. Prognostic value of procalcitonin in adult patients with sepsis: A systematic review and meta-analysis. *PLoS One.* 2015; 10(6): e0129450. doi: 10.1371/journal.pone.0129450.

42. Wu CC, Lan HM, Han ST *et al.* Comparison of diagnostic accuracy in sepsis between presepsin, procalcitonin, and C-reactive protein: A systematic review and meta-analysis. *Annals of Intensive Care.* 2017; 7(1): 91. doi: 10.1186/ s13613-017-0316-z.

43. Tan M, Lu Y, Jiang H, Zhang L. The diagnostic accuracy of procalcitonin and C-reactive protein for sepsis: A systematic review and meta-analysis. *Journal of Cellular Biochemistry.* 2019; 120(4): 5852–9. doi: 10.1002/jcb.27870.

Chapter 32 **Adult Septic Arthritis**

Ian T. Ferguson and Christopher R. Carpenter

Department of Emergency Medicine, Washington University School of Medicine, St. Louis, MO, USA

Highlights

- The accuracy of history, physical exam, and labs differ for gonococcal and nongonococcal septic arthritis.
- Similarly, native joint septic arthritis exhibits different patient demographics, serum, and synovial features than prosthetic joint septic arthritis.
- For the diagnosis of a nongonococcal septic joint, the most useful findings on history and physical exam are cellulitis overlying a prosthetic joint (LR+ 15) and recent (<3 months) joint surgery (LR+ 7).
- Peripheral WBC does not accurately distinguish nongonococcal native joint septic arthritis from other etiologies of monoarticular arthritis, but procalcitonin may rule in septic arthritis.
- Synovial white blood cell counts >100,000 (LR+ 28) or >50,000 (LR+ 8) and Gram stain (LR+ 21) are the most useful tests to rule in the diagnosis of nongonococcal native joint septic arthritis.

Background

Acute monoarticular arthritis presenting to the emergency department (ED) can be due to a number of etiologies as summarized in Table 32.1.[1] Septic (bacterial) arthritis has an annual incidence of 10 per 100,000 individuals but is more common among those with rheumatoid arthritis or a prosthetic joint (up to 70 cases per 100,000).[2,3] Among patients in whom clinically concerning monoarticular arthritis is evaluated, the prevalence of

---

Evidence-Based Emergency Care: Diagnostic Testing and Clinical Decision Rules, Third Edition.
Edited by Jesse M. Pines, Fernanda Bellolio, Christopher R. Carpenter, and Ali S. Raja.
© 2023 John Wiley & Sons Ltd. Published 2023 by John Wiley & Sons Ltd.

Table 32.1 Differential diagnosis of monoarticular arthritis

Infection (bacterial, fungal, mycobacterial, viral, and spirochete)
Rheumatoid arthritis
Gout/pseudogout
Lupus
Lyme disease
Sickle cell disease
Dialysis-related amyloidosis
Transient synovitis
Plant thorn synovitis
Metastatic carcinoma
Hemarthrosis
Pigmented villonodular synovitis
Neuropathic arthropathy
Intra-articular injury

Source: Data from [1].

septic arthritis across ED studies ranges from 7% to 27%.[4,5] Septic arthritis most commonly affects the knees, which account for 50% of cases. In decreasing order of frequency, septic arthritis also occurs in the hip, shoulder, and elbow. However, any articular surface can become infected.[6] Most cases result from hematogenous spread since bacterial organisms can easily enter the synovial fluid through synovial tissue, which lacks a basement membrane. Although native joint surgery for septic arthritis need not occur emergently, prompt diagnosis, and appropriate antibiotic management are essential in the ED since cartilage can be destroyed within days and the in-hospital mortality of treated infections can reach 15%.[7,8] The incidence of prosthetic joint infections is increasing.[9] Important differences exist in the diagnosis and management of native joint versus prosthetic joint septic arthritis (Table 32.2).[10,11]

Staphylococcal and streptococcal species produce 70% of nongonococcal (GC) septic arthritis cases. These Gram-positive species are isolated in both blood and synovial fluid in only 48% of cases.[6,12] Methicillin-resistant *Staphylococcus aureus* septic arthritis is being increasingly reported, particularly in older adults and in those with intravenous drug abuse.[13–15] Gram-negative septic arthritis more often involves the knee with pseudomonas species and *Escherichia coli* the most common organisms.[16] Patients with human immunodeficiency virus (HIV) are not at increased risk for septic arthritis.[17] Less common causes of septic arthritis include mycobacterium tuberculosis, brucella from unvaccinated livestock or unpasteurized milk, penetrating injuries from thorny plants, and Whipple disease.[18]

Table 32.2 Differences between native joint and prosthetic joint septic arthritis

Risk factor	Septic arthritis	Prosthetic joint infection
Incidence (%)	0.006–0.010	1–3
Common age (years)	<3 and >55	>65
Synovial WBC cutoff	>50,000 cells/μL	Acute >10,000 cells/μL Chronic >3,000 cells/μL
Management recommendation	Needle lavage, arthroscopic lavage, or open arthrotomy lavage	Open surgical debridement or implant removal and 1- or 2-stage reimplantation
Antibiotic duration	6 weeks	Up to 3 months

Source: Data from [10].

Table 32.3 Risk factors for gonococcal arthritis

Female
Pregnancy
Menses
Multiple sexual partners
Low socioeconomic status
Intravenous drug abuse
Mucosal infection (asymptomatic)
HIV
Lupus
Complement deficiencies
Gonococcal organism factors

Source: Data from [19].

With an annual incidence of 3 per 100,000, GC arthritis is a less common cause of septic arthritis in the United States. Unlike non-GC septic arthritis, GC joint infections respond rapidly to appropriate antimicrobial management. GC septic arthritis is frequently accompanied by a tenosynovitis and, in the absence of pelvic symptoms, can be difficult to distinguish from non-GC septic arthritis. GC septic arthritis is more common in younger adults, with a 4:1 female-to-male predominance. Risk factors for GC arthritis are listed in Table 32.3. Gram stain (<50%), blood (<50%), and synovial cultures (~50%) are less often positive in GC septic arthritis, but genitourinary specimens will be positive in up about 90% of cases.[19]

Table 32.4 Historical risk factors for nongonococcal septic arthritis

Risk factor	Positive likelihood ratio	Negative likelihood ratio
Age > 80 years	3.5 (1.7–6.4)	0.86 (0.70–0.96)
Diabetes mellitus	2.7 (1.1–6.2)	0.93 (0.79–1.0)
Rheumatoid arthritis	2.5 (1.9–2.9)	0.45 (0.27–0.67)
Recent joint surgery	6.9 (3.7–11.6)	0.78 (0.63–0.90)
Prior same joint surgery	2.3 (1.0–5.1)	0.55 (0.18–1.6)
Prior septic arthritis	0 (0–5.9)	1.1 (0.55–1.4)
Hip or knee prosthesis	3.1 (1.9–4.5)	0.73 (0.55–0.88)
Skin infection	2.8 (1.7–4.2)	0.76 (0.58–0.91)
Prosthesis *and* skin infection	15.0 (8.0–26)	0.77 (0.62–0.88)
HIV infection	1.7 (0.76–1.5)	0.64 (0.23–1.37)

Source: Data from [5].

Clinical question

Can history or physical exam accurately and reliably distinguish non-GC septic arthritis from other causes of monoarticular symptoms?

History and physical exam alone are inadequate to rule in or rule out septic arthritis.[5] The prevalence of non-GC septic arthritis in ED patients with concerning monoarticular symptoms ranges from 7% to 27%.[4,20,21] Table 32.4 summarizes septic arthritis risk factors from the medical history, along with estimates of their diagnostic accuracy.[1,3,5] Notably, none of these findings, when absent, significantly reduced the probability of septic arthritis. A single-center prospective study found chills to have the highest LR+ among all clinical features evaluated (2.2, CI 1.2–7.3) although given a pretest probability of 27%, this would only change the posttest probability to 45%.[21] Objective fever has a reported LR+/LR− of 1.13/0.88 in one study and 0.67/1.7 in another, making it unhelpful to rule in or out the diagnosis of septic arthritis.[21,22]

Table 32.5 summarizes physical exam accuracy from one small single-center prospective study.[4] Global clinician intuition prior to lab testing most accurately rules-in septic arthritis, but the confidence intervals from this study are too wide to be convincing. Interrater reliability for physical exam findings was good for erythema ($\kappa = 0.83$), fair for palpation pain ($\kappa = 0.41$), and poor for palpable effusion ($\kappa = 0$).[4,23]

Clinical question

Can serum labs accurately and reliably distinguish septic arthritis from other causes of monoarticular symptoms?

White blood cell (WBC) over 10,000 cells is not useful acutely in ruling in or ruling out the diagnosis of septic arthritis (Table 32.6).[5] On the other hand,

Table 32.5 Physical exam accuracy for nongonococcal septic arthritis

Risk factor	Positive likelihood ratio	Negative likelihood ratio
Clinician gestalt		
>20% likelihood	3 (2–4)	0
>50% likelihood	6.6 (2–19)	0.44 (0.15–1.3)
>80% likelihood	2.6 (0.38–18.5)	0.87 (0.56–1.3)
Joint erythema	1.7 (0.77–3.7)	0.62 (0.21–1.8)
Joint pain with movement	1.0 (0.58–1.1)	0 (0–15)
Joint pain at rest	0.68 (0.33–1.4)	3.2 (0.93–11.4)
Joint pain with palpation	1.0 (0.38–1.1)	0 (0–17)
Joint swelling	1.0 (0.99–1.04)	0 (0–222)

Source: Data from [4].

Table 32.6 Serum inflammatory markers for nongonococcal septic arthritis

Serum marker	Positive likelihood ratio	Negative likelihood ratio
WBC>10,000/mm^3	1.1–1.7	0.28–0.84
ESR>30mm/hour	1.3–3.5	0.17–0.60
CRP>100mg/L	1.6–4.5	0–0.70
Procalcitonin>0.3ng/mL	5–infinity	0.30–0.80

Source: Adapted from [4, 5].

some studies demonstrate a role for erythrocyte sedimentation rate (ESR) and C-reactive protein (CRP) in adults with monoarticular arthritis. Li et al.[24,25] assessed only cases of confirmed septic arthritis and demonstrated a sensitivity of 96% for ESR>30mm/hour. Given the possibility of selection bias, this sensitivity may be falsely elevated. In contrast, Li et al.[26] demonstrated a ESR sensitivity of 75% and a specificity of 11% using the same definition of abnormal and Carpenter et al.[4] demonstrated a sensitivity of 75% with specificity of 78% for ESR>49mm/hour. Hariharan[27] only assessed confirmed septic arthritis cases and, using a threshold of ESR>10mm/hour and CRP≥20mg/L, noted sensitivities of 98% and 92%, respectively. Using ESR>15mm/hour and CRP>0.8mg/L, Ernst et al.[28] demonstrated sensitivities of 66% and 90%, respectively. A meta-analysis by Shen et al. demonstrated summary LR+ 5 (CI 2–11) for procalcitonin with LR− 0.40 (CI 0.16–1.0), while a meta-analysis by Zhao quantified LR+ 11 (CI 5–26) and LR− 0.49 (CI 0.38–0.62).[29,30] These likelihood ratios imply a role for procalcitonin to rule in the diagnosis of septic arthritis.

A handful of serum tests remain experimental and unavailable, such as CD64.[31] In addition, novel serum inflammatory markers such as Alpha-defensin and IL-6 are being explored to diagnose peri-prosthetic joint infections.[32,33]

Clinical question

Can synovial labs accurately and reliably distinguish septic arthritis from other causes of monoarticular symptoms?

An ED meta-analysis in 2011 identified no studies evaluating likelihood ratios for synovial Gram stain.[5] More recently, rheumatology research indicated that Gram stain does not accurately rule in or rule out non-GC septic arthritis,[18] whereas ED research implies otherwise with ranges of LR+ 32 to infinity and LR– 0–0.6.[4,21]

For native joint infections, the synovial WBC count (sWBC) >50,000 cells/mm^3 optimizes LR+ and LR–, but approximately 30–50% of patients with septic arthritis will have WBC levels under the 50,000 threshold.[18] The interval likelihood ratio (iLR, see Chapter 3) for sWBC: for the range of 0–25,000 cells/mm^3, the iLR is 0.33; for the range of 25,000–50,000 cells/mm^3, the iLR is 1.06; for the range of 50,000–100,000 cells/mm^3, the iLR is 3.59; and for the sWBC >100,000 cells/mm^3, the iLR is infinity.[5] Research to quantify the diagnostic accuracy of synovial WBC in immunocompromised patients is nonexistent and as previously noted prosthetic joint infections demonstrate lower thresholds.[5] Although synovial fluid should be evaluated for uric acid or calcium pyrophosphate crystals (diagnostic of crystalloid arthropathies) septic arthritis can coexist with gout or pseudogout in 1.5% of cases.[34] In one cohort, microcrystals identified in the synovial fluid did not decrease the probability of septic arthritis in multivariate regression models because 24% of the patients with septic arthritis had synovial microcrystals.[21]

Older research suggested that synovial lactate offered a promising approach to rule in or rule out septic arthritis.[5,35-38] These early studies generally neglected to report whether D-lactate or L-lactate was evaluated. Some recent ED research demonstrates much less impressive synovial fluid accuracy for L-lactate[4,39] and no detectable D-lactate.[4] However, other research suggests synovial L-lactate accurately rules-in septic arthritis.[40] Other synovial fluids labs including glucose, protein, lactate dehydrogenase (LDH), and tumor necrosis factor-alpha (TNFα)[20,22,41-43] are not helpful, generally unavailable, or remain unproven in the diagnosis of septic arthritis (Table 32.7).[5] Novel synovial fluid tests under investigation include interleukin-6,[40] leukocyte esterase,[44] acridine orange staining,[45] and mid-infrared spectroscopy.[46]

To date, no clinical decision instruments exist to assist clinicians' risk stratification of adult patients for septic arthritis[5] and physician gestalt alone is likely inadequate to accurately determine patients most likely to benefit from synovial fluid testing.[4] Arthrocentesis is painful and not risk-free but can be safely performed even in patients with therapeutic warfarin anticoagulation with a risk of clinically significant hemorrhage below 10%.[47] Based

Table 32.7 Synovial fluid tests for nongonococcal septic arthritis

Test	Positive likelihood ratio	Negative likelihood ratio
sWBC > 100,000 cell/mL	4.7–42.0	0.61–0.84
sWBC > 50,000	2.2–19.0	0.33–0.57
sWBC > 36,000	22.8 (4–53)	0.50 (0.17–1.5)
sWBC > 25,000	1.7–4.0	0.17–0.47
PMN > 90%	1.8–4.2	0.10–0.63
Low glucose	2.5–4.2	0.43–0.74
Protein > 3 g/dL	0.89–0.93	1.10
LDH > 250 U/L	1.9	0.09–0.11
TNFα > 36.2 pg/mL	3.3	0.07
L-Lactate > 5 mmol/L	2.7 (0.68–4.7)	0.52 (0.09–1.1)
Polymerase chain reaction	3 (1.3–7.2)	0.50 (0.17–1.5)
Gram stain	32 (8–125)	0 (0–0.52)

Source: Adapted from [4, 5].

upon these estimates of synovial fluid accuracy and evidence-based estimates of diagnostic test risk and treatment risk and benefit, the theoretical thresholds below which emergency physicians should contemplate not performing an arthrocentesis is 5% and the threshold above which treatment should ensue without an arthrocentesis is 39% (see Chapter 1).[5,48]

Comment

The risk factors and findings for GC and non-GC septic arthritis differ. In addition, the findings and management of native joint septic arthritis differ from prosthetic joint cases. History, physical exam, and clinician gestalt are inaccurate in isolation to rule in or rule out septic arthritis. Elevated procalcitonin may increase the probability of septic arthritis. On the other hand, nonelevated ESR and CRP may weakly reduce the probability of septic arthritis. Evaluation of synovial WBC and Gram stain remain the *sine qua non* to distinguish septic arthritis from other causes of acute monoarticular pain in the ED. The presence of a synovial WBC >100,000 will significantly increase the probability of septic arthritis and >50,000 should raise concern. Test- and treatment thresholds quantify patients most likely to benefit from arthrocentesis. The diagnostic accuracy for synovial lactate differs between studies and should not be used to risk stratify suspected septic arthritis patients at this time. Combinations of findings from the history and physical exam, serum, and synovial fluid labs may be more accurate than any single finding, so deriving and validating clinical decision aids is one approach that remains unexplored. In the meantime, clinicians should be aware of the risk factors for GC and non-GC septic arthritis and expeditiously select appropriate diagnostic and therapeutic options while consulting orthopedic surgery for early operative management in cases where the clinical evaluation remains less than definitive.

Recent ED-based studies demonstrate surprising differences in diagnostic accuracy compared with older research in septic arthritis.[4,5,21] Most notably, synovial polymerase chain reaction and L-lactate now seem far less accurate than initially believed. One explanation for these disparate findings might be adherence to more recent studies to enhancing the quality and transparency of health research (EQUATOR) network reporting standards for diagnostic studies, which increases the clarity and uniformity of manuscripts.[49,50] Emergency medicine diagnostics researchers often failed to adhere to EQUATOR reporting standards, which increases the risk of biased accuracy estimates.[51,52] For example, whereas older studies defined the presence of any bacterial growth as a case of septic arthritis whether or not Infectious Disease or Orthopedics ultimately deemed the organism a contaminant or a true infection, more recent studies differentiated false positives from true positives based upon operative or antimicrobial response to the culture. The distinction between the presence/absence of septic arthritis may include outcome assessors' awareness of many of the serum or synovial results, increasing the risk for incorporation bias that skews observed estimates of sensitivity and specificity upward.[25] As another example, some suspected septic arthritis patients may refuse arthrocentesis or have an inadequate aspiration and require clinical follow-up rather than synovial culture to rule in or rule out septic arthritis. As discussed in Chapter 6, this situation increases the risk of differential verification bias, which lowers observed sensitivity and specificity for diseases like septic arthritis that only become detectable during follow-up.[25]

References

1. Margaretten ME, Kohlwes J, Moore D, Bent S. Does this adult patient have septic arthritis? *JAMA*. 2007; 297(13): 1478–88.
2. Goldenberg DL. Septic arthritis. *Lancet*. 1998; 351(9097): 197–202.
3. Kaandorp CJ, Van Schaardenburg D, Krijnen P, Habbema JD, van de Laar MA. Risk factors for septic arthritis in patients with joint disease. A prospective study. *Arthritis and Rheumatism*. 1995; 38(12): 1819–25.
4. Carpenter CR, Vandenberg J, Solomon M *et al.* Diagnostic accuracy of synovial lactate, polymerase chain reaction, or clinical examination for suspected adult septic arthritis. *The Journal of Emergency Medicine*. 2020; 59(3): 339–47.
5. Carpenter CR, Schuur JD, Everett WW, Pines JM. Evidence-based diagnostics: Adult septic arthritis. *Academic Emergency Medicine*. 2011; 18(8): 781–96.

6. Kaandorp CJ, Dinant HJ, van de Laar MA, Moens HJ, Prins AP, Dijkmans BA. Incidence and sources of native and prosthetic joint infection: A community based prospective survey. *Annals of the Rheumatic Diseases.* 1997; 56(8): 470–5.
7. Gupta MN, Sturrock RD, Field M. A prospective 2-year study of 75 patients with adult-onset septic arthritis. *Rheumatology (Oxford).* 2001; 40(1): 24–30.
8. Lauper N, Davat M, Gijka E et al. Native septic arthritis is not an immediate surgical emergency. *The Journal of Infection.* 2018; 77(1): 47–53.
9. Huotari K, Peltola M, Jämsen E. The incidence of late prosthetic joint infections: A registry-based study of 112,708 primary hip and knee replacements. *Acta Orthopaedica.* 2015; 86(3): 321–5.
10. Roerdink RL, Huijbreqts HJTAM, van Lieshout AWT, Dietvorst M, van der Zwaard BC. The difference between native septic arthritis and prosthetic joint infections: A review of literature. *Journal of Orthopaedic Surgery.* 2019; 27(2): 2309499019860468.
11. De Fine M, Giavaresi G, Fini M, Illuminati A, Terrando S, Pignatti G. The role of synovial fluid analysis in the detection of periprosthetic hip and knee infections: A systematic review and meta-analysis. *International Orthopaedics.* 2018; 42(5): 983–94.
12. Gupta MN, Sturrock RD, Field M. Prospective comparative study of patients with culture proven and high suspicion of adult onset septic arthritis. *Annals of the Rheumatic Diseases.* 2003; 62(4): 327–31.
13. Frazee BW, Fee C, Lambert L. How common is MRSA in adult septic arthritis? *Annals of Emergency Medicine.* 2009; 54(5): 695–700.
14. Lin WT, Wu CD, Cheng SC et al. High prevalence of methicillin-resistant *Staphylococcus aureus* among patients with septic arthritis caused by *Staphylococcus aureus.* *PLoS One.* 2015; 10(5): e0127150.
15. Peterson TC, Pearson C, Zekaj M, Hudson I, Fakhouri G, Vaidya R. Septic arthritis in intravenous drug abusers: A historical comparison of habits and pathogens. *The Journal of Emergency Medicine.* 2014; 47(6): 723–8.
16. Lin WT, Tang HJ, Lai CC, Chao CM. Clinical manifestations and bacteriological features of culture-proven Gram-negative bacterial arthritis. *Journal of Microbiology, Immunology, and Infection.* 2017; 50(4): 527–31.
17. Saraux A, Taelman H, Blanche P et al. HIV infection as a risk factor for septic arthritis. *British Journal of Rheumatology.* 1997; 36(3): 333–7.
18. Ross JJ. Septic arthritis of native joints. *Infectious Disease Clinics of North America.* 2017; 31(2): 203–18.
19. Bardin T. Gonococcal arthritis. *Best Practice & Research. Clinical Rheumatology.* 2003; 17(2): 201–8.
20. Jeng GW, Wang CR, Liu ST et al. Measurement of synovial tumor necrosis factor-alpha in diagnosing emergency patients with bacterial arthritis. *The American Journal of Emergency Medicine.* 1997; 15(7): 626–9.
21. Couderc M, Pereira B, Mathieu S et al. Predictive value of the usual clinical signs and laboratory tests in the diagnosis of septic arthritis. *CJEM.* 2015; 17(4): 403–10.
22. Kortekangas P, Aro HT, Tuominen J, Toivanen A. Synovial fluid leukocytosis in bacterial arthritis vs. reactive arthritis and rheumatoid arthritis in the adult knee. *Scandinavian Journal of Rheumatology.* 1992; 21(6): 283–8.

23. Byrt T. How good is that agreement? *Epidemiology.* 1996; 7: 561.
24. Li SF, Henderson J, Dickman E, Darzynkiewicz R. Laboratory tests in adults with monoarticular arthritis: Can they rule out a septic joint? *Academic Emergency Medicine.* 2004; 11(3): 276–80.
25. Kohn MA, Carpenter CR, Newman TB. Understanding the direction of bias in studies of diagnostic test accuracy. *Academic Emergency Medicine.* 2013; 20(11): 1194–206.
26. Li SF, Cassidy C, Chang C, Gharib S, Torres J. Diagnostic utility of laboratory tests in septic arthritis. *Emergency Medicine Journal.* 2007; 24(2): 75–7.
27. Hariharan P, Kabrhel C. Sensitivity of erythrocyte sedimentation rate and C-reactive protein for the exclusion of septic arthritis in emergency department patients. *The Journal of Emergency Medicine.* 2011; 40(4): 428–31.
28. Ernst AA, Weiss SJ, Tracy LA, Weiss NR. Usefulness of CRP and ESR in predicting septic joints. *Southern Medical Journal.* 2010; 103(6): 522–6.
29. Shen CJ, Wu MS, Lin KH et al. The use of procalcitonin in the diagnosis of bone and joint infection: A systemic review and meta-analysis. *European Journal of Clinical Microbiology & Infectious Diseases.* 2013; 32(6): 807–14.
30. Zhao J, Zhang S, Zhang L et al. Serum procalcitonin levels as a diagnostic marker for septic arthritis: A meta-analysis. *The American Journal of Emergency Medicine.* 2017; 35(8): 1166–71.
31. Oppegaard O, Skodvin B, Halse AK, Langeland N. CD64 as a potential biomarker in septic arthritis. *BMC Infectious Diseases.* 2013; 13: 278.
32. Yuan J, Yan Y, Zhang J, Wang B, Feng J. Diagnostic accuracy of alpha-defensin in periprosthetic joint infection: A systematic review and meta-analysis. *International Orthopaedics.* 2017; 41(12): 2447–55.
33. Yoon JR, Yang SH, Shin YS. Diagnostic accuracy of interleukin-6 and procalcitonin in patients with periprosthetic joint infection: A systematic review and meta-analysis. *International Orthopaedics.* 2018; 42(6): 1213–26.
34. Shah K, Spear J, Nathanson LA, McCauley J, Edlow JA. Does the presence of crystal arthritis rule out septic arthritis? *The Journal of Emergency Medicine.* 2007; 32(1): 23–6.
35. Brook I, Reza MJ, Bricknell KS, Bluestone R, Finegold SM. Synovial fluid lactic acid. A diagnostic aid in septic arthritis. *Arthritis and Rheumatism.* 1978; 21(7): 774–9.
36. Mossman SS, Coleman JM, Gow PJ. Synovial fluid lactic acid in septic arthritis. *The New Zealand Medical Journal.* 1981; 93(678): 115–7.
37. Riordan T, Doyle D, Tabaqchali S. Synovial fluid lactic acid measurement in the diagnosis and management of septic arthritis. *Journal of Clinical Pathology.* 1982; 35(4): 390–4.
38. Gratacós J, Vila J, Moyá F et al. D-lactic acid in synovial fluid. A rapid diagnostic test for bacterial synovitis. *The Journal of Rheumatology.* 1995; 22(8): 1504–8.
39. Shu E, Farshidpour L, Young M, Darracq M, Ives Tallman C. Utility of point-of-care synovial lactate to identify septic arthritis in the emergency department. *The American Journal of Emergency Medicine.* 2019; 37(3): 502–5.

40. Lenski M, Scherer MA. The significance of interleukin-6 and lactate in the synovial fluid for diagnosing native septic arthritis. *Acta Orthopaedica Belgica*. 2014; 80(1): 18–25.
41. Krey PR, Bailen DA. Synovial fluid leukocytosis. A study of extremes. *The American Journal of Medicine*. 1979; 67(3): 436–42.
42. Shmerling RH, Delbanco TL, Tosteson AN, Trentham DE. Synovial fluid tests. What should be ordered? *JAMA*. 1990; 264(8): 1009–14.
43. Soderquist B, Jones I, Fredlund H, Vikerfors T. Bacterial or crystal-associated arthritis? Discriminating ability of serum inflammatory markers. *Scandinavian Journal of Infectious Diseases*. 1998; 30(6): 591–6.
44. Tarabichi M, Fleischman AN, Shahi A, Tian S, Parvizi J. Interpretation of leukocyte esterase for the detection of periprosthetic joint infection based on serologic markers. *The Journal of Arthroplasty*. 2017; 32(9s): S97–S100.e1.
45. Cunningham G, Seghrouchni K, Ruffieux E *et al.* Gram and acridine orange staining for diagnosis of septic arthritis in different patient populations. *International Orthopaedics*. 2014; 38(6): 1283–90.
46. Albert JD, Monbet V, Jolivet-Gougeon A *et al.* A novel method for a fast diagnosis of septic arthritis using mid infrared and deported spectroscopy. *Joint, Bone, Spine*. 2016; 83(3): 318–23.
47. Thumboo J, O'Duffy JD. A prospective study of the safety of joint and soft tissue aspirations and injections in patients taking warfarin sodium. *Arthritis and Rheumatism*. 1998; 41(4): 736–9.
48. Pauker SG, Kassirer JP. The threshold approach to clinical decision making. *The New England Journal of Medicine*. 1980; 302(20): 1109–17.
49. Simel DL, Rennie D, Bossuyt PM. The STARD statement for reporting diagnostic accuracy studies: Application to the history and physical examination. *Journal of General Internal Medicine*. 2008; 23(6): 768–74.
50. Bossuyt PM, Reitsma JB, Bruns DE *et al.* STARD 2015: An updated list of essential items for reporting diagnostic accuracy studies. *BMJ*. 2015; 351: h5527.
51. Gallo L, Hua N, Mercuri M, Silveira A, Worster A. Adherence to standards for reporting diagnostic accuracy in emergency medicine research. *Academic Emergency Medicine*. 2017; 24(8): 914–9.
52. Carpenter CR, Meisel ZF. Overcoming the tower of babel in medical science by finding the "EQUATOR": Research reporting guidelines. *Academic Emergency Medicine*. 2017; 24(8): 1030–3.

Chapter 33 **Osteomyelitis**

Ian T. Ferguson and Christopher R. Carpenter

Department of Emergency Medicine, Washington University School of Medicine, St. Louis, MO, USA

Highlights

- Scant research exists on the diagnosis of nondiabetic foot osteomyelitis.
- Charcot neuropathy mimics diabetic foot ulcers and is treated quite differently.
- Ulcer size >2 cm, a positive probe-to-bone test, or erythrocyte sedimentation rate >70 mm/hour each independently increases the likelihood of the diagnosis of diabetic osteomyelitis.
- Negative MRI and SPECT both significantly decrease the likelihood of diabetic foot osteomyelitis.
- Single findings from history, physical exam, and laboratory results do not significantly reduce the posttest probability for diabetic foot osteomyelitis although the combination of laboratory or imaging with physical exam findings may be useful to reduce the likelihood of osteomyelitis.

Background

Osteomyelitis is an infectious, inflammatory process that results in bony destruction. The infection can be isolated to the cortex or involve the periosteum and surrounding soft tissues.[1] The symptoms of acute osteomyelitis are typically noted over weeks, while chronic osteomyelitis (Figure 33.1) can evolve over months or years.

Lew and Waldvogel divide osteomyelitis etiologies into three categories: (i) hematogenous osteomyelitis; (ii) direct inoculation from trauma, surgery, prostheses, or soft tissue spread; or (iii) vascular insufficiency seen most

---

Evidence-Based Emergency Care: Diagnostic Testing and Clinical Decision Rules, Third Edition.
Edited by Jesse M. Pines, Fernanda Bellolio, Christopher R. Carpenter, and Ali S. Raja.
© 2023 John Wiley & Sons Ltd. Published 2023 by John Wiley & Sons Ltd.

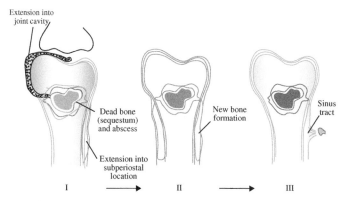

Figure 33.1 The progression of chronic osteomyelitis. Phase I: An area of devascularized dead bone is sequestered into an abscess cavity. Note that extension of intramedullary infection into an intracapsular location can result in septic arthritis, while progression into a periosteal location may produce periosteal elevation. Phase II: New bone formation results from periosteal elevation. Phase III: Extension of the abscess and necrotic material through cortical bone creates a fistula. Reproduced from Jauregui LE *et al.* Diagnosis and management of bone infections (1995)[2]

often in diabetes.[2] Risk factors for osteomyelitis include intravascular catheters, intravenous drug abuse, and nonbone foci of infections such as cellulitis, cutaneous abscesses, and urinary tract infections.[3] Hematogenous spread to the long bones is the most common etiology in children with more than half of cases occurring in children less than 5 years old. Risk factors include indwelling catheters, skin or soft tissue infection, or abnormal urinary anatomy.[4] Sickle cell disease is another risk factor for osteomyelitis in children with an estimated incidence of 8 cases per 100,000 children per year. Direct inoculation is more common in adults, often as a result of trauma which can complicate 25% of open fractures.[4]

Staphylococcal species are the most commonly isolated organisms, but the specific infective agent depends upon the site of infection, whether the spread is hematogenous or contiguous, and whether the joint is prosthetic or native (Figure 33.2). Osteomyelitis is a heterogeneous disease and no uniform treatment algorithm exists although antibiotic therapy is the mainstay of treatment in all cases.[5] The general approach to management involves a combination of intravenous antibiotics often with surgical debridement, followed by an additional extended course of oral antibiotics.[6] Local antibiotic delivery using antibiotic-containing beads or cement spacers may be used in some cases.[7]

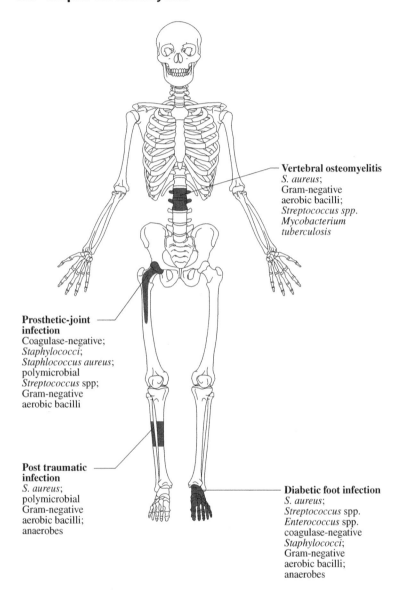

Figure 33.2 The microbiology of osteomyelitis. The microorganisms of osteomyelitis in order of prevalence from high to low by site of infection. (Reproduced from [1]/ With permission of Elsevier.)

One frequently encountered emergency department scenario in which osteomyelitis is a concern is foot ulcers. Foot ulcers can be venous, arterial, or diabetic, and the distinction can be challenging.[8] Generally, venous ulcers are proximal to the malleoli with irregular borders, whereas arterial ulcers involve the toes or shins with a pale and punched-out appearance. By comparison, diabetic ulcers typically occur in areas of increased pressure, such as the soles. Charcot neuropathy is a severe complication of peripheral neuropathy and can mimic diabetic osteomyelitis with a very similar clinical presentation, but the management for the two conditions is vastly different. Charcot neuropathy is treated with a cast and non-weight-bearing status rather than antibiotics and debridement. The prevalence of Charcot neuropathy in diabetic patients ranges from 0.08% to 13% in high-risk patients.[9] Distinguishing Charcot neuropathy from diabetic osteomyelitis is important for emergency physicians since catastrophic bony collapse in the ankle joint can occur in a short timeframe in Charcot neuropathy.[10]

Despite the fact that osteomyelitis of the foot or ankle is the primary or secondary reason for 75,000 hospitalizations in the United States each year, clinicians often underestimate the likelihood of diabetic foot osteomyelitis.[11] The pretest probability for osteomyelitis in a diabetic foot wound ranges from 15% to 20%.[12] Foot-related complications account for 20% of diabetes-related admissions in North America[8] and as many as 15% of patients with diabetic foot ulcers ultimately require amputations. One study found that, over a 3-year period, 61% of diabetic foot ulcers are likely to recur, 10% of ulcers will lead to amputation, and the overall survival rate for diabetic patients with foot ulcers was only 72% (compared to 87% for age- and gender-matched diabetic control patients).[13] The presence of diabetic foot osteomyelitis increases the risk of amputation and the 30-day postamputation perioperative mortality ranges from 7% to 15%.[14-16]

Clinical question

Can history, physical exam, or labs, accurately differentiate acute osteomyelitis from other causes of musculoskeletal or infectious symptoms?

One 2008 diagnostic meta-analysis concluded that no single laboratory or physical exam finding can significantly decrease the likelihood of diabetic osteomyelitis[17] (Table 33.1), although using a combination of findings may significantly reduce the negative likelihood ratio (LR−). A case-control study combining ulcer depth >3 mm with C-reactive protein (CRP) > 3.2 mg/dL (or erythrocyte sedimentation rate [ESR] > 60 mm/hour) reported LR− 0.009 for osteomyelitis.[18] Ulcer size >2 cm, bone exposure, a positive probe-to-bone

Table 33.1 Diagnostic test characteristics for diabetic osteomyelitis

Diagnostic test	LR+ (95% confidence interval)	LR– (95% confidence interval)
Bone exposure	9.2 (0.57–146)	0.70 (0.53–0.92)
Probe to bone test	6.4 (3.6–11)	0.39 (0.20–0.76)
Ulcer area >2 cm^2	7.2 (1.1–49)	0.48 (0.31–0.76)
Ulcer inflammation	1.5 (0.51–4.7)	0.84 (0.56–1.3)
Clinical judgment	9.2 (0.57–147)	0.70 (0.53–0.92)
Wagner >2	5.5 (1.8–17)	0.54 (0.30–0.97)
ESR >70 mm/hour	11.0 (1.6–79)	0.34 (0.06–1.9)
Swab culture	1.0 (0.65–79)	1.0 (0.08–13)

Note: Wagner grading scale:
- Grade 0 = No open lesions; may have evidence of healed lesions or deformities
- Grade 1 = Superficial ulcer
- Grade 2 = Deeper ulcer to tendon, bone, or joint capsule
- Grade 3 = Deeper tissues involved, with abscess, osteomyelitis, or tendonitis
- Grade 4 = Localized gangrene of toe or forefoot
- Grade 5 = Gangrene of foot.

Source: Data from [19].

test, a Wagner grade >2, or ESR >70 mm/hour each significantly *increases* the likelihood of diabetic osteomyelitis (Table 33.1).[19–23]

A systematic review on the utility of the probe-to-bone test in diagnosing diabetic osteomyelitis reported a pooled LR+ of 5.12 and a LR– 0.16.[24] These systematic review authors concluded, in conjunction with the current international working group on the diabetic foot guidelines,[25] that the probe-to-bone test should be used to rule in osteomyelitis in high-risk patients (positive predictive value [PPV] >90% if pretest probability >60%), and used to rule out osteomyelitis in low risk, outpatient settings (negative predictive value [NPV] >95% at pretest probability below 20%). To conduct this test, the clinician should use either a sterile blunt end probe or mosquito forceps to explore the entire depth of the wound: a positive test is one in which a grinding sensation is appreciated as the object is moved across the bony surface (Figure 33.3).[26]

Laboratory values that have been investigated to aid the diagnosis of osteomyelitis include ESR, CRP, white blood cells (WBC), and procalcitonin. With the exception of ESR, all the other markers return to baseline within 7 days while ESR has been shown to remain elevated in patients with sustained infection.[27] A retrospective study of 102 patients found ESR and CRP were not helpful in diagnosing osteomyelitis in nondiabetic patients with foot ulcers.[28] Optimal cut-off values determined by Youden's index were an ESR of 45.5 mm/hour and CRP of 3.45 mg/dL. At these values, the sensitivity

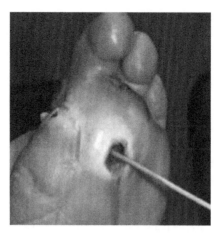

Figure 33.3 Example of the probe-to-bone test on a foot ulcer. (Michael S. Pinzur M.D./Springer Link.)

of ESR and CRP were 49% and 45%, respectively. The gold standard for osteomyelitis in this study was a positive bacterial culture from bone specimens and/or histopathologic changes consistent with osteomyelitis and ruled out if the above criteria were negative or the patient had a negative magnetic resonance imaging (MRI) or single-photon emission computed tomography (SPECT). While there is little reported research in the laboratory diagnosis of osteomyelitis in nondiabetic patients, one study reported mean ESR in non-diabetic patients without osteomyelitis to be nonsignificantly different from diabetic patients with confirmed osteomyelitis (72.3 versus 77.4 mm/hour with $p = 0.66$).[29] An ESR < 70 mm/hour had a NPV of 30.5% in those with diabetes mellitus (DM) and 58.3% without DM, suggesting ESR is poor at discriminating osteomyelitis in both DM and non-DM groups.

Clinical question

Can X-ray, nuclear imaging, computed tomography (CT), or MRI distinguish nondiabetic osteomyelitis from other causes of musculoskeletal symptoms?

There are far fewer studies on imaging in nondiabetic osteomyelitis than in diabetic osteomyelitis. Plain films can demonstrate joint space widening or narrowing, periosteal reaction, and bone destruction, although the latter is not apparent for up to 21 days after the onset of infection.[30] When metal is in close proximity to an area of osteomyelitis, image resolution is suboptimal due to beam-hardening artifact.[31] Narrative reviews have reported unreferenced sensitivities for conventional X-ray of 43–75% and specificities of 75–83% for *acute* osteomyelitis.[31] Two studies totaling 33 patients summarized in one meta-analysis evaluated plain radiography for *chronic* osteomyelitis and found that sensitivity ranged from 60% to 78% and specificity from 67% to 100%.[32–34] One 2005 systematic review found and summarized only one study assessing CT to diagnosis chronic osteomyelitis of the vertebra demonstrating LR+ 1.34 and LR– 0.66.[33,34]

A Health Technology Assessment systematic review of 69 studies reported on the diagnostic accuracy of CT, MRI, positron emission tomography (PET), scintigraphy, SPECT, and X-ray in the subset of patients without diabetes.[35] The report diagnostic odds ratio (DOR), which is a summary measure that incorporates both sensitivity and specificity and is similar to accuracy but does not depend on prevalence (diagnostic odds ratio [DOR] = [True Positive/False Positive] ÷ [False Negative/True Negative]). SPECT had the highest DOR of 95.8 (21.9–419.3), while plain radiography had the lowest DOR of 7.07 (2.7–18.1). MRI had a DOR of 30.3 (10.6–86.2); CT 9.74 (3.3–28.5); Scintigraphy 9.3 (4.1–21). Scintigraphy depends on the type performed with technetium-99m hexamethylpropylene amine oxime (^{99m}Tc HMPAO) WBC scintigraphy reporting similar accuracy to PET. MRI had the highest reported sensitivity at 95% (87.5–98). Plain radiography had similar reported sensitivity and specificity to CT (Sens 60.3% versus 67.9% and Spec 89.8% versus 90.8%). Albeit based on limited data, the diagnostic accuracy of any imaging study does not appear to vary based on chronicity (acute versus chronic) or location (hip, long bone, axial skeleton). Both PET-CT and MRI are excellent modalities to rule out vertebral osteomyelitis. A prospective study compared fluorine-18 fluorodeoxyglucose (^{18}F-FDG)-PET/CT and MRI and found that both modalities had 100% sensitivity and NPV for vertebral osteomyelitis when defined by the Infectious Disease Society of America guidelines as new back pain plus positive blood or tissue culture plus one positive imaging outcome.[36,37] MRI had a higher sensitivity for small epidural abscesses, while PET was superior in identifying infectious loci in locations other than the spine. One benefit of PET is that metallic objects are not a contraindication.[37]

Clinical question

What is the diagnostic accuracy of X-ray, nuclear imaging, or MRI for the diagnosis of diabetic osteomyelitis?

X-ray criteria for osteomyelitis include periosteal reaction, cortical disruption (loss of cortex with bony erosion), sequestrum (devitalized bone that is radiodense compared to normal bone), and affected bone marrow (focal loss

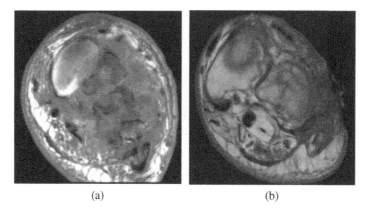

(a)   (b)

Figure 33.4 MRI appearance of (a) Charcot neuropathy compared with (b) osteomyelitis. (a) Neuropathic arthropathy. MRI demonstrating diffuse soft tissue swelling without an ulcer. Constellation of findings (soft tissue swelling, no ulcer, joint disorganization, and bone fragmentation) characteristic of neuropathic arthropathy. (b) Osteomyelitis: MRI demonstrating large soft tissue ulcer in continuity with cuboid bone marrow edema and destruction, diagnostic of osteomyelitis on MRI. In the radiology of diabetic feet, no ulcer = no osteomyelitis. (Courtesy of Dr. Jennifer Demertzis.)

of trabecular pattern or marrow radiolucency).[38] Of these, cortical disruption is the most sensitive finding.[38] MRI criteria for osteomyelitis are generally defined as focally decreased marrow signal intensity in T1-weighted images and a focally increased signal intensity in fat-suppressed T2-weighted or short tau inversion recovery images (Figure 33.4a, b).

Clinical question

Can X-ray, nuclear imaging, CT, or MRI accurately differentiate diabetic osteomyelitis from other foot ulcers?

Radiography has a reported specificity that is similar to MRI from a recent systematic review (78% [confidence interval (CI) 63.7–87.8]), but with inferior sensitivity compared with MRI, PET, Scintigraphy, and SPECT (68.9% [CI 57.6–78.4]).[35] Another systematic review concluded that diagnosis from plain radiographs is based on highly variable data with sensitivities ranging from 28% to 75%, and a pooled LR+ and LR− 1.69 and 0.68, respectively.[12] Combining the probe-to-bone test with plain radiography had a LR+ of 12.8 (6.3–26.2) and LR− of 0.02 (0.01–0.05) in one study, although the probe-to-bone test was performed by a surgeon with significant experience.[39]

Table 33.2 Imaging test characteristics for diabetic osteomyelitis

Diagnostic test	Positive likelihood ratio (LR+)	Negative likelihood ratio (LR−)	Diagnostic odds ratio (DOR)
Plain film (X-ray)	3.1	0.40	5.97
MRI	5.3	0.05	51.08
PET	11.7	0.17	33.91
SPECT	2.1	0.08	22.91
Scintigraphy	3.3	0.21	8.66

MRI = magnetic resonance imaging; PET = positron emission tomography;
SPECT = single photon emission computed tomograph. DOR = [TP/FP]/[FN/TN].
LR+ = sensitivity/1-specificity. LR− = 1-sensitivity/specificity.
Source: Data from [36].

In a systematic review of 35 studies in which at least 60% of patients had diabetic foot ulcers, MRI and SPECT had the highest sensitives reported with 95.8% (CI 91.8–97.8) and 95.5% (CI 75.9–99.3), respectively (Table 33.2).[35] PET had the highest specificity (92.8% [CI 75.7–98.2]) but a wider CI of sensitivities than MRI or SPECT (84.3% [CI 52.8–96.3]). Scintigraphy had a sensitivity slightly better than PET (84.7% [CI 65.9–94.1]) and moderate specificity (74% [CI 55–86.9]), although there is also variation with the specific isotope used. ^{99m}Tc HMPAO WBC is reported as having the highest sensitivity and specificity among this type of scintigraphy. However, bone scintigraphy can yield false-positive results with Charcot arthropathy, gout, trauma, or surgery.[1] Ultrasound had a sensitivity and specificity with CIs that ranged from around 2% to 99%, so ultrasound is not useful in the diagnosis of osteomyelitis.

Comment

Although the probe-to-bone test offers one potential, biologically plausible, and low-cost option to quickly rule in or rule out osteomyelitis of diabetic foot ulcers, further research is needed to verify the reliability and diagnostic accuracy of this test in the hands of emergency providers. In addition, the willingness of emergency physicians and specialists to incorporate the results of probe testing into diagnostic and therapeutic algorithms to obviate the need for expensive and time-consuming imaging modalities such as bone scan and MRI would be determined only by a randomized controlled trial.[40] If consultants require an MRI regardless of the results of the probe-to-bone

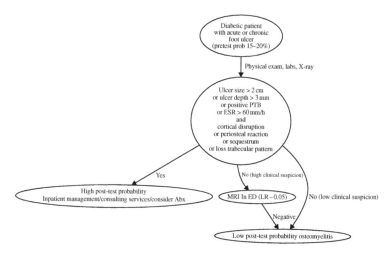

Figure 33.5 Diagnostic algorithm for diabetic foot osteomyelitis in the emergency department.

test, then there would be minimal value to performing the probe test. Figure 33.5 provides an algorithm based upon the best available evidence to guide the diagnostic evaluation of suspected osteomyelitis in the emergency department.

Future research is needed to understand the usefulness and reliability of combinations of history, physical exam, labs, and imaging tests for the risk stratification of osteomyelitis in ED patients with diabetic foot lesions. Ultimately, a clinical decision rule may help to efficiently and reliably risk-stratify diabetic foot lesions for osteomyelitis in the ED.

References

1. Lew DP, Waldvogel FA. Osteomyelitis. *Lancet.* 2004; 364(9431): 369–79.
2. Lew DP, Waldvogel FA. Osteomyelitis. *The New England Journal of Medicine.* 1997; 336(14): 999–1007.
3. Wald ER. Risk factors for osteomyelitis. *The American Journal of Medicine.* 1985; 78(6B): 206–12.
4. Schmitt SK. Osteomyelitis. *Infectious Disease Clinics of North America.* 2017; 31(2): 325–38.
5. Castellazzi L, Mantero M, Esposito S. Update on the management of pediatric acute osteomyelitis and septic arthritis. *International Journal of Molecular Sciences.* 2016; 17(6): 855.

6. Conterno LO, Turchi MD. Antibiotics for treating chronic osteomyelitis in adults. *Cochrane Database of Systematic Reviews.* 2013; (9): CD004439. doi: 10.1002/14651858. CD004439.pub3.

7. Qiu XS, Zheng X, Shi HF *et al.* Antibiotic-impregnated cement spacer as definitive management for osteomyelitis. *BMC Musculoskeletal Disorders.* 2015; 16: 254.

8. London NJ, Donnelly R. ABC of arterial and venous disease. Ulcerated lower limb. *BMJ.* 2000; 320(7249): 1589–91.

9. Womack J. Charcot arthropathy versus osteomyelitis: Evaluation and management. *The Orthopedic Clinics of North America.* 2017; 48(2): 241–7.

10. van der Ven A, Chapman CB, Bowker JH. Charcot neuroarthropathy of the foot and ankle. *The Journal of the American Academy of Orthopaedic Surgeons.* 2009; 17(9): 562–71.

11. Newman LG, Waller J, Palestro CJ *et al.* Unsuspected osteomyelitis in diabetic foot ulcers. Diagnosis and monitoring by leukocyte scanning with indium in 111 oxyquinoline. *JAMA.* 1991; 266(9): 1246–51.

12. Dinh MT, Abad CL, Safdar N. Diagnostic accuracy of the physical examination and imaging tests for osteomyelitis underlying diabetic foot ulcers: Meta-analysis. *Clinical Infectious Diseases.* 2008; 47(4): 519–27.

13. Apelqvist J, Larsson J, Agardh CD. Long-term prognosis for diabetic patients with foot ulcers. *Journal of Internal Medicine.* 1993; 233(6): 485–91.

14. Bamberger DM, Daus GP, Gerding DN. Osteomyelitis in the feet of diabetic patients. Long-term results, prognostic factors, and the role of antimicrobial and surgical therapy. *The American Journal of Medicine.* 1987; 83(4): 653–60.

15. Subramaniam B, Pomposelli F, Talmor D, Park KW. Perioperative and long-term morbidity and mortality after above-knee and below-knee amputations in diabetics and nondiabetics. *Anesthesia and Analgesia.* 2005; 100(5): 1241–7, table of contents.

16. Stone PA, Flaherty SK, Aburahma AF *et al.* Factors affecting perioperative mortality and wound-related complications following major lower extremity amputations. *Annals of Vascular Surgery.* 2006; 20(2): 209–16.

17. Butalia S, Palda VA, Sargeant RJ, Detsky AS, Mourad O. Does this patient with diabetes have osteomyelitis of the lower extremity? *JAMA.* 2008; 299(7): 806–13.

18. Fleischer AE, Didyk AA, Woods JB, Burns SE, Wrobel JS, Armstrong DG. Combined clinical and laboratory testing improves diagnostic accuracy for osteomyelitis in the diabetic foot. *The Journal of Foot and Ankle Surgery.* 2009; 48(1): 39–46.

19. Grayson ML, Gibbons GW, Balogh K, Levin E, Karchmer AW. Probing to bone in infected pedal ulcers. A clinical sign of underlying osteomyelitis in diabetic patients. *JAMA.* 1995; 273(9): 721–3.

20. Wagner FW Jr. The dysvascular foot: A system for diagnosis and treatment. *Foot & Ankle.* 1981; 2(2): 64–122.

21. Enderle MD, Coerper S, Schweizer HP *et al.* Correlation of imaging techniques to histopathology in patients with diabetic foot syndrome and clinical suspicion of chronic osteomyelitis. The role of high-resolution ultrasound. *Diabetes Care.* 1999; 22(2): 294–9.

22. Vesco L, Boulahdour H, Hamissa S *et al.* The value of combined radionuclide and magnetic resonance imaging in the diagnosis and conservative management of

minimal or localized osteomyelitis of the foot in diabetic patients. *Metabolism.* 1999; 48(7): 922–7.

23. Kapoor A, Page S, Lavalley M, Gale DR, Felson DT. Magnetic resonance imaging for diagnosing foot osteomyelitis: A meta-analysis. *Archives of Internal Medicine.* 2007; 167(2): 125–32.

24. Lam K, van Asten SA, Nguyen T, La Fontaine J, Lavery LA. Diagnostic accuracy of probe to bone to detect osteomyelitis in the diabetic foot: A systematic review. *Clinical Infectious Diseases.* 2016; 63(7): 944–8.

25. Lipsky BA, Berendt AR, Cornia PB *et al.* 2012 infectious diseases society of america clinical practice guideline for the diagnosis and treatment of diabetic foot infections. *Journal of the American Podiatric Medical Association.* 2013; 103(1): 2–7.

26. Malhotra R, Chan CS, Nather A. Osteomyelitis in the diabetic foot. *Diabetic Foot & Ankle.* 2014; 5. doi: 10.3402/dfa.v5.24445.

27. Michail M, Jude E, Liaskos C *et al.* The performance of serum inflammatory markers for the diagnosis and follow-up of patients with osteomyelitis. *The International Journal of Lower Extremity Wounds.* 2013; 12(2): 94–9.

28. Ryan EC, Ahn J, Wukich DK, Kim PJ, La Fontaine J, Lavery LA. Diagnostic utility of erythrocyte sedimentation rate and C-reactive protein in osteomyelitis of the foot in persons without diabetes. *The Journal of Foot and Ankle Surgery.* 2019; 58(3): 484–8.

29. Rabjohn L, Roberts K, Troiano M, Schoenhaus H. Diagnostic and prognostic value of erythrocyte sedimentation rate in contiguous osteomyelitis of the foot and ankle. *The Journal of Foot and Ankle Surgery.* 2007; 46(4): 230–7.

30. Gold RH, Hawkins RA, Katz RD. Bacterial osteomyelitis: Findings on plain radiography, CT, MR, and scintigraphy. *AJR. American Journal of Roentgenology.* 1991; 157(2): 365–70.

31. Pineda C, Espinosa R, Pena A. Radiographic imaging in osteomyelitis: The role of plain radiography, computed tomography, ultrasonography, magnetic resonance imaging, and scintigraphy. *Seminars in Plastic Surgery.* 2009; 23(2): 80–9.

32. Alsheikh W, Sfakianakis GN, Mnaymneh W *et al.* Subacute and chronic bone-infections - diagnosis using In-111, Ga-67 and Tc-99m MDP bone-scintigraphy, and radiography. *Radiology.* 1985; 155(2): 501–6.

33. Whalen JL, Brown ML, Mcleod R, Fitzgerald RH. Limitations of indium leukocyte imaging for the diagnosis of spine infections. *Spine.* 1991; 16(2): 193–7.

34. Termaat MF, Raijmakers PG, Scholten HJ, Bakker FC, Patka P, Haarman HJ. The accuracy of diagnostic imaging for the assessment of chronic osteomyelitis: A systematic review and meta-analysis. *The Journal of Bone and Joint Surgery. American Volume.* 2005; 87(11): 2464–71.

35. Llewellyn A, Jones-Diette J, Kraft J, Holton C, Harden M, Simmonds M. Imaging tests for the detection of osteomyelitis: A systematic review. *Health Technology Assessment.* 2019; 23(61): 1–128.

36. Berbari EF, Kanj SS, Kowalski TJ *et al.* 2015 Infectious Diseases Society of America (IDSA) clinical practice guidelines for the diagnosis and treatment of native vertebral osteomyelitis in adults. *Clinical Infectious Diseases.* 2015; 61(6): e26–46.

37. Kouijzer IJE, Scheper H, de Rooy JWJ *et al.* The diagnostic value of (18)F-FDG-PET/CT and MRI in suspected vertebral osteomyelitis - a prospective study. *European Journal of Nuclear Medicine and Molecular Imaging.* 2018; 45(5): 798–805.

38. Alvaro-Afonso FJ, Lazaro-Martinez JL, Garcia-Morales E, Garcia-Alvarez Y, Sanz-Corbalan I, Molines-Barroso RJ. Cortical disruption is the most reliable and accurate plain radiographic sign in the diagnosis of diabetic foot osteomyelitis. *Diabetic Medicine.* 2019; 36(2): 258–9.

39. Aragon-Sanchez J, Lipsky BA, Lazaro-Martinez JL. Diagnosing diabetic foot osteomyelitis: Is the combination of probe-to-bone test and plain radiography sufficient for high-risk inpatients? *Diabetic Medicine.* 2011; 28(2): 191–4.

40. Lord SJ, Irwig L, Simes RJ. When is measuring sensitivity and specificity sufficient to evaluate a diagnostic test, and when do we need randomized trials? *Annals of Internal Medicine.* 2006; 144(11): 850–5.

Chapter 34 **Sexually Transmitted Infections (STIs)**

Jonathan Sheele[1] and Christopher R. Carpenter[2]

[1] Department of Emergency Medicine, Mayo Clinic, Jacksonville, FL, USA
[2] Department of Emergency Medicine, Washington University School of Medicine, St. Louis, MO, USA

Highlights

- Sexually transmitted infections (STIs) are usually underdiagnosed and overtreated in emergency medicine.
- Urinary tract infections (UTIs) cannot be accurately differentiated from STIs in at-risk patients based on the history or physical exam.
- Clinical gestalt of emergency physicians to distinguish STI from UTI is inaccurate.
- Adolescent and young adult females presenting with genital-urinary complaints should receive testing for STIs and a urine culture.
- Nucleic acid amplification tests (NAATs) are the preferred testing method for *Neisseria gonorrhoeae*, *Chlamydia trachomatis*, and *Trichomonas vaginalis*.
- NAATs for *N. gonorrhoeae*, *C. trachomatis*, and *T. vaginalis* should be ordered for at-risk males and females presenting to the ED with genitourinary complaints.

Background

Sexually transmitted infections (STIs) are caused by organisms acquired through sexual activity.[1] The most common STIs diagnosed in the emergency department (ED) include *Neisseria gonorrhoeae*, *Chlamydia trachomatis*, *Trichomonas vaginalis*, syphilis, herpes viruses, human immunodeficiency virus (HIV), and human

---

Evidence-Based Emergency Care: Diagnostic Testing and Clinical Decision Rules, Third Edition.
Edited by Jesse M. Pines, Fernanda Bellolio, Christopher R. Carpenter, and Ali S. Raja.
© 2023 John Wiley & Sons Ltd. Published 2023 by John Wiley & Sons Ltd.

papillomaviruses. STIs in the ED can range from asymptomatic to having vaginal or penile discharge, genital-urinary pain, abdominal pain, urethritis, cervicitis, tubo-ovarian abscesses, orchitis, and epididymitis.[1-4] Long-term complications for some untreated STIs can include pelvic inflammatory disease (PID), infertility, increased risk for ectopic pregnancy, acquisition of HIV, and continued community transmission of the infection.

Screening for STIs can occur in the ED for at-risk patients who may have limited outpatient access to medical care.[4] Assessing patients' risk for STIs in the ED can be challenging because ED providers may not ask for detailed sexual histories and patients may not provide honest answers about their sexual behavior. Obtaining an accurate STI risk assessment can be particularly difficult with nonemancipated adolescents or in the setting of unrecognized human trafficking or spousal abuse.[5] Pad-based screening allowing patients to respond nonverbally while awaiting ED evaluation could be an approach to overcome socially difficult interactions.[6,7] Race and gender are associated with disparities in STI testing and treatment in ED settings.[8] ED physicians often fail to adhere to Centers for Disease Control (CDC) Guidelines for the diagnosis and treatment of STIs, a trend that has continued for almost two decades.[9,10] The CDC recommended diagnostic tests for *N. gonorrhoeae, C. trachomatis,* and *T. vaginalis* are the nucleic acid amplification tests (NAATs).[11] NAAT testing can occur from genital swab or be obtained from the urine. While urine specimens are easier to obtain and provide 99% specificity, sensitivities range from 88% to 93% for Chlamydia and 88% for gonorrhea compared with endocervical specimens.[12,13] Unfortunately, the results of the NAATs are usually not available during the clinical encounter resulting in significant under- and overtreatment of ED patients for STIs.[14-16] In addition, some settings lack access to NAAT or other STI testing that provides faster results.[17] Nonetheless, the future of STI testing likely includes rapid diagnostic tests where the results can be available during the patient encounter.[18]

In this chapter, we focus on *N. gonorrhoeae, C. trachomatis,* and *T. vaginalis.* We do not address HIV, herpes, or syphilis. For additional information, readers are referred to the CDC, "Sexually Transmitted Diseases Treatment Guidelines, 2015."[11]

Clinical question

Can a urinary tract infection (UTI) be reliably differentiated from a STI based on history and physical exam?

Urinary symptoms such as dysuria and frequency are common chief complaints in the ED, and the differential diagnoses include both UTIs and STIs (see Chapter 32).[19] UTIs predominantly affect women and occur in all ages, whereas *N. gonorrhoeae* and *C. trachomatis* are predominantly seen in nonwhite younger male or female sexually active patients. When urinary symptoms are reported a pelvic exam is less likely to be performed.[20] A prospective cohort study of 92 adult female ED patients with urinary frequency, urgency, dysuria, and no new or changes in their vaginal discharge found that combining the history, physical examination finding, and urine dip was 50% sensitive (CI 23–77%) and 86% specific (CI 76–93%) for an STI.[21] Sexual histories obtained in the ED are often inadequately documented, patients may not provide accurate information, and ED providers perform insufficient STI testing even when the medical history suggests a STI.[20,22–26]

Reed *et al.*[27] analyzed 250 adolescent females who received STI testing and found that being of black race (odds ratio [OR] = 3.2), having a new partner within the last 3 months (OR = 1.9), cervical discharge (OR = 2.0), absence of yeast (OR = 3.3), and >10 white blood cells (OR = 2.5) on vaginal Gram stain predicted a STI. The model was only 75% sensitive and 71% specific, with a negative predictive value of 85%. There have been two clinical prediction tools developed for STIs in the ED though neither has been externally validated.[28] The first model for estimating risk of *N. gonorrhoeae* and *C. trachomatis* in men in the ED included: ≤24 years of age, penile discharge, and contact with someone infected with *N. gonorrhoeae* or *C. trachomatis*, and lack of health insurance status.[29] The other model utilized a point-system and the following variables: age, marital status, education, new sex partner within past 2 years, non-ED as a primary source for health care, nonantibiotic use past month, dysuria, or discharge in the past 3 months.[28] The latter prediction model had area under the receiver operating curve (ROC) of 0.64 for females and 0.72 for males.[28] Other models derived and validated outside ED settings seek to guide testing for asymptomatic gonorrhea or chlamydia.[30,31] Before widespread incorporation into ED practice, these STI models must better define discrimination, calibration, reliability, external validity, comparative usefulness, and viable implementation strategies.[32] The components of an adequate sexual history in the ED are highlighted in Table 34.1. Risk factors for STI acquisition and high-risk groups are summarized in Tables 34.2 and 34.3.

Clinical question

Are the history and physical exam useful for diagnosing STIs?
The CDC considers the clinicians' history and physical examination "foundational" for diagnosing and treating STIs.[43,44] Sexual histories can identify patients that are at high risk for STIs, but the history and physical exams done in the ED do not accurately differentiate between patients that have

Table 34.1 Elements of an adequate sexual history in the ED

The following are elements of a sexual history that can be used to risk stratify patients for STI testing, and possibly treatment, during their clinical encounter:

1. Number of sexual partners
2. Date of last sexual intercourse
3. Sexual orientation
4. Type of contraception and frequency of use
5. Birth control methods
6. Types of sexual practices
7. History of previous STIs
8. Risk factors for the patient's sexual partner(s)

Source: Data from [26, 33].

Table 34.2 Risk factors for STI acquisition

New sex partner in past 60 days
Multiple sex partners or sex partner with multiple concurrent sex partners
Sex with a partner recently treated for an STI
Transactional sex
Sexual contact with sex worker
Meeting a partner for sex on the internet
Group sex

Source: Data from [34–39].

Table 34.3 High-risk groups (higher prevalence or higher morbidity from STIs)

Young age (15–24 years old)
Men who have sex with men
History of a prior STI
HIV-positive status
Pregnant women
Incarcerated or juvenile detention center
Illicit drug use

Source: Data from [34, 36, 38, 40–42].

STI or UTI.[14,20,23,44] Sexual histories obtained by ED providers are frequently inadequate, and patients might provide incorrect information.[22–24,26,45] ED providers often perform insufficient testing for STI even when the history suggests a possible STI.[22–24,26] Self-collected vaginal swabs are not inferior to provider-performed endocervical sampling for ED diagnosis of *N. gonorrhoeae* and *C. trachomatis* and improve patient acceptability.[46] Pelvic exams are routinely performed on women in the ED with genital-urinary complaints, although the utility of the exam for diagnosing STIs has recently been called into question.[20,23,27,47] Pelvic exams in the ED make women uncomfortable, increase their lengths of stay, and do not usually change clinical management.[20,23,27,47,48] ED pelvic exams should be considered in certain circumstances including when there is a possibility of a retained foreign body or laceration.

Comment

Patients in the ED are paradoxically overtreated for and underdiagnosed with STIs. NAATs are the preferred testing modality for *N. gonorrhoeae*, *C. trachomatis*, and *T. vaginalis*, although many healthcare settings lack access to rapid testing with the consequence of healthcare inequities around the diagnosis and treatment of STIs.[49,50] The signs and symptoms of UTIs can overlap with those infected with *N. gonorrhoeae* and *C. trachomatis*. Neither the history nor the physical exam in the ED can reliably differentiate patients with UTIs or STIs. Reliability studies in ED settings quantifying the reproducibility of subjective physical exam findings such as vaginal odor, cervical motion tenderness, or adnexal fullness do not exist. Sufficiently accurate STI clinical decision aids await derivation and validation.

References

1. Pfennig CL. Sexually transmitted diseases in the emergency department. *Emergency Medicine Clinics of North America.* 2019; 37: 165–92.
2. Mehta SD, Shahan J, Zenilman JM. Ambulatory STD management in an inner-city emergency department: Descriptive epidemiology, care utilization patterns, and patient perceptions of local public STD clinics. *Sexually Transmitted Diseases.* 2000; 27: 154–8.
3. Mills BB. Vaginitis: Beyond the basics. *Obstetrics and Gynecology Clinics of North America.* 2017; 44: 159–77.
4. Schneider K, FitzGerald M, Byczkowski T, Reed J. Screening for asymptomatic gonorrhea and Chlamydia in the pediatric emergency department. *Sexually Transmitted Diseases.* 2016; 43: 209–15.
5. Tracy EE, Macias-Konstantopoulos W. Identifying and assisting sexually exploited and trafficked patients seeking women's health care services. *Obstetrics and Gynecology.* 2017; 130: 443–53.
6. Ahmad FA, Jeffe DB, Plax K et al. Computerized self-interviews improve Chlamydia and gonorrhea testing among youth in the emergency department. *Annals of Emergency Medicine.* 2014; 64: 376–84.
7. Ahmad FA, Jeffe DB, Carpenter CR et al. Emergency department directors are willing to expand reproductive health services for adolescents. *Journal of Pediatric and Adolescent Gynecology.* 2019; 32: 170–4.
8. Dretler AW, Trolard A, Bergquist EP et al. The influence of race and sex on gonorrhea and Chlamydia treatment in the emergency department. *The American Journal of Emergency Medicine.* 2020; 38: 566–70.

9. Kane BG, Degutis LC, Sayward HK, D'Onofrio G. Compliance with the Centers for Disease Control and Prevention recommendations for the diagnosis and treatment of sexually transmitted diseases. *Academic Emergency Medicine*. 2004; 11: 371–7.

10. Evans EM, Goyke TE, Cohrac SA *et al*. Compliance with Centers for Disease Control guidelines for ED patients with sexually transmitted diseases. *The American Journal of Emergency Medicine*. 2016; 34: 1727–9.

11. Workowski KA, Bolan GA. Centers for Disease C, Prevention. Sexually transmitted diseases treatment guidelines, 2015. *MMWR - Recommendations and Reports*. 2015; 64: 1–137.

12. Airell A, Ottosson L, Bygdeman SM *et al*. *Chlamydia trachomatis* PCR (Cobas Amplicor) in women: endocervical specimen transported in a specimen of urine versus endocervical and urethral specimens in 2-SP medium versus urine specimen only. *International Journal of STD & AIDS*. 2000; 11: 651–8.

13. Lunny C, Taylor D, Hoang L *et al*. Self-collected versus clinician-collected sampling for Chlamydia and gonorrhea screening: A systemic review and meta-analysis. *PLoS One*. 2015; 10: e0132776.

14. Sheele JM, Smith J, Niforatos JD *et al*. History, physical examination, and laboratory findings associated with infection and the empiric treatment of gonorrhea and Chlamydia of women in the emergency department. *Cureus*. 2019; 11: e6482.

15. Krivochenitser R, Jones JS, Whalen D, Gardiner C. Underrecognition of cervical *Neisseria gonorrhoeae* and *Chlamydia trachomatis* infections in pregnant patients in the ED. *The American Journal of Emergency Medicine*. 2013; 31: 661–3.

16. Pattishall AE, Rahman SY, Jain S, Simon HK. Empiric treatment of sexually transmitted infections in a pediatric emergency department: Are we making the right decisions? *The American Journal of Emergency Medicine*. 2012; 30: 1588–90.

17. Wi TE, Ndowa FJ, Ferreyra C *et al*. Diagnosing sexually transmitted infections in resource-constrained settings: Challenges and ways forward. *Journal of the International AIDS Society*. 2019; 22: e25343.

18. Adamson PC, Loeffelholz MJ, Klausner JD. Point-of-care testing for sexually transmitted infections: A review of recent developments. *Archives of Pathology & Laboratory Medicine*. 2020; 144: 1344–51.

19. Bent S, Nallamothu BK, Simel DL, Fihn SD, Saint S. Does this woman have an acute uncomplicated urinary tract infection? *JAMA*. 2002; 287: 2701–10.

20. Wilbanks MD, Galbraith JW, Geisler WM. Dysuria in the emergency department: Missed diagnosis of *Chlamydia trachomatis*. *The Western Journal of Emergency Medicine*. 2014; 15: 227–30.

21. Shapiro T, Dalton M, Hammock J, Lavery R, Matjucha J, Salo DF. The prevalence of urinary tract infections and sexually transmitted disease in women with symptoms of a simple urinary tract infection stratified by low colony count criteria. *Academic Emergency Medicine*. 2005; 12: 38–44.

22. Goyal MK, Shea JA, Hayes KL *et al*. Development of a sexual health screening tool for adolescent emergency department patients. *Academic Emergency Medicine*. 2016; 23: 809–15.

23. Farrukh S, Sivitz AB, Onogul B, Patel K, Tejani C. The additive value of pelvic examinations to history in predicting sexually transmitted infections for young female patients with suspected cervicitis or pelvic inflammatory disease. *Annals of Emergency Medicine.* 2018; 72: 703–12 e1.

24. Sequeira S, Morgan JR, Fagan M, Hsu KK, Drainoni ML. Evaluating quality of care for sexually transmitted infections in different clinical settings. *Sexually Transmitted Diseases.* 2015; 42: 717–24.

25. Banas DA, Cromer BA, Santana M *et al.* Comparison of clinical evaluation of genitourinary symptoms in female adolescents among primary care versus emergency department physicians. *Journal of Pediatric and Adolescent Gynecology.* 2010; 23: 71–6.

26. Niforatos JD, Nowacki AS, Cavendish J, Gripshover BM, Yax JA. Emergency provider documentation of sexual health risk factors and its association with HIV testing: A retrospective cohort study. *The American Journal of Emergency Medicine.* 2019; 37: 1365–7.

27. Reed JL, Mahabee-Gittens EM, Huppert JS. A decision rule to identify adolescent females with cervical infections. *Journal of Women's Health (2002).* 2007; 16: 272–80.

28. Al-Tayyib AA, Miller WC, Rogers SM *et al.* Evaluation of risk score algorithms for detection of chlamydial and gonococcal infections in an emergency department setting. *Academic Emergency Medicine.* 2008; 15: 126–35.

29. Merchant RC, DePalo DM, Liu T, Rich JD, Stein MD. Developing a system to predict laboratory-confirmed chlamydial and/or gonococcal urethritis in adult male emergency department patients. *Postgraduate Medicine.* 2010; 122: 52–60.

30. Falasinnu T, Gilbert M, Gustafson P, Shoveller J. Deriving and validating a risk estimation tool for screening asymptomatic Chlamydia and gonorrhea. *Sexually Transmitted Diseases.* 2014; 41: 706–12.

31. Falasinnu T, Gilbert M, Gustafson P, Shoveller J. A validation study of a clinical prediction rule for screening asymptomatic Chlamydia and gonorrhoea infections among heterosexuals in British Columbia. *Sexually Transmitted Infections.* 2016; 92: 12–8.

32. Falasinnu T, Gustafson P, Hottes TS, Gilbert M, Ogilvie G, Shoveller J. A critical appraisal of risk models for predicting sexually transmitted infections. *Sexually Transmitted Diseases.* 2014; 41: 321–30.

33. Pakpreo P. Why do we take a sexual history? *The Virtual Mentor.* 2005; 7. doi: 10.1001/virtualmentor.2005.7.10.medu1-0510.

34. Torrone E, Papp J, Weinstock H. Prevalence of *Chlamydia trachomatis* genital infection among persons aged 14–39 years–United States, 2007–2012. *MMWR. Morbidity and Mortality Weekly Report.* 2014; 63: 834–8.

35. Ness RB, Smith KJ, Chang CCH, Schisterman EF, Bass DC. Prediction of pelvic inflammatory disease among young, single, sexually active women. *Sexually Transmitted Diseases.* 2006; 33: 137–42.

36. Niccolai LM, Ethier KA, Kershaw TS, Lewis JB, Meade CS, Ickovics JR. New sex partner acquisition and sexually transmitted disease risk among adolescent females. *The Journal of Adolescent Health.* 2004; 34: 216–23.

37. Jones J, Salazar LF, Crosby R. Contextual factors and sexual risk behaviors among young, black men. *American Journal of Men's Health*. 2017; 11: 508–17.

38. Lofy KH, Hofmann J, Mosure DJ, Fine DN, Marrazzo JM. Chlamydial infections among female adolescents screened in juvenile detention centers in Washington State, 1998–2002. *Sexually Transmitted Diseases*. 2006; 33: 63–7.

39. Lewnard JA, Berrang-Ford L. Internet-based partner selection and risk for unprotected anal intercourse in sexual encounters among men who have sex with men: A meta-analysis of observational studies. *Sexually Transmitted Infections*. 2014; 90: 290–6.

40. Chernick LS, Chun TH, Richards R *et al.* Sex without contraceptives in a multicenter study of adolescent emergency department patients. *Academic Emergency Medicine*. 2020; 27: 283–90.

41. Klausner JD, Kent CK, Wong W, McCright J, Katz MH. The public health response to epidemic syphilis, San Francisco, 1999-2004. *Sexually Transmitted Diseases*. 2005; 32: S11–8.

42. Beymer MR, Weiss RE, Bolan RK *et al.* Sex on demand: Geosocial networking phone apps and risk of sexually transmitted infections among a cross-sectional sample of men who have sex with men in Los Angeles County. *Sexually Transmitted Diseases*. 2014; 90: 567–72.

43. Barrow RY, Ahmed F, Bolan GA, Workowski KA. Recommendations for providing quality sexually transmitted diseases clinical services, 2020. *MMWR - Recommendations and Reports*. 2020; 68: 1–20.

44. Jenkins WD, LeVault KR. Sexual history taking in the emergency department - more specificity required. *The Journal of Emergency Medicine*. 2015; 48: 143–51.

45. Territo HM, Wrotniak BH, Bouton S, Burstein GR. A new strategy for trichomonas testing female adolescents in the emergency department. *Journal of Pediatric and Adolescent Gynecology*. 2016; 29: 378–81.

46. Chinnock B, Yore M, Mason J *et al.* Self-obtained vaginal swabs are not inferior to provider-performed endocervical sampling for emergency department diagnosis of *Neisseria gonorrhoeae* and *Chlamydia trachomatis*. *Academic Emergency Medicine*. 2021; 28: 612–20.

47. Tucker P, Evans DD. Are pelvic exams necessary anymore? *Advanced Emergency Nursing Journal*. 2019; 41: 282–9.

48. Brown J, Fleming R, Aristzabel J, Gishta R. Does pelvic exam in the emergency department add useful information? *The Western Journal of Emergency Medicine*. 2011; 12: 208–12.

49. Murray-Horwitz ME, Pace LE, Ross-Degnan D. Trends and disparities in sexual and reproductive health behaviors and service use among young adult women (aged 18-25 years) in the United States, 2002-2015. *American Journal of Public Health*. 2018; 108: S336–43.

50. Lieberman JA, Cannon CA, Bourassa LA. Laboratory perspective on racial disparities in sexually transmitted infections. *The Journal of Applied Laboratory Medicine*. 2021; 6: 264–73.

Chapter 35 **Influenza**

Ali S. Raja[1] and Christopher R. Carpenter[2]

[1] Department of Emergency Medicine, Massachusetts General Hospital, Harvard Medical School, Boston, MA, USA
[2] Department of Emergency Medicine, Washington University School of Medicine, St. Louis, MO, USA

Highlights

- Assessing the current regional pretest probability of influenza is essential in distinguishing influenza from influenza-like illness mimics.
- Taken alone, no signs or symptoms accurately rule in or rule out the diagnosis of influenza.
- Rapid influenza tests can effectively rule in, but not rule out, the diagnosis of influenza. Both digital immunoassay and rapid nucleic acid amplification tests are more sensitive than rapid influenza tests.

Background

In typical years, up to 20% of residents in the United States develop influenza, resulting in between 140,000 and 710,000 annual hospitalizations between 2010 and 2020.[1] While the incidence of influenza has been significantly less during the coronavirus disease 2019 (COVID-19) pandemic,[2] once mask restrictions and physical distancing recommendations are withdrawn, influenza rates will likely return to their baseline levels. Influenza increases morbidity and mortality for a number of specific patient populations, including the very young and older adults and those with chronic lung disease.[3,4] Geriatric patients (>65 years) account for 71–85% of annual influenza deaths

---

Evidence-Based Emergency Care: Diagnostic Testing and Clinical Decision Rules, Third Edition.
Edited by Jesse M. Pines, Fernanda Bellolio, Christopher R. Carpenter, and Ali S. Raja.
© 2023 John Wiley & Sons Ltd. Published 2023 by John Wiley & Sons Ltd.

in the United States.[5] In general, healthy children and young adults do not experience life-threatening complications from influenza, but antigenic shifts in 1918, 1957, and 1968 were associated with viral pneumonia, acute respiratory distress syndrome, and multiorgan failure in these populations. Interpandemic influenza is an extremely unpleasant experience even for healthy individuals, with significant costs accrued due to diminished productivity, absenteeism, and related healthcare expenditures. In the United States, influenza results in between $2.0 and $5.8 billion in direct healthcare costs and $16.3 billion in lost earnings each year.[6,7]

Historically, emergency department (ED) resources have been occasionally strained by influenza-like illness (ILI) pandemics such as severe acute respiratory syndrome (SARS) in 2003 and H1N1 swine flu in 2009. The sustained multiyear COVID-19 pandemic has, of course, fundamentally changed the this into a long-term and devastating stress rather than an occasional periodic strain. Since infectious patients need to be sequestered during such pandemics in order to limit the exposure of the general population, diagnostic testing may be unavailable, emphasizing the importance of emergency clinicians' understanding of the diagnostic accuracy of bedside testing to distinguish influenza from ILI.[8] ILI is defined by the Centers for Disease Control (CDC) as a temperature higher than 37.8 °C with a cough or sore throat, but patients with influenza may present to the ED with a variety of atypical manifestations including delirium, falls, vomiting, incontinence, or diarrhea. Clinicians must integrate the chief complaint with a thorough review of systems within the context of their own regional influenza prevalence.[9]

Two strains of influenza exist (Type A and Type B) and are clinically indistinguishable. However, the distinction remains relevant because older antiviral agents (amantadine and rimantadine) are effective for Type A only – and even then, only somewhat. Many strains of influenza A, including the 2009 H1N1 variant, have been found to be resistant to these medications.[10] More modern antiviral medications like oseltamivir may be effective against both types – especially in high-risk populations – but only if used within 48 hours of symptom onset, emphasizing the importance of early diagnosis.[11] Unfortunately, the "viral syndrome" is not unique to influenza and may be the presentation for a variety of viral (coronavirus, rhinovirus, adenovirus, and parainfluenza virus) and bacterial (Legionella, Mycoplasma, and Streptococcal) respiratory infections that do not respond to anti-influenza therapy.

The prevalence of influenza is in a constant state of flux, influenced by the geographical region, time of year, and patient population. In the United States, the CDC maintains a weekly report of influenza activity stratified by region and influenza subtype (http://www.cdc.gov/flu/weekly/). Although these estimates are derived from office-based practices rather than the ED, they can be used to estimate regional influenza pretest probabilities while interpreting physical exam findings and contemplating viral testing and therapy. For example, in the week of 26 February 2022, the proportion of tested specimens that demonstrated influenza was 4.1% and ILI represented 1.5% of office visits. Therefore, the prevalence of influenza was $4.1\% \times 1.5\% = 0.062\%$ (the pretest probability). Similar influenza epidemiological data outside the United States are also available at the World Health Organization's Global Influenza Surveillance and Response System (https://www.who.int/ initiatives/global-influenza-surveillance-and-response-system).

Clinical question

What is the diagnostic accuracy of the history and physical exam for influenza?
One diagnostic meta-analysis, which intentionally neglected manuscripts in the immediate post-SARS period, focusing instead on influenza. Based upon six studies of 7105 patients (five prospective, none ED based), they reported the summary estimates as shown in Table 35.1.[12] Another systematic review that included two additional studies reported several more elements of the history that may be useful to rule in (rigors LR+ 7.2, fever and presenting within 3 days LR+ 4.0, and sweating LR+ 3.0) or rule out (any systemic symptoms LR− 0.36, coughing LR− 0.38, and inability to cope with daily activities LR− 0.39) influenza.[13]

Another systematic review evaluated the accuracy of clinical decision rules or combinations of signs and symptoms.[14] They were able to find 10 heterogeneous studies that presented 14 clinical decision rules. Only one of the rules (the Flu-Score) had been validated prospectively and externally,[15] with an area under the curve (AUC) of only 0.66 (confidence interval [CI] 0.63–0.70) in the validation study, limiting its clinical utility.

Stein *et al.* evaluated 258 consecutive adult ED or urgent care patients with respiratory tract infections during flu season, testing clinician gestalt against the "cough and fever" heuristic and using polymerase chain reaction (PCR) as the criterion standard. The prevalence of influenza was 21%. The heuristic had LR+ 5.1 and LR− 0.7 versus gestalt LR+ 3.6 and LR− 0.77. However, when stratified by how soon patients presented after symptom onset, clinical gestalt had LR+ 17.3 and LR− 0.4 if symptom onset was less than 48 hours prior to evaluation.[16] Friedman and Attia evaluated 128 children (ages 0–17 years) with ILI, defined as a temperature >38 °C in the ED and at least one additional symptom (coryza, cough, headache, sore throat, or muscle aches). The prevalence of influenza in their population was 35%, and the

Table 35.1 Diagnostic accuracy of signs or symptoms for influenza

Sign or symptom	Positive likelihood ratio	Negative likelihood ratio
Chills		
All ages	1.1	0.68
Only ≥60 years	2.6	0.66
Cough		
All ages	1.1	0.42
Only ≥60 years	2.0	0.57
Fever		
All ages	1.8	0.40
Only ≥60 years	3.8	0.72
Fever and cough		
All ages	1.9	0.54
Only ≥60 years	5.0	0.75
Fever, cough, and acute onset		
All ages	2.0	0.54
Only ≥60 years	5.4	0.77
Headache		
All ages	1.0	0.75
Only ≥60 years	1.9	0.70
Malaise		
All ages	0.98	1.1
Only ≥60 years	2.6	0.55
Myalgia		
All ages	0.93	1.2
Only ≥60 years	2.4	0.68
Sneezing		
All ages	1.2	0.87
Only ≥60 years	0.47	2.1
Sore throat		
All ages	1.0	0.96
Only ≥60 years	1.4	0.77
Vaccine history		
All ages	0.63	1.1

Source: Data from [12].

heuristic of cough–headache–pharyngitis was evaluated using viral cultures as the criterion standard, yielding LR+ 3.7 (CI 2.3–6.3) and LR– 0.26 (CI 0.14–0.44).[17] Another prediction rule has been derived to estimate the probability of hospitalization or all-cause mortality in community-dwelling older adults with the diagnosis of influenza. This score-based rule assesses age, gender, preillness outpatient visit rate, comorbidities, and prior pneumonia or influenza hospitalizations, yielding LR+ 8.1 (CI 5.0–13.3) and LR– 0.12 (CI 0.08–0.2) with a cutoff score of 50.[18]

Table 35.2 Diagnostic accuracy of influenza tests

Index test type	Influenza A: pooled sensitivity (CI)	Influenza A: pooled specificity (CI)	Influenza B: pooled sensitivity (CI)	Influenza B: pooled specificity (CI)
RIDT	54.4 (48.9–59.8)	99.4 (99.1–99.7)	53.2 (41.7–64.4)	99.8 (99.7–99.9)
DIA	80.0 (73.4–85.6)	98.3 (97.4–98.9)	76.8 (65.4–85.4)	98.7 (97.5–99.4)
Rapid NAAT	91.6 (84.9–95.9)	99.2 (98.6–99.7)	95.4 (87.3–98.7)	99.4 (98.9–99.8)

Source: Data from [19].

Clinical question

What is the diagnostic accuracy of rapid influenza tests compared to digital immunoassays (DIAs) and nucleic acid amplification tests (NAATs)?

The CDC maintains a summary of diagnostic accuracy information on rapid influenza tests for lab directors and clinicians (https://www.cdc.gov/flu/professionals/diagnosis/clinician_guidance_ridt.htm). A 2017 meta-analysis compared the traditional rapid influenza diagnostic tests (RIDTs), DIAs, and NAATs in both children and adults with suspected influenza.[19] The meta-analysis included a total of 162 studies, of which 130 focused on RIDTs (four different commercial brands), 19 focused on DIAs (two different commercial brands), and 13 focused on NAATs (also two different commercial brands). The majority of samples were via nasopharyngeal swab or aspirate, although some studies included throat swabs. Nine studies included samples from EDs. Pooled test characteristics for the three types of tests are included in Table 35.2. In general, a negative RIDT result or DIA result may not exclude the diagnosis in areas of high prevalence, but a negative NAAT result likely does. However, specificity for all three test types was high enough to rule the diagnosis in with any positive results. Another evidentiary review also focused on the impact of RIDT testing and found that the tests reduced overall diagnostic testing, antibiotic use, ED length of stay, and increased antiviral prescribing.[20]

Comment

History and physical exam are insufficient to rule in or rule out the diagnosis of influenza. Rapid tests are available, but they cannot be used to rule out the diagnosis in areas of high prevalence. This diagnostic challenge highlights the importance of emergency clinicians understanding their regional influenza prevalence while deciding upon ancillary influenza testing, antiviral therapy, or symptom management. Various patient-specific factors should influence antiviral treatment thresholds including symptom duration, vaccination status and anticipated vaccine efficacy, comorbid illness burden, and age-related susceptibility to suboptimal outcomes.

References

1. CDC. Burden of Influenza [Internet]. Centers for Disease Control and Prevention. Available from: https://www.cdc.gov/flu/about/burden/index.html. 2022. Accessed March 10, 2022.

2. Olsen SJ, Winn AK, Budd AP *et al.* Changes in influenza and other respiratory virus activity during the COVID-19 pandemic — United States, 2020–2021. *MMWR. Morbidity and Mortality Weekly Report.* 2021; 70(29): 1013–9.

3. Griffin MR, Coffey CS, Neuzil KM, Mitchel EF Jr, Wright PF, Edwards KM. Winter viruses: influenza- and respiratory syncytial virus–related morbidity in chronic lung disease. *Archives of Internal Medicine.* 2002; 162(11): 1229–36.

4. Hansen CL, Chaves SS, Demont C, Viboud C. Mortality associated with influenza and respiratory syncytial virus in the US, 1999-2018. *JAMA Network Open.* 2022; 5(2): e220527.

5. Reed C, Chaves SS, Kirley PD *et al.* Estimating influenza disease burden from population-based surveillance data in the United States. *PLoS One.* 2015; 10(3): e0118369.

6. Yan S, Weycker D, Sokolowski S. US healthcare costs attributable to type A and type B influenza. *Human Vaccines & Immunotherapeutics.* 2017; 13(9): 2041–7.

7. Molinari N-AM, Ortega-Sanchez IR, Messonnier ML *et al.* The annual impact of seasonal influenza in the US: Measuring disease burden and costs. *Vaccine.* 2007; 25(27): 5086–96.

8. Lee TC, Taggart LR, Mater B, Katz K, McGeer A. Predictors of pandemic influenza infection in adults presenting to two urban emergency departments, Toronto, 2009. *CJEM.* 2011; 13(1): 7–12.

9. Monmany J, Rabella N, Margall N, Domingo P, Gich I, Vázquez G. Unmasking influenza virus infection in patients attended to in the emergency department. *Infection.* 2004; 32(2): 89–97.

10. Research C for DE and. Influenza (Flu) Antiviral Drugs and Related Information. FDA [Internet]. Available from: https://www.fda.gov/drugs/information-drug-class/influenza-flu-antiviral-drugs-and-related-information. 2022. Accessed March 10, 2022.

11. Shim S-J, Chan M, Owens L, Jaffe A, Prentice B, Homaira N. Rate of use and effectiveness of oseltamivir in the treatment of influenza illness in high-risk populations: A systematic review and meta-analysis. *Health Science Reports.* 2021; 4(1): e241.

12. Call SA, Vollenweider MA, Hornung CA, Simel DL, McKinney WP. Does this patient have influenza? *Journal of the American Medical Association.* 2005; 293(8): 987–97.

13. Ebell MH, White LL, Casault T. A systematic review of the history and physical examination to diagnose influenza. *The Journal of the American Board of Family Practice.* 2004; 17(1): 1–5.

14. Ebell MH, Rahmatullah I, Cai X *et al.* A systematic review of clinical prediction rules for the diagnosis of influenza. *Journal of American Board of Family Medicine.* 2021; 34(6): 1123–40.

15. van Vugt SF, Broekhuizen BD, Zuithoff NP *et al.* Validity of a clinical model to predict influenza in patients presenting with symptoms of lower respiratory tract infection in primary care. *Family Practice.* 2015; 32(4): 408–14.

16. Stein J, Louie J, Flanders S *et al.* Performance characteristics of clinical diagnosis, a clinical decision rule, and a rapid influenza test in the detection of influenza infection in a community sample of adults. *Annals of Emergency Medicine.* 2005; 46(5): 412–9.

17. Friedman MJ, Attia MW. Clinical predictors of influenza in children. *Archives of Pediatrics & Adolescent Medicine.* 2004; 158(4): 391–4.

18. Hak E, Wei F, Nordin J, Mullooly J, Poblete S, Nichol KL. Development and validation of a clinical prediction rule for hospitalization due to pneumonia or influenza or death during influenza epidemics among community-dwelling elderly persons. *The Journal of Infectious Diseases.* 2004; 189(3): 450–8.

19. Merckx J, Wali R, Schiller I *et al.* Diagnostic accuracy of novel and traditional rapid tests for influenza infection compared with reverse transcriptase polymerase chain reaction: A systematic review and meta-analysis. *Annals of Internal Medicine.* 2017; 167(6): 394–409.

20. Petrozzino JJ, Smith C, Atkinson MJ. Rapid diagnostic testing for seasonal influenza: An evidence-based review and comparison with unaided clinical diagnosis. *The Journal of Emergency Medicine.* 2010; 39(4): 476–90.e1.

Chapter 36 **Fever without a Source 3–36 Months**

Jana L. Anderson and Fernanda Bellolio

Department of Emergency Medicine, Mayo Clinic, Rochester, MN, USA

Highlights

- Well appearing children, 3–36 months of age who are fully immunized for age, with fever ≥39 °C and no source, no longer require an empiric fever without source (FWS) evaluation, and should be assessed based on their risk of urinary tract infection and occult pneumonia.
- Well appearing, unimmunized or under-immunized children who present with FWS, warrant a FWS evaluation which includes a CBC with differential, procalcitonin, and urinalysis and possible blood culture and chest X-ray.
- Ill-appearing children require a full sepsis evaluation, antibiotics, and admission.

Background

The fever without a source (FWS) evaluation in children, 3–36 months of age with a temperature ≥39 °C, has a long history that starts prior to routine *Haemophilus influenzae* type b (Hib) and the conjugated pneumococcal vaccination. Back in the 1980s, occult bacteremia was common with a prevalence estimated at 3–12% of well-appearing children with FWS.[1,2] The concern was progression of occult bacteremia to serious bacterial infections (SBI) such as pneumonia, septic arthritis, cellulitis, sepsis, or meningitis. Hib is a very invasive bacterium, with a 12 times higher likelihood of causing meningitis than *Streptococcus pneumoniae* when bacteremia is present.[3] This led to the

---

Evidence-Based Emergency Care: Diagnostic Testing and Clinical Decision Rules, Third Edition.
Edited by Jesse M. Pines, Fernanda Bellolio, Christopher R. Carpenter, and Ali S. Raja.
© 2023 John Wiley & Sons Ltd. Published 2023 by John Wiley & Sons Ltd.

routine FWS work-up for well-appearing children, 3–36 months, with fever ≥39 °C and no source on physical examination. This evaluation included a complete blood count (CBC) and differential, and if elevated, a blood culture was sent, and antibiotics were administered. If the white blood cell (WBC) count was ≥20,000 a chest X-ray was performed.[2] Since the introduction of the Hib vaccination in 1987, the rate invasive *H. influenzae* infections has decreased to the point of near elimination of the disease.[4] The rate of occult bacteremia for FWS children after widespread Hib vaccination was then estimated at 1.9%, with the majority being due to *S. pneumoniae*.[5,6] In 2000, the first conjugated pneumococcal vaccine was introduced, and the rate of bacteremia in FWS children declined markedly to 0.25% in 2009.[7] Because the rate of occult bacteremia is so low, routine FWS evaluations are no longer recommended in fully vaccinated children.[8] Now, in the well-appearing, vaccinated child with FWS one must evaluate them for their risk for urinary tract infection (UTI) and occult pneumonia. Exceptions are children who are un- or under-vaccinated, who warrant assessment for occult bacteremia in addition to UTI and occult pneumonia. Also, children with FWS for ≥5 days warrant an evaluation for possible Kawasaki Syndrome, and in fever present for ≥7 days without a source, a fever of unknown origin evaluation should be performed.

In the child that is under-immunized due to age (2–6 months), it appears that risk for *S. pneumoniae* and *H. influenzae* bacteremia is not significantly increased and remarkably low at <1%. This low rate of bacteremia is likely due to maternal antibodies and herd immunity. Traditionally, the practice of drawing a CBC was performed while holding the blood culture and if WBC was >15,000 then sending the blood culture. One reason this was performed was the high rate of contamination of the blood culture, the ratio of blood culture contaminants is 7.6–1 for detecting one positive blood culture.[7] Now that inflammatory markers are available in a timely fashion, C-reactive protein (CRP) or procalcitonin may be helpful in detecting the child with possible bacteremia. In a systematic review and meta-analysis of over 7000 children with FWS, a procalcitonin >0.5 ng/mL was found to have a sensitivity of 82% and specificity of 86% for detecting invasive bacterial infection.[9] Procalcitonin has been found to be more sensitive and specific than CRP or WBC count.[10] In the older under- or un-vaccinated child (6–36 months) the rate of bacteremia was found to be low but up to 1.4%. Given the low rate of bacteremia in the under- or un-vaccinated child, inflammatory markers can be helpful to detect children at risk for SBI, and one must weigh the risk and benefits of workup on this population.

Most children with FWS that are well-appearing, have a self-limited viral illness.[11] UTIs are the most common occult bacterial infection in children presenting with FWS with a prevalence rate that differs by age, race, sex, and circumcision status.[12] The estimated prevalence of UTI for girls with FWS in the first year of life is between 5.7% and 8.5%, then declines to 2.1% between 12 and 24 months of age. The rate of UTI in febrile, uncircumcised boys 6–12 months of age is similar to girls, with a prevalence of 7.3%.[13] This is in stark contrast to circumcised boys, aged 6–12 months, where the prevalence of UTI is 0.3%; with an even lower estimate after 1 year. Given the relatively high prevalence of UTI as a source of FWS, current recommendations are to obtain a urinalysis and (if urinalysis is positive) urine culture, on all girls, age <24 months, uncircumcised boys <12 months of age, and circumcised boys <6 months.[14–16] Factors that increase the likelihood of a UTI are previous UTI, fever ≥39 °C, fever duration >2 days, nonblack race, uncircumcised male status, and suprapubic pain.[17] Once a UTI has been detected, the estimated rate of bacteremia in an older infant or child is 2–5% compared to up to 9% in an infant <3 months.[12,18,19] In a recent case-controlled study of young infants with febrile UTIs, the procalcitonin level was found to be elevated to 36.5 ng/mL (95% confidence interval [CI] 15–28) in the bacteremic group compared to nonbacteremic febrile UTIs with a procalcitonin of 5 ng/mL (95% CI 0.9–9).[20] These levels of procalcitonin are higher than the screening level for SBI in neonates at 0.5 ng/mL.

Occult pneumonia, having a focal lung infiltrate on chest-X-ray despite no cough or focal lung findings on examination, is an entity that was first recognized when chest X-rays were routinely performed on children with leukocytosis of ≥20,000/μL in the FWS work-up.[21] Even in the era of pneumococcal vaccination, occult pneumonia continues to be present in children with an elevated WBC count, with a prevalence of 15% prepneumococcal vaccine compared to 9% postpneumococcal vaccination. Routine CBC and blood culture are not recommended in the immunized child anymore. In a post-conjugate pneumococcal vaccine study of 146 patients with WBC ≥25,000/μL, the prevalence of pneumonia was 28%. In an immunized child with fever for 5 days, an empiric chest X-ray should be performed to evaluate for occult pneumonia, labs do not need to routinely be performed. In the un-immunized or under-immunized child, a CBC and blood culture would routinely be performed and if ≥20,000, chest X-ray should be performed. Other factors to help determine when a chest X-ray should be considered are when the oxygen saturation is <95% and there is tachypnea despite defervescence.

Clinical question

Does a well-appearing, vaccinated 3-month-old infant with fever of 39 °C for 2 days and no source of infection on examination require a CBC and blood culture?
If the child is well-appearing and has a negative urine, no lab work is necessary, close follow-up, and consideration of viral testing is all that is needed. The rate

of bacteremia in a well-appearing infant without a UTI is very low and estimated at <1%.[8] This infant, if vaccinated at 2 months, would have one dose of the conjugated pneumococcal vaccine and Hib, and therefore some protection from invasive infections, in addition, there is herd and maternal immunity at this age.[22,23] The use of procalcitonin to evaluate for risk for bacteremia in children is still unclear but has outperformed WBC, absolute neutrophil count (ANC), and CRP in the detection of SBI in children with a sensitivity of 83% and specificity of 69%.[10] In a meta-analysis the cut-off of 0.5 ng/mL has been suggested, this level is similar to the Step-by-Step febrile infant protocol suggested by Gomez *et al.*[24-26] and lower than the Pediatric Emergency Care Applied Research Network (PECARN) febrile infant protocol (1.71 ng/mL). This cut-off is much lower than the procalcitonin levels found in infants with bacteremic (36 ng/mL) versus nonbacteremic febrile (5 ng/mL) UTIs.

If the infant has a UTI, given the young age of 3 months, the risk of bacteremia in the setting of UTI is higher. A conservative approach will be to send a CBC, procalcitonin, and a blood culture. The decision to admit depends on how the infant is feeding and the ability to take oral antibiotics, also the comfort of the parents and transportation should be considered.[27] Another approach is to treat the UTI with an oral third-generation cephalosporin and have close follow-up within 1–2 days.

Clinical question

What work-up does an unimmunized, uncircumcised 2-year-old male require with fever of 39 °C for 5 days who appears well?
Being unimmunized places this child with FWS at substantial risk for bacteremia and sequelae from *H. influenzae* and *S. pneumoniae* at an estimated rate of 2.8%.[2] In addition a child with fever for 5 days should be assessed for the risk of Kawasaki. A CBC with differential, inflammatory markers, and blood culture should be sent. An X-ray should be obtained to evaluate for pneumonia. If the child has not had a previous UTI, even though he is uncircumcised, he is at low risk of UTI estimated <1%.[17,28] If no source is found on the chest X-ray for the fever and leukocytosis, shared decision-making about the risk for UTI would be the next step.

References

1. Fleisher GR, Rosenberg N, Vinci R *et al.* Intramuscular versus oral antibiotic therapy for the prevention of meningitis and other bacterial sequelae in young, febrile children at risk for occult bacteremia. *The Journal of Pediatrics.* 1994; 124: 504–12.

2. Jaffe DM, Tanz RR, Davis AT, Henretig F, Fleisher G. Antibiotic administration to treat possible occult bacteremia in febrile children. *The New England Journal of Medicine.* 1987; 317: 1175–80.

3. Shapiro ED, Aaron NH, Wald ER, Chiponis D. Risk factors for development of bacterial meningitis among children with occult bacteremia. *The Journal of Pediatrics.* 1986; 109: 15–9.

4. Centers for Disease Control and Prevention. Progress toward elimination of *Haemophilus influenzae* type b disease among infants and children – United States, 1987-1995. *MMWR. Morbidity and Mortality Weekly Report.* 1996; 45: 901–6.

5. Alpern ER, Alessandrini EA, Bell LM, Shaw KN, McGowan KL. Occult bacteremia from a pediatric emergency department: Current prevalence, time to detection, and outcome. *Pediatrics.* 2000; 106: 505–11.

6. Lee GM, Harper MB. Risk of bacteremia for febrile young children in the post-*Haemophilus influenzae* type b era. *Archives of Pediatrics & Adolescent Medicine.* 1998; 152: 624–8.

7. Wilkinson M, Bulloch B, Smith M. Prevalence of occult bacteremia in children aged 3 to 36 months presenting to the emergency department with fever in the postpneumococcal conjugate vaccine era. *Academic Emergency Medicine.* 2009; 16: 220–5.

8. Carstairs KL, Tanen DA, Johnson AS, Kailes SB, Riffenburgh RH. Pneumococcal bacteremia in febrile infants presenting to the emergency department before and after the introduction of the heptavalent pneumococcal vaccine. *Annals of Emergency Medicine.* 2007; 49: 772–7.

9. Trippella G, Galli L, De Martino M, Lisi C, Chiappini E. Procalcitonin performance in detecting serious and invasive bacterial infections in children with fever without apparent source: A systematic review and meta-analysis. *Expert Review of Anti-Infective Therapy.* 2017; 15: 1041–57.

10. Yo CH, Hsieh PS, Lee SH *et al.* Comparison of the test characteristics of procalcitonin to C-reactive protein and leukocytosis for the detection of serious bacterial infections in children presenting with fever without source: A systematic review and meta-analysis. *Annals of Emergency Medicine.* 2012; 60: 591–600.

11. Finkelstein JA, Christiansen CL, Platt R. Fever in pediatric primary care: Occurrence, management, and outcomes. *Pediatrics.* 2000; 105: 260–6.

12. Hoberman A, Chao HP, Keller DM, Hickey R, Davis HW, Ellis D. Prevalence of urinary tract infection in febrile infants. *The Journal of Pediatrics.* 1993; 123: 17–23.

13. Marild S, Jodal U. Incidence rate of first-time symptomatic urinary tract infection in children under 6 years of age. *Acta Paediatrica.* 1998; 87: 549–52.

14. Newman TB. The new American Academy of Pediatrics urinary tract infection guideline. *Pediatrics.* 2011; 128: 572–5.

15. Newman TB. Evidence basis for individualized evaluation and less imaging in febrile urinary tract infection: An editorial commentary. *Pediatric Clinics of North America.* 2012; 59: 923–6.

16. Subcommittee on Urinary Tract Infection SCoQI, Management, Roberts KB. Urinary tract infection: Clinical practice guideline for the diagnosis and management of the initial UTI in febrile infants and children 2 to 24 months. *Pediatrics.* 2011; 128: 595–610.

17. Shaikh N, Morone NE, Bost JE, Farrell MH. Prevalence of urinary tract infection in childhood: A meta-analysis. *The Pediatric Infectious Disease Journal.* 2008; 27: 302–8.

18. Megged O. Bacteremic vs nonbacteremic urinary tract infection in children. *The American Journal of Emergency Medicine.* 2017; 35: 36–8.

19. Pitetti RD, Choi S. Utility of blood cultures in febrile children with UTI. *The American Journal of Emergency Medicine.* 2002; 20: 271–4.

20. Goeller C, Desmarest M, Garraffo A, Bonacorsi S, Gaschignard J. Management of febrile urinary tract infection with or without bacteraemia in children: A French case-control retrospective study. *Frontiers in Pediatrics.* 2020; 8: 237.

21. Bachur R, Perry H, Harper MB. Occult pneumonias: Empiric chest radiographs in febrile children with leukocytosis. *Annals of Emergency Medicine.* 1999; 33: 166–73.

22. Loo JD, Conklin L, Fleming-Dutra KE *et al.* Systematic review of the indirect effect of pneumococcal conjugate vaccine dosing schedules on pneumococcal disease and colonization. *The Pediatric Infectious Disease Journal.* 2014; 33(Suppl 2): S161–71.

23. Whitney CG, Goldblatt D, O'Brien KL. Dosing schedules for pneumococcal conjugate vaccine: Considerations for policy makers. *The Pediatric Infectious Disease Journal.* 2014; 33(Suppl 2): S172–81.

24. Gomez B, Mintegi S, Bressan S *et al.* Validation of the "step-by-step" approach in the management of young febrile infants. *Pediatrics.* 2016; 138: e20154381.

25. Jones AE, Fiechtl JF, Brown MD, Ballew JJ, Kline JA. Procalcitonin test in the diagnosis of bacteremia: A meta-analysis. *Annals of Emergency Medicine.* 2007; 50: 34–41.

26. Kuppermann N, Dayan PS, Levine DA *et al.* A clinical prediction rule to identify febrile infants 60 days and younger at low risk for serious bacterial infections. *JAMA Pediatrics.* 2019; 173: 342–51.

27. Hoberman A, Wald ER, Hickey RW *et al.* Oral versus initial intravenous therapy for urinary tract infections in young febrile children. *Pediatrics.* 1999; 104: 79–86.

28. Shaikh N, Morone NE, Lopez J *et al.* Does this child have a urinary tract infection? *JAMA.* 2007; 298: 2895–904.

SECTION 5
Surgical and Abdominal Complaints

Chapter 37 **Acute, Nonspecific, Nontraumatic Abdominal Pain**

Lucas Oliveira Junqueira e Silva[1,2] and Fernanda Bellolio[2]

[1] Department of Emergency Medicine, Hospital de Clínicas de Porto Alegre, Porto Alegre, Brazil
[2] Department of Emergency Medicine, Mayo Clinic, Rochester, MN, USA

Highlights

- Plain abdominal X-rays are not helpful in ruling out serious abdominal diagnoses in patients with abdominal pain.
- Noncontrast abdominal CT identifies intra-abdominal pathologies with high sensitivity and specificity.
- Ultrasound has a role in ruling out specific etiologies of abdominal pain like gallstones, hydronephrosis, cholecystitis, and appendicitis.
- The threshold for ordering an abdominopelvic CT in older adults presenting with acute, nonspecific, nontraumatic abdominal pain should be low given the low diagnostic yield of history and physical exam in this population and high rates of underlying serious diagnoses.

Background

Acute abdominal pain is one of the most common presenting complaints to the emergency department (ED), accounting for up to 8.8% of all ED visits in 2018.[1] A study using the National Hospital Ambulatory Medical Care Survey (NHAMCS)[2] estimated 23 million visits for abdominal pain in 2013. Computerized tomography (CT) scans were used in 30.1% of the visits in 2010 and 28.6% in 2013. More than 50% of the visits received diagnostic imaging, and less than 20% became hospital admissions.[2]

Evidence-Based Emergency Care: Diagnostic Testing and Clinical Decision Rules, Third Edition.
Edited by Jesse M. Pines, Fernanda Bellolio, Christopher R. Carpenter, and Ali S. Raja.
© 2023 John Wiley & Sons Ltd. Published 2023 by John Wiley & Sons Ltd.

Developments in imaging techniques have dramatically changed the ED evaluation of abdominal pain, with CT and ultrasound (US) widely used in current practice. Most presentations of acute abdominal pain fall into one of eight diagnoses: appendicitis, bowel obstruction, cholecystitis, renal colic, peptic ulcer disease, pancreatitis, diverticular disease, and nonspecific abdominal pain. With such a wide array of potential etiologies for abdominal pain, the clinician must decide how to rationally use diagnostic tests and not to miss any serious diagnoses against concerns for costs of testing, length of stay, and adverse effects of imaging. Concerns for overuse, incidental findings, and radiation risks have been raised, and a consensus conference was convened in 2015 resulting in a research agenda to optimize diagnostic imaging in the ED.[3]

Laboratory tests, such as complete blood count, urinalysis, liver function tests, and tests for pancreatic enzymes are ordered on approximately 70% of ED patients with acute nontraumatic abdominal pain.[2,4] While many studies have evaluated the usefulness of laboratory tests in the diagnosis of specific conditions (e.g., appendicitis), few studies evaluated laboratory tests among all acute undifferentiated abdominal pain. None of these studies reliably determined whether a laboratory test changed the diagnosis, so we will not discuss lab testing for undifferentiated abdominal pain patients in this chapter.

Imaging modalities available include plain abdominal radiography, CT (with or without intravenous and oral contrast), US, and magnetic resonance imaging (MRI), leaving clinicians with a choice of which tests to order and in what sequence. While it seems that a clinical decision rule could be helpful with this decision, nontraumatic abdominal pain is a heterogeneous presenting complaint, and to date, no rule has been validated.[5] In this chapter, we will address the role of imaging in acute undifferentiated abdominal pain, including comments on special populations such as older adults. In subsequent chapters, we address tests for the most common causes of acute nontraumatic abdominal pain.

Clinical question

Which diagnostic imaging modality is most sensitive in diagnosing patients with acute undifferentiated abdominal pain?

Several studies have evaluated how abdominal CT changes diagnoses, the admission decision, and the need for surgery in ED patients. One randomized study concluded that early CT scanning in patients with acute abdominal pain improves diagnostic accuracy, and might reduce the duration of hospitalization and mortality.[6] A prospective study evaluated the added value of CT in 536 consecutive patients with nontraumatic acute abdominal pain.[7] Physicians responded to five questions prior to ordering the CT scan, including their pretest diagnostic impression and level of certainty about intended management before CT results were available. Pre and posttest diagnoses were concordant for only 37% of the patients. CT scanning was associated with a reduction in rates of planned immediate surgical intervention from 13% to 5% and reduced the perceived need for admission by 17%. The authors concluded that ED use of CT was associated with increased diagnostic certainty, reduced unnecessary surgery, and hospital admissions, and that the value of CT is greater than its direct costs. Barksdale *et al.*[8] in a prospective cohort of 547 ED patients with nontraumatic abdominal pain, found that 54% had a significant change in their diagnosis based on the CT scanning.

Plain abdominal radiography has limited value in the ED setting and several studies have demonstrated its lower accuracy than other diagnostic modalities. A small study compared noncontrast abdominal CT with three-view plain abdominal radiography in patients with abdominal pain within the previous 7 days.[9] Among 103 patients, CT had a sensitivity of 96% (95% confidence interval [CI] 86–100%), specificity of 95% (95% CI 83–99%), and accuracy of 96%. The abdominal X-ray series had a sensitivity of 30% (95% CI 18–45%), specificity of 88% (95% CI 74–96%), and accuracy of 56%. Noncontrast abdominal CT revealed the cause of acute abdominal pain, including many of the concerning surgical or medically emergent or urgent causes, significantly better than plain films, and CT led to the discovery of pathology that was not identified using plain radiography. This study also supported that noncontrast CT has sufficiently high sensitivity, specificity, and accuracy to make it a clinically useful study.[9] Another study of undifferentiated acute abdominal pain compared the diagnostic yield of abdominal plain radiography and abdominal CT scanning.[10] Out of 1000 patients, only 120 had both plain abdominal imaging and abdominal CTs performed. Plain abdominal radiography had sensitivities of 0% (95% CI ranges 0–84%) for the diagnosis of urolithiasis, appendicitis, pyelonephritis, pancreatitis, and diverticulitis. X-rays had sensitivity of 33% (95% CI 25–42%) for bowel obstruction. The specificity for all the diagnoses was 100% (95% CI range 96–100%). The authors concluded that plain abdominal radiography was insufficiently sensitive in the evaluation of acute nontraumatic abdominal pain.[10] Gerhardt *et al.*[11] examined 165 patients with acute nontraumatic nonspecific abdominal pain undergoing abdominal imaging. The need for urgent intervention within 24 hours was 13%, and 34% underwent elective interventions that mitigated morbidity or mortality. They found that noncontrast abdominal CT was the most accurate variable for prediction of an acute medical or surgical intervention. In a classification and regression tree analysis, the combination of history, physical exam, acute abdominal series imaging, and noncontrast abdominal CT imaging yielded the best test characteristics to predict the need for medical or surgical intervention (sensitivity 92%, specificity 90%, a LR+ of 9.2, and a LR− of 0.09). Other models that did not include CT imaging had lower sensitivities and specificities and were felt to be clinically unacceptable. The authors of this derivation study concluded that noncontrast abdominal CT was useful and the imaging study of choice when faced with nonspecific abdominal pain.[11]

A systematic review by Alshamari *et al.*[12] compared the use of low-dose CT scanning with abdominal radiography in diagnosing patients who present with nontraumatic acute abdominal pain. The sensitivity of low-dose CT ranged from 75% to 96%, while the sensitivity of abdominal radiography ranged from 30% to 77%.

A prospective study in the Netherlands evaluated eleven possible diagnostic strategies in 1021 nonpregnant adults with acute abdominal pain.[13] The strategies included clinical evaluation alone or in combination with plain X-rays, US, and/or CT scanning. Physician reviewers later classified the patients as having had an urgent or a nonurgent condition (treatment within 24 hours not required) based on 6-month follow-up. The prevalence of urgent conditions was 65%. Clinical evaluation alone was 88% sensitive and 41% specific for an "urgent" condition. US to all patients would have been less sensitive (70%), but more specific (85%). Two strategies that involved doing US in all patients were the most sensitive: US followed by CT scanning if the US is negative or inconclusive (sensitivity 94%, specificity 68%), or CT only if the US is negative (sensitivity 85%, specificity 76%). These two strategies would result in the lowest use of CT (49% and 27% of patients, respectively). The authors concluded that in nonpregnant adults with acute abdominal pain, if a clinician thinks imaging is required, then US should be the initial modality, followed by CT, as US has high sensitivity and can reduce the use of CT by about half.[13]

Subsequent studies concluded that CT and US have been shown to increase diagnostic accuracy substantially and have decreased the added diagnostic value of plain abdominal radiography and that there is no place for plain abdominal radiography in the workup of ED adult patients with acute nonspecific abdominal pain in current practice.[14]

The decision to order a CT should be based on clinical judgment. However, there is a high variability in the use of CT between emergency physicians. Cross *et al.*[15] performed a retrospective study including 6409 ED visits for nontraumatic abdominal pain to evaluate physician- and patient-level factors. They found that among physician-level factors, only those with more than 21 years of experience after medical school graduation were less likely to order a CT. After adjusting for physician-level factors, they found that patient-visit factors (e.g., age, arrival model, admission team, prior CT, ED arrival time, US, and white blood cell [WBC] count) were key reasons behind CT ordering practice.

Diagnostic US has been widely studied for specific abdominal diagnoses (e.g., gallstones). However, its use in acute nonspecific abdominal pain by emergency physicians has not been comprehensively studied. Hasani et al.[16] prospectively compared the diagnostic accuracy of emergency physicians with radiologists when using point-of-care US in patients presenting to the ED with acute nontraumatic abdominal pain. Emergency physicians had a diagnostic accuracy of 78%, sensitivity of 76%, and specificity of 81%. The radiologists had similar performance with accuracy of 78.6%, sensitivity of 82%, and specificity of 73%. They found that emergency physicians had better results in diagnosing some entities (abdominal aortic aneurysm [AAA] and renal stones) than others (acute appendicitis, cholelithiasis, and cholecystitis). A systematic review of the diagnostic characteristics of point-of-care US in the ED for diagnosing AAA, included seven high-quality studies[17] and showed excellent performance (pooled sensitivity 99% [95% CI 96–100%], specificity 98% [95% CI 97–99%]). In unstable patients presenting with undifferentiated abdominal pain in which AAA is suspected, point-of-care US should be the initial study of choice.

Jang et al.[18] performed a pilot study to assess the impact of emergency physician-performed US on diagnostic testing and decision-making in ED patients presenting with nonspecific abdominal pain. A total of 128 patients were included, of which 58 (45%) had an improvement in diagnostic accuracy and planned diagnostic workup with emergency physician-performed US.

While different imaging modalities are used to evaluate the undifferentiated patient with abdominal pain in the ED, a systematic review published in 2018 found 10 studies evaluating diagnostic pathways to be used in this population.[19] Only five studies developed their pathways based on prospective studies, however, none of these studies have evaluated the impact on complication rates, hospital length of stay, or cost. Although based on low-quality evidence, most studies recommend the use of routine US followed by CT scan when there is still diagnostic uncertainty. The authors highlight the fact that sensitivity and accuracy of US are operator and hospital dependent, and this should be considered when developing diagnostic protocols in the ED.

Lastly, there are few diagnoses that are infrequent as the cause of acute nontraumatic abdominal pain in the ED. Acute mesenteric ischemia is such example and it has an estimated annual incidence of 0.09–0.2% per patient-year. However, the mortality associated with this condition is very high and it is often a concern of emergency physicians. This diagnosis is not further discussed in other chapters, and we will briefly discuss it here. A systematic review and meta-analysis by Cudnik et al.[20] evaluated the diagnostic characteristics of history, physical exam, laboratory, and imaging modalities for the diagnosis of acute mesenteric ischemia. They included a total of 23 studies in their analysis. While no characteristics of history and physical exam had good discriminatory ability, acute abdominal pain was present in 60–100% of patients, and a history of atrial fibrillation was present in up to 79% of patients. Laboratory modalities including lactate and D-dimer had poor sensitivity and specificity. However, multidetector CT had a pooled sensitivity of 94% (95% CI 90–97) and specificity of 95% (95% CI 93–97), with a pooled LR+ of 17.5 and LR– of 0.09. The authors also calculated a test threshold of 2.1% and a treatment threshold of 74%. Although difficult to estimate pretest probabilities given limited data, this would translate to order a CT in all but the very low pretest probability patients and consider immediate surgical consultation for those with high pretest probability (higher than 74%).

Older adults

Older adults with abdominal pain are at higher risk for adverse events as they are more likely to have life-threatening etiologies, confounding overlying comorbidities, and often present later in the course of disease with nonspecific symptoms. For this reason, emergency physicians should have a low threshold for ordering imaging in this population.

In a retrospective cohort study, Henden Çam et al.[21] evaluated 336 older adults who presented with abdominal pain to the ED. A total of 164 (48.8%) patients were hospitalized and 59 (17.6%) received a surgical treatment. While 258 (76.8%) had a diagnosis established for the origin of the abdominal pain, in 9.8% of patients the pain was related to malignancy. In a large registry-based cohort study in Sweden,[22] Ferlander et al. examined the percentage of patients being diagnosed with *de novo* cancer within a year after ED discharge for a visit in which they received a diagnosis of nonspecific abdominal pain. Among 24,801 patients discharged from the ED with "nonspecific abdominal pain," 556 (2.2%) were diagnosed with malignancy within 1 year. Among these 556 patients, 352 (63.3%) were 60 years or older.

Esses et al. prospectively studied the value of CT in 104 stable older adults with abdominal pain in the ED.[23] They asked ordering clinicians questions about the need for admission, surgery, and antibiotics and compared the answers to the post-CT management. They found that the post-CT decisions around admission were changed for 26% of the patients, decisions about a need for surgery were changed for 12%, and decisions about antibiotic therapy were changed for 21% of the patients. Hustey et al.[24] prospectively evaluated a cohort of 337 patients aged 60 years and older. Among older adults with acute nontraumatic abdominal pain, 37% had abdominal CT. The leading diagnoses were diverticulitis (18%), bowel obstruction (18%), nephrolithiasis (10%), and gallbladder disease (10%). CT was diagnostic in 57% of patients overall, in 75% of patients requiring acute intervention, and 85% of patients requiring acute surgical intervention. In an older population aged ≥80, Gardner et al.[25] performed a retrospective cohort study to evaluate patients who presented to the ED with acute nontraumatic abdominal symptoms and underwent abdominal CT. They classified the CT as negative or positive for "actionable" findings, defined as those potentially requiring a change in surgical or medical management. Among 464 patients, the abdominal CT was positive in 255 (55%) patients. The most common diagnosis was small bowel obstruction (18%). Among all diagnoses made with the CT, there were 43% who were clinically unsuspected prior to CT, highlighting the difficulty of history and physical exam on determining pretest probabilities in this population. In this study, the CT results significantly influenced management in 36% of all patients (166/464). Among the 55 who required operative management, 49 (89%) were influenced by the CT findings.

Based on the idea that early CT for this population is often beneficial, Millet et al.[26] published a prospective cohort study evaluating the impact of early systematic unenhanced abdominal CT scan for all older adults (age ≥ 75) presenting to the ED with acute nontraumatic abdominal symptoms. Among 401 older adults included, mechanical bowel obstruction (11.5%), fecal impaction (12.2%), and nonspecific abdominal pain (10.7%) were the most common diagnoses. Although the CT was requested by the emergency physician in 312 cases (77.8%), all patients received an abdominal noncontrast CT in the ED. In the group for which CT was not requested by the emergency physician, noncontrast CT led to a diagnosis of acute unsuspected disorders in 30.3% of cases, and it changed the management in 37.1% of cases. Among the acute unsuspected pathologies that the CT led to, 3.4% had to undergo surgical management.[26]

The authors of all studies abovementioned concluded that the increase in diagnostic certainty and improved management support the early use of CT in the ED for older adults with abdominal pain.

Clinical question

Is contrast necessary for CT imaging for diagnosing patients presenting with acute nontraumatic abdominal pain?

The widespread use of CT and progress in the quality of images provided by new scanners have raised questions about the utility of enhanced imaging with contrast in this era. Obtaining an initial noncontrast CT is associated with short-term repeat CT imaging for abdominal pain.[27] In a prospective cohort study including 118 patients presenting to the ED with acute abdominal pain, Lee et al.[28] compared the agreement between noncontrast CT with oral contrast-enhanced CT. There was an agreement of 79% between these two methods, and for only one patient did the radiologists agree that there was a definite discordant result. Payor et al.[29] studied 72 consecutive patients with acute nontraumatic abdominal pain who underwent noncontrast CT in the ED. None of the patients included in their study had a clinically important result missed by the noncontrast CT. Barat et al.[30] compared the use of unenhanced CT with contrast-enhanced CT for older adults (age ≥ 75) presenting to the ED with acute nontraumatic abdominal pain. Patients were included if they had abdominopelvic CT with both pre- and postcontrast acquisitions. Three independent radiologists reviewed all images and diagnostic accuracy of both methods were compared to the standard reference defined as a final diagnosis based on clinical, laboratory, and radiological evaluations. The diagnostic accuracy for unenhanced CT ranged from 64% to 68%, while it ranged from 68% to 71% when the contrast-enhanced images were included. The inter-reader agreement was substantial for unenhanced images (kappa 0.74–0.78). The authors concluded that unenhanced CT alone is accurate and associated with a high inter-reader agreement for evaluating acute nontraumatic abdominal pain in older adults presenting to the ED.[30]

Although noncontrast CT seems to have good diagnostic accuracy on this population, several protocols require the use of IV and oral contrast for patients presenting to the ED with acute nontraumatic abdominal pain. The administration of oral contrast often leads to a prolonged ED length of stay. Razavi et al.[31] investigated the impact of implementing a protocol without oral contrast for abdominopelvic CT evaluations on radiology turnaround time and ED length of stay. The study included 6409 abdominopelvic CTs for evaluation of acute nontraumatic abdominal pain. The protocol without oral contrast had significantly decreased radiology turnaround time (36-minutes reduction) and reduced ED length of stay (43-minutes reduction). Schuur et al.[32] performed a similar study with a before–after design to evaluate the impact of change in the protocol of oral contrast use. There was an absolute reduction of 30.3% of oral contrast use and the median ED length of stay decreased by 30 minutes after the implementation of the protocol. Basile et al.[33] performed a small before–after study to evaluate the implementation of a protocol that a specified oral contrast should only be used for abdominopelvic CT scans if body mass index (BMI) < 25 (with less intra-abdominal fat) or young patients (age < 30), or if there was a history of inflammatory bowel disease, gastrointestinal surgery, or suspected bowel malignancy.

The mean ED length of stay decreased by 29 minutes from the pre-(365 minutes) to the postimplementation (336 minutes) period.

Uyeda et al.[34] specifically evaluated whether using a BMI-based criterion is appropriate to make the decision about the use of oral contrast when evaluating acute nontraumatic abdominal pain. BMI is a surrogate marker of intra-abdominal fat as greater degrees of intra-abdominal fat may ease diagnostic evaluation by providing an inherent intra-abdominal contrast.[34] Among 1992 patients with BMI > 25 undergoing abdominopelvic CT with IV contrast and without oral contrast for nontraumatic acute abdominal pain, they found that only four patients (0.2%) had to undergo repeat CT studies directly related to the absence of oral contrast in the original imaging acquisition. Similarly, Wu et al.[35] found that 97% of the patients with BMI ≥ 25 had sufficient intraabdominal and intrapelvic fat to allow delineation of anatomic structures without the use of oral contrast material. Kessner et al.[36] performed a retrospective cohort study in Israel comparing patients presenting to the ED with acute nontraumatic abdominal pain who received IV contrast-enhanced abdominal CT either with or without oral contrast. Among 348 patients, 174 received IV contrast only, and 174 received both IV and oral contrast. There were no significant differences between distribution of clinical diagnoses and no differences in technical adequacy measured by radiologists. In fact, among the patients who received oral contrast, the material reached the area of pathology in only 42 of 61 (68.9%) patients who had a bowel-related disease. The radiologists determined that the oral contrast was useful only in eight patients and that only six patients who did not receive oral contrast would benefit from it.

Other studies focus on CT for specific pathologies and are detailed in other chapters, for example, a systematic review looking at the role of IV and oral contrast for acute appendicitis included six studies with 1949 patients and demonstrated no benefit of oral contrast when compared to no oral contrast. The same review included eight studies with 1297 patients and concluded no benefit of IV contrast when compared to noncontrast CT for appendicitis.[37]

Comments

Acute abdominal pain is a common presenting complaint in the ED, frequently represents serious pathology, and is difficult to diagnose clinically. A thorough history and physical exam are critical for clinicians to develop a differential diagnosis and corresponding pretest probabilities. While laboratory tests can be useful for the diagnosis of specific disorders, the routine use of broad laboratory panels (e.g., "belly labs") for patients with nontraumatic abdominal pain is costly and it has not been proven to increase diagnostic accuracy.[38] Rather, clinicians should tailor their laboratory ordering to specific diagnoses for which they have a moderate to high pretest probability.

Multiple studies show that CT scanning is the most sensitive and specific diagnostic imaging modality for acute abdominal pain, and it is likely to be the most useful initial test in patients in whom there is not a clear leading diagnosis and in high-risk patient populations, such as older adults and the immunosuppressed. Due to its diagnostic accuracy and availability, CT use has increased exponentially in EDs, leading to concerns that it is used inappropriately.[27] Further research is needed to define a subset of abdominal pain patients that can safely be evaluated without CT. Some centers may adopt protocols using US as a first imaging modality of choice, followed by CT when the US is equivocal or negative. While this will reduce the use of CT, the vast majority of EDs do not have access to skilled ultrasonographers at all times of day and night. For now, individual clinicians will continue to use their judgment in ordering CT. Additionally, it is important that clinicians avoid premature closure when working up patients with acute abdominal pain, especially in those with recurrent abdominal pain in which psychiatric disorders are frequent and may lead to stop thinking about other potential causes of abdominal pain.[39]

The role of imaging in patients with recurrent abdominal pain was recently evaluated in the Guidelines for Reasonable and Appropriate Care in the Emergency department (GRACE).[40] A patient with a normal or nondiagnostic CT of the abdomen and pelvis might have the final diagnosis of nonspecific abdominal pain. If the abdominal pain is recurrent, the GRACE-2 guidelines found insufficient evidence to accurately identify populations in whom repeat CT imaging can be safely avoided or routinely advocated.[41] The guidelines also reported that CT of abdomen and pelvis, particularly if performed with IV contrast, is very sensitive for abdominal and pelvic surgical pathology, and US after a negative CT rarely (<0.3%) identifies pathology that requires immediate intervention. US may be beneficial in cases of suspected female pelvic pathology and/or gallbladder disease, which could improve diagnostic certainty in less than 10% of the cases.[42-45] The GRACE-2 recommendation advises against routine US after a normal CT, unless there is specific ongoing concern for pelvic or biliary pathology.[41]

References

1. National Center for Health Statistics. NAMCS and NHAMCS Web Tables: NHAMCS - Emergency Department Summary Tables. https://www.cdc.gov/nchs/ahcd/web_tables.htm. Accessed December 2, 2021.

2. Meltzer AC, Pines JM, Richards LM, Mullins P, Mazer-Amirshahi M. US emergency department visits for adults with abdominal and pelvic pain (2007–13): Trends in demographics, resource utilization and medication usage. *The American Journal of Emergency Medicine.* 2017; 35(12): 1966–9. doi: 10.1016/j.ajem.2017.06.019.

3. Marin JR, Mills AM. Developing a research agenda to optimize diagnostic imaging in the emergency department: An executive summary of the 2015 Academic Emergency Medicine consensus conference. *Academic Emergency Medicine.* 2015; 22(12): 1363–71. doi: 10.1111/acem.12818.

4. Nagurney JT, Brown DFM, Chang Y, Sane S, Wang AC, Weiner JB. Use of diagnostic testing in the emergency department for patients presenting with non-traumatic abdominal pain. *The Journal of Emergency Medicine.* 2003; 25(4): 363–71. doi: 10.1016/s0736-4679(03)00237-3.

5. Finnerty NM, Rodriguez RM, Carpenter CR *et al.* Clinical decision rules for diagnostic imaging in the emergency department: A research agenda. *Academic Emergency Medicine.* 2015; 22(12): 1406–16. doi: 10.1111/ACEM.12828.

6. Ng CS, Watson CJE, Palmer CR *et al.* Evaluation of early abdominopelvic computed tomography in patients with acute abdominal pain of unknown cause: Prospective randomised study. *BMJ.* 2002; 325(7377): 1387. doi: 10.1136/bmj.325.7377.1387.

7. Rosen MP, Siewert B, Sands DZ, Bromberg R, Edlow J, Raptopoulos V. Value of abdominal CT in the emergency department for patients with abdominal pain. *European Radiology.* 2003; 13(2): 418–24. doi: 10.1007/s00330-002-1715-5.

8. Barksdale AN, Hackman JL, Gaddis M, Gratton MC. Diagnosis and disposition are changed when board-certified emergency physicians use CT for non-traumatic abdominal pain. *The American Journal of Emergency Medicine.* 2015; 33(11): 1646–50. doi: 10.1016/j.ajem.2015.07.082.

9. MacKersie AB, Lane MJ, Gerhardt RT *et al.* Nontraumatic acute abdominal pain: Unenhanced helical CT compared with three-view acute abdominal series. *Radiology.* 2005; 237(1): 114–22. doi: 10.1148/radiol.2371040066.

10. Ahn SH, Mayo-Smith WW, Murphy BL, Reinert SE, Cronan JJ. Acute nontraumatic abdominal pain in adult patients: Abdominal radiography compared with CT evaluation. *Radiology.* 2002; 225(1): 159–64. doi: 10.1148/radiol.2251011282.

11. Gerhardt RT, Nelson BK, Keenan S, Kernan L, MacKersie A, Lane MS. Derivation of a clinical guideline for the assessment of nonspecific abdominal pain: The Guideline for Abdominal Pain in the ED Setting (GAPEDS) Phase 1 Study. *The American Journal of Emergency Medicine.* 2005; 23(6): 709–17. doi: 10.1016/j.ajem.2005.01.010.

12. Alshamari M, Norrman E, Geijer M, Jansson K, Geijer H. Diagnostic accuracy of low-dose CT compared with abdominal radiography in non-traumatic acute abdominal pain: Prospective study and systematic review. *European Radiology.* 2016; 26(6): 1766–74. doi: 10.1007/s00330-015-3984-9.

13. Laméris W, Van Randen A, Wouter Van Es H *et al.* Imaging strategies for detection of urgent conditions in patients with acute abdominal pain: Diagnostic accuracy study. *BMJ.* 2009; 339(7711): 29–33. doi: 10.1136/bmj.b2431.

14. Gans SL, Pols MA, Stoker J, Boermeester MA. Guideline for the diagnostic pathway in patients with acute abdominal pain. *Digestive Surgery*. 2015; 32(1): 23–31. doi: 10.1159/000371583.

15. Cross R, Bhat R, Li Y, Plankey M, Maloy K. Emergency department computed tomography use for non-traumatic abdominal pain: Minimal variability. *The Western Journal of Emergency Medicine*. 2018; 19(5): 782–96. doi: 10.5811/westjem.2018.6.37381.

16. Hasani SA, Fathi M, Daadpey M, Zare MA, Tavakoli N, Abbasi S. Accuracy of bedside emergency physician performed ultrasound in diagnosing different causes of acute abdominal pain: A prospective study. *Clinical Imaging*. 2015; 39(3): 476–9. doi: 10.1016/j.clinimag.2015.01.011.

17. Rubano E, Mehta N, Caputo W, Paladino L, Sinert R. Systematic review: Emergency department bedside ultrasonography for diagnosing suspected abdominal aortic aneurysm. *Academic Emergency Medicine*. 2013; 20(2): 128–38. doi: 10.1111/acem.12080.

18. Jang T, Chauhan V, Cundiff C, Kaji AH. Assessment of emergency physician-performed ultrasound in evaluating nonspecific abdominal pain. *The American Journal of Emergency Medicine*. 2014; 32(5): 457–60. doi: 10.1016/j.ajem.2014.01.004.

19. De Burlet KJ, Ing AJ, Larsen PD, Dennett ER. Systematic review of diagnostic pathways for patients presenting with acute abdominal pain. *International Journal for Quality in Health Care*. 2018; 30(9): 678–83. doi: 10.1093/intqhc/mzy079.

20. Cudnik MT, Darbha S, Jones J, Macedo J, Stockton SW, Hiestand BC. The diagnosis of acute mesenteric ischemia: A systematic review and meta-analysis. *Academic Emergency Medicine*. 2013; 20(11): 1087–100. doi: 10.1111/acem.12254.

21. Henden Çam P, Baydin A, Yürüker S, Erenler AK, Şengüldür E. Investigation of geriatric patients with abdominal pain admitted to emergency department. *Current Gerontology & Geriatrics Research*. 2018; 2018: 9109326. doi: 10.1155/2018/9109326.

22. Ferlander P, Elfström C, Göransson K, Von Rosen A, Djärv T. Nonspecific abdominal pain in the emergency department: Malignancy incidence in a nationwide Swedish cohort study. *European Journal of Emergency Medicine*. 2018; 25(2): 105–9. doi: 10.1097/MEJ.0000000000000409.

23. Esses D, Birnbaum A, Bijur P, Shah S, Gleyzer A, Gallagher EJ. Ability of CT to alter decision making in elderly patients with acute abdominal pain. *The American Journal of Emergency Medicine*. 2004; 22(4): 270–2. doi: 10.1016/j.ajem.2004.04.004.

24. Hustey FM, Meldon SW, Banet GA, Gerson LW, Blanda M, Lewis LM. The use of abdominal computed tomography in older ED patients with acute abdominal pain. *The American Journal of Emergency Medicine*. 2005; 23(3): 259–65. doi: 10.1016/j.ajem.2005.02.021.

25. Gardner CS, Jaffe TA, Nelson RC. Impact of CT in elderly patients presenting to the emergency department with acute abdominal pain. *Abdominal Imaging*. 2015; 40(7): 2877–82. doi: 10.1007/s00261-015-0419-7.

26. Millet I, Sebbane M, Molinari N et al. Systematic unenhanced CT for acute abdominal symptoms in the elderly patients improves both emergency department diagnosis and prompt clinical management. *European Radiology*. 2017; 27(2): 868–77. doi: 10.1007/s00330-016-4425-0.

27. Carpenter CR, Griffey RT, Mills A *et al.* Repeat computed tomography in recurrent abdominal pain: An evidence synthesis for guidelines for reasonable and appropriate care in the emergency department. *Academic Emergency Medicine.* 2022; 29(5): 630–48. doi: 10.1111/ACEM.14427.

28. Lee SY, Coughlin B, Wolfe JM, Polino J, Blank FS, Smithline HA. Prospective comparison of helical CT of the abdomen and pelvis without and with oral contrast in assessing acute abdominal pain in adult emergency department patients. *Emergency Radiology.* 2006; 12(4): 150–7. doi: 10.1007/s10140-006-0474-z.

29. Payor A, Jois P, Wilson J *et al.* Efficacy of noncontrast computed tomography of the abdomen and pelvis for evaluating nontraumatic acute abdominal pain in the emergency department. *The Journal of Emergency Medicine.* 2015; 49(6): 886–92. doi: 10.1016/j.jemermed.2015.06.062.

30. Barat M, Paisant A, Calame P *et al.* Unenhanced CT for clinical triage of elderly patients presenting to the emergency department with acute abdominal pain. *Diagnostic and Interventional Imaging.* 2019; 100(11): 709–19. doi: 10.1016/j.diii.2019.05.004.

31. Razavi SA, Johnson JO, Kassin MT, Applegate KE. The impact of introducing a no oral contrast abdominopelvic CT examination (NOCAPE) pathway on radiology turn around times, emergency department length of stay, and patient safety. *Emergency Radiology.* 2014; 21(6): 605–13. doi: 10.1007/s10140-014-1240-2.

32. Schuur JD, Chu G, Sucov A. Effect of oral contrast for abdominal computed tomography on emergency department length of stay. *Emergency Radiology.* 2010; 17(4): 267–73. doi: 10.1007/s10140-009-0847-1.

33. Basile J, Kenny JF, Khodorkovsky B *et al.* Effects of eliminating routine use of oral contrast for computed tomography of the abdomen and pelvis: A pilot study. *Clinical Imaging.* 2018; 49: 159–62. doi: 10.1016/j.clinimag.2018.03.002.

34. Uyeda JW, Yu H, Ramalingam V, Devalapalli AP, Soto JA, Anderson SW. Evaluation of acute abdominal pain in the emergency setting using computed tomography without oral contrast in patients with body mass index greater than 25. *Journal of Computer Assisted Tomography.* 2015; 39(5): 681–6. doi: 10.1097/RCT.0000000000000277.

35. Wu Y, Ali I, Teunissen B *et al.* Using body mass index and bioelectric impedance analysis to assess the need for positive oral contrast agents before abdominopelvic CT. *American Journal of Roentgenology.* 2018; 211(2): 340–6. doi: 10.2214/AJR.17.19127.

36. Kessner R, Barnes S, Halpern P, Makrin V, Blachar A. CT for acute nontraumatic abdominal pain—Is oral contrast really required? *Academic Radiology.* 2017; 24(7): 840–5. doi: 10.1016/j.acra.2017.01.013.

37. Soucy Z, Cheng D, Vilke GM, Childers R. Systematic review: The role of intravenous and oral contrast in the computed tomography evaluation of acute appendicitis. *The Journal of Emergency Medicine.* 2020; 58(1): 162–6. doi: 10.1016/j.jemermed.2019.10.034.

38. Carpenter CR, Raja AS, Brown MD. Overtesting and the downstream consequences of overtreatment: Implications of "preventing overdiagnosis" for emergency medicine. *Academic Emergency Medicine.* 2015; 22(12): 1484–92. doi: 10.1111/ACEM.12820.

39. Oliveira J. e Silva L, Prakken SD, Meltzer AC *et al.* Depression and anxiety screening in emergency department patients with recurrent abdominal pain: An evidence synthesis for a clinical practice guideline. *Academic Emergency Medicine.* 2022; 29(5): 615–29. doi: 10.1111/acem.14394.

40. Carpenter CR, Bellolio MF, Upadhye S, Kline JA. Navigating uncertainty with GRACE: Society for Academic Emergency Medicine's guidelines for reasonable and appropriate care in the emergency department. *Academic Emergency Medicine.* 2021; 28(7): 821–5. doi: 10.1111/ACEM.14297.

41. Broder JS, Oliveira J. e Silva L, Bellolio F *et al.* Guidelines for Reasonable and Appropriate Care in the Emergency Department (GRACE) 2 2: Low-risk, recurrent abdominal pain in the emergency department. *Academic Emergency Medicine;* 29(5): 526–60.

42. Harfouch N, Stern J, Chowdhary V *et al.* Utility of ultrasound after a negative CT abdomen and pelvis in the emergency department. *Clinical Imaging.* 2020; 68: 29–35. doi: 10.1016/J.CLINIMAG.2020.06.007.

43. Motuzko E, Solis M, Kazi M, Gefen R. Non-visualization of the ovary on CT or ultrasound in the ED setting: Utility of immediate follow-up imaging. *Abdominal Radiology (New York).* 2018; 43(9): 2467–73. doi: 10.1007/S00261-017-1438-3.

44. Gao Y, Lee K, Camacho M. Utility of pelvic ultrasound following negative abdominal and pelvic CT in the emergency room. *Clinical Radiology.* 2013; 68(11): e586–92. doi: 10.1016/J.CRAD.2013.05.101.

45. Hiatt KD, Ou JJ, Childs DD. Role of ultrasound and CT in the workup of right upper quadrant pain in adults in the emergency department: A retrospective review of more than 2800 cases. *AJR. American Journal of Roentgenology.* 2020; 214(6): 1305–10. doi: 10.2214/AJR.19.22188.

Chapter 38 **Small Bowel Obstruction**

Amr Gharib[1] and Christopher R. Carpenter[2]

[1] Department of Emergency Medicine, University of Pittsburgh Medical Center, Harrisburg, PA, USA
[2] Department of Emergency Medicine, Washington University School of Medicine, St. Louis, MO, USA

Highlights

- The best history/physical exam predictors of small bowel obstruction are previous history of abdominal surgery, constipation, abnormal bowel sounds, and abdominal distension.
- Abdominal CT is superior to clinical exam, X-rays, ultrasound, or MRI to rule in or rule out small bowel obstruction.
- Abdominal CT has the advantages over X-ray and US to identify the location, severity, and cause of the obstruction, as well as distinguishing small bowel obstruction from common mimics.
- MRI and US provide radiation-free alternatives to CT which may be important in some populations.
- Emergency physicians can use point-of-care ultrasound (POCUS) to rapidly rule in small bowel obstruction.

Background

Mechanical small bowel obstruction (SBO) is a surgical disorder of the small intestine responsible for 2% of emergency department (ED) visits for abdominal pain and represents 15% of all surgery admissions from the ED.[1,2] Approximately 75% of SBO cases result from intra-abdominal adhesions.[3] Bowel strangulation, which occurs when bowel wall edema compromises perfusion to the intestine and necrosis ensues, is the most severe complication of SBO and occurs in up to 10%.[4] The rate of nonviable bowel with strangulation

---

Evidence-Based Emergency Care: Diagnostic Testing and Clinical Decision Rules, Third Edition.
Edited by Jesse M. Pines, Fernanda Bellolio, Christopher R. Carpenter, and Ali S. Raja.
© 2023 John Wiley & Sons Ltd. Published 2023 by John Wiley & Sons Ltd.

increases with patient age and treatment delays.[5] If untreated, strangulated bowel may perforate, leading to peritonitis with a high rate of mortality. Over 300,000 patients undergo surgery every year in the United States for adhesion-induced SBO; however, SBOs also occur for other reasons including hernias, malignancies, volvulus, inflammatory conditions, foreign bodies, gallstones, pancreatitis, and intussusceptions.[3] SBO typically presents as abdominal pain, distension, vomiting, and sometimes constipation.[6]

Clinical question

What elements of the history and physical examination are best predictors of SBO?

A diagnostic meta-analysis in 2013 quantified the accuracy of history and physical examination for the diagnosis of SBO based on two publications meeting their inclusion criteria.[6-8] The criterion standard for SBO included surgical findings, X-ray, or diagnosis at the time of discharge. The meta-analysis identified the most accurate predictors of SBO to be history of abdominal surgery (+LR range = 2.7–3.9 and −LR range = 0.19–0.42) and a history of constipation (+LR range = 3.7–8.8 and −LR range = 0.59–0.70). The most accurate physical exam findings were abdominal distension (+LR range = 5.6–16.8 and −LR range = 0.34–0.43) and abnormal bowel sounds (+LR = 6.33 and −LR = 0.27).[6] Table 38.1 summarizes the accuracy of history and Table 38.2 summarizes the accuracy of physical exam.

Table 38.1 Diagnostic accuracy of history for SBO

Finding	+LR	−LR
Age > 50	2.2	0.55
Constipation	3.7–8.8	0.59–0.70
Intermittent pain	1.6–2.8	0.35–0.85
Intolerable pain	1.2	0.57
Nausea	1.4	0.35
No appetite	1.3	0.25
No aggravating factor	1.4	0.85
Pain duration > 6 hours	1.4	0.79
Pain increased with eating	2.8	0.88
Pain worsening	1.2	0.65
Previous abdominal surgery	2.6–3.9	0.19–0.42
Previous similar pain	1.2	0.91
Relieved with vomiting	2.7–4.5	0.78–0.87
Vomiting	2.1	0.38

Source: Data from [6].

Table 38.2 Diagnostic accuracy of physical exam for SBO

Finding	+LR	−LR
Abnormal bowel sounds	6.3	0.27
Abdominal mass	2.1	0.89
Abdominal scar	3.7	0.19
Abnormal abdominal movement	3.0–3.7	0.80–0.87
Decreased bowel sounds	3.3	0.83
Distention	5.6–16.8	0.34–0.43
Increased bowel sounds	3.6	0.67
No rebound	1.1	0.85
Rigidity	3.0	0.89
Temperature < 37.1 °C	1.4	0.45
Tenderness (generalized)	2.6–5.0	0.42–0.70
Visible peristalsis	∞	0.94

Source: Data from [6].

Clinical question

Which diagnostic imaging modality is most sensitive in diagnosing SBO?
SBOs can be categorized as either partial or complete obstructions, depending on whether any gas or liquid can pass through the point at which the small bowel is narrowed.[9] The American Association for the Surgery of Trauma recommends a computed tomography (CT) of the abdomen and pelvis with water-soluble contrast follow through to distinguish partial from complete obstruction.[10] Oral contrast CT can predict SBO complications and indications for surgery.[11] Water soluble contrast administered orally or by nasogastric tube may also be therapeutic by alleviating the obstruction nonoperatively.[12-14] Oral contrast did not significantly decrease operative intervention across eight studies (relative rate [RR] 0.84; 95% confidence interval [CI] 0.53–1.3) but did decrease the average length of stay by 3.6 hours.[15] A systematic review of 13 studies and 947 patients evaluating the diagnostic role of hyperosmotic contrast reported that the presence of oral contrast in the right colon, had sensitivity of 92% (CI 90–94%), specificity of 93% (CI 88–96%), positive predictive value (PPV) of 98% (CI 97–99%), negative predictive value (NPV) of 75% (CI 70–81%), positive likelihood ratio (LR+) 12.78 (CI 7.7–21.2), and negative likelihood ratio (LR−) of 0.08 (CI 0.06–0.10) for the diagnosis of SBO.[11]

Other imaging modalities include abdominal X-rays, magnetic resonance imaging (MRI), and ultrasound (US). X-rays are generally unhelpful in the evaluation of SBO and rarely indicated.[16] In fact, over 20 years ago 55% of suspected SBO patients with abdominal X-rays proceeded to CT.[17] Nonetheless, abdominal X-rays for possible SBO continue to be ordered (Figures 38.1 and 38.2).[18]

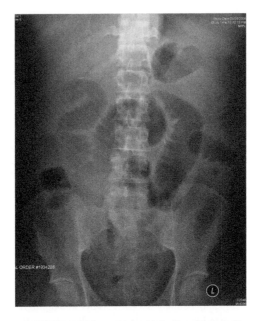

Figure 38.1 Supine abdominal X-ray with multiple dilated loops of bowel.

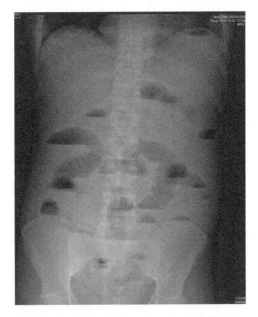

Figure 38.2 Upright abdominal X-ray with multiple air-fluid levels in dilated loops of bowel.

Table 38.3 Test characteristics for bowel obstruction evaluation using X-ray, computed tomography (CT), and ultrasound

Imaging	+LR	−LR
X-ray	1.6 (1.1–2.5)	0.43 (0.24–0.79)
CT		
5–10 mm slice	3.6 (2.3–5.4)	0.18 (0.09–0.35)
0.75 mm slice	∞	0.04
MRI	6.7 (2.1–21.5)	0.11 (0.04–0.26)
Ultrasound	27.5–∞	0.08–0.17

Note: 95% confidence intervals are not provided in source study.
Source: Data from [6, 19].

ED physicians can obtain point-of-care ultrasound (POCUS) or obtain formal radiology US. Two recent systematic reviews demonstrate the accuracy of US to rule in or rule out SBO (Table 38.3).[6,19] Although only three studies had ED physician POCUS, US accuracy is similar whether obtained by minimally trained emergency medicine physicians (as little as 10-minute training) or radiology (Table 38.4).[20-22] POCUS may be particularly valuable in austere settings without immediate access to CT or MRI. The advantage of CT over US is that CT can often identify the location, severity, and operative urgency of SBO, albeit at the cost of increased medical radiation exposure. Surgical guidelines do not recommend any role for or against US in SBO (Figure 38.3).[10]

MRI also avoids medical radiation exposure. In a prospective cross-sectional study of patients with clinical evidence of bowel obstruction, Two studies evaluated MRI for suspected SBO and demonstrate similarly superb accuracy to rule in or rule out SBO.[23,24] Evaluation of suspected SBO in pregnancy is a scenario where US or MRI may be preferred over CT to minimize fetal radiation exposure. The American College of Obstetricians and Gynecologists' guidelines recommend alternatives to CT during pregnancy if safer alternatives with similar diagnostic accuracy exist.[25]

Table 38.4 Test characteristics of bedside ultrasound for the evaluation of bowel obstruction, performed by both emergency medicine (EM) and radiology residents

	Positive likelihood ratio (LR+)	Negative likelihood ratio (LR−)
EM residents	9.5 (2.1–42.2)	0.04 (0.01–0.13)
Radiology	14.1 (3.6–55.6)	0.13 (0.08–0.20)

Source: Data from [6].

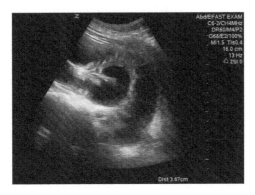

Figure 38.3 Dilated bowel loops indicative of small bowel obstruction seen on ultrasound. (Used with permission of Elke Platz, Heidi Kimberly & Dorothea Hempel, Department of Emergency Medicine, Brigham and Women's Hospital.)

Comment

Few high-quality comparative accuracy studies of clinical exam or different imaging modalities for suspected SBO exist. Many of the studies suffer from the lack of uniform diagnostic criterion standards, making broad comparisons of several similar studies difficult.

Understanding these limitations, several take-home points are reasonable. Abdominal X-rays have little role in the evaluation of suspected SBO. Exceptions probably include prolonged delay or absolute unavailability of CT or US imaging to expedite gastric decompression, especially if a time-sensitive etiology such as volvulus is suspected. Plain radiography is still used in other acute abdominal pain situations like foreign body ingestions, but its use is diminishing.[26] MRI and POCUS provide alternatives to avoid medical radiation exposure. CT remains the superior imaging approach for SBO and surgical guidelines favor oral contrast CT for nonoperative management of SBO in selected patients.

References

1. Foster NM, McGory ML, Zingmond DS, Ko CY. Small bowel obstruction: A population-based appraisal. *Journal of the American College of Surgeons.* 2006; 203: 170–6.
2. Hastings RS, Powers RD. Abdominal pain in the ED: A 35 year retrospective. *The American Journal of Emergency Medicine.* 2011; 29: 711–6.
3. Miller G, Boman J, Shrier I, Gordon PH. Etiology of small bowel obstruction. *American Journal of Surgery.* 2000; 180: 33–6.

4. Jancelewicz T, Vu LT, Shawo AE, Yeh B, Gasper WJ, Harris HW. Predicting strangulated small bowel obstruction: An old problem revisited. *Journal of Gastrointestinal Surgery.* 2009; 13: 93–9.

5. Fevang BT, Fevang J, Stangeland L, Soreide O, Svanes K, Viste A. Complications and death after surgical treatment of small bowel obstruction: A 35-year institutional experience. *Annals of Surgery.* 2000; 231: 529–37.

6. Taylor MR, Lalani N. Adult small bowel obstruction. *Academic Emergency Medicine.* 2013; 20: 528–44.

7. Eskelinen M, Ikonen J, Lipponen P. Contributions of history-taking, physical examination, and computer assistance to diagnosis of acute small-bowel obstruction. A prospective study of 1333 patients with acute abdominal pain scand. *Journal of Gastroenterology.* 1994; 29: 715–21.

8. Böhner H, Yang Q, Franke C, Verreet PR, Ohmann C. Simple data from history and physical examination help to exclude bowel obstruction and to avoid radiographic studies in patients with acute abdominal pain. *The European Journal of Surgery.* 1998; 164: 777–84.

9. Long B, Robertson J, Koyfman A. Emergency medicine evaluation and management of small bowel obstruction: Evidence-based recommendations. *The Journal of Emergency Medicine.* 2019; 56: 166–76.

10. Schuster KM, Holena DN, Salim A, Savage S, Crandall M. American Association for the Surgery of Trauma Emergency General Surgery Guideline Summaries 2018: Acute appendicitis, acute cholecystitis, acute diverticulitis, acute pancreatitis, and small bowel obstruction. *Trauma Surgery & Acute Care Open.* 2019; 4: e000281.

11. Ceresoli M, Coccolini F, Catena F *et al.* Water-soluble contrast agent in adhesive small bowel obstruction: A systematic review and meta-analysis of diagnostic and therapeutic value. *American Journal of Surgery.* 2016; 211: 1114–25.

12. Abbas S, Bissett IP, Parry BR. Oral water soluble contrast for the management of adhesive small bowel obstruction. *Cochrane Database of Systematic Reviews.* 2007; 2007: CD004651.

13. Syrmis W, Richard R, Jenkins-Marsh S, Chia SC, Good P. Oral water soluble contrast for malignant bowel obstruction. *Cochrane Database of Systematic Reviews.* 2018; 3: CD012014.

14. Zielinski MD, Haddad NN, Cullinane DC *et al.* Multi-institutional, prospective, observational study comparing the Gastrografin challenge versus standard treatment in adhesive small bowel obstruction. *Journal of Trauma and Acute Care Surgery.* 2017; 83: 47–54.

15. Koh A, Adiamah A, Chowdhury A, Mohiuddin MK, Bharathan B. Therapeutic role of water-soluble contrast media in adhesive small bowel obstruction: A systematic review and meta-analysis. *Journal of Gastrointestinal Surgery.* 2020; 24: 473–83.

16. Carpenter CR, Pines JM. The end of X-rays for suspected small bowel obstruction? Using evidence-based diagnostics to inform best practices in emergency medicine. *Academic Emergency Medicine.* 2013; 20: 618–20.

17. Nagurney JT, Brown DF, Novelline RA, Kim J, Fischer RH. Plain abdominal radiographs and abdominal CT scans for nontraumatic abdominal pain – added value? *The American Journal of Emergency Medicine.* 1999; 17: 668–71.

18. Jackson K, Taylor D, Judkins S. Emergency department abdominal X-rays have a poor diagnostic yield and their usefulness is questionable. *Emergency Medicine Journal.* 2011; 28: 745–9.

19. Gottlieb M, Peksa GD, Pandurangadu AV, Nakitende D, Takhar S, Seethala RR. Utilization of ultrasound for the evaluation of small bowel obstruction: A systematic review and meta-analysis. *The American Journal of Emergency Medicine.* 2018; 36: 234–42.

20. Lin CK, Chiu HM, Lien WC, Liu YP, Chang CY, Wang HP. Ultrasonographic bisection approximation method for gastrointestinal obstruction in ER. *Hepato-Gastroenterology.* 2006; 53: 547–51.

21. Unlüer EE, Yavaşi O, Eroğlu O, Yilmaz C, Akarca FK. Ultrasonography by emergency medicine and radiology residents for the diagnosis of small bowel obstruction. *European Journal of Emergency Medicine.* 2010; 17: 260–4.

22. Jang TB, Schindler D, Kaji AH. Bedside ultrasonography for the detection of small bowel obstruction in the emergency department. *Emergency Medicine Journal.* 2011; 28: 676–8.

23. Regan F, Beall DP, Bohlman ME, Khazan R, Sufi A, Schaefer DC. Fast MR imaging and the detection of small-bowel obstruction. *American Journal of Roentgenology.* 1998; 170: 1465–9.

24. Beall DP, Fortman BJ, Lawler BC, Regan F. Imaging bowel obstruction: A comparison between fast magnetic resonance imaging and helical computed tomography. *Clinical Radiology.* 2002; 57: 719–24.

25. The American College of Obstetrics and Gynecology Committee on Obstetric Practice, Committee opinion No. 723: Guidelines for diagnostic imaging during pregnancy and lactation. *Obstetrics and Gynecology.* 2017; 130: e210–6.

26. Raja AS, Mortele KJ, Hanson R, Sodickson AD, Zane R, Khorasani R. Abdominal imaging utilization in the emergency department: Trends over two decades. *International Journal of Emergency Medicine.* 2011; 4: 19.

Chapter 39 **Acute Pancreatitis**

Lucas Oliveira Junqueira e Silva[1,2] and Fernanda Bellolio[2]

[1] Department of Emergency Medicine, Hospital de Clínicas de Porto Alegre, Porto Alegre, Brazil
[2] Department of Emergency Medicine, Mayo Clinic, Rochester, MN, USA

Highlights

- Acute pancreatitis accounts for about one in 350 emergency department (ED) visits, is commonly associated with alcohol use and gallstones, and carries an approximate 1–5% mortality rate.
- Even though lipase is likely better than amylase for the diagnosis of acute pancreatitis, both tests are imperfect and should not be used alone when making the diagnosis of acute pancreatitis.
- Clinical and CT-based scoring systems have limited use when trying to predict severe pancreatitis or mortality in ED patients with acute pancreatitis.

Background

Acute pancreatitis is an inflammatory process of the pancreas, which typically presents with severe upper abdominal pain and elevated serum pancreatic enzymes. Most adult cases are related to gallstones or alcohol use. Other causes include medications, hyperlipidemia, and hypercalcemia. In children, abdominal trauma is the most common cause of acute pancreatitis. In 2003, about one in 350 (0.3%) emergency department (ED) visits were for acute pancreatitis.[1] Similarly, in 2018, "diseases of the pancreas" accounted for 0.2% of total ED visits in the United States.[2] In 2012, the incidence of ED visits for acute pancreatitis was 13.6 per 10,000 US adult population, and

---

72.7% of these visits resulted in hospitalization.[3] The incidence of acute pancreatitis has been increasing worldwide secondary to an increase in obesity.[4]

Pancreatitis remains a frustrating and humbling condition to treat. While most patients will have a mild, self-limited course, a subset become significantly ill. In a review of acute pancreatitis by Banks *et al.*[5], overall mortality was approximately 5%, increasing to 17% in cases of necrotizing pancreatitis due to systemic inflammatory response syndrome (SIRS). To date, no interventions, including antibiotics, enzymatic treatments, or surgery, have been definitively shown to improve morbidity and mortality. The mainstay of therapy is excellent supportive care. For this reason, the ability to accurately prognosticate is clinically useful and of interest to patients and families. Correspondingly, several scoring systems have been developed to predict the severity of acute pancreatitis. In this chapter, we review the diagnostic characteristics of laboratory tests and the accuracy of prognostic systems for acute pancreatitis. As the diagnosis of chronic pancreatitis is largely clinical, we do not address chronic pancreatitis in this chapter.

Clinical question

What is the role of serum amylase and lipase in the diagnosis of acute pancreatitis?

Serum amylase and lipase are the most frequently used diagnostic tests for pancreatitis in the ED. Lipases are enzymes secreted from pancreatic acinar cells that hydrolyze triglycerides into metabolic substrates. Normally, 99% of lipases are secreted into the pancreatic ductal system, while less than 1% makes its way into the serum, giving the serum lipase level the theoretical advantage of being specific to pancreatic pathology.[6] Amylase is a small enzyme that cleaves starches into smaller carbohydrates. There are two major sources of amylase, the pancreas, and salivary glands, but the many physiologic and pathologic causes of amylase elevation give amylase lower specificity for pancreatitis.[7]

Studies evaluating laboratory tests for pancreatitis have several weaknesses. First, there is no clear criterion standard for acute pancreatitis. Currently, the diagnosis of acute pancreatitis is made by 2 of the following: clinical presentation suggestive of pancreatitis, elevation in serum lipase or amylase three times or more than the upper limit of normal, or findings of acute pancreatitis on imaging. Earlier studies often used the laboratory test in question (usually amylase) as the sole marker or as one of the diagnostic criteria of pancreatitis, inflating the sensitivity of the test (incorporation bias). Better constructed studies use several factors, including lab tests, computed tomography (CT) results, surgical findings, and discharge diagnoses, to define the population with pancreatitis. Second, "normal limits" defined in a sample of healthy young men may differ from the population at risk for pancreatitis.

Butler *et al.*[8] conducted a rapid review to determine whether lipase was better than amylase in the diagnosis of pancreatitis in patients presenting with abdominal pain. They identified seven studies that compared the tests head-to-head and included almost 2000 patients. The studies demonstrated that serum amylase (sensitivity 72–95%, specificity 85–99%) had worse test characteristics than serum lipase (sensitivity 86–100%, specificity 95–99%) for pancreatitis.

In 2017, a Cochrane systematic review compared the diagnostic accuracy of serum amylase and serum lipase for acute pancreatitis in adult patients presenting with abdominal pain to the ED.[9] The authors have also evaluated the use of urinary trypsinogen, but this test is usually not available in the ED. Case-control studies were excluded from this review due to the inappropriateness of this design to address diagnostic accuracy. In this meta-analysis using the traditional threshold of above three times the normal values, lipase had slightly higher sensitivity than amylase, but similar specificity and number of false negatives (Table 39.1). The median prevalence (pretest probability) of acute pancreatitis (defined as lipase or amylase three times the normal value) among the included studies was 22.6%. This means that 7 (95% confidence interval [CI] 3–15) out of 100 patients with negative lipase, and eight patients with a negative amylase would have acute pancreatitis (false negatives) (Table 39.1). This highlights the importance of having high

Table 39.1 Pooled sensitivity and specificity of amylase and lipase for acute pancreatitis in adults obtained from a Cochrane diagnostic test accuracy meta-analysis

Test	Pooled sensitivity, % (95% CI)	Pooled specificity, % (95% CI)	Number of false positives per 100 people having a positive test	Number of false negatives per 100 people having a negative test
Serum amylase (threshold: >3 times normal) on admission, three studies (605 participants)				
	72% (59–82%)	93% (66–99%)	26 (6–67)	8 (5–12)
Serum lipase (threshold: >3 times normal) on admission, four studies (678 participants)				
	79% (54–92%)	89% (46–99%)	32 (6–79)	7 (3–15)

Source: Data from [9].

clinical suspicion if the symptoms are highly suggestive of acute pancreatitis, even after negative amylase or lipase. Also, the specificity of these tests is good but imperfect and one should also consider alternative diagnoses even if these tests are positive.

It is important to note that lipase elevations occur earlier and last longer than amylase elevations in the setting of acute pancreatitis,[7] which likely explains the higher sensitivity of lipase. In fact, the authors of the Cochrane review also looked at the sensitivity of amylase and lipase 2–3 days after admission and 4–5 days after admission.[9] The sensitivity of both tests decreased significantly over time, but the decrease in amylase's sensitivity was greater, which is aligned with the classic understanding that amylase has a shorter half-life than lipase. With that said, we often do not know the exact timing of symptom onset for patients presenting to the ED, which favors the use of lipase in the setting of suspected acute pancreatitis.

Overall, studies show serum lipase to be slightly more sensitive as a diagnostic marker when used to rule out pancreatitis, and elevations start earlier in the course of the condition. The specificity of these tests appears to be somewhat similar in the context of an undifferentiated patient with abdominal pain in the ED and suspected pancreatitis, despite the physiology-based understanding that lipase should be more specific than amylase. Although lipase is likely better for the diagnosis of acute pancreatitis, these tests are imperfect and should be used in the appropriate clinical context.

Clinical question

Can clinical prediction rules accurately predict the severity of pancreatitis based on features present in the ED?

Acute pancreatitis can be divided into mild (75–85%) and severe or necrotizing pancreatitis (15–25%).[10] Severe pancreatitis is associated with local complications such as pseudocysts and abscesses, organ failure, respiratory failure, and an approximately 15% mortality.[4,5] Early identification of high-risk patients is difficult, as clinical features such as pain severity, vital signs, and diagnostic test values (such as serum lipase) do not correlate with severity. Numerous rating scales incorporating clinical features, laboratory test values, and imaging have been developed to prognosticate the severity of acute pancreatitis; however, several well-known scales are not useful to the emergency clinician. Of note, Ranson's score requires values at 48 hours and the CT severity index (CTSI or Balthazar score) requires a contrast-enhanced CT, which is not indicated for all ED patients with acute pancreatitis.[1]

Scoring systems that can be calculated in the ED include the acute physiology and chronic health examination (APACHE) II score,[11] the SIRS score,[12] and the bedside index of severity in acute pancreatitis (BISAP) score.[13] The APACHE II score was originally developed for critically ill patients in intensive care units (ICUs) and has been the most studied in acute pancreatitis after the Ranson's score. The APACHE II score includes 12 physiologic measures, age, and chronic disease, making it cumbersome and most easily calculated using a computerized calculator, available in common online textbooks and websites.[14] The SIRS score includes: temperature >38.5 °C or <35.0 °C; heart rate of >90 beats/minute; respiratory rate of >20 breaths/minute or $PaCO_2$ of <32 mmHg; and white blood cell (WBC) count of >12,000 cells/mL, <4000 cells/mL, or >10% bands. The BISAP score includes blood urea nitrogen (BUN) >25 mg/dL, impaired mental status, SIRS, age >60 years, and pleural effusions.

Gravante et al.[15] conducted a systematic review of studies of prognostic scores for acute pancreatitis and their relationship to mortality. They excluded studies that analyzed factors associated with the severity of disease or the presence of disease-related complications. They identified 195 relevant studies and included 58; however, due to heterogeneous populations and variable test cutoffs, they were unable to calculate pooled diagnostic test characteristics. Among the scores investigated, APACHE II had the greatest positive predictive value (PPV) for mortality (maximum 69%), with sensitivities from 65% to 81% and specificities from 77% to 91%. No scores had high PPV (>80%). While most prognostic variables and scores showed high negative predictive values (NPVs) for mortality (>90%), this was heavily weighted by the relatively low mortality rates. In many studies, clinical assessment for severe pancreatitis (including shock, respiratory distress, or signs of peritonitis) was as accurate as the scoring systems. The authors conclude that despite the number of scoring systems for grading acute pancreatitis, none are ideal for the prediction of mortality. A similar conclusion was reached in a more recent systematic review evaluating prediction models of mortality in adults with acute pancreatitis.[16] The authors included 94 studies evaluating 18 different scores in 53,547 patients. Data were highly heterogeneous across studies and the authors were not able to perform a meta-analysis. There were 13 studies (2452 patients) looking at APACHE II, and using a threshold of >7, the median sensitivity and specificity were 100% (range 67.7–100%) and 63.4% (range 21.4–95.9%), respectively. As for BISAP, there were 17 studies (21,733 patients) included and using a threshold of >2, the median sensitivity and specificity were 71.4% (range 33.3–100%) and 87.6% (range 62.9–97.6%), respectively. SIRS score was evaluated by nine studies (1227 patients) using a threshold of >1 and the median sensitivity and specificity were 100% (range 33.3–100%) and 59.6% (range 15.5–78.2%). These scores had relatively low specificities, translating to high false positive rates. Most importantly, however, is that the quality of studies was low. Key concerns involved selection bias and selective reporting with insufficient information in the manuscripts. Also, the authors of this systematic review attempted to find studies evaluating clinical utility, effect on patient outcomes, or cost-effectiveness of the scoring systems, and they did not find any relevant studies. They concluded that test characteristics and utility of acute pancreatitis severity scores remain uncertain.

Our ability to predict mortality in patients with acute pancreatitis using available scoring systems is limited. As an alternative, researchers have been looking at the ability of scoring systems to predict two key determinants of severity: persistent organ failure, and infected pancreatic and/or peripancreatic necrosis. Both outcomes are tightly correlated with mortality.

Mounzer et al.[17] conducted a prospective study to evaluate the accuracy of different scoring systems for predicting persistent organ failure, defined as organ failure lasting ≥48 hours and involving the cardiovascular, pulmonary, and/or renal systems. Data were separated into two cohorts from different medical centers: 256 prospectively enrolled patients in the first cohort and 397 prospectively enrolled patients in the second cohort. Only patients admitted to the hospital with acute pancreatitis were included. In the 256 patients from the first cohort, 62 (24%) developed persistent organ failure and 10 (3.9%) patients died during hospitalization, all of whom had developed persistent organ failure. In the 397 patients from the second cohort, 34 (9%) developed persistent organ failure and 14 (3.5%) died during hospitalization, 10 of whom had developed persistent organ failure. Using data obtained at admission (as close to the ED as it could be), none of the evaluated scoring systems performed with high predictive accuracy. The score with highest area under the curve was the Glasgow score, which is a scoring system developed in 1984 that includes the following parameters: age (>55 years), WBC (>15,000/mL), glucose (>180 mg/dL), BUN (>45 mg/dL), PaO_2 (<60 mmHg), calcium (<8 g/dL), albumin (<3.2 g/dL), and lactate dehydrogenase (LDH) (>600 IU/L). The sensitivity and specificity of this score in both cohorts, however, were not ideal (first cohort: sensitivity of 85% and specificity of 83%; second cohort: sensitivity of 65% and specificity of 82%). Despite an attempt to combine different rules in order to increase predictive accuracy, the authors concluded that the ability to predict severity of acute pancreatitis cannot be expected to improve unless new approaches are developed.

Papachristou et al.[18] compared BISAP with the "traditional" multifactorial scoring systems: Ranson's, APACHE-II, and CTSI in predicting severity, pancreatic necrosis, and mortality in a prospective cohort of patients with pancreatitis. They studied 185 consecutive patients over 4 years, of whom 73% underwent contrast-enhanced CT scan. Forty patients (22%) developed organ failure and were classified as having severe acute pancreatitis, 36 (19%) developed pancreatic necrosis, and seven died (3.8%). The sensitivity and specificity of the scoring systems for severe disease ranged from 38% to 86% and from 71% to 92% respectively, and using areas under the curve, no system was better at consistently predicting any of the outcomes.

Bollen *et al.*[19] compared the accuracy of CT and clinical scoring systems for predicting the severity of acute pancreatitis on admission. They studied 346 consecutive patients, of whom 159 received a contrast-enhanced CT scan. Seven CT scoring systems as well as two clinical scoring systems (APACHE-II and BISAP) were evaluated regarding their ability to predict the severity of acute pancreatitis on admission (first 24 hours of hospitalization). Clinically severe acute pancreatitis (defined as one or more of the following: mortality, persistent organ failure, and/or the presence of local pancreatic complications that require intervention) was diagnosed in 18% of patients, and 6% of patients died. The sensitivity and specificity of the scoring systems ranged from 59% to 87% and from 58% to 85%, respectively, and using areas under the curve, there were no statistically significant differences between the predictive accuracies of CT and clinical scoring systems. Therefore, the authors concluded that a CT on admission solely for severity assessment in acute pancreatitis is not recommended.

Lastly, a systematic review published in 2014 evaluated predictors of persistent organ failure, infected pancreatic necrosis, or both.[20] For the prediction of persistent organ failure, the authors found that when using data obtained within 48 hours of admission (as close to the ED as it could be), the APACHE-II with a cutoff of 7 had the highest sensitivity at 84%. The Japanese Severity Scale with a cutoff of 1 had the highest specificity at 90%. The Japanese Severity Scale includes base excess (≤ 3 mEq/L), PaO_2 (≤ 60 mmHg or respiratory failure), BUN (≥ 40 mg/dL) or Cr (≥ 2 mg/dL), LDH ($\geq 2\times$ upper limit of normal), platelet ($\leq 100,000/mm^3$), calcium (≤ 7.5 mg/dL), C-reactive protein (CRP) (≥ 15 mg/dL), SIRS (≥ 3), and age (≥ 70 years). The positive likelihood ratio (LR+) of this complex score to predict persistent organ failure was the highest at 5.19 yet similar to the use of simpler predictors alone such as CRP (LR+ 4.85) and BUN (LR+ 3.64). This study also evaluated the evidence for the prediction of infected pancreatic necrosis specifically. Overall, the included studies enrolled a total of 1533 patients with an incidence of infected pancreatic necrosis of 20%. Among predictors in all patients with acute pancreatitis, the accuracy of procalcitonin and CRP was the most frequently evaluated. The pooled (5 studies, 327 patients) test characteristics of procalcitonin for the prediction of infected pancreatic necrosis were the following: sensitivity 85%, specificity 78%, LR+ 4.54, and negative likelihood ratio [LR−] 0.13. As for CRP, the pooled (4 studies, 227 patients) test characteristics were: sensitivity 64%, specificity 82%, LR+ 3.34, and LR− 0.49.

More recently, another Cochrane review evaluated the diagnostic accuracy of serum CRP, procalcitonin, and LDH for the diagnosis of pancreatic necrosis among patients with acute pancreatitis.[21] The ability to identify pancreatic necrosis is important because this is a key marker of severity. The authors found only three studies, all of which had several methodological flaws, and it was not possible to arrive at any conclusions regarding the diagnostic test accuracy of these three biomarkers. Further research needs to elucidate the usefulness of these biomarkers in detecting pancreatic necrosis in patients with acute pancreatitis, which may or may not help in the decision to upgrade the level of care in these patients.

Comments

Acute pancreatitis can present as a mild, self-limited illness with no sequelae, or as fulminant multiple-organ failure with circulatory collapse. When evaluating patients in whom there is a clinical suspicion for acute pancreatitis, serum lipase should be used as the routine initial serum test, as it is more sensitive and as specific as serum amylase. Lipase elevations occur earlier and last longer than amylase elevations in the setting of acute pancreatitis. If lipase is not available, amylase should be used. The outcome for an individual patient diagnosed with acute pancreatitis in the ED is difficult to predict. Most patients with acute pancreatitis will need admission, although a subset who are well appearing and can reliably follow dietary instructions, and whose pain is controlled with oral analgesics, may be appropriate for outpatient management. There is no evidence to support the ED use of any clinical or CT-based scoring system to predict severity of disease, local complications, or death, and therefore determine disposition. We recommend that clinicians use their clinical judgment as they would for other potentially critically ill patients to determine the need for ICU placement. This includes vital signs, patient comfort, signs of sepsis, and respiratory status.

References

1. Fagenholz PJ, Fernández-del Castillo C, Harris NS, Pelletier AJ, Camargo CA. National study of United States emergency department visits for acute pancreatitis, 1993-2003. *BMC Emergency Medicine.* 2007; 7: 1. doi: 10.1186/1471-227X-7-1.
2. National Center for Health Statistics. National Hospital Ambulatory Medical Care Survey: 2018 Emergency Department Summary Tables. https://www.cdc.gov/nchs/data/nhamcs/web_tables/2018-ed-web-tables-508.pdf. 2018. Accessed December 7, 2021.

3. Garg SK, Sarvepalli S, Campbell JP *et al.* Incidence, admission rates, and predictors, and economic burden of adult emergency visits for acute pancreatitis: Data from the national emergency department sample, 2006 to 2012. *Journal of Clinical Gastroenterology.* 2019; 53(3): 220–5. doi: 10.1097/MCG.0000000000001030.

4. Yadav D, Lowenfels AB. The epidemiology of pancreatitis and pancreatic cancer. *Gastroenterology.* 2013; 144(6): 1252–61. doi: 10.1053/j.gastro.2013.01.068.

5. Banks PA, Freeman ML, Fass R *et al.* Practice guidelines in acute pancreatitis. *The American Journal of Gastroenterology.* 2006; 101(10): 2379–400. doi: 10.1111/j.1572-0241.2006.00856.x.

6. Tietz NW, Shuey DF. Lipase in serum - The elusive enzyme: An overview. *Clinical Chemistry.* 1993; 39(5): 746–56. doi: 10.1093/clinchem/39.5.746.

7. Vissers RJ, Abu-Laban RB, McHugh DF. Amylase and lipase in the emergency department evaluation of acute pancreatitis. *The Journal of Emergency Medicine.* 1999; 17(6): 1027–37. doi: 10.1016/S0736-4679(99)00136-5.

8. Butler J, Mackay-Jones K. Serum amylase or lipase to diagnose pancreatitis in patients presenting with abdominal pain. *Emergency Medicine Journal.* 2002; 19(5): 430–1. doi: 10.1136/emj.19.5.430.

9. Rompianesi G, Hann A, Komolafe O, Pereira SP, Davidson BR, Gurusamy KS. Serum amylase and lipase and urinary trypsinogen and amylase for diagnosis of acute pancreatitis. *Cochrane Database of Systematic Reviews.* 2017; 2017(4): CD012010. doi: 10.1002/14651858.CD012010.pub2.

10. Bradley EL. A clinically based classification system for acute pancreatitis: Summary of the International Symposium on Acute Pancreatitis, Atlanta, GA, September 11 through 13, 1992. *Archives of Surgery.* 1993; 128(5): 586–90. doi: 10.1001/archsurg.1993.01420170122019.

11. Ho KM, Dobb GJ, Knuiman M, Finn J, Lee KY, Webb SAR. A comparison of admission and worst 24-hour Acute Physiology and Chronic Health Evaluation II scores in predicting hospital mortality: A retrospective cohort study. *Critical Care.* 2005; 10(1): R4. doi: 10.1186/cc3913.

12. Annane PD, Bellissant PE, Cavaillon JM. Septic shock. *Lancet.* 2005; 365: 63–78. doi: 10.1016/S0140-6736(04)17667-8.

13. Wu BU, Johannes RS, Sun X, Tabak Y, Conwell DL, Banks PA. The early prediction of mortality in acute pancreatitis: A large population-based study. *Gut.* 2008; 57(12): 1698–703. doi: 10.1136/gut.2008.152702.

14. MDCalc website, APACHE II Score, https://www.mdcalc.com/calc/1868/apache-ii-score.

15. Gravante G, Garcea G, Ong SL *et al.* Prediction of mortality in acute pancreatitis: A systematic review of the published evidence. *Pancreatology.* 2009; 9(5): 601–14. doi: 10.1159/000212097.

16. Di MY, Liu H, Yang ZY, Bonis PAL, Tang JL, Lau J. Prediction models of mortality in acute pancreatitis in adults: A systematic review. *Annals of Internal Medicine.* 2016; 165(7): 482–90. doi: 10.7326/M16-0650.

17. Mounzer R, Langmead CJ, Wu BU *et al.* Comparison of existing clinical scoring systems to predict persistent organ failure in patients with acute pancreatitis. *Gastroenterology.* 2012; 142(7): 1476–82. doi: 10.1053/j.gastro.2012.03.005.

18. Papachristou GI, Muddana V, Yadav D *et al.* Comparison of BISAP, Ranson's, APACHE-II, and CTSI scores in predicting organ failure, complications, and mortality in acute pancreatitis. *The American Journal of Gastroenterology.* 2010; 105(2): 435–41. doi: 10.1038/ajg.2009.622.
19. Bollen TL, Singh VK, Maurer R *et al.* A comparative evaluation of radiologic and clinical scoring systems in the early prediction of severity in acute pancreatitis. *The American Journal of Gastroenterology.* 2012; 107(4): 612–9. doi: 10.1038/ajg.2011.438.
20. Yang CJ, Chen J, Phillips ARJ, Windsor JA, Petrov MS. Predictors of severe and critical acute pancreatitis: A systematic review. *Digestive and Liver Disease.* 2014; 46(5): 446–51. doi: 10.1016/j.dld.2014.01.158.
21. Komolafe O, Pereira SP, Davidson BR, Gurusamy KS. Serum C-reactive protein, procalcitonin, and lactate dehydrogenase for the diagnosis of pancreatic necrosis. *Cochrane Database of Systematic Reviews.* 2017; 4(4): CD012645. doi: 10.1002/14651858.CD012645.

Chapter 40 **Acute Appendicitis**

Marianna M. Fischmann[1] and Fernanda Bellolio[2]

[1] Department of Surgery, Pontifical Catholic University of Rio Grande do Sul, Porto Alegre, Brazil
[2] Department of Emergency Medicine, Mayo Clinic, Rochester, MN, USA

Highlights

- The diagnosis of acute appendicitis is clinically challenging as the classic presentation of periumbilical pain followed by nausea and vomiting, with migration of pain to the right lower quadrant, occurs in only about half of patients with appendicitis.
- White blood cell count and other laboratory tests are not useful to rule in or rule out the diagnosis of acute appendicitis.
- Clinical decision rules such as the Alvarado Score are not accurate enough to rule in or rule out appendicitis.
- Abdominal CT is more sensitive than abdominal ultrasound in diagnosing appendicitis and is the preferred imaging study in nonpregnant adults. Oral contrast does not improve diagnostic performance of CT. Low-dose CT is accurate, and it is being implemented to reduce radiation exposure.
- Protocols using ultrasound first and CT for equivocal cases are being used more frequently to reduce radiation exposure and cost.
- Increased use of CT has been associated with lower negative appendectomy rates, but clinicians should be aware that false-positive CTs are possible and negative appendectomy rates are still reported to be at least 5%.
- For pediatric patients, a positive point-of-care ultrasound (POCUS) is diagnostic, but a negative POCUS is not sufficient to rule out disease.
- Abdominopelvic ultrasound or MRI are appropriate options for primary imaging in pregnant women with suspected appendicitis.

Evidence-Based Emergency Care: Diagnostic Testing and Clinical Decision Rules, Third Edition.
Edited by Jesse M. Pines, Fernanda Bellolio, Christopher R. Carpenter, and Ali S. Raja.
© 2023 John Wiley & Sons Ltd. Published 2023 by John Wiley & Sons Ltd.

Background

Acute appendicitis is frequently in the differential diagnosis of patients presenting to the emergency department (ED) with acute abdominal pain. Approximately one in every 4000 ED visits (0.03%) is for acute appendicitis,[1] and appendectomy is the most commonly performed emergency surgical procedure. Yet, the diagnosis of appendicitis remains challenging, as the classic presentation of periumbilical pain followed by nausea and vomiting, with migration of pain to the right lower quadrant (RLQ), occurs in only 50–60% of patients with appendicitis.[2] Appendicitis remains a commonly missed diagnosis and one of the five most frequent conditions leading to malpractice claims against emergency physicians. Potentially missed appendicitis is reported to be as frequent as 6% in adults and 4.4% in children.[3]

The usefulness of specific lab tests and imaging studies in aiding with the diagnosis has been questioned. Traditionally, a surgical consultant was engaged early during the evaluation in patients with any suspicion for having appendicitis. However, in the last decade, with the increasing use of computed tomography (CT), point-of-care ultrasound (POCUS), and magnetic resonance imaging (MRI) to both rule out and rule in appendicitis, many emergency physicians involve a surgeon only after a confirmed diagnosis of appendicitis.

Clinical question

What is the role of the white blood cell (WBC) count and other laboratory tests in the diagnosis of acute appendicitis?

Traditional surgical teaching highlights the importance of leukocytosis in the diagnosis of acute abdominal pathology, including appendicitis. A systematic review of clinical and laboratory values for adult patients admitted to the hospital with acute appendicitis[2] found 24 articles with enough information to calculate likelihood ratios (LR) and/or receiver operator characteristic (ROC) curves. Studies based on unselected patients with abdominal pain, patients taken to surgery for suspected appendicitis, or comparisons of patients with verified appendicitis with healthy controls were excluded. Diagnostic performance was determined using weighted pooled estimates of the area under the ROC curves and LRs for diagnostic variables of interest. Results for elevated WBC count are in Table 40.1. While increasing WBC count correlates with the diagnosis of acute appendicitis, there is a clear trade-off between sensitivity and specificity; no cutoff exists with test characteristics that would change clinical practice.

A more recent systematic review without meta-analysis performed by Shogilev *et al.*[4] included 19 studies and found a representative approximation

Table 40.1 Pooled likelihood ratios of elevated WBC in diagnosing acute appendicitis

White blood cell (WBC) count ($\times 10^9$/L)	Positive likelihood ratio LR+/ confidence interval (CI)	Negative likelihood ratio LR−/(CI)
WBC ≥ 10	2.5 (2.1–3.0)	0.3 (0.2–0.4)
WBC ≥ 12	2.8 (2.0–3.8)	0.5 (0.4–0.6)
WBC ≥ 14	3.0 (2.5–3.5)	0.7 (0.6–0.9)
WBC ≥ 15	3.5 (1.6–7.8)	0.8 (0.7–1.0)

Source: Data from [2].

of the true sensitivity and specificity of a WBC >10,000 cells/mm³ of 83% and 67%, respectively. The discriminatory power of an elevated WBC count, expressed as an area under the curve (AUC), ranged from 0.72 to 0.80, representing modest discriminatory power. The study ratifies that a WBC >10,000 cell/mm³ is insufficient for diagnosis.

The authors identified 12 studies, including two large meta-analyses, assessing C-reactive protein (CRP) as a predictor of appendicitis. A CRP cutoff of >10 mg/L yielded a sensitivity between 65% and 85% and specificity between 59% and 73%. They found that CRP serves as a strong predictor for appendiceal perforation but its use is limited as a diagnostic tool. Novel markers including interleukin 6, serum amyloid A, granulocyte colony-stimulating factor, urine leucine-rich 16 α-2 glycoprotein, and calprotectin were also evaluated, but although all of them seem to contribute to the presentation of appendicitis, none of them has been proven to change the diagnostic management of suspected appendicitis on their own.

Clinical question

Are clinical decision rules useful in the diagnosis of acute appendicitis?
Several clinical decision rules that incorporate elements of the patient's history, physical exam, and lab findings have been developed to aid in the diagnosis of acute appendicitis. Individual values from the history and physical exam are associated with acute appendicitis, but none is individually predictive enough to alter clinical judgment. Andersson[2] calculated pooled LRs for history and physical exam findings and found that none of the findings had a LR+ above 3 and that direct tenderness and rebound tenderness had LR− below 0.4.

The clinical decision rule for acute appendicitis that has been most studied in the ED was developed by Alvarado.[5] He derived the rule retrospectively on a group of 305 hospitalized patients with abdominal pain suggestive of

Table 40.2 Alvarado Score for acute appendicitis

Feature	Points
Migration of pain	1
Anorexia	1
Nausea	1
Tenderness in right lower quadrant	2
Rebound pain	1
Elevated temperature (>37.3 °C or >99.1 °F)	1
Leukocytosis (>10,000)	2
"Left shift" of white blood cell count (e.g., >75% neutrophils)	1

Source: Data from [4].

appendicitis and identified eight factors predictive of acute appendicitis. Based on the weight of their association, each factor was given a score that, when summed, makes up the Alvarado Score (Table 40.2).

The American College of Emergency Physicians (ACEP) Clinical Policy on acute appendicitis reviewed the literature on the Alvarado Score and concluded that imaging can be warranted even in patients with low Alvarado Scores.[6] They noted that in three studies, a significant proportion (9%, 36%, and 72%) of patients with low-risk Alvarado Scores (<5) ultimately had appendicitis.

In 2017, Kularatna et al.[7] published a systematic review comparing 12 different clinical decision rules available and assessed how they perform for the diagnosis of appendicitis. Twenty-two validation studies were also part of the analysis. The best decision rule was the Appendicitis Inflammatory Response Score (AIR),[8] which showed a high sensitivity (92%) and moderate specificity (63%) at a cutoff value above five. This score is depicted in Table 40.3. The original derivation study set a cutoff value above eight. In fact, when this cutoff was analyzed, the sensitivity was only 20% and specificity increased up to 97%. The AUC values generated for AIR ranged from 0.805 to 0.97, with an average value of 0.872.

The same study compared the Alvarado Score with the modified Alvarado Score, which was first described in 1994 by Kalan and differs from the original one by not including the left shift of WBC.[9] The average AUC value for the Alvarado Score ranged between 0.74 and 0.88; higher than the modified Alvarado Score which had an AUC of 0.69 based on a single study. The sensitivity of the Alvarado Score ranged from 67.7% to 96.3%, while specificity ranged from 58.2 to 89.4% when the originally recommended cutoff of 7 was used. This variability was also seen in Kalan's modified Alvarado Score where

Table 40.3 Appendicitis inflammatory response score (AIR)

Predictor factors	Points (0–12)
Vomiting	1
Pain in right inferior fosse	1
Rebound tenderness of muscular defense – light	1
Rebound tenderness of muscular defense – medium	2
Rebound tenderness of muscular defense – strong	3
Body temperature > 38.5 °C	1
Polymorphonuclear leukocytes – 70–84%	1
Polymorphonuclear leukocytes – ≥85%	2
WBC count – 10.0–14.9×10^9/L	1
WBC count – ≥15.0–9×10^9/L	2
CRP concentration – 10–49 g/L	1
CRP concentration – ≥50 g/L	2

Interpretation: AIR 0–4 low risk; AIR 5–8 indeterminate risk; AIR 9–12 high risk of appendicitis

Source: Data from [7].

the sensitivity ranged from 53.8% to 97.6%, and specificity ranged from 28.6% to 80% for the same cutoff value. The variability remained regardless of the quality of the studies. It is important to note that significant heterogeneity across the studies precluded the authors from performing a meta-analysis. Overall, the AIR score outperformed other scores, but it has been validated in only a small number of studies.

Of note, most studies do not answer the question if any of the existing clinical decision rules add diagnostic utility beyond the decision-making of an emergency clinician.

Clinical question

Which diagnostic imaging modality is best for diagnosing acute appendicitis?
Three common imaging studies are used in the setting of suspected acute appendicitis: ultrasound, CT, and MRI. CT is widely available and rapid but employs both intravenous (IV) contrast and ionizing radiation. Ultrasound does not employ ionizing radiation or IV contrast but requires the availability of a technician, radiologist, or trained emergency medicine physician, and is operator dependent. MRI has been increasingly used in recent years, especially to avoid the effects of radiation in some groups of people like pregnant patients, although there are limiting factors including high cost and availability.

Table 40.4 Comparison of different modalities of imaging for suspected acute appendicitis

Imaging modality	Sensitivity (95% CI)	Specificity (95% CI)
CT	96% (95–97)	96% (93–97)
Ultrasound	85% (79–90)	90% (83–95)
MRI	95% (88–98)	92% (87–95)

Source: Data from [9].

Dahabreh *et al.*[10] performed a meta-analysis comparing the three modalities of imaging. CT had high sensitivity (96–100%) and specificity (91–100%); MRI had high sensitivity (94–100%) but appeared to have variable specificity (86–100%), mainly because of the smaller number of studies. In adult populations, ultrasound had lower sensitivity (85%) and specificity (90%) than CT and MRI and led to more nondiagnostic scans (Table 40.4).

Many studies have assessed the population effects of widespread use of CT on the diagnosis of and outcomes for acute appendicitis. Coursey *et al.*[11] evaluated patients with suspected appendicitis at one institution over 10 years to determine how many patients received CT for diagnosis and whether changes in CT utilization were associated with changes in the negative appendectomy rate. The percentage of patients undergoing CT prior to appendectomy increased from 18.5% in the first year of the study to 94.2% one decade later ($p < 0.0001$). During this same time period, the negative appendectomy rate at the institution declined from 16.7% to 8.7%, but the decrease was only seen in females.

In 2018, the American College of Radiology published the most recent edition of an evidence-based guideline to determine appropriate imaging for diagnosing acute appendicitis.[12] CT of abdomen and pelvis with IV contrast was recommended as the preferred test for imaging evaluation. The results of the appropriateness of initial imaging for nonpregnant adults with suspected appendicitis are shown in Table 40.5.

Clinical question

Can ultrasound be used first to reduce the use of CT in the diagnosis of acute appendicitis?

Several studies have evaluated pathways that first use ultrasound, followed by CT, to diagnose acute appendicitis. The studies have generally found similar diagnostic characteristics for ultrasound and CT as described in this chapter. A Dutch study evaluated a diagnostic imaging protocol consisting of initial

Table 40.5 Appropriateness of initial imaging for nonpregnant adults with suspected appendicitis

Procedure	Appropriateness category	Adult effective dose estimate range (mSv) of radiation
CT abdomen and pelvis with intravenous (IV) contrast	Usually appropriate	1–10
CT abdomen and pelvis without IV contrast	May be appropriate	1–10
US abdomen	May be appropriate	0
MRI abdomen and pelvis	May be appropriate	0
US pelvis	May be appropriate	0
CT abdomen and pelvis without and with IV contrast	Usually not appropriate	10–30
Radiography abdomen	Usually not appropriate	0.1–1
Fluoroscopy contrast enema	Usually not appropriate	1–10
Tc-99m WBC scan abdomen and pelvis	Usually not appropriate	10–30

Source: Data from [12].

graded compression ultrasound followed by selective IV contrast-enhanced CT scanning in 151 adults with suspected acute appendicitis.[13] Patients diagnosed with appendicitis on ultrasound went directly to surgery, and those with negative or equivocal ultrasound underwent CT. The criterion standard was the result of surgery or observation for those with negative CTs. Ultrasound was consistent with appendicitis in 79 patients (52%), all of whom had surgery; the negative appendectomy rate was 10%. CT scanning was performed in 60 patients with negative or inconclusive ultrasound and diagnosed appendicitis in 21 patients, none of whom had a negative appendectomy. None of the 39 patients observed following negative ultrasound and CT required surgical intervention. The authors concluded that the protocol is safe and avoided CT in about half of patients.

Considering ultrasound as the first modality, a large meta-analysis was performed evaluating which would be the best second-line imaging after an initial inconclusive ultrasound.[14] The sensitivity and specificity were all high and not statistically different among CT, MRI, or a second ultrasound as a second-line imaging. Since ultrasound is a highly operator-dependent exam and given the fact that some hospitals do not have a radiologist available 24/7, POCUS has become more commonly used in the ED. Recent studies have found similar performance between radiologists and emergency physicians. A recent meta-analysis of 17 studies evaluated the sensitivity and specificity of POCUS performed by emergency physicians.[15] The authors found excellent diagnosing rates for acute appendicitis in both adults (sensitivity: 84%, specificity: 91%), and in children (sensitivity: 95%, specificity: 95%). They directly compared radiologists and emergency physicians' interpretations which showed similar diagnostic performances. The pooled sensitivity and specificity of emergency medicine doctors were 81% (confidence interval [CI] 61–90%) and 89% (CI 77–95%), respectively, while for radiologists, the pooled sensitivity and specificity were 74% (CI 65–81%) and 97% (CI 93–98%), respectively. The results were not significantly different for sensitivity ($p = 0.18$) or specificity ($p = 0.85$), and the diagnostic performances were also not significantly different ($p = 0.24$).

Clinical question

Is oral or IV contrast useful when performing CT scans for acute appendicitis? Is low-dose CT as accurate as standard-dose CT?

The traditional protocol for abdominal CT for undifferentiated abdominal pain includes the use of oral contrast prior to the study and IV contrast during the study. Alternative protocols for appendicitis have been developed using rectal contrast in lieu of oral contrast. Some centers perform noncontrast CTs for appendicitis, which eliminates several hours of waiting as well as the risks of IV contrast. Anderson *et al.*[16] performed a systematic review of 23 studies and found that the diagnostic performance of CT with and without oral contrast material for the diagnosis of appendicitis in adults was similar (sensitivity, 95% versus 92%; and specificity, 97% versus 94%).

Soucy *et al.*[17] performed a systematic review showing that there is no direct evidence that IV contrast CT is better than CT without contrast in the evaluation of acute appendicitis, although the available literature is consistent with slightly better test characteristics for IV contrast. The sensitivity and specificity of noncontrast CT ranged from 87% to 97% and 92% to 100%, respectively. The authors concluded that if CT with IV contrast is not easily obtained in a timely manner, unenhanced CT would also be very accurate.

The same study assessed whether adding oral contrast to a CT protocol that already includes IV contrast could improve the diagnosis of acute appendicitis. Six studies met the inclusion criteria for this analysis. All of the studies found that CT with IV contrast has excellent test characteristics for diagnosing appendicitis and that the addition of oral contrast does not improve diagnostic rates. Also, considering the additional time required to use oral contrast, as well as the patient discomfort it causes, it is hard to justify its use.

Table 40.6 Summary analysis of accuracy of type of contrast and radiation dose (CT) for diagnosing acute appendicitis

Enhancement and dose (CT)	Sensitivity (95% CI)	Specificity (95% CI)	LR+	LR−
Unenhanced	91% (87–93%)	94% (90–96%)	15 (9–24)	0.10 (0.07–0.14)
IV contrast	96% (92–98%)	93% (90–95%)	14 (9–20)	0.04 (0.02–0.08)
Rectal contrast	97% (93–99%)	95% (90–98%)	21 (9–51)	0.04 (0.02–0.08)
IV and oral contrast	96% (93–98%)	94% (92–96%)	17 (12–26)	0.04 (0.02–0.07)
Low-dose CT	94 (90–97%)	94% (91–96%)	16 (10–24)	0.06 (0.03–0.11)
Standard-dose CT	95 (93–96%)	94% (92–95%)	15.6 (12.3–19.7)	0.05 (0.04–0.07)

Source: Data from [18].

A Cochrane Review published in 2019 compared the accuracy of contrast versus no contrast and low dose versus standard dose CT for the diagnosis of acute appendicitis (Table 40.6).[18] Sixty-four studies were included. In a subgroup analysis according to contrast enhancement, summary sensitivity was higher for CT with IV contrast (96%, CI 92–98%), CT with rectal contrast (97%, CI 93–99%), and CT with IV and oral contrast enhancement (96%, CI 93–0.98%) than for unenhanced CT (91%, CI 87–93%). Results showed no significant differences in specificity, which varied from 93% to 95% between subgroups. Regarding the use of standard dose versus low-dose CT, the summary sensitivity was 94% (CI 90–97%) and 95% (CI 93–96%), respectively. The summary specificity did not differ between low-dose and standard-dose CT when the objective was to diagnose acute appendicitis. According to these results, it seems that, in adults, low-dose CT should be preferred over standard-dose CT as a first-line imaging test, with standard-dose CT reserved for persons with inconclusive findings on low-dose CT.

Clinical question

What is the best diagnostic approach for suspected appendicitis in children?
Although acute appendicitis is the most common surgical emergency in children, the diagnosis remains challenging due to atypical presentations and the difficulty in obtaining a reliable history and physical examination. In clinical practice, the diagnosis is often based on clinical suspicion and, if deemed

Table 40.7 The pediatric appendicitis score

Item	Score (0–10 points)
Anorexia	1
Nausea or vomiting	1
Migration of pain	1
Fever >38 °C (100.5 °F)	1
Pain with cough, percussion, or hopping	2
RLQ tenderness	2
WBC count >10,000 cells/mm^3	1
Neutrophils plus band forms >7500 cells/mm^3	1

Interpretation: PAS ≤ 3 low risk; PAS of 3–7 indeterminate risk; PAS ≥ 8 high risk of appendicitis

Source: Data from [19].

appropriate, laboratory exams and imaging. Some scoring systems such as the pediatric appendicitis score (PAS)[19] and pediatric appendicitis risk calculator (pARC)[20] have the ability to categorize patients into groups that are at low, moderate, and high risk of appendicitis. However, they have limited ability as diagnostic tools.

The use of the pARC requires the use of an online calculator, which may be a barrier to implementation in some EDs. This clinical decision rule is based upon patient age, sex, duration of pain, migration of pain to the RLQ, maximal tenderness in the RLQ, abdominal guarding, and absolute neutrophil count.

Regarding the use of PAS (Table 40.7) as a clinical decision rule, one prospective observational study with 196 children with abdominal pain suggested a clinical pathway based upon the PAS to determine discharge (PAS ≤ 3), emergency ultrasonography (PAS 4–7), or surgery consult (PAS 8–10).[21] The sensitivity and specificity of the pathway for appendicitis were 92% and 95%, respectively. Perforated appendicitis occurred in 15% of patients and the negative appendectomy rate was 4.4%. No child with a PAS ≤ 3 had appendicitis.

In a prospective validation study performed in 11 community EDs, the authors evaluated 2089 patients with suspected appendicitis of whom 353 (16.9%) had confirmed appendicitis.[22] They compared both PAS and pARC scores and found that the pARC score had higher discrimination for appendicitis than the PAS (AUC 0.89 [CI 0.87–0.92] versus AUC 0.80 [CI 0.77–0.82], respectively).

Benabbas *et al.*[23] conducted a systematic review and meta-analysis to determine the utility of each predictor in the diagnosis of acute appendicitis

Table 40.8 Summary findings in children with suspected acute appendicitis

Predictor of pediatric appendicitis	LR+ (95% CI)	LR– (95% CI)
Fever	1.13 (0.99–1.29)	0.94 (0.89–1.00)
Nausea/vomiting	1.30 (1.19–1.41)	0.65 (0.57–0.73)
Anorexia	1.33 (1.26–1.40)	0.58 (0.52–0.65)
Pain migration to RLQ	1.75 (1.58–1.94)	0.70 (0.62–0.79)
Cough/hop pain	1.61 (1.42–1.83)	0.52 (0.45–0.61)
RLQ rebound tenderness	2.19 (1.91–2.51)	NR*
Guarding	2.09 (1.83–2.37)	0.47 (0.39–0.56)
Periumbilical tenderness	1.00 (0.72–1.39)	1.00 (0.86–1.17)
Rovsing's sign	3.52 (2.65–4.68)	0.72 (0.66–0.78)
WBC count ≥10,000 cells/mm³	2.01 (1.86–2.17)	0.21 (0.19–0.25)
Neutrophils ≥75%	2.02 (1.85–2.21)	0.35 (0.28–0.43)
PAS ≥8	4.40 (3.26–5.95)	0.49 (0.42–0.57)
PAS ≥9	5.26 (3.34–8.29)	0.72 (0.62–0.83)
PAS ≥10	5.80 (1.97–17.11)	0.92 (0.89–0.95)
Positive ED-POCUS result	9.24 (6.42–13.28)	0.17 (0.09–0.30)

* Pooled data not reported because of high heterogeneity (I-squared >50%).
Source: Data from [23].

in ED pediatric patients. The results are shown in Table 40.8. POCUS had a sensitivity of 86% (CI 79–90%), specificity of 91% (CI 87–94%), LR+ = 9.24 (CI 6.42–13.28), and LR– = 0.17 (CI 0.09–0.30), making positive ED-POCUS a good predictor of appendicitis. The author concluded that no single history, physical exam, laboratory findings, or PAS cutoff point is sufficient to rule out acute appendicitis without the need for imaging. A positive POCUS might be diagnostic, while a negative POCUS is not sufficient to rule out the disease without performing a CT or MRI.

The American College of Radiology recommends that imaging in children with atypical or equivocal clinical findings for appendicitis begin with ultrasonography.[12] If the first imaging exam is not diagnostic, the patient may either be observed with serial physical examinations or have repeat imaging performed at a later time (either ultrasound, CT, or MRI).

Considering that imaging is crucial to diagnose appendicitis in children, several studies have evaluated ultrasound as the first choice for imaging to avoid the ionizing radiation of CT scans. A prospective cohort study developed in Canada aimed to evaluate the diagnostic accuracy of a serial ultrasound pathway to detect appendicitis in previously healthy children 4–17 years of age presenting to the ED with suspected appendicitis.[24] The clinical pathway consisted of an initial ultrasound followed by a clinical reassessment in all patients and an interval ultrasonography in patients with equivocal initial imaging and persistent concern about appendicitis on reassessment. They also examined the diagnostic performance of the initial and interval ultrasound and compared the accuracy of the initial ultrasound to that of the series of imaging. Of the 294 patients enrolled and using the serial ultrasound clinical diagnostic pathway, 274 children (93%, CI 90–96%) had diagnostically accurate results; 108 of 111 appendicitis cases were identified without CT scans (two were missed and one had a CT scan), for a sensitivity of 97% (CI 94–100%), and 166 of 183 negative cases were successfully ruled out without CT scans (14 underwent negative operations and three had CT scans), for a specificity of 91% (CI 87–95%). The positive predictive value was 86% (108 of 125, CI 79–92%) and the negative predictive value was 98% (166 of 169, CI 96–100%). In a subanalysis of the initial ultrasound, a total of 54% were diagnostically accurate, with a sensitivity of 80%, specificity of 39%, and 42% equivocal rate. This study highlights that a combination of ultrasonography and clinical reassessment is very helpful in diagnosing appendicitis and that the reassessment represents a powerful tool in identifying children at high risk of appendicitis.

Clinical question

What is the best diagnostic approach for suspected acute appendicitis in pregnant women?

Imaging of the pregnant patient can be difficult, particularly with respect to minimizing radiation exposure and risk. The incidence of appendicitis in pregnancy is 101 cases per 100,000 births in the United States.[25]

Segev *et al.*[26] performed a retrospective study comparing pregnant versus not pregnant women at reproductive age who underwent appendectomy. Two hundred patients of both groups underwent preoperative ultrasound (73% of pregnant and 27% of nonpregnant). There was no significant difference in the predictive performance of ultrasound for acute appendicitis between the pregnant and nonpregnant patients (AUC 0.76 and 0.73 respectively, $p = 0.78$). A subgroup analysis of each trimester showed that no significant difference in the diagnostic performance of ultrasound by trimester, with first trimester ($n = 23$) AUC 0.73, second trimester ($n = 32$) AUC 0.67, and third trimester ($n = 12$) AUC 0.86 ($p = 0.4$). The positive predictive value of ultrasound was 0.94 in the pregnant group and 0.91 in the nonpregnant group; the negative predictive values were 0.40 and 0.43, respectively.

A systematic review and meta-analysis published in 2019 showed that the use of MRI for pregnant women with suspected appendicitis had a sensitivity of 91.8% (CI 87.7–94.9%) and specificity of 97.9% (CI 97.2–100%).[27] The positive and negative LRs for MRI in diagnosing appendicitis in pregnant women were 31.0 (CI 21.3–45.0) and 0.10 (CI 0.03–0.32), respectively. Also, MRI can be performed at any stage of pregnancy, with no evidence of adverse effects on fetal outcomes as it is currently being used. The American College of Radiology guideline for imaging in patients with suspected appendicitis suggests for pregnant women both MRI of abdomen and pelvis without IV contrast, or ultrasound of abdomen, as the primary modality of imaging.[12]

Comment

Appendicitis remains a challenging diagnosis in emergency medicine. Clinicians are pulled in several directions when considering diagnostic tests: pressure to not miss the diagnosis, avoiding unnecessary use of CT and its associated radiation, efficiently treating such patients, and pressure from consultants and radiologists about which tests to order. After developing a clinical suspicion of appendicitis, clinicians should not use laboratory tests to alter their suspicion as no laboratory tests, including WBC count and CRP, have high LRs; a clinician is more likely to falsely anchor his or her diagnostic reasoning on a laboratory value than improve the accuracy of diagnosis. Additionally, the clinical decision rules available, which combine historical features, physical findings, and laboratory test results, are not accurate enough to rule in or rule out appendicitis.

Over the years, EDs have developed protocols around imaging patients with suspected appendicitis in order to reduce interphysician variability and practice a consistent standard. In children and young patients, ultrasound-first protocols reduce the number of CTs but require the availability of skilled ultrasonographers and surgeons willing to operate based on their findings. In adults, CT remains the diagnostic test of choice in the United States, while in other countries more centers are adopting ultrasound-first pathways. The safety of these protocols has been shown in several studies, especially for children and pregnant women. MRI has been more studied as a safe first-line imaging, but there are still limitations to its use due to availability and high costs.

References

1. Tsze DS, Asnis LM, Merchant RC, Amanullah S, Linakis JG. Increasing computed tomography use for patients with appendicitis and discrepancies in pain management between adults and children: An analysis of the NHAMCS. *Annals of Emergency Medicine.* 2012; 59(5): 395–403.
2. Andersson REB. Meta-analysis of the clinical and laboratory diagnosis of appendicitis. *The British Journal of Surgery.* 2004; 91(1): 28–37.

3. Mahajan P, Basu T, Pai CW *et al.* Factors associated with potentially missed diagnosis of appendicitis in the emergency department. *JAMA Network Open.* 2020; 3(3): e200612.

4. Shogilev DJ, Duus N, Odom SR, Shapiro NI. Diagnosing appendicitis: Evidence-based review of the diagnostic approach in 2014. *The Western Journal of Emergency Medicine.* 2014; 15(7): 859–71.

5. Alvarado A. A practical score for the early diagnosis of acute appendicitis. *Annals of Emergency Medicine.* 1986; 15(5): 557–64.

6. Howell JM, Eddy OL, Lukens TW, Thiessen MEW, Weingart SD, Decker WW. Clinical policy: Critical issues in the evaluation and management of emergency department patients with suspected appendicitis. *Annals of Emergency Medicine.* 2010; 55(1): 71–116.

7. Kularatna M, Lauti M, Haran C *et al.* Clinical prediction rules for appendicitis in adults: Which is best? *World Journal of Surgery.* 2017; 41(7): 1769–81.

8. Andersson M, Andersson RE. The appendicitis inflammatory response score: A tool for the diagnosis of acute appendicitis that outperforms the Alvarado score. *World Journal of Surgery.* 2008; 32(8): 1843–9.

9. Kalan M, Talbot D, Cunliffe WJ, Rich AJ. Evaluation of the modified Alvarado score in the diagnosis of acute appendicitis: A prospective study. *Annals of the Royal College of Surgeons of England.* 1994; 76(6): 418–9.

10. Dahabreh I, Adam G, Halladay C, *et al.* Diagnosis of Right Lower Quadrant Pain and Suspected Acute Appendicitis. Agency for Healthcare Research and Quality (US).https://www.effectivehealthcare.ahrq.gov/ehc/products/528/2158/appendicitis-report-151214.pdf. 2015. Accessed February 17, 2020.

11. Coursey CA, Nelson RC, Patel MB *et al.* Making the diagnosis of acute appendicitis: Do more preoperative CT scans mean fewer negative appendectomies? A 10-year study. *Radiology.* 2010; 254(2): 460–8.

12. Garcia EM, Camacho MA, Karolyi DR *et al.* ACR appropriateness criteria® right lower quadrant pain-suspected appendicitis. *Journal of the American College of Radiology.* 2018; 15(11): S373–87.

13. Poortman P, Oostvogel HJM, Bosma E *et al.* Improving diagnosis of acute appendicitis: Results of a diagnostic pathway with standard use of ultrasonography followed by selective use of CT. *Journal of the American College of Surgeons.* 2009; 208(3): 434–41.

14. Eng KA, Abadeh A, Ligocki C *et al.* Acute appendicitis: A meta-analysis of the diagnostic accuracy of US, CT, and MRI as second-line imaging tests after an initial US. *Radiology.* 2018; 288(3): 717–27.

15. Lee SH, Yun SJ. Diagnostic performance of emergency physician-performed point-of-care ultrasonography for acute appendicitis: A meta-analysis. *The American Journal of Emergency Medicine.* 2019; 37(4): 696–705.

16. Anderson BA, Salem L, Flum DR. A systematic review of whether oral contrast is necessary for the computed tomography diagnosis of appendicitis in adults. *American Journal of Surgery.* 2005; 190(3): 474–8.

17. Soucy Z, Cheng D, Vilke GM, Childers R. Systematic review: The role of intravenous and oral contrast in the computed tomography evaluation of acute appendicitis. The Journal of Emergency Medicine. 2020; 58(1): 162–6. doi: 10.1016/j.jemermed.2019.10.034.

18. Rud B, Vejborg TS, Rappeport ED, Reitsma JB, Wille-Jørgensen P. Computed tomography for diagnosis of acute appendicitis in adults. *Cochrane Database of Systematic Reviews.* 2019; 2019(11): CD009977.

19. Samuel M. Pediatric appendicitis score. *Journal of Pediatric Surgery.* 2002; 37(6): 877–81.

20. Kharbanda AB, Vazquez-Benitez G, Ballard DW *et al.* Development and validation of a novel pediatric appendicitis risk calculator (pARC). *Pediatrics.* 2018; 141(4): e20172699.

21. Saucier A, Huang EY, Emeremni CA, Pershad J. Prospective evaluation of a clinical pathway for suspected appendicitis. *Pediatrics.* 2014; 133(1): e88–95.

22. Cotton DM, Vinson DR, Vazquez-Benitez G *et al.* Validation of the pediatric appendicitis risk calculator (pARC) in a community emergency department setting. *Annals of Emergency Medicine.* 2019; 74(4): 471–80.

23. Benabbas R, Hanna M, Shah J, Sinert R. Diagnostic accuracy of history, physical examination, laboratory tests, and point-of-care ultrasound for pediatric acute appendicitis in the emergency department: A systematic review and meta-analysis. *Academic Emergency Medicine.* 2017; 24(5): 523–51.

24. Schuh S, Chan K, Langer JC *et al.* Properties of serial ultrasound clinical diagnostic pathway in suspected appendicitis and related computed tomography use. In: *Academic Emergency Medicine.* Vol. 22: Blackwell Publishing Inc.; 2015: 406–14.

25. Abbasi N, Patenaude V, Abenhaim HA. Management and outcomes of acute appendicitis in pregnancy-population-based study of over 7000 cases. *BJOG : An International Journal of Obstetrics and Gynaecology.* 2014; 121(12): 1509–14.

26. Segev L, Segev Y, Rayman S, Nissan A, Sadot E. The diagnostic performance of ultrasound for acute appendicitis in pregnant and young nonpregnant women: A case-control study. *International Journal of Surgery.* 2016; 34: 81–5.

27. Kave M, Parooie F, Salarzaei M. Pregnancy and appendicitis: A systematic review and meta-analysis on the clinical use of MRI in diagnosis of appendicitis in pregnant women. *World Journal of Emergency Surgery: WJES.* 2019; 14(1): 37.

Chapter 41 **Acute Cholecystitis**

Marianna M. Fischmann[1] and Fernanda Bellolio[2]

[1] Department of Surgery, Pontifical Catholic University of Rio Grande do Sul, Porto Alegre, Brazil
[2] Department of Emergency Medicine, Mayo Clinic, Rochester, MN, USA

Highlights

- History, physical exam findings, and laboratory values are not sensitive predictors of acute cholecystitis.
- The most appropriate initial imaging technique for patients with suspected cholecystitis is ultrasound. CT and MRI are preferred if the differential is broad. HIDA scans can be used if the diagnosis remains uncertain.
- Emergency physician-performed ultrasound has favorable test characteristics and can obviate further testing, but it is operator dependent.

Background

Acute cholecystitis is a common concern in patients presenting for the evaluation of abdominal pain, accounting for approximately 7% of patients presenting to the emergency department (ED) with abdominal pain.[1] Patients typically present with pain localized to the right upper quadrant (RUQ), and the disease involves inflammation of the gallbladder, most commonly due to cystic duct obstruction by a gallstone. Gallstones themselves are relatively common, with a prevalence between 9% and 29% in United States patients, depending on ethnicity and gender.[2] Risk factors for gallstones include age (>40 years), gender (women are more than twice as likely as men to have the disease), obesity (>120% of ideal body weight), pregnancy, and the use of oral contraceptives or estrogen replacement therapy.

Evidence-Based Emergency Care: Diagnostic Testing and Clinical Decision Rules, Third Edition.
Edited by Jesse M. Pines, Fernanda Bellolio, Christopher R. Carpenter, and Ali S. Raja.
© 2023 John Wiley & Sons Ltd. Published 2023 by John Wiley & Sons Ltd.

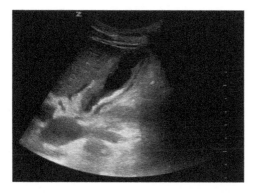

Figure 41.1 Acute cholecystitis with a thickened gallbladder wall and pericholecystic fluid seen on ultrasound. (Used with permission of Elke Platz, Heidi Kimberly & Dorothea Hempel, Department of Emergency Medicine, Brigham and Women's Hospital.)

Once present, gallstones can obstruct the cystic duct leading to the gallbladder inflammation that defines cholecystitis. Acute cholecystitis is typically diagnosed using ultrasound (with presence of gallstones, thickened gallbladder wall, pericholecystic fluid, and a sonographic Murphy sign; Figure 41.1), hepatobiliary cholescintigraphy (HIDA scan, with a lack of isotope accumulation in the gallbladder, indicating cystic duct obstruction), computed tomography (CT, with gallbladder wall thickening, pericholecystic fluid, and inflammation in the pericholecystic fat), or magnetic resonance imaging (MRI, with pericholecystic high signal intensity and visualization of the biliary tract).[3] Secondary infection due to bile stasis commonly occurs, making empiric antibiotic therapy a mainstay of treatment.[4] Definitive treatment requires cholecystectomy, and either percutaneous cholecystostomy[5] or endoscopic gallbladder drainage via endoscopic retrograde cholangiopancreatography in patients thought to be too high risk for surgery. Acalculous cholecystitis, which occurs in up to 10% of cases of cholecystitis in adults and more than 50% of cases in children, can occur due to a number of infectious causes and has a higher morbidity and mortality.[6]

Clinical question

What is the accuracy of the history, physical examination, and laboratory testing for the diagnosis of acute cholecystitis?

Trowbridge *et al.*[7] conducted a review of studies comparing the physical exam, medical history, and lab tests in diagnosing acute cholecystitis. They included 17 studies that evaluated a total of 12 findings in the history and physical examination as well as five laboratory tests. They found that none of the tested findings, which included fever, Murphy sign, rebound tenderness, total bilirubin, liver function tests, and leukocytosis, had sufficient positive likelihood ratio (LR+) or negative likelihood ratio (LR−) to rule in or rule out the disease. Even RUQ tenderness, which had a summary LR− of 0.4, had a 95% confidence interval (CI) of 0.2–1.1.

In a more recent systematic review, Jain *et al.*[1] evaluated the diagnostic test accuracy of history, physical exam, and laboratory tests to predict if any of those elements would allow the diagnosis without utilizing imaging resources. When comparing point estimates, none of the characteristics including fever, RUQ mass, pain, tenderness or rebound, jaundice, Murphy's sign, or vomiting had sufficiently low LR−'s to decrease the probability of cholecystitis. When evaluating laboratory findings, only one study met the inclusion criteria. The study analyzed the test characteristics of total bilirubin, showing that an elevated bilirubin increased the probability of the disease (LR+ = 5.8), but was not robust enough to significantly decrease the probability of cholecystitis (LR− = 0.64). The sensitivity and specificity of the test were 40% (95% CI 12–74%) and 93% (95% CI 77–99%), respectively. The authors suggested that the development of a clinical decision rule with multiple parameters (not including imaging) could be useful for the correct diagnosis, since no single predictor of history, physical examination, or laboratory test is sufficient to diagnose or rule out acute cholecystitis.

The last update of the Tokyo Guideline for the management of acute cholecystitis (TG18) utilized an expert consensus methodology to integrate the diagnostic modalities.[8] They suggest that if at least one of the local signs of inflammation (Murphy's sign, RUQ mass/pain/tenderness) and one systemic sign of inflammation (fever, elevated C-reactive protein, elevated white blood cell count) are present, the patient should be classified as suspected cholecystitis. However, a confirming imaging (ultrasound, HIDA, CT, or MRI) is necessary to achieve definite diagnosis. Validation studies found that the diagnostic accuracy from this diagnostic criterion ranges from 60% to 94%.

Clinical question

What is the accuracy of CT, MRI, ultrasound, or nuclear medicine scans for the diagnosis of acute cholecystitis?
Ultrasound is the first imaging option for patients with suspected cholecystitis.[3] HIDA was considered the criterion standard for diagnosing acute cholecystitis for a long time. In a single-center retrospective analysis of patients suspected of having acute cholecystitis (who had both ultrasound and HIDA scan tests ordered simultaneously), the performance characteristics of the two tests

were compared.[9] It was standard practice at the study hospital for both studies to be ordered together when the diagnosis was considered. Consecutive patients were included, and patients were excluded if a test was ordered based on a prior test to minimize bias based on the initial tests' results. The final diagnosis was determined using surgical, pathology, autopsy reports, or a clinical diagnosis for those who did not undergo surgery. A total of 107 patients were examined, 32 (30%) of whom had a final diagnosis of acute cholecystitis. Using data provided in their study, the performance characteristics of the two tests are shown in Table 41.1.

The authors concluded that HIDA was superior to ultrasound in diagnosing acute cholecystitis. They suggest that, since the costs of each of these studies at the time in their institution were similar, the decision should be based on availability and diagnostic performance.

A systematic review and meta-analysis were performed by Kiewiet et al.[10] to obtain summary estimates of diagnostic accuracy for different imaging modalities (Table 41.2). Data regarding CT accuracy could not be summarized because only one study met the inclusion criteria. In that study, CT had a sensitivity of 94% (95% CI 73–99%) and a specificity of 59% (95% CI 42–74%) for the detection of acute cholecystitis. For MRI, the summary estimate of sensitivity was 85% (95% CI 66–95%) and specificity was 81% (95% CI 69–90%). Ultrasound had a sensitivity and specificity of 81% (95% CI 75–87%) and 83% (95% CI 74–89%), respectively. HIDA had a sensitivity of 96% (95% CI 94–97%) and specificity of 90% (95% CI 86–93%). The summarized estimates were significantly higher for HIDA than for ultrasound

Table 41.1 Test characteristics of hepatobiliary scintigraphy (HIDA) scan and ultrasound for cholecystitis

	Acute biliary disease (+)	Acute biliary disease (−)	Totals
HIDA (+)	28	5	33
HIDA (−)	4	70	74
Totals	32	75	107
Ultrasound (+)	16	9	25
Ultrasound indeterminate or (−)	16	66	82
Totals	32	75	107

Note: HIDA: positive likelihood ratio (LR+) 12.6, negative likelihood ratio (LR−) 0.13, sensitivity 88% (95% CI 71–97%), and specificity 93% (95% CI 85–98%). Ultrasound: LR+ 4.2, LR− 0.57, sensitivity 50% (95% CI 32–68%), and specificity 88% (95% CI 78–94%). Source: Data from [9].

Table 41.2 Summarized estimates of different imaging modalities for the diagnosis of acute cholecystitis

Imaging modality	Sensitivity (95% CI)	Specificity (95% CI)
HIDA	96% (94–94%)	90% (86–93%)
Ultrasound	81% (75–87%)	83% (74–89%)
MRI	85% (66–95%)	81% (69–90%)
CT*	94% (73–99%)	59% (42–74%)

*Reported summary of only one study that met inclusion criteria. Source: Data from [10].

and the authors suggested that HIDA cholescintigraphy has the highest diagnostic accuracy of all imaging modalities. Because of its lower availability, and associated radiation and contrast dye use, HIDA should only be considered in clinically equivocal cases.[11,12]

Given the lack of HIDA availability in most EDs as well as the rapid proliferation of bedside ultrasound, several studies have evaluated the test characteristics of emergency physician-performed point-of-care ultrasound (POCUS) for the diagnosis of acute cholecystitis. A 2011 systematic review by Ross *et al.*[13] found eight prospective studies with appropriate reference standards (radiologist-performed ultrasound or surgical and pathology reports). This pooled dataset contained 710 patients and found an overall sensitivity of 90% (95% CI 86–93%) and a specificity of 88% (95% CI 84–91%). The resultant pooled LR+ was 7.5 and the pooled LR− was 0.11, and the individual studies are described in Table 41.3.

Table 41.3 Individual and pooled test characteristics of emergency physician-performed ultrasound to diagnose acute cholecystitis

Study	Sample size	Sensitivity (95% CI)	Specificity (95% CI)
Alexander *et al.*[14]	50	86% (67–96%)	95% (77–100%)
Davis *et al.*[15]	105	81% (69–90%)	86% (72–95%)
Ha *et al.*[16]	59	94% (71–100%)	95% (84–99%)
Kendall and Shimp[17]	109	96% (87–100%)	88% (77–95%)
Miller *et al.*[18]	127	94% (88–97%)	96% (80–100%)
Rosen *et al.*[19]	110	92% (83–97%)	78% (63–89%)
Rowland *et al.*[20]	35	75% (48–93%)	84% (60–97%)
Summers *et al.*[21]	115	89% (79–95%)	86% (73–95%)
Pooled	710	90% (86–93%)	88% (84–91%)

Source: Data from [14–21].

While a number of these studies were based on convenience samples, had relatively small sample sizes, and were susceptible to partial verification bias (see Chapter 6)[1], the pooled analysis demonstrates favorable test characteristics and relatively narrow CIs. The authors concluded that emergency physician-performed bedside ultrasound can be useful in both making the diagnosis of acute cholecystitis and, if negative, justifying broadening a patient's evaluation to include other possible etiologies for his or her acute symptomatology. A 2017 systematic review also evaluated the use of ED bedside ultrasonography to diagnose acute cholecystitis. The LR+ ranged from 2.68 to 4.72, while the LR− ranged from 0.13 to 0.21. Ranges for sensitivity and specificity were 82–91% and 66–95%, respectively.[1] The authors defined a pretest probability of cholecystitis by the weighted prevalence (31%) across the reviewed studies. The calculated range of posttest probabilities after a positive ED ultrasound was 55–68%, and after a negative ED, ultrasound was 6–7%. They concluded that if the bedside ultrasound is positive for cholecystitis further tests could be obviated, while if the test is negative, it is not sufficient to rule out the disease (the posttest probability would decrease from 31% to 6%), and continued testing is required.

Villar *et al.*[22] (using the same cohort as Summers *et al.*[21]) evaluated if the absence of gallstones on point of care ultrasound would be sufficient to rule out acute cholecystitis. The test characteristics of POCUS for acute cholecystitis using gallstones alone had a sensitivity of 100% (95% CI 85.7–100%), specificity of 54.6% (95% CI 46.8–62.6%), negative predictive value of 100% (95% CI 92.2–100%), and positive predictive value of 26.4% (95% CI 18.3–36.6%). The LR− was <0.01. The results suggest that using only the presence of gallstones in POCUS as a simplified definition for acute cholecystitis could be adopted as a screening test. A negative test could exclude cholecystitis if the patient does not have risk factors for acalculous cholecystitis.

A retrospective study of 283 patients who underwent biliary POCUS by emergency physicians, showed that the presence of any of these: gallstones, sonographic Murphy's sign, or gallbladder wall thickness, resulted in a sensitivity of 63% (95% CI 48–78%) and a specificity of 89% (95% CI 84–93%) to predict cholecystectomy.[23] In a multivariate regression, the presence of gallstones in POCUS had an odds ratio (OR) of 13.1 (95% CI 5.6–30.9), and was the strongest predictor for surgery. Patients referred for radiology-based imaging had longer ED length of stay compared with those who had POCUS alone and were discharged (433 ± 50 minutes versus 309 ± 30 minutes, respectively, $p < 0.001$). Among the patients referred to general surgery, only 43% had a cholecystectomy, and 95% of the patients underwent radiology department imaging prior to surgery,[23] questioning the value added of POCUS. Surgical pathology (or clinical follow-up for patients who do not undergo surgery) is the reference standard for acute cholecystitis, and in this study, not all patients underwent the reference standard, and patients who had POCUS and were dismissed, were not followed up to ensure there was not missed cholecystitis.

Trowbridge et al.[24] reported that the combination of bedside ultrasonographic with evidence of gallstones and a positive sonographic Murphy sign had a LR+ of 2.7 (95% CI 1.7–4.1) and a LR– 0.13 (95% CI 0.04–0.39) for acute cholecystitis. The authors conclude that the evaluation of patients with abdominal pain suggestive of cholecystitis relies on the clinical gestalt and the use of diagnostic imaging like ultrasound.

All the aforementioned bedside ultrasonography studies were performed on adults. Acute cholecystitis is not a common diagnosis in children, and most of the cases are associated with predisposing conditions or infectious diseases. Acalculous cholecystitis represents more than 50% of the acute cholecystitis cases during childhood.[25] A retrospective review of 223 pediatric patients who underwent cholecystectomy, reported a sensitivity and specificity of 82% and 16%, respectively for ultrasound as the first imaging modality.[26] In this study, only 8% of patients had acute cholecystitis, and 83% of children had chronic cholecystitis, which might explain a lower diagnostic accuracy of ultrasound in children.

Comment

There are no aspects of the history, physical examination, or laboratory test results that can accurately diagnose or rule out acute cholecystitis. In patients in whom the diagnosis is suspected, an ultrasound should be the first imaging tool. While emergency physician-performed bedside ultrasound is well supported by the literature and taught in most emergency medicine residencies, its ability to detect acute cholecystitis is operator dependent, a limitation acknowledged both by the individual studies cited in this chapter as well as by systematic review authors. Theoretically, bedside scores incorporating elements of history, physical exam, and sonographic findings could reduce variations in ultrasonography interpretation, but these scores await further validation.[27] Acknowledging these factors, bedside ultrasonography by emergency physicians can reduce ED length-of-stay and time-to-consultant.[23] Nonetheless, emergency medicine bedside sonography research is susceptible to partial verification bias and too often neglects standards for reporting of diagnostic accuracy studies (STARD) reporting guidelines (see Chapter 6), so additional research is still required.[1, 28, 29]

Brook *et al.*[30] reviewed cases of missed cholecystitis at their institution and determined that most of them were due to lack of recognition of the radiological findings of gallbladder wall edema and gallbladder wall thickening, whether on CT and ultrasound. With improved training and quality assurance mechanisms for emergency physician-performed ultrasound, we should continue to see improvements in test characteristics and reliability.[31] Until then, its use should be site and user dependent and based on a well-orchestrated ultrasound quality assurance program involving education, image review, and routine feedback and evaluation.[32]

References

1. Jain A, Mehta N, Secko M *et al.* History, physical examination, laboratory testing, and emergency department ultrasonography for the diagnosis of acute cholecystitis. *Academic Emergency Medicine.* 2017; 24(3): 281–97. doi: 10.1111/acem.13132.

2. Everhart JE, Khare M, Hill M, Maurer KR. Prevalence and ethnic differences in gallbladder disease in the United States. *Gastroenterology.* 1999; 117(3): 632–9. doi: 10.1016/s0016-5085(99)70456-7.

3. Peterson CM, McNamara MM, Kamel IR *et al.* ACR appropriateness criteria right upper quadrant pain. *Journal of the American College of Radiology.* 2019; 16(5S): S235–43. doi: 10.1016/J.JACR.2019.02.013.

4. Young Kim E, Ho Hong T. Empirical antibiotics for acute cholecystitis-what generation of antibiotics is an appropriate choice? A prospective, randomized controlled study. *Journal of Hepato-Biliary-Pancreatic Sciences.* 2021; 28(10): 848–55. doi: 10.1002/JHBP.926.

5. Huang H, Zhang H, Yang D, Wang W, Zhang X. Percutaneous cholecystostomy versus emergency cholecystectomy for the treatment of acute calculous cholecystitis in high-risk surgical patients: A meta-analysis and systematic review. *Updates in Surgery.* 2022; 74(1): 55–64. doi: 10.1007/S13304-021-01081-9.

6. Jones MW, Ferguson T. Acalculous Cholecystitis - PubMed. StatPearls. https://pubmed.ncbi.nlm.nih.gov/29083717/. 2021. Accessed December 22, 2021.

7. Trowbridge RL, Rutkowski NK, Shojania KG. Does this patient have acute cholecystitis? *Journal of the American Medical Association.* 2003; 289(1): 80–6. doi: 10.1001/jama.289.1.80.

8. Yokoe M, Hata J, Takada T *et al.* Tokyo Guidelines 2018: Diagnostic criteria and severity grading of acute cholecystitis (with videos). *Journal of Hepato-Biliary-Pancreatic Sciences.* 2018; 25(1): 41–54. doi: 10.1002/jhbp.515.

9. Chatziioannou SN, Moore WH, Ford PV, Dhekne RD. Hepatobiliary scintigraphy is superior to abdominal ultrasonography in suspected acute cholecystitis. *Surgery.* 2000; 127(6): 609–13. doi: 10.1067/msy.2000.105868.

10. Kiewiet JJS, Leeuwenburgh MMN, Bipat S, Bossuyt PMM, Stoker J, Boermeester MA. A systematic review and meta-analysis of diagnostic performance of imaging in acute cholecystitis. *Radiology.* 2012; 264(3): 708–20. doi: 10.1148/radiol.12111561.

11. Kaoutzanis C, Davies E, Leichtle SW *et al*. Abdominal ultrasound versus hepato-imino diacetic acid scan in diagnosing acute cholecystitis–what is the real benefit? *The Journal of Surgical Research*. 2014; 188(1): 44–52. doi: 10.1016/J. JSS.2014.01.004.

12. Rodriguez LE, Santaliz-Ruiz LE, De La Torre-Bisot G *et al*. Clinical implications of hepatobiliary scintigraphy and ultrasound in the diagnosis of acute cholecystitis. *International Journal of Surgery*. 2016; 35: 196–200. doi: 10.1016/J. IJSU.2016.09.084.

13. Ross M, Brown M, McLaughlin K *et al*. Emergency physician-performed ultrasound to diagnose cholelithiasis: A systematic review. *Academic Emergency Medicine*. 2011; 18(3): 227–35. doi: 10.1111/j.1553-2712.2011.01012.x.

14. Alexander D, Ragg M, Stella J. Emergency department ultrasound for the investigation of right upper quadrant abdominal pain. *Emergency Medicine Australasia*. 2008; 20(Suppl 1): A21.

15. Davis DP, Campbell CJ, Poste JC, Ma G. The association between operator confidence and accuracy of ultrasonography performed by novice emergency physicians. *The Journal of Emergency Medicine*. 2005; 29(3): 259–64. doi: 10.1016/j. jemermed.2005.02.008.

16. Ha Y-R, Kim H, Yoo S, Chung S-P, Kim S-H, Yoo I-S. Accuracy of emergency ultrasonography for biliary parameters by physicians with limited training. Journal of the Korean Society of Emergency Medicine. 2002; 13: 407–10. http://jksem.org/m/makeCookie. php?url=/m/journal/view.php?number=1422. Accessed February 23, 2020.

17. Kendall JL, Shimp RJ. Performance and interpretation of focused right upper quadrant ultrasound by emergency physicians. *The Journal of Emergency Medicine*. 2001; 21(1): 7–13. doi: 10.1016/s0736-4679(01)00329-8.

18. Miller AH, Pepe PE, Brockman CR, Delaney KA. ED ultrasound in hepatobiliary disease. *The Journal of Emergency Medicine*. 2006; 30(1): 69–74. doi: 10.1016/j. jemermed.2005.03.017.

19. Rosen CL, Brown DFM, Chang Y *et al*. Ultrasonography by emergency physicians in patients with suspected cholecystitis. *The American Journal of Emergency Medicine*. 2001; 19(1): 32–6. doi: 10.1053/ajem.2001.20028.

20. Rowland JL, Kuhn M, Bonnin RLL, Davey MJ, Langlois SLP. Accuracy of emergency department bedside ultrasonography. *Emergency Medicine*. 2001; 13(3): 305–13. doi: 10.1046/j.1035-6851.2001.00233.x.

21. Summers SM, Scruggs W, Menchine MD *et al*. A prospective evaluation of emergency department bedside ultrasonography for the detection of acute cholecystitis. *Annals of Emergency Medicine*. 2010; 56(2): 114–22. doi: 10.1016/j. annemergmed.2010.01.014.

22. Villar J, Summers SM, Menchine MD, Fox JC, Wang R. The absence of gallstones on point-of-care ultrasound rules out acute cholecystitis. *The Journal of Emergency Medicine*. 2015; 49(4): 475–80. doi: 10.1016/j.jemermed.2015.04.037.

23. Hilsden R, Leeper R, Koichopolos J *et al*. Point-of-care biliary ultrasound in the emergency department (BUSED): Implications for surgical referral and emergency department wait times. *Trauma Surgery & Acute Care Open*. 2018; 3(1): e000164. doi: 10.1136/tsaco-2018-000164.

24. Trowbridge RLSK. Acute cholecystitis. In: Simel DL, Rennie D, editors. The rational clinical examination: evidence-based clinical diagnosis JAMAevidence. New York: McGraw-Hill Medical. https://jamaevidence.mhmedical.com/content. aspx?bookid=845&sectionid=61357499. Accessed February 20, 2020.

25. Poddighe D, Sazonov V. Acute acalculous cholecystitis in children. *World Journal of Gastroenterology*. 2018; 24(43): 4870–9. doi: 10.3748/wjg.v24.i43.4870.

26. Tsai J, Sulkowski JP, Cooper JN, Mattei P, Deans KJ, Minneci PC. Sensitivity and predictive value of ultrasound in pediatric cholecystitis. *The Journal of Surgical Research*. 2013; 184(1): 378–82. doi: 10.1016/j.jss.2013.03.066.

27. Graglia S, Shokoohi H, Loesche MA *et al.* Prospective validation of the bedside sonographic acute cholecystitis score in emergency department patients. *The American Journal of Emergency Medicine*. 2021; 42: 15–9. doi: 10.1016/J. AJEM.2020.12.085.

28. Kohn MA, Carpenter CR, Newman TB. Understanding the direction of bias in studies of diagnostic test accuracy. *Academic Emergency Medicine*. 2013; 20(11): 1194–206. doi: 10.1111/ACEM.12255.

29. Prager R, Bowdridge J, Kareemi H, Wright C, McGrath TA, McInnes MDF. Adherence to the standards for reporting of diagnostic accuracy (STARD) 2015 guidelines in acute point-of-care ultrasound research. *JAMA Network Open*. 2020; 3(5): e203871. doi: 10.1001/JAMANETWORKOPEN.2020.3871.

30. Brook OR, Kane RA, Tyagi G, Siewert B, Kruskal JB. Lessons learned from quality assurance: Errors in the diagnosis of acute cholecystitis on ultrasound and CT. *American Journal of Roentgenology*. 2011; 196(3): 597–604. doi: 10.2214/ AJR.10.5170.

31. Schleifer J, Haney RM, Shokoohi H *et al.* Longitudinal accuracy analysis of ultrasound performed during a four-year emergency medicine residency. AEM Education and Training. 2021; 5(3): e10574. doi: 10.1002/AET2.10574.

32. ACEP Clinical Policy. Ultrasound guidelines: Emergency, point-of-care and clinical ultrasound guidelines in medicine. *Annals of Emergency Medicine*. 2017; 69(5): e27–54. doi: 10.1016/J.ANNEMERGMED.2016.08.457.

Chapter 42 **Aortic Emergencies**

Ali S. Raja[1] and Jesse M. Pines[2,3]

[1] Department of Emergency Medicine, Massachusetts General Hospital, Harvard Medical School, Boston, MA, USA
[2] US Acute Care Solutions, Canton, OH, USA
[3] Department of Emergency Medicine, Drexel University, Philadelphia, PA, USA

Highlights

- Physical examination findings are insufficiently sensitive to rule out either thoracic aortic dissections or abdominal aortic aneurysms (AAA).
- Chest X-ray cannot rule out the presence of aortic dissection.
- The Aortic Dissection Detection Risk Score, with the addition of a D-dimer value, can be used to rule out the disease.
- Emergency clinician-performed bedside ultrasound is accurate for screening for AAA, given appropriate training.
- Magnetic resonance angiography (MRA) can be used to evaluate for aortic dissection in patients who cannot undergo computed tomography angiography (CTA).

Background

Thoracic aortic dissection and abdominal aortic aneurysm (AAA) are the two aortic emergencies most commonly seen in emergency department (ED) patients. Rupture of AAA is typically a concern in patients presenting with acute abdominal or flank pain, as 4–8% of older men (and slightly fewer women) have occult aneurysms. Similarly, thoracic aortic dissection is a differential diagnostic consideration for patients presenting to the ED with

---

Evidence-Based Emergency Care: Diagnostic Testing and Clinical Decision Rules, Third Edition.
Edited by Jesse M. Pines, Fernanda Bellolio, Christopher R. Carpenter, and Ali S. Raja.
© 2023 John Wiley & Sons Ltd. Published 2023 by John Wiley & Sons Ltd.

chest pain. Given the low frequency (but high morbidity and mortality) of aortic emergencies, ED evaluation should appropriately focus on screening modalities with high accuracy. While computed tomography angiography (CTA) has become the current criterion standard for both disease processes (replacing traditional angiography due to its greater availability), it carries with it the potential risks of contrast-induced nephropathy, allergy, and radiation-induced malignancy, as well as the time delay involved with its use in a busy ED. As a result, plain chest radiography and D-dimer have been considered as risk-stratification tools for the presence of an aortic dissection, and the use of bedside ultrasound has been advocated to screen for AAA.

Clinical question

Which findings on the history or physical examination increase or decrease the likelihood of a patient with chest pain having an acute aortic dissection? Is chest radiography or D-dimer testing appropriate for excluding aortic dissection in patients presenting with chest pain?

A meta-analysis by Klompas[1] in 2002 reviewed the test characteristics of physical examination and radiographic findings for aortic dissection. As few studies met criteria for inclusion, the author was only able to develop pooled data for 1553 patients and analyze one historical factor (history of hypertension), one symptom (sudden chest pain), two signs (pulse deficit and a diastolic murmur), and one radiographic finding (enlarged aorta or wide mediastinum). The results (Table 42.1) demonstrate that, while the presence of a pulse deficit increases the likelihood for aortic dissection, no element in the history or physical exam is sensitive enough to reliably rule out the disease.

A more recent meta-analysis by Ohle[2] in 2018 delved further into whether there were physical examination findings that might increase or decrease the

Table 42.1 Accuracy of clinical findings for thoracic aortic dissection

Symptom or sign	Positive likelihood ratio (LR+) (CI)	Negative likelihood ratio (LR−) (CI)
History of hypertension	1.6 (1.2–2.0)	0.5 (0.3–0.7)
Sudden chest pain	1.6 (1.0–2.4)	0.3 (0.2–0.4)
Pulse deficit	5.7 (1.4–23.0)	0.7 (0.6–0.9)
Diastolic murmur	1.4 (1.0–2.0)	0.9 (0.8–1.0)
Enlarged aorta or wide mediastinum	2.0 (1.4–3.1)	0.3 (0.2–0.4)

Source: Data from [1].

likelihood of aortic dissection. The authors included nine studies with a total of 2400 patients; the prevalence of aortic dissection in the studies varied from 22% to 76%. They concluded that the presence of either a neurological deficit (LR+ 4.4, confidence interval [CI] 3.3–5.7) or hypotension (LR+ 2.9, CI 1.8–4.6) significantly increased the likelihood of disease in patients suspected of having aortic dissection.

Similarly, while a chest X-ray finding of a widened mediastinum was 90% sensitive for thoracic aortic dissection, given the significant morbidity of the disease it was not an appropriate screening exam in patients with a high pretest probability of disease. A study by von Kodolitsch et al.[3] in 2004 confirmed the poor sensitivity of chest X-ray for aortic dissection, finding that it had a sensitivity of only 67% for dissections later verified by either computed tomography (CT) or surgery, and a 2019 study by Nazerian et al.[4] reaffirmed this, finding that chest X-ray had only a 54% sensitivity for acute aortic syndromes. The Ohle meta-analysis confirmed that chest X-rays could not rule out aortic dissections, finding a sensitivity that ranged from 76% to 95% for a chest X-ray finding of a widened mediastinum.[2]

A 2021 meta-analysis of 1135 patients from 16 studies evaluated the use of D-dimer for the exclusion of aortic dissection.[5] A cutoff of 500 ng/mL was used because it is commonly used as the cutoff for the exclusion of pulmonary emboli. All of the studies used CT angiography as the criterion standard and were performed from 2004 to 2017. The results of the pooled analysis demonstrated a D-dimer sensitivity of 96% (CI 91–98%) and a LR− 0.06 (CI 0.03–0.12). However, given the number of pathologic situations that can result in an elevated D-dimer, specificity (70%, CI 57–81%) and positive predictive and LR+ (3.25) were low. Additionally, these studies are at risk of spectrum bias, as D-dimer testing was not performed on all patients with a suspected aortic dissection. Rather the studies evaluated a group of disease-positive patients in whom the test had been performed.

Clinical question

Can the Aortic Dissection Detection Risk Score (ADD-RS), with or without D-dimer measurement, be reliably used to evaluate for and rule out aortic aneurysm?
Given the aforementioned lack of sensitivity for history and physical exam findings for the evaluation of aortic dissection, Rogers et al.[6] developed the ADD-RS in 2011 to risk stratify patients with chest pain. Their initial study evaluated patients with known aortic dissection enrolled in the International Registry of Acute Aortic Dissection and resulted in a three-point decision instrument with a sensitivity of 95.7% for a score >0 (Table 42.2). Specificity could not be calculated given that all patients had known dissections.

Table 42.2 The Aortic Dissection Detection Risk Score

History, symptom, or sign	Definition
Any high-risk condition (1 point)	Marfan syndrome Family history of aortic disease Known aortic valve disease Recent aortic manipulation Known thoracic aortic aneurysm
Any high-risk pain feature (1 point)	Chest, back, or abdominal pain described as any of the following: Abrupt onset Severe intensity Ripping or tearing
Any high-risk exam feature (1 point)	Evidence of perfusion deficit (pulse deficit, systolic blood pressure differential, or focal neurological deficit in conjunction with pain) New murmur of aortic insufficiency (with pain)

Source: Data from [4].

A 2020 systematic review and meta-analysis by Bima *et al.*[7] evaluated the test characteristics of the ADD-RS combined with D-dimer, using both a cutoff of 500 ng/mL as well as an age-adjusted threshold of 10× age (with patients older than 50 years). They included four studies with a total of 3804 patients. Sensitivity for aortic dissection for an ADD-RS = 0 with a D-dimer cutoff < 500 ng/mL was 99% (CI 98–100%), while the sensitivity for the combination of an ADD-RS = 0 with an age-adjusted D-dimer cutoff was 98% (CI 96–99%).

Clinical question

Can abdominal ultrasound be reliably used by emergency clinicians to evaluate for and rule out AAAs?

The addition of abdominal ultrasound to the emergency clinicians' diagnostic toolkit allowed for point-of-care diagnostic capabilities to a disease that previously required cross-sectional imaging (Figure 42.1). A 2013 systematic review and meta-analysis by Rubano *et al.*[8] reviewed the operatic characteristics of ED ultrasonography for AAA, including seven studies with a total of 655 patients. Reference standards used included radiologist review of ED images, radiology-performed ultrasound, and/or CT. The authors note the wide range of ultrasound experience and skill in the reviewed studies, as well as the fact that skill in both obtaining and interpreting images is

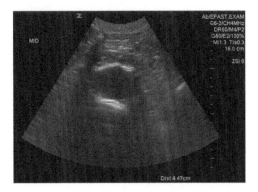

Figure 42.1 Abdominal aortic aneurysm seen on ultrasound. (Used with permission of Elke Platz, Heidi Kimberly & Dorothea Hempel, Department of Emergency Medicine, Brigham and Women's Hospital.)

necessary, making the observer variability and inter-rater reliability important caveats. Nevertheless, they calculated an overall sensitivity of ED ultrasound for AAA of 99% (CI 95–100%) and an LR– of 0.00–0.025, as well as a specificity of 99% (CI 97–99%) and a LR+ of 10.8 to infinity.

Clinical question

Can magnetic resonance angiography (MRA) be used to evaluate for and rule out aortic dissection in ED patients?

While CT imaging is typically the cross-sectional imaging study of choice to diagnose patients suspected of having aortic dissection in the ED, some patients may not be appropriate for CT. In these patients, the use of MRA may be considered. While this has not been widely studied, a 2017 study by Wang *et al.*[9] reviewed 50 ED patients who had MRA imaging for suspected aortic dissection due to iodinated contrast allergy, renal insufficiency, the desire to spare ionizing radiation, or further workup after CTA. While one patient was unable to tolerate the exam, 49 were – of which 47 were negative and allowed for the disease to be ruled out.

Comment

Most emergency physicians evaluate patients with possible aortic emergencies every day, and it is important to use tests that demonstrate acceptable accuracy. However, reliance on historical characteristics, physical examination findings, or chest radiography is inadequate; while a wide mediastinum on chest X-ray should lead to further consideration of the possibility of aortic dissection, a normal chest X-ray cannot rule out the disease. The 2014 American College of Emergency Physicians Clinical Policy regarding the diagnosis of aortic dissection reaffirms this, stating that neither risk scores nor D-dimer testing alone should be used to rule out aortic dissection.[10] However, this policy was published prior to much of the work combining the ADD-RS score with a D-dimer measurement.

The use of the ADD-RS score, especially with the addition of a D-dimer measurement, is highly sensitive and appropriate for use for the rule out of aortic dissection in patients in whom clinicians suspect the disease. However, the poor specificity of this decision instrument argues against its widespread or indiscriminate use in all patients who present with chest pain, as it will invariably lead to overtesting given its poor specificity.[11]

The use of bedside ultrasound as a screening modality for AAA in ED patients with suspected AAA should be part of every emergency physician's armamentarium. However, as the meta-analysis by Rubano reminds us, the effective use of ultrasound is operator dependent and requires both adequate training and quality assurance. Finally, MRA can be used to rule out aortic dissection in patients who cannot undergo CT, although some patients may not be able to tolerate the exam.

References

1. Klompas M. Does this patient have an acute thoracic aortic dissection? *JAMA: The Journal of the American Medical Association.* 2002; 287(17): 2262–72.
2. Ohle R, Kareemi HK, Wells G, Perry JJ. Clinical examination for acute aortic dissection: A systematic review and meta-analysis. *Academic Emergency Medicine.* 2018; 25(4): 397–412.
3. von Kodolitsch Y, Nienaber CA, Dieckmann C *et al.* Chest radiography for the diagnosis of acute aortic syndrome. *The American Journal of Medicine.* 2004; 116(2): 73–7.
4. Nazerian P, Pivetta E, Veglia S *et al.* Integrated use of conventional chest radiography cannot rule out acute aortic syndromes in emergency department patients at low clinical probability. *Academic Emergency Medicine.* 2019; 26(11): 1255–65.
5. Yao J, Bai T, Yang B, Sun L. The diagnostic value of D-dimer in acute aortic dissection: A meta-analysis. *Journal of Cardiothoracic Surgery.* 2021; 16(1): 343.
6. Rogers AM, Hermann LK, Booher AM *et al.* Sensitivity of the Aortic Dissection Detection Risk Score, a novel guideline-based tool for identification of acute aortic dissection at initial presentation. *Circulation.* 2011; 123(20): 2213–8.
7. Bima P, Pivetta E, Nazerian P *et al.* Systematic review of Aortic Dissection Detection Risk Score plus D-dimer for diagnostic rule-out of suspected acute aortic syndromes. *Academic Emergency Medicine.* 2020; 27(10): 1013–27.

8. Rubano E, Mehta N, Caputo W, Paladino L, Sinert R. Systematic review: Emergency department bedside ultrasonography for diagnosing suspected abdominal aortic aneurysm. *Academic Emergency Medicine.* 2013; 20(2): 128–38.

9. Wang GX, Hedgire SS, Le TQ *et al.* MR angiography can guide ED management of suspected acute aortic dissection. *The American Journal of Emergency Medicine.* 2017; 35(4): 527–30.

10. American College of Emergency Physicians Clinical Policies Subcommittee (Writing Committee) on Thoracic Aortic Dissection, Diercks DB, Promes SB *et al.* Clinical policy: Critical issues in the evaluation and management of adult patients with suspected acute nontraumatic thoracic aortic dissection. *Annals of Emergency Medicine.* 2015; 65(1): 32–42.e12.

11. Hill JM, Murphy TG, Fermann GJ. Aortic Dissection Detection Risk Score: A clinical decision rule that needs some parenting. *Academic Emergency Medicine.* 2019; 26(6): 695–7.

Chapter 43 **Ovarian Torsion**

Amr Gharib[1] and Christopher R. Carpenter[2]

[1] Department of Emergency Medicine, University of Pittsburgh Medical Center, Harrisburg, PA, USA
[2] Department of Emergency Medicine, Washington University School of Medicine, St. Louis, MO, USA

Highlights

- The majority of ovarian torsion cases are missed on initial evaluation.
- Prior diagnostic research on elements of the history and physical exam for ovarian torsion has only assessed disease-positive patients, so specificities and likelihood ratios remain unknown.
- No findings on history or physical exam are sufficiently sensitive to rule out the diagnosis of ovarian torsion.
- Ultrasound is the most sensitive tool for ovarian torsion. The use of Doppler does not affect the sensitivity, and slightly increases the specificity for detecting torsion.
- The most sensitive ultrasound finding to diagnose ovarian torsion is the absence of ovarian venous flow which is more sensitive than the absence of ovarian arterial flow (67% versus 46%)
- Within 1 day of symptom onset, the sensitivity of absent venous flow is 85% for ovarian torsion diagnosis.
- Diagnostic certainty for ovarian torsion can be obtained only via direct visualization through laparoscopy.

Background

Adnexal torsion, commonly referred to as *ovarian torsion*, occurs when the vascular pedicle twists and may involve the Fallopian tubes and ovaries. The most common initial symptom is sudden onset intermittent unilateral lower

---

Evidence-Based Emergency Care: Diagnostic Testing and Clinical Decision Rules, Third Edition.
Edited by Jesse M. Pines, Fernanda Bellolio, Christopher R. Carpenter, and Ali S. Raja.
© 2023 John Wiley & Sons Ltd. Published 2023 by John Wiley & Sons Ltd.

quadrant abdominal pain. Thirty percent of cases occur in females under the age of 20 and younger individuals often present with a longer delay since pain began (24 versus 8 hours).[1] The majority of patients with ovarian torsion present for initial evaluation to the emergency department (ED) (75%) rather than the primary care or gynecology clinic – and usually within 12 hours of symptom onset.[2] Ovarian torsion is commonly misdiagnosed and only considered in the differential diagnosis in 47% of cases.[2] Up to 80% of ovarian torsion cases are associated with usually benign ovarian tumors or cysts, but only 25% of patients with ovarian torsion report a history of a known ovarian cyst or mass.[2] Additional risk factors for ovarian torsion include both first-trimester pregnancy and chemical induction of ovulation.[2,3] Although ovarian torsion is the fifth most common reason for emergent surgery in women presenting with abdominal pain (Figure 43.1), the diagnosis is still quite rare, with an annual prevalence of about 3%.[4] Consequently, diagnostic research is limited to retrospective case series.

The ovaries have a dual blood supply from the uterine and ovarian arteries, so complete arterial obstruction is rare. Attempts at surgical salvage via detorsion are therefore warranted even if the diagnosis is made at 72 hours (or later) in the disease course because ovarian function is preserved in 93% of laparoscopically detorsed cases.[5–7] If detorsion is unsuccessful, one ovary is sufficient to maintain fertility.[8] In pediatric (and probably adult) patients, optimal ovarian salvage rates are obtained in those who are taken to the operating room within 8 hours of diagnosis. In cases where operative detorsion has been delayed for over 24 hours, salvage rates approach zero.[9]

The differential diagnosis of atraumatic abdominal pain in women includes appendicitis, ovarian cysts, ectopic pregnancy, renal colic, urinary

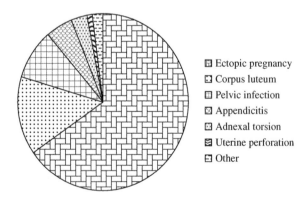

Figure 43.1 Etiology of female abdominal pain requiring emergent surgery. (Data from [4].)

tract infection, pelvic inflammatory disease, malignancy, and diverticulitis.[10] In the evaluation of acute female abdominal pain, the choice of which initial imaging modality to obtain should be based upon the most likely etiology after a careful history and physical exam, including a pelvic exam. Ultrasound is generally considered the imaging technique of choice for ovarian torsion. Computed tomography (CT) is only 34% sensitive for the diagnosis of ovarian torsion (specificity unknown) and agrees with ultrasound results only 50% of the time.[11,12] Magnetic resonance imaging (MRI) may be considered in pregnant patients or as an alternative imaging strategy if ultrasound is unavailable or indeterminant.[13]

Clinical question

What is the diagnostic accuracy of physical exam findings for ovarian torsion in women with abdominal pain?

Right-sided ovarian torsion is more common (55.8%) than left-sided ovarian torsion, possibly due to a stabilizing effect of the sigmoid colon on the left.[14] Other common symptoms of ovarian torsion include nausea (57–77%) and lower quadrant abdominal pain (90%), which can be characterized as sharp or stabbing in 70% and of moderate to severe intensity in 82% of patients with ovarian torsion.[15] However, only half of patients present with the classical pain and up to 30% will not have tenderness on exam.[16] Other clinical findings are not sufficiently sensitive to be useful in the ED (Table 43.1). Suspected ovarian torsion is confirmed operatively in only half of the cases.[17]

Table 43.1 Sensitivity of history and physical exam findings for ovarian torsion

Finding	Sensitivity (%)
Sudden onset pain	87
Constant pain	65
Palpable abdominal mass	62
Nausea	59
Vomiting	54
Any pain	44
Any ovarian torsion risk factors	31
Leukocytosis (WBC > 15,000)	21
Fever	20
Nonmenstrual vaginal bleeding	4

Source: Data from [14].

Table 43.2 Huchon risk prediction score

Finding	Score points
Absence of leukorrhea and metrorrhagia	25
Cyst >5 cm on ultrasound	25
Pain duration <8 hours	20
Vomiting	20
Spontaneous unilateral abdominal or lumbar pain	15
Ovarian torsion score	Predicted risk (95% CI)
0–40	4% (0–8%)
45–60	20% (4–36%)
>60	69% (53–84%)

Source: Data from [18].

A clinical decision rule to assess the likelihood of adnexal torsion has been derived (Table 43.2). The findings most indicative of ovarian torsion include absence of leukorrhea (adjusted odds ratio 12.6 [95% confidence interval [CI] 2.3–67.6]) and an ovarian cyst >5 cm by ultrasound (adjusted odds ratio 10.6 [95% CI 2.9–38.8]), but these results await validation.[18,19]

The specificity of history and physical exam findings, as well as their reproducibility, remains undefined,[2,14] so Bayesian clinicians cannot quantify the impact of any finding (in isolation or combination) upon a patient's post-test probability for Ovarian torsion (see Chapter 3). Therefore, emergency physicians must include ovarian torsion in the differential diagnosis of all women with abdominal pain (who still have their ovaries) to maintain a sufficiently safe threshold for further imaging and prompt gynecological consultation to optimize ovarian salvage. Future diagnostic research on consecutive patients with suspected ovarian torsion is needed to fully understand the epidemiology of ovarian torsion as well as the specificity, likelihood ratios, and reproducibility for elements of history and physical exam.

Clinical question

What is the diagnostic accuracy for adnexal sonography for ovarian torsion in women with abdominal pain?

Ultrasound can be used to evaluate both ovary size and Doppler arterial and venous blood flow, but should not be relied upon as the sole diagnostic test to rule out ovarian torsion.[20] Color Doppler evaluation may increase the post-test probability of ovarian torsion if abnormal (however, "abnormal" was not defined by the investigators) with a positive likelihood ratio (LR+) of 5.3, but the absence of an abnormal Doppler signal does not decrease (negative likelihood ratio [LR–] 0.61) the likelihood of ovarian torsion.[17] In adult patients with lower quadrant abdominal pain of less than 3 days duration, the absence of ovarian venous flow is more sensitive for the diagnosis of ovarian torsion than is the absence of arterial flow (67% versus 46%, respectively) with LR+ 50 (95% CI 11–50) and LR– 0 (95% CI 0–0.2).[21] The sensitivity of absent venous flow diminishes with time since symptom onset: 1-day 85%, 2-days, 75%, ≥3 days, 43%.

As judged by ultrasound, all ovarian torsion patients have enlarged ovaries (mean volume 957 cm^3 in adults with ovarian torsion versus normal nonovarian torsion mean 15 cm^3 in reproductive-aged adults) and 56% have an associated cyst or benign mass.[5] In fact, maximum ovarian diameter (MOD) has been proposed as a screening tool for ovarian torsion in females presenting to the ED with pelvic pain. MOD > 3 cm LR+ 1.4 (95% CI 1.3–1.7) and LR– of 0. MOD > 5 cm LR+ 11.2 (95% CI 5.5–22.9) and LR– 0.09 (95% CI 0.04–0.19).[22]

A systematic review evaluating diagnostic test accuracy of ultrasound for adnexal torsion, reported a pooled sensitivity (n = 1187 patients) of 79% (CI 63–92%), specificity of 76% (CI 54–93%), LR– of 0.29 (CI 0.13–0.66) and LR+ of 4.35 (95% CI 2.03–9.32). Using Doppler (n = 7845) had a sensitivity of 80% (CI 67–93%) and specificity of 88% (CI 72–100%).[23]

Prospective studies of consecutive patients with and without ovarian torsion are essential to further quantify the diagnostic accuracy and reproducibility of ultrasound in addition to history and physical exam for the diagnosis of ovarian torsion.

Clinical question

Can other imaging modalities aid in the evaluation for ovarian torsion?
Because ovarian torsion mimics multiple other more common conditions such as appendicitis and renal colic, CT is frequently obtained on adults with undifferentiated abdominal pain that is ultimately diagnosed as ovarian torsion. However, compared with ultrasound or Doppler ultrasound, CT is the least accurate imaging choice for ovarian torsion in adolescents and probably in adults.[24] Although a normal CT cannot exclude ovarian torsion, some CT findings should raise concern.[16] These findings include asymmetric ovarian enlargement, peripheral follicles surrounding an enlarged ovary, free pelvic fluid, ovarian hemorrhage, inflammatory fat stranding adjacent to the ovary, thickened uterine tube, uterine deviation toward the side of torsion, and a twisted vascular pedicle (the latter, if present, is pathognomonic for ovarian torsion). If these findings are present in the appropriate clinical context, an ovarian US is essential to diagnose ovarian torsion.

A systematic review evaluating diagnostic test accuracy of MRI for adnexal torsion, reported pooled sensitivity (n = 99) of 81% (CI 63–91%) and specificity of 91% (CI 80–96%). Pooling data for CT were not possible because data were obtained from two case-control and one cohort study (n = 232), with sensitivity from 74% to 95% and specificity from 80% to 90%.[23]

Comment

History and physical exam alone can neither rule in nor rule out the diagnosis of ovarian torsion. Although clinical decision instruments to quantify the risk of ovarian torsion are emerging, these await external validation, and ultrasound with Doppler remains the most frequent imaging choice. MRI is a reasonable alternative.

The entirety of the ovarian torsion history and physical exam diagnostic accuracy research consists of case series. In other words, only disease-positive (confirmed ovarian torsion) cases were assessed. Therefore, critical readers *can only estimate the sensitivity* for these findings. Clinicians cannot estimate specificity, LR+ or LR– for findings such as pelvic pain, palpable adnexal mass, and vaginal bleeding. We have no empirical data by which to know whether the presence or absence of these findings increase, decrease, or do not change the posttest probability of ovarian torsion. In general, diagnostic studies that evaluate only disease-positive patients overestimate sensitivity point estimates.[25]

Another limitation of the ovarian torsion diagnostic trials is that they focus only upon accuracy. Future studies should use the Standards for the Reporting of Diagnostic Accuracy Studies (STARD) criteria, which are too often neglected in ED research.[26–28] These studies should quantify diagnostic accuracy and reproducibility across heterogeneous ED settings (rural/urban, academic/community) for each element of history, physical exam, lab testing, and sonography before eventually assessing patient-important outcomes.[29] Based upon the available evidence, emergency physicians should include ovarian torsion in the differential diagnosis of women of all ages with abdominal pain (as long as they still have their ovaries) and maintain a low threshold for further imaging and gynecologic consultation while recognizing that each of those modalities is also imperfect for this sometimes challenging diagnosis.

References

1. Ashwal E, Hiersch L, Krissi H *et al.* Characteristics and management of ovarian torsion in premenarchal compared with postmenarchal patients. *Obstetrics and Gynecology.* 2015; 126(3): 514–20.

2. Houry D, Abbott JT. Ovarian torsion: A fifteen-year review. *Annals of Emergency Medicine*. 2001; 38(2): 156–9.

3. Hasson J, Tsafrir Z, Azem F *et al.* Comparison of adnexal torsion between pregnant and nonpregnant women. *American Journal of Obstetrics and Gynecology*. 2010; 202(6): 536.e1–6.

4. Hibbard LT. Adnexal torsion. *American Journal of Obstetrics and Gynecology*. 1985; 152(4): 456–61.

5. Shadinger LL, Andreotti RF, Kurian RL. Preoperative sonographic and clinical characteristics as predictors of ovarian torsion. *Journal of Ultrasound in Medicine*. 2008; 27(1): 7–13.

6. Cohen SB, Oelsner G, Seidman DS, Admon D, Mashiach S, Goldenberg M. Laparoscopic detorsion allows sparing of the twisted ischemic adnexa. *The Journal of the American Association of Gynecologic Laparoscopists*. 1999; 6(2): 139–43.

7. Abraham M, Keyser EA. ACOG Committee Opinion: Adnexal torsion in adolescents. *Obstetrics and Gynecology*. 2019; 134(2): e56–63.

8. Lass A. The fertility povarian torsionential of women with a single ovary. *Human Reproduction Update*. 1999; 5(5): 546–50.

9. Anders JF, Powell EC. Urgency of evaluation and outcome of acute ovarian torsion in pediatric patients. *Archives of Pediatrics & Adolescent Medicine*. 2005; 159(6): 532–5.

10. Nichols DH, Julian PJ. Torsion of the adnexa. *Clinical Obstetrics and Gynecology*. 1985; 28(2): 375–80.

11. Hiller N, Appelbaum L, Simanovsky N, Lev-Sagi A, Aharoni D, Sella T. CT features of adnexal torsion. *AJR. American Journal of Roentgenology*. 2007; 189(1): 124–9.

12. Moore C, Meyers AB, Capotasto J, Bokhari J. Prevalence of abnormal CT findings in patients with proven ovarian torsion and a proposed triage schema. *Emergency Radiology*. 2009; 16(2): 115–20.

13. Masselli G, Brunelli R, Casciani E *et al.* Acute abdominal and pelvic pain in pregnancy: MR imaging as a valuable adjunct to ultrasound? *Abdominal Imaging*. 2011; 36(5): 596–603.

14. White M, Stella J. Ovarian torsion: 10-year perspective. *Emergency Medicine Australasia*. 2005; 17(3): 231–7.

15. Rey-Bellet Gasser C, Gehri M, Joseph JM, Pauchard JY. Is it ovarian torsion? A systematic literature review and evaluation of prediction signs. *Pediatric Emergency Care*. 2016; 32(4): 256–61.

16. Robertson JJ, Long B, Koyfman A. Myths in the evaluation and management of ovarian torsion. *The Journal of Emergency Medicine*. 2017; 52(4): 449–56.

17. Bar-On S, Maschiach R, Stockheim D *et al.* Emergency laparoscopy for suspected ovarian torsion: Are we too hasty to operate? *Fertility and Sterility*. 2010; 93(6): 2012–5.

18. Huchon C, Staraci S, Fauconnier A. Adnexal torsion: A predictive score for preoperative diagnosis. *Human Reproduction*. 2010; 25(9): 2276–80.

19. Damigos E, Johns J, Ross J. An update on the diagnosis and management of ovarian torsion. *The Obstetrician and Gynaecologist*. 2012; 14: 229–36.
20. Grunau GL, Harris A, Buckley J, Todd NJ. Diagnosis of ovarian torsion: Is it time to forget about Doppler? *Journal of Obstetrics and Gynaecology Canada*. 2018; 40(7): 871–5.
21. Ben-Ami M, Perlitz Y, Haddad S. The effectiveness of spectral and color Doppler in predicting ovarian torsion. A prospective study. *European Journal of Obstetrics, Gynecology, and Reproductive Biology*. 2002; 104: 64–6.
22. Budhram G, Elia T, Dan J et al. A case-control study of sonographic maximum ovarian diameter as a predictor of ovarian torsion in emergency department females with pelvic pain. *Academic Emergency Medicine*. 2019; 26(2): 152–9.
23. Wattar B, Rimmer M, Rogozinska E, Macmillian M, Khan KS, Wattar BHA. Accuracy of imaging modalities for adnexal torsion: A systematic review and meta-analysis. *BJOG: An International Journal of Obstetrics and Gynaecology*. 2021; 128(1): 37–44.
24. Bronstein ME, Pandya S, Snyder CW, Shi Q, Muensterer OJ. A meta-analysis of B-mode ultrasound, Doppler ultrasound, and computed tomography to diagnose pediatric ovarian torsion. *European Journal of Pediatric Surgery*. 2015; 25(1): 82–6.
25. Kohn MA, Carpenter CR, Newman TB. Understanding the direction of bias in studies of diagnostic test accuracy. *Academic Emergency Medicine*. 2013; 20(11): 1194–206.
26. Bossuyt PMM, Reitsma JB, Bruns DE et al. STARD 2015: An updated list of essential items for reporting diagnostic accuracy studies. *BMJ*. 2015; 351: h5527.
27. Simel DL, Rennie D, Bossuyt PM. The STARD statement for reporting diagnostic accuracy studies: Application to the history and physical examination. *Journal of General Internal Medicine*. 2008; 23(6): 768–74.
28. Gallo L, Hua N, Mercuri M, Silveira A, Worster A. Adherence to standards for reporting diagnostic accuracy in emergency medicine research. *Academic Emergency Medicine*. 2017; 24(8): 914–9.
29. El Dib R, Tikkinen KAO, Akl EA et al. Systematic survey of randomized trials evaluating the impact of alternative diagnostic strategies on patient-important outcomes. *Journal of Clinical Epidemiology*. 2017; 84: 61–9.

SECTION 6
Urology

Chapter 44 **Nephrolithiasis**

Jesse M. Pines[1,2] and Christopher R. Carpenter[3]

[1] US Acute Care Solutions, Canton, OH, USA
[2] Department of Emergency Medicine, Drexel University, Philadelphia, PA, USA
[3] Department of Emergency Medicine, Washington University School of Medicine, Saint Louis, MO, USA

Highlights

- Nephrolithiasis should be considered in patients presenting with acute flank pain, hematuria, groin pain, and/or vomiting.
- Unenhanced CT imaging should be considered the gold standard when diagnosing nephrolithiasis in the emergency department.
- Unenhanced CT, radiology-performed ultrasound, and point-of-care ultrasound are reasonable choices for diagnostic imaging with one randomized controlled trial demonstrating no significant differences in outcomes or costs between the three imaging options.
- The test of choice in renal colic should be determined based on the patient's presentation and risk factors, such as whether the patient is presenting with their first stone where there is a high rate of alternative diagnoses.
- Repeat CT scanning in patients with a previously documented history of nephrolithiasis results in a change in urgent management in a minority (7%) of cases.

Background

There are about two million annual emergency department (ED) visits in the United States with suspected renal colic.[1] The lifetime risk of nephrolithiasis (i.e., kidney stones) is 10.6% in men and 7.1% in women in the United States.[2]

Evidence-Based Emergency Care: Diagnostic Testing and Clinical Decision Rules, Third Edition.
Edited by Jesse M. Pines, Fernanda Bellolio, Christopher R. Carpenter, and Ali S. Raja.
© 2023 John Wiley & Sons Ltd. Published 2023 by John Wiley & Sons Ltd.

Patients frequently seek emergency care for the pain associated with nephrolithiasis because it is typically severe and refractory to over-the-counter analgesics. Notably, pain severity does not correlate with the kidney stone size or likelihood of spontaneous passage.[3,4] Clinical features of symptomatic nephrolithiasis include acute flank pain radiating to the groin, nausea, vomiting, and either gross or microscopic hematuria. However, the presence of hydronephrosis on imaging is more specific for obstructing kidney stone than any of these clinical findings.[5] Standard imaging modalities for the initial diagnosis of nephrolithiasis are either noncontrast spiral computed tomography (CT) scan or ultrasound (US) with no significant difference in cost noted when selecting CT or US.[6] Healthcare disparities and/or practice variability have been identified in suspected renal colic CT imaging associated with geographic locale and socioeconomic strata.[7,8] Of patients with known nephrolithiasis, almost 50% will develop additional stones within 5–7 years.[9]

Clinical question

How do different diagnostic modalities (unenhanced CT, US, and other diagnostic modalities) compare when it comes to diagnosing nephrolithiasis?
Modern emergency care involves choosing between different options when it comes to the diagnosis of nephrolithiasis in patients with suspected renal colic, in particular the use of unenhanced standard or low-dose CT, radiology or emergency medicine point-of-care in the US, or no imaging. A recent study showed that CT scanning is the predominant test used and is performed in more than 90% of patients diagnosed with kidney stones.[10] Each imaging type gives specific information. In general, unenhanced CT is viewed as the gold standard and can give the most detailed information including the diagnosis of nephrolithiasis, the size of the stone which guides whether intervention is needed (i.e., is ≥10 mm in size), whether hydronephrosis is present, and of overall stone burden.[11] In addition, CT can also detect other intraabdominal abnormalities that may be causing symptoms including aortic aneurysm and appendicitis. By contrast, the US is used to detect the presence and degree of hydronephrosis and can also detect anatomical issues or other signs of kidney infection. US is less sensitive in the ability to detect the specific size of the stone.[12] Historically older diagnostic modalities that have been used to diagnose nephrolithiasis have included intravenous (IV) urography, renal tomography, and plain radiography.

An early study on the topic in the late 1980s investigated the sensitivity of the US to detect renal calculi in a three-phase study in 100 patients.[13] In the first phase, US was performed after reviewing abdominal radiography and renal tomograms in 30 patients who had undergone extracorporeal shock wave lithotripsy (ESWL), and the sensitivity for detecting stones was 98%. In the second phase, US was performed in 30 post-ESWL patients without any prior review of radiographs or tomograms. In the second group, the sensitivity of US for stone detection was 95%. In the third phase, 40 patients had the US performed in a blinded way in a random mix of post-ESWL patients and patients who had undergone urography for other reasons. In this group, the sensitivity of the US was 91%. In combined data, the authors reported an overall sensitivity of the US of 96%.

A 2003 randomized trial compared CT to IV urography for patients with suspected nephrolithiasis enrolled 122 patients with acute flank pain.[14] A total of 59 of them were randomized to CT and 63 to IV urography. The radiographic studies were independently interpreted by four radiologists. Of patients receiving IV urography, mild to moderate adverse reactions from contrast material were seen in three (5%) patients. The mean radiation dose was 3.3 mSv for urography and 6.5 mSv for CT scan. Sensitivity and specificity of CT were 94% and 94%, respectively. For urography, sensitivity and specificity were lower at 85% and 90%, respectively.

Another study investigated the sensitivity of radiology performed diagnostic US compared to CT for the detection of kidney stones in 46 patients with acute flank pain, using a combination of tests and clinical follow-up as the criterion standard.[15] CT imaging detected 22 of 23 ureteral calculi (sensitivity: 96%), and US detected 14 of 23 ureteral calculi (sensitivity: 61%). The specificity for each technique was 100%. When modalities were compared for the detection of any clinically relevant abnormality, the sensitivities of US and CT were 92% and 100%, respectively.

An additional study was performed in a Spanish hospital and published in 2010.[16] The authors enrolled patients with "persistent renoureteral colic" after standard care. The patients were blindly evaluated by US and CT and, in the 124 patients studied, nephrolithiasis was present in 60%. The specificity and positive predictive value (PPV) of US for nephrolithiasis were 100%, but its sensitivity was only 30%.

Another study determined the test characteristics of US for any ureteral stone and for stones ≥5 mm in size.[17] In 117 patients, the sensitivity for the US was 77% (CI 59–88%) and the specificity was 86% (CI 74–93%) for any stone disease. For stones ≥5 mm, the sensitivity was 90% (CI 54–100%) and the specificity was 64% (CI 53–73%).

A more recent study has examined the sensitivity and specificity of radiology-performed US for the detection of nephrolithiasis.[18] It also assessed the accuracy to determine the size of calculi and whether this information may help in decisions around counseling patients. In a retrospective study, patients who had undergone an US followed by a noncontrast CT within 60 days were followed at the Cleveland Clinic. Notably, patients were enrolled across a variety of settings, including asymptomatic patients. In 552 patients, the sensitivity and specificity of the US were 54% and 91%. The sensitivity of US increased as stone size increased but was not affected by the location of the stone. When divided by stone size of 0–4 mm (which involve observation) compared to stones ≥5 mm (where intervention is commonly required), there were 54/384 (14%) of cases where US would have led to a recommendation for observation while CT would suggest intervention was needed. In addition, when CT would suggest an intervention, the US would suggest observation in 65/168 (39%) of cases. The authors concluded that by performing US that 119/552 (22%) would be inappropriately counseled with 43% of stones in the 5–10 mm by US having the management recommendation changes when CT was performed.

Clinical question

In ED patients presenting with suspected uncomplicated renal colic which diagnostic strategy should be pursued to optimize patient outcomes?

A large multicenter pragmatic comparative effectiveness clinical trial has demonstrated that there are no differences in serious adverse events when patients were randomized to point-of-care ultrasound (POCUS) performed by emergency physicians, US interpreted by radiologists, or unenhanced CT.[19] Specifically, in 2759 patients undergoing randomization to the three interventions, serious adverse events were 12.4%, 10.8%, and 11.2% ($p = 0.50$), respectively. Pain scores were similar across all three groups and there were no differences in return ED visits, hospitalizations, or diagnostic accuracy. The US groups notably did have less cumulative exposure to radiation at 6 months.

A group of ED physicians, urologists, and radiologists recently convened to answer this question using a systematic review methodology as well as group consensus that was subsequently published in each specialty's journals.[20] The systematic review covered the dates 1995–2018. Following the systematic review of the sensitivity of different imaging studies for renal colic, a series of 29 clinical scenarios was presented with the goal of reaching consensus on the optimal initial imaging. The focus was on scenarios where either standard or reduced-radiation-dose CT may not be the clear, initial approach, and other approaches could be taken such as point-of-care or radiology-performed US or no imaging. The authors gained consensus using a modified Delphi process with three rounds of anonymous voting and group discussions with nine members voting.

In 43 articles that compared radiology-performed US and POCUS, the sensitivity of radiology-performed US for most studies ranged from 57% to 91%. Several studies were identified that demonstrated that US would not miss stones requiring intervention.[21,22] When it came to POCUS performed by emergency physicians, the diagnostic accuracy in 15 studies was assessed based on the presence of hydronephrosis rather than direct stone visualization. The sensitivity was 70.2% and the specificity of 75.4%.[23] Based on the results of the voting among the nine clinicians, there was an excellent agreement based on the Delphi results with different recommendations that should be tailored to the individual circumstance.[21]

For example, the scenario, "35-year-old man with no prior history of kidney stones presents with an acute onset of flank pain over the last 3 hours. He reports nausea with vomiting and has hematuria on urine dip. He has no abdominal tenderness. His pain is relieved after IV analgesics" was voted as POCUS by all nine of the clinicians. By contrast, the scenario "A 75-year-old man with no prior history of kidney stones presents with an acute onset of flank pain over the last 3 hours. He reports nausea with vomiting and has hematuria on urine dip. He has no abdominal tenderness. His pain is relieved after IV analgesics" was voted as CT by all nine. The authors concluded that CT is some common clinical scenarios when uncomplicated renal colic is suspected. For the scenario, "A 35-year-old woman who is 10 weeks pregnant with no prior history of kidney stones presents with acute onset right flank pain over the last 3 hours. She reports nausea with vomiting and has hematuria on urine dip. She has no abdominal tenderness. Her pain is relieved after IV analgesics. An US is performed; there is hydronephrosis on the side of the pain, and a stone is not visualized," all nine agreed that no additional imaging was required.

Clinical question

Is it important to use unenhanced CT to diagnose kidney stones on the first visit for presumed ureteral colic?

Several studies have examined this question. A prospective observational study assessed the impact of helical CT in 132 patients with a first episode of suspected nephrolithiasis (see Figures 44.1 and 44.2).[25] Patients with a known history of nephrolithiasis were excluded. Prior to the CT, emergency physicians completed questionnaires detailing their diagnostic certainty of nephrolithiasis as well as the patient's anticipated disposition. The primary study outcome was a comparison of physician diagnostic certainty to CT results. The secondary outcome measure was an alternate diagnosis. Pre-CT diagnostic certainty was divided into four groups (0–49%, 50–74%, 75–90%, and

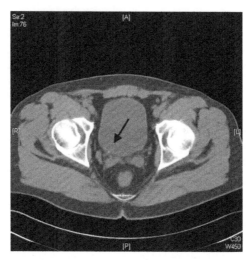

Figure 44.1 Unenhanced computed tomography (CT) scan showing 1–2 mm calculus at the right ureterovesical junction.

90–100%), and these groups each had a diagnosis of urinary calculi made in 28.6%, 45.7%, 74.2%, and 80.5% of their patients, respectively. An alternative diagnosis was revealed on CT scan in 40 cases (33%), 19 of whom had another significant pathology. The majority of these other significant diagnoses were previously unrecognized cancers, and some were less significant (such as adrenal adenomas). Prior to CT scanning, physicians planned to discharge 115 patients and admit six patients. The authors concluded that patients presenting with a first episode of clinically suspected nephrolithiasis should undergo a CT scan because it enhances diagnostic accuracy and identifies clinically significant alternative diagnoses.

Another study examined the incidence and clinical relevance of alternate diagnoses in a large series of 1500 patients with acute flank pain and suspected urinary calculi who received a CT scan.[26] In this study, patients with a history of urinary tract calculi were not excluded. Alternate findings on CT were classified as to whether they required immediate or delayed treatment or were of little or no clinical importance. They found that 69% of their patients had urinary tract calculi, including 30% with nephrolithiasis, 36% with ureterolithiasis, and 34% with both conditions. Of all patients, 1064 (71%) had other or additional CT findings, 207 (14%) had nonnephrolithiasis related CT findings requiring immediate or deferred treatment, 464 (31%) had pathological conditions of little clinical importance, and 393 (26%) had pathological conditions of no clinical relevance. The authors concluded that

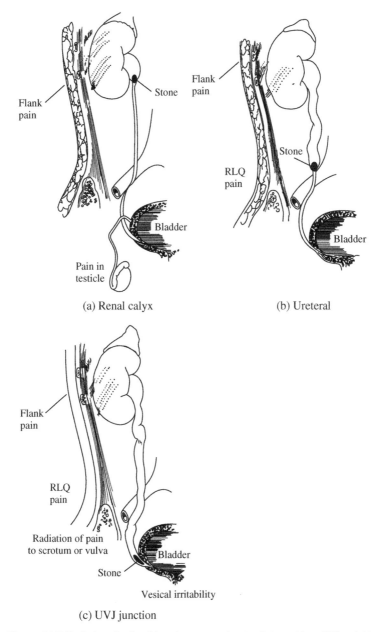

(a) Renal calyx

(b) Ureteral

(c) UVJ junction

Figure 44.2 Radiation of pain with various types of ureteral stone. Note: RLQ = right lower quadrant. Tanagho and McAninch[24]

CT in patients with acute flank pain allows for the accurate diagnosis of urinary stone disease and can provide further important information leading to emergency treatment in a substantial number of patients.

Clinical question

Is it helpful to repeat CT imaging in patients with known urinary calculi when they re-present with acute flank pain, similar to previous episodes of nephrolithiasis?

A study sought to determine the incidence of "alternative diagnoses" in patients with a history of prior documented nephrolithiasis who underwent repeat CT imaging when they returned to the ED in a single tertiary care hospital.[27] In 231 patients who had been rescanned for similar symptoms of renal colic, 181 (82%) had no change in their diagnosis as a result of the repeat CT scan, 27 (12%) had an alternative diagnosis that did not require an additional intervention, and 15 (7%) were diagnosed with a condition that required an urgent intervention. In the 27 patients with an alternative diagnosis, the most common diagnosis was musculoskeletal pain (18 patients). In the 15 patients who required urgent intervention, the most common diagnosis was acute pyelonephritis (seven patients), followed by diverticulitis (two), appendicitis (two), small bowel obstruction (one), pneumonia (one), pelvic inflammatory disease (one), and cholecystitis (one).

Clinical question

Can a predicted rule identify patients with uncomplicated ureteral stones?

A 2014 study aimed to derive and validate a clinical prediction rule to identify the presence of uncomplicated ureteral stones in ED patients who otherwise undergo unenhanced CT.[28] Data were gathered from an urban, tertiary care ED and a suburban freestanding ED. The derivation cohort was a random selection of 1040 patients who underwent CT from 2005 to 2010, and the validation cohort was prospectively enrolled from 2011 to 2013. In the derivation cohort, the top five factors associated with a ureteral stone were male gender, short duration of pain, nonblack race, presence of nausea or vomiting, and microscopic hematuria. Together, the sex, timing, origin, nausea, erythrocytes (STONE) score was developed (see Table 44.1). In the derivation and validation cohorts, a ureteral stone was present in 8.3% and 9.2% of the low probability cohort (STONE score 0–5), 51.6%, and 51.3% of the moderate probability cohort (STONE score 6–9), and 89.6% and 88.6% of the high probability cohort (STONE score 10–13). In the high probability group, important alternative findings were present in 0.3% of the derivation and 1.6% of the validation cohorts.

Table 44.1 The STONE score to detect
symptomatic ureteral stones

Factor	Points
Sex:	
Female	0
Male	2
Pain duration:	
>24 hours	0
6–24 hours	1
<6 hours	3
Race:	
Black	0
Nonblack	3
Nausea and vomiting:	
None	0
Nausea alone	1
Vomiting	2
Hematuria:	
Absent	0
Present	3

Score interpretation:
Score 0–5 – low risk for stones
Score 6–9 – moderate risk for stones
Score 10–13 – high risk for stones.

In an external validation study, 845 patients were included, of which 331 (30%) had a ureteral stone.[29] The performance of the STONE score was found to be superior to physician gestalt with an area under the receiver operating characteristic (AUROC) = 0.78, compared to 0.68. In low-, moderate, and high-score groups, the prevalence of a ureteral stone on CT scan was 14% in the low score group and 73% in the high score group. The sensitivity and specificity of a high score were 53% and 87% respectively, and the authors concluded that it lacked sufficient accuracy to defer CT scan in cases of suspected ureteral stone.

This prompted the creators of the STONE score to assess whether the addition of renal point-of-care limited ultrasonography (PLUS), along with the STONE score variables could help identify patients with uncomplicated stones or who needed urological intervention.[30] In particular, the Renal PLUS was assessed for the presence of hydronephrosis. In 835 patients, there were ureteral stones in 53%, while 6.5% had an acutely important alternative finding on CT scan. Renal PLUS modestly increased the sensitivity for symptomatic stone among the low and moderate STONE categories. Moderate or more than moderate hydronephrosis improved the specificity from 67% to 98%, and 42% to 92% in low and moderate risk patients by the STONE score. By comparison, test characteristics were unchanged among the high-risk patients. Any hydronephrosis was 66% sensitive for urological intervention while moderate or more than moderate hydronephrosis was 86% specific and 81% sensitive. The authors concluded that hydronephrosis on Renal PLUS the STONE criteria improved the risk stratification of low- and moderate-risk STONE score patients. In addition, the presence or absence of hydronephrosis among high-risk patients did not change the likelihood of a symptomatic stone but can help identify patients who are more likely to need urological intervention.

Comment

There are differences in test characteristics between US and unenhanced CT when it comes to detecting nephrolithiasis in patients with suspected renal colic. Unenhanced CT provides more information and is a better indicator of stone size and can detect alternative diagnoses. However, there are clinical scenarios where either diagnostic US performed by radiologists or emergency physicians are a safe alternative, suggesting that a customized diagnostic approach based on the clinical question is a reasonable approach. As noted in Chapter 6, one approach to definitely evaluate whether varying diagnostic approaches yield different patient-centric outcomes is by a randomized controlled trial, which are rare. The ED renal colic scenario is one diagnostic question that has been evaluated by a randomized controlled trial and despite the differences in diagnostic accuracy between US and CT, patient outcomes were the same.

In addition, the STONE score exists to help ED clinicians weigh the value of imaging for individual patients. A high STONE score can reduce the need for an immediate CT scan in otherwise healthy patients, where an alternative diagnosis is not suspected. A moderate STONE score plus the finding of hydronephrosis suggests a very high likelihood of stones in otherwise healthy patients, can may reduce the need for immediate unenhanced CT scan. By contrast, a low score should prompt clinicians to seek an alternative diagnosis. Nevertheless, what is clear from these nuanced ways to use STONE and ED US together is that additional research is needed in this area. The 2015 Society for Academic Emergency Medicine Consensus Conference identified implementation of flank pain clinical decision rules as a top priority research domain to optimize diagnostic imaging in ED settings.[31] Ultimately, ED clinical practice guidelines that incorporate GRADE criteria of the balance between benefits/ harms, costs, and health equity while incorporating patient values will be essential to align renal colic imaging decisions with the best evidence.

References

1. Dai JC, Chang HC, Holt SK, Harper JD. National trends in CT utilization and estimated CT-related radiation exposure in the evaluation and follow-up of stone patients. *Urology*. 2019; 133: 50–6.

2. Scales CD Jr, Smith AC, Hanley JM, Saigal CS. Urologic diseases in America project. Prevalence of kidney stones in the United States. *European Urology*. 2012; 62(1): 160–5.

3. Sasmaz Mİ, Kirpat V. The relationship between the severity of pain and stone size, hydronephrosis and laboratory parameters in renal colic attack. *The American Journal of Emergency Medicine*. 2019; 37(11): 2107–10.

4. Gourlay K, Splinter G, Hayward J, Innes G. Does pain severity predict stone characteristics or outcomes in emergency department patients with acute renal colic? *The American Journal of Emergency Medicine*. 2021; 45: 37–41.

5. Saw JT, Imeri NN, Aldridge ES, Buntine PG. Predictive values of haematuria and hydronephrosis in suspected renal colic: An emergency department retrospective audit. *Emergency Medicine Australasia*. 2020; 32(4): 573–7.

6. Melnikow J, Xing G, Cox G et al. Cost analysis of the STONE randomized trial: Can health care costs be reduced one test at a time? *Medical Care*. 2016; 54(4): 337–42.

7. Hyams ES, Matlaga BR, Korley FK. Practice patterns in the emergency care of kidney stone patients: An analysis of the National Hospital Ambulatory Medical Care Survey (NHAMCS). *The Canadian Journal of Urology*. 2012; 19(4): 6351–9.

8. Balthazar P, Sadigh G, Hughes D, Rosenkrantz AB, Hanna T, Duszak R Jr. Increasing use, geographic variation, and disparities in emergency department CT for suspected urolithiasis. *Journal of the American College of Radiology*. 2019; 16(11): 1547–53.

9. Rule AD, Lieske JC, Li X, Melton LJ 3rd, Krambeck AE, Bergstralh EJ. The ROKS nomogram for predicting a second symptomatic stone episode. *Journal of the American Society of Nephrology*. 2014; 25(12): 2878–86.

10. Fwu CW, Eggers PW, Kimmel PL, Kusek JW, Kirkali Z. Emergency department visits, use of imaging, and drugs for urolithiasis have increased in the United States. *Kidney International*. 2013; 83(3): 479–86.

11. Assimos D, Krambeck A, Miller NL et al. Surgical management of stones: American Urological Association/Endourological Society Guideline, Part II. *The Journal of Urology*. 2016; 196(4): 1161–9.

12. Moore CL, Carpenter CR, Heilbrun ME et al. Imaging in suspected renal colic: Systematic review of the literature and multispecialty consensus. *Journal of the American College of Radiology*. 2019; 16(9 Pt A): 1132–43.

13. Middleton WD, Dodds WJ, Lawson TL. Foley WD renal calculi: Sensitivity for detection with US. *Radiology*. 1988; 167: 239–44.

14. Pfister SA, Deckart A, Laschke S et al. Unenhanced helical computed tomography vs intravenous urography in patients with acute flank pain: Accuracy and economic impact in a randomized prospective trial. *European Radiology*. 2003; 13: 2513–20.

15. Sheafor DH, Hertzberg BS, Freed KS *et al.* Nonenhanced helical CT and US in the emergency evaluation of patients with renal colic: Prospective comparison. *Radiology.* 2000; 217: 792–7.

16. Rengifo Abbad D, Rodríguez Caravaca G, Barreales Tolosa L *et al.* Diagnostic validity of helical CT compared to ultrasonography in renal-ureteral colic. *Archivos Españoles de Urología.* 2010; 63: 139–44.

17. Moak JH, Lyons MS, Lindsell CJ. Bedside renal ultrasound in the evaluation of suspected ureterolithiasis. *American Journal of Emergency Medicine.* 2012; 30: 218–21.

18. Ganesan V, De S, Greene D, Torricelli FC, Monga M. Accuracy of ultrasonography for renal stone detection and size determination: Is it good enough for management decisions? *BJU International.* 2017; 119(3): 464–9.

19. Smith-Bindman R, Aubin C, Bailitz J *et al.* Ultrasonography versus computed tomography for suspected nephrolithiasis. *The New England Journal of Medicine.* 2014; 371(12): 1100–10.

20. Moore CL, Carpenter CR, Heilbrun ME *et al.* Imaging in suspected renal colic: Systematic review of the literature and multispecialty consensus. *Annals of Emergency Medicine.* 2019; 74(3): 391–9.

21. Ekici S, Sinanoglu O. Comparison of conventional radiography combined with ultrasonography versus nonenhanced helical computed tomography in evaluation of patients with renal colic. *Urological Research.* 2012; 40(5): 543–7.

22. Kobayashi T, Nishizawa K, Watanabe J, Ogura K. Clinical characteristics of ureteral calculi detected by nonenhanced computerized tomography after unclear results of plain radiography and ultrasonography. *The Journal of Urology.* 2003; 170(3): 799–802.

23. Wong C, Teitge B, Ross M, Young P, Robertson HL, Lang E. The accuracy and prognostic value of point-of-care ultrasound for nephrolithiasis in the emergency department: A systematic review and meta-analysis. *Academic Emergency Medicine.* 2018; 25(6): 684–98.

24. Tanagho EA, McAninch JW. *Smith's General Urology.* 16th ed. New York: McGraw-Hill; 2003.

25. Ha M, MacDonald RD. Impact of CT scan in patients with first episode of suspected nephrolithasis. *Journal of Emergency Medicine.* 2004; 27: 225–31.

26. Hoppe H, Studer R, Kessler TM *et al.* Alternate or additional findings to stone disease on unenhanced computerized tomography for acute flank pain can impact management. *Journal of Urology.* 2006; 175: 1725–30.

27. Goldstone A, Bushnell A. Does diagnosis change as a result of repeat renal colic computed tomography scan in patients with a history of kidney stones? *American Journal of Emergency Medicine.* 2010; 28: 291–5.

28. Moore CL, Bomann S, Daniels B *et al.* Derivation and validation of a clinical prediction rule for uncomplicated ureteral stone–the STONE score: Retrospective and prospective observational cohort studies. *BMJ.* 2014; 348: g2191.

29. Wang RC, Rodriguez RM, Moghadassi M *et al.* External validation of the STONE score, a clinical prediction rule for ureteral stone: An observational multi-institutional study. *Annals of Emergency Medicine.* 2016; 67(4): 423–32.e2.

30. Daniels B, Gross CP, Molinaro A *et al.* STONE PLUS: Evaluation of emergency department patients with suspected renal colic, using a clinical prediction tool combined with point-of-care limited ultrasonography. *Annals of Emergency Medicine.* 2016; 67(4): 439–48.

31. Finnerty NM, Rodriguez RM, Carpenter CR *et al.* Clinical decision rules for diagnostic imaging in the emergency department: A research agenda. *Academic Emergency Medicine.* 2015; 22(12): 1406–16.

Chapter 45 **Testicular Torsion**

Ali S. Raja[1] and Jesse M. Pines[2,3]

[1] Department of Emergency Medicine, Massachusetts General Hospital, Harvard Medical School, Boston, MA, USA
[2] US Acute Care Solutions, Canton, OH, USA
[3] Department of Emergency Medicine, Drexel University, Philadelphia, PA, USA

Highlights

- Acute testicular torsion is a urological emergency and should be considered in males presenting with testicular or scrotal pain.
- The combination of pain, nausea or vomiting, ipsilateral scrotal skin changes, and the absence of the ipsilateral cremasteric reflex is highly concerning for torsion, especially in the pediatric population.
- Testicular ultrasound is widely available and highly accurate but does not definitively rule out torsion in patients with classic symptomatology.

Background

The patient with testicular pain presents a diagnostic challenge for emergency physicians. While there are multiple causes for testicular pain, including infectious and inflammatory reasons, neoplasms, hernias, and trauma, torsion is one of the most concerning due to the possibility of organ loss which may be prevented by emergent intervention.[1,2] Torsion should be considered in the differential diagnosis for every male presenting with testicular, scrotal, or lower abdominal pain, but it is predominately a condition of the young and very young, occurring in approximately one in 4000 males under the age of 25. Notably, while adult testicular torsion is rare, adult patients may

---

Evidence-Based Emergency Care: Diagnostic Testing and Clinical Decision Rules, Third Edition.
Edited by Jesse M. Pines, Fernanda Bellolio, Christopher R. Carpenter, and Ali S. Raja.
© 2023 John Wiley & Sons Ltd. Published 2023 by John Wiley & Sons Ltd.

be more likely to have delayed presentations and diagnoses, and thus lower testicular salvage rates.[3]

Testicular torsion is a urological emergency, as twisting of the spermatic cord compromises first venous, and then arterial blood flow causing acute pain and testicular ischemia. Ruling out testicular torsion is important and time-sensitive because delays in diagnosis and therapy can result in problems with fertility, organ loss, and a poor cosmetic outcome. Viability and salvage-ability of the torsed testicle decrease as time from onset of symptoms (e.g., pain) increases, with approximately 90% salvageability with detorsion in <6 hours, nearly 50% viability after 12 hours, and close to 10% after 24 hours. A 20-year review of cases by Yang et al.[2] included 118 cases with a median duration of symptoms of 64 hours, only 39% of whom had viable testes at surgery. The median duration of symptoms for those with viable testes was 12 hours, while those in whom testes could not be salvaged had a median duration of 90 hours. Due to the importance that time plays in the treatment of testicular torsion, patients with historical and physical exam findings suggestive of the disease should have emergent urologic evaluation. In unclear cases, imaging may be helpful and, in the emergency department (ED), ultra-sound has replaced scintigraphy as the standard imaging modality for diagnosing testicular torsion due to its widespread availability and the limited availability of nuclear imaging.

Clinical question

Which historical and physical exam findings can help diagnose or exclude testicular torsion?

Two pediatric studies have focused on the diagnostic utility of the history and physical exam findings for testicular torsion. Beni-Israel et al.[4] conducted a retrospective review of 523 patients with scrotal pain presenting to their pediatric ED, using ultrasound and surgical findings as their criterion standard. In a population with a mean age of 10 years and 9 months, the authors found an incidence of testicular torsion of 3.3% and, on univariate analysis, determined that five clinical variables were associated with testicular torsion: duration of symptoms <24 hours (odds ratio [OR] 6.7, confidence interval [CI] 1.6–33), nausea and/or vomiting (OR 8.9, CI 2.6–30), abdominal pain (OR 3.2, CI 1.2–8.9), high position of the testes (OR 58.8, CI 19–167), and abnormal cremasteric reflex (OR 27.8, CI 7.5–100). However, it should be noted that patients who were discharged without ultrasound were not followed up and may have presented elsewhere with missed testicular torsion. This lack of an acceptable criterion standard or meaningful estimates of diagnostic accuracy such as positive likelihood ratio (LR+) or negative likelihood

Table 45.1 Test characteristics of combinations of absence of the ipsilateral cremasteric reflex, presence of nausea or vomiting, and scrotal skin changes

	Sensitivity (%)	Specificity (%)	Positive predictive value (PPV) (%)	Negative predictive value (NPV) (%)
0 positive	100	76	32	100
1 positive	44	80	20	93
2 positive	25	97	50	92
3 positive	25	100	100	92

Source: Data from [5].

ratio (LR−), as well as the retrospective nature of this study, preclude any possibility of using these associated symptoms to rule out or rule in torsion.

Srinivasan et al.[5] performed a prospective study on 79 consecutive pediatric patients with a mean age of 11 years who were evaluated in the ED by urology residents. There was an inherent selection bias (see Chapter 6) in that not all patients presenting to the ED with scrotal pain were included (urologic consultation had to be obtained), but they were able to follow up with all patients enrolled and used either this clinical follow-up or surgical findings as their criterion standards. Using multivariate regression with 11 historical and 12 physical examination parameters, they found three that were predictive of testicular torsion: absence of the ipsilateral cremasteric reflex ($p < 0.001$) presence of nausea or vomiting ($p < 0.05$), and scrotal skin changes ($p < 0.001$) (Table 45.1).[5] They then developed a decision rule using these three parameters, finding that the absence of all three resulted in a negative predictive value (NPV) of 100% while the presence of all three resulted in a positive predictive value (PPV) of 100%. While this retrospectively derived rule needs validation before it can be used with confidence (see Chapter 4), it may someday form the basis for a decision rule for testicular torsion.

A prospective study of 338 children with acute scrotal pain, including 51 with testicular torsion, proposed a clinical scoring system. All patients had physical exam performed by a urologist and underwent ultrasound. The score included: testicular swelling (2 points), hard testicle (2), absent cremasteric reflex (1), nausea/vomiting (1), and high riding testis (1). A score ≤2 could exclude testicular torsion with a sensitivity of 100% (CI 91–100), specificity 82% (CI 77–86), and NPV 100% (CI 98–100); however, further validation is needed before this can be implemented Barbosa et al.[6]

While the two studies noted in this chapter evaluated all patients with suspected torsion, Eaton et al.[7] focused primarily on pediatric patients with diagnosed intermittent testicular torsion (ITT) in order to determine whether there were historical or physical examination findings suggestive of the disease. After reviewing the charts of 50 patients with a mean age of 12 years and who had a mean number of 4.3 painful episodes prior to surgery, they found that the only finding suggestive of ITT on exam was a testis with a horizontal lie ($p < 0.05$). While this finding cannot rule in or rule out torsion, ITT should be considered in patients with rapid onset and resolution of testicular pain.

It should be noted, however, that none of these three studies commented on the reliability of the physical examination findings that were tested and their presence may very well be practitioner dependent. In addition, there are no studies of similar quality in the adult population and so these findings should be extrapolated with caution to nonpediatric patients.

Clinical question

What is the diagnostic accuracy of testicular scintigraphy compared to testicular ultrasound for the diagnosis of testicular torsion?

Several studies have compared testicular scintigraphy with testicular ultrasound. Scintigraphy is typically considered positive if a photopenic central area is present and ultrasound is considered positive when arterial flow is either absent or markedly decreased. Unlike ovarian torsion (see Chapter 43), there have been no studies specifically evaluating the utility of absent venous flow on ultrasound in the diagnosis of testicular torsion. A retrospective pediatric study of 41 boys with acute scrotal pain and equivocal physical exams from 1990 to 1996 compared the performance of color Doppler ultrasound with testicular scintigraphy for the diagnosis of testicular torsion.[8] Patients were followed through surgery or clinically until symptom resolution. A total of 11 cases of torsion (27%) were diagnosed, and several studies were interpreted as nondiagnostic. The authors presented two sets of performance tables, one that treated indeterminate studies as positive for torsion (Table 45.2) and another that treated indeterminate cases as negative for torsion (Table 45.3). The data presented in this way comprise a sensitivity analysis of sorts, showing the effect that indeterminate cases have on the diagnostic performance of the tests.

The weaknesses of the retrospective design of this study prompted a prospective study of children comparing the same diagnostic studies.[9] Forty-six children with acute scrotal pain received both testicular scintigraphy by pediatric nuclear medicine radiologists and ultrasound performed by pediatric sonographers. Final diagnoses were determined surgically in 16 cases and by assessing for clinical resolution in 30 cases. A total of 14 cases of torsion were diagnosed in this study (incidence 34%). Twelve had testicular torsion proven

Table 45.2 Performance of color Doppler ultrasound and scintigraphy for diagnosing testicular torsion when the indeterminate studies were considered positive for torsion

resence of nausea or vomiting, and scrotal skin ch	Torsion (+)	Torsion (−)	Totals
Color Doppler ultrasound (+)/ scintigraphy (+)	11/11	7/1	18/12
Color Doppler ultrasound (−)/ scintigraphy (−)	0/0	23/29	23/29
Totals	11	30	41
Sensitivity (CI)	Ultrasound 100% (72–100%), scintigraphy 100% (72–100%)		
Specificity (CI)	Ultrasound 77% (58–90%), scintigraphy 97% (83–100%)		

Source: Data from [8].

Table 45.3 Performance of color Doppler ultrasound and scintigraphy for diagnosing testicular torsion when the indeterminate studies were considered negative for torsion

	Torsion (+)	Torsion (−)	Totals
Doppler ultrasound (+)/ scintigraphy (+)	9/10	1/0	10
Doppler ultrasound (−)/ scintigraphy (−)	2/1	29/30	31
Totals	11	30	41
Sensitivity (CI)	Ultrasound 82% (48–98%), scintigraphy 91% (59–100%)		
Specificity (CI)	Ultrasound 97% (83–100%), scintigraphy 100% (88–100%)		

Source: Data from [8].

at surgery, one case was detected based on an antecedent torsion and testicular atrophy, and one case of late testicular torsion was detected at follow-up.

The correct diagnosis of torsion was made by ultrasound in 11 of 14 cases (sensitivity 79%, CI 49–95%), and the correct diagnosis of nonsurgical conditions was made in 31 of 32 cases (specificity 97%, CI 84–100%). The PPV and NPV using ultrasound were 92% (CI 62–100%) and 91% (CI 76–98%), respectively. Using ultrasound yielded a diagnostic accuracy of 91%. The correct diagnosis of torsion was made by scintigraphy in 11 of 14 cases (sensitivity 79%, CI 49–96%), and the correct diagnosis of nonsurgical conditions was made in 29 of 32 cases (specificity 91%, CI 75–98%). The PPV and NPV using scintigraphy were 79% (CI 49–95%) and 91% (CI 75–98%), respectively. Scintigraphy resulted in a diagnostic accuracy of 87%.

The lack of a true criterion standard imaging test is demonstrated by the false negatives seen in this study. The authors noted that one of the difficulties in diagnosing normal arterial flow, not to mention detection of abnormal or absent flow, was the small size of the prepubescent testicles.

From 1999 to 2005, European researchers studying the diagnosis of testicular torsion examined 61 infants and children ranging in age from 1 day to 17 years presenting with acute scrotal pain, swelling, and redness.[10] Fifteen cases of torsion were detected (prevalence 25%; 14 by the absence of both arterial and venous flow, and one by the absence of venous flow coupled with decreased arterial pulsation) and all were surgically confirmed with no missed cases at 2-year follow-up. Forty-six nontorsion cases were also diagnosed correctly. Table 45.4 shows the performance using Doppler ultrasound for diagnosing testicular torsion. Within the same manuscript, these authors also performed a retrospective analysis of 75 acute scrotum cases from 1985 to 1994, prior to the start of the study described here. All cases of suspected testicular torsion were explored surgically. Only 25 of the 75 cases (33%) were confirmed as torsion. These data were used as supporting evidence to demonstrate that using testicular ultrasound decreased unnecessary surgical explorations.

A 2011 large retrospective database study reviewed 1228 cases of patients presenting with scrotal pain to one children's hospital over 18 years.[2] There were 103 diagnosed cases of testicular torsion, of which ultrasound correctly identified decreased arterial flow in 96 (93.2%). The seven cases missed by ultrasound were explored operatively due to character and duration of the

Table 45.4 Performance Doppler ultrasound for diagnosing acute testicular torsion in pediatric patients

	Torsion (+)	Torsion (−)	Totals
Color Doppler ultrasound (+)	15	0	15
Color Doppler ultrasound (−)	0	46	46
Totals	15	46	61
Sensitivity (CI)	100% (78–100%)		
Specificity (CI)	100% (92–100%)		
Positive predictive value (PPV) (CI)	100% (78–100%)		
Negative predictive value (NPV) (CI)	100% (92–100%)		

Source: Data from [10].

symptoms, highlighting that patients with classic symptomatology should be explored regardless of initial ultrasound results. As the study was retrospective with no follow-up or criterion standard, it is unknown whether other patients with negative ultrasound were subsequently found to have torsion.

While most studies evaluating the use of ultrasound to diagnose suspected testicular torsion have used color Doppler ultrasound to visualize the absence of testicular arterial flow, a 2008 Irish study by Shaikh *et al.*[11] used a handheld Doppler (HHD, typically used to detect fetal heartbeats and monitor peripheral arterial and venous flow). They evaluated 25 patients (median age 15 years, interquartile range 9–23 years) with acute scrotal pain who presented to a general ED. The HHD evaluation was performed by the surgical resident, and torsion was suspected with either weak or absent audible signals. The results of the HHD were not used in clinical decision-making, and patients received color Doppler ultrasound, surgical exploration, or conservative management based on clinical suspicion of torsion. Of the 25 patients evaluated, nine were diagnosed with torsion, 13 with epididymitis, and three with other disease processes. All patients were followed up at both 6 weeks and 3 months. Sensitivity and specificity of HHD were both 100%, with no signal present in seven of the nine cases of torsion and only weak signals present in the other two cases, providing support for the notion that HHD may be an appropriate evaluative tool for patients with suspected torsion, especially if color Doppler ultrasound is unavailable.

The most recent modality to be tested for the diagnosis of testicular torsion is high-resolution ultrasonography (HRUS). This technique images the spermatic cord to directly visualize and detect twisting of the cord. In a European multicenter study, children with acute scrotal pain were studied with both color Doppler ultrasound as well as HRUS.[12] The study enrolled 919 patients from 1992 to 2005 (age range 1 day–18 years). Spermatic cord torsion was diagnosed in 208 patients (prevalence 23%). The use of color Doppler ultrasound detected 158 of the 208 cases (sensitivity 76%, CI 70–82%), whereas HRUS demonstrated 199 of the 208 cases (sensitivity 96%, CI 92–98%). Data were not presented to permit calculation of the specificity for color Doppler ultrasound, however, the specificity for HRUS was 99% (CI 98–100%), with 705 of 711 cases revealing a linear (normal) spermatic cord. The PPV and NPV for HRUS were 97% (CI 94–99%) and 99% (CI 98–99%), respectively.

Comment

The current practice environment for evaluation of acute scrotal pain requires either prompt surgical evaluation or a diagnostic imaging study to evaluate for testicular torsion. Patients presenting with "classic" findings of acute onset of pain, absence of the ipsilateral cremasteric reflex, presence of nausea and/or vomiting, and scrotal skin changes should be explored surgically, as a normal ultrasound demonstrating the presence of arterial flow does not rule out the disease given an imperfect sensitivity and a high pretest clinical probability. It is those cases in which the history, the physical findings, or both are equivocal that should prompt the use of a diagnostic imaging study. While no studies have specifically evaluated adult patients with torsion, it seems reasonable to extrapolate pediatric findings to the adult population with the caveat that adults typically present later and have a greater elapsed time between presentation and operative intervention.[3]

The array of studies presented demonstrates several key findings. First, regardless of the type of imaging study, none have been shown in any large studies to be perfectly sensitive or specific. Technological advances and newer uses of the existing diagnostic equipment continue to advance the diagnostic thresholds, and these have to be considered when conducting a review of the literature. Cases for which the clinical suspicion is great enough to warrant ordering a study, and cases in which the study results are indeterminate or poor quality, warrant a urological consultation. Secondly, while none of the studies described specifically addressed this issue, clinicians should consider the experience of the ultrasonographer and radiologist interpreting the study. Finally, while this discussion has focused on using the imaging studies to rule out testicular torsion, ultrasound has the added advantage of identifying other related diagnoses, such as epididymitis, orchitis, and torsion of the testicular appendages.

The availability of ultrasound is greater than that of nuclear scintigraphy, making ultrasound the study of choice. As there have not yet been studies performed evaluating emergency physician-performed scrotal ultrasound, clinicians without appropriate imaging available should arrange to transfer the patient to a medical facility capable of performing both the diagnostic study and the surgical procedure that a positive study would necessitate. Notably, the recent 25-patient study by Shaikh *et al.* demonstrates that HHD sonography may be an appropriate screening tool in low-resource settings, but its results warrant corroboration prior to generalization.

References

1. Molokwu CN, Somani BK, Goodman CM. Outcomes of scrotal exploration for acute scrotal pain suspicious of testicular torsion: A consecutive case series of 173 patients. *BJU International* 2011; 107(6): 990–3.
2. Yang C, Song B, Tan J, Liu X, Wei G. Testicular torsion in children: A 20-year retrospective study in a single institution. *The Scientific World Journal* 2011; 11: 362–8.

3. Cummings JM, Boullier JA, Sekhon D, Bose K. Adult testicular torsion. *Journal of Urology* 2002; 167(5): 2109–10.

4. Beni-Israel T, Goldman M, Bar Chaim S, *et al.* Clinical predictors for testicular torsion as seen in the pediatric ED. *The American Journal of Emergency Medicine* 2010; 28(7): 786–9.

5. Srinivasan A, Cinman N, Feber KM, Gitlin J, Palmer LS. History and physical examination findings predictive of testicular torsion: An attempt to promote clinical diagnosis by house staff. *Journal of Pediatric Urology* 2011; 7(4): 470–4.

6. João A. Barbosa, Bruno Camargo Tiseo, Ghassan A. Barayan, et al. (2013). Development and initial validation of a scoring system to diagnose testicular torsion in children. *Journal of Urology* 189(5): 1859–1864.

7. Eaton SH, Cendron MA, Estrada CR *et al.* Intermittent testicular torsion: Diagnostic features and management outcomes. *Journal of Urology* 2005; 174(4Pt 2): 1532–5; discussion 1535.

8. Paltiel HJ, Connolly LP, Atala A *et al.* Acute scrotal symptoms in boys with an indeterminate clinical presentation: Comparison of color Doppler sonography and scintigraphy. *Radiology* 1998; 207(1): 223–31.

9. Nussbaum Blask AR, Bulas D, Shalaby-Rana E *et al.* Color Doppler sonography and scintigraphy of the testis: A prospective, comparative analysis in children with acute scrotal pain. *Pediatric Emergency Care* 2002; 18(2): 67–71.

10. Gunther P, Schenk JP, Wunsch R *et al.* Acute testicular torsion in children: The role of sonography in the diagnostic workup. *European Radiology* 2006; 16(11): 2527–32.

11. Shaikh FM, Giri SK, Flood HD, Drumm J, Naqvi SA. Diagnostic accuracy of hand-held Doppler in the management of acute scrotal pain. *Irish Journal of Medical Science* 2008; 177(3): 279–82.

12. Kalfa N, Veyrac C, Lopez M *et al.* Multicenter assessment of ultrasound of the spermatic cord in children with acute scrotum. *Journal of Urology* 2007; 177(1): 297–301; discussion 301.

SECTION 7
Neurology

Chapter 46 **Nontraumatic Subarachnoid Hemorrhage**

Ian T. Ferguson and Christopher R. Carpenter

Department of Emergency Medicine, Washington University School of Medicine, St. Louis, MO, USA

Highlights

- In isolation, no signs or symptoms accurately rule in or rule out nontraumatic subarachnoid hemorrhage (SAH).
- The "Ottawa SAH Rule" identifies low-risk headache patients who do not require additional testing, including CT or lumbar puncture (LP).
- Regardless of whether "Ottawa SAH Rule" is used, when no SAH findings are evident on a CT scan within 6 hours of symptom onset, most patients do not benefit from additional imaging or LP to rule out SAH.
- Initial implementation studies demonstrate a safe reduction in post-CT LPs and admission rates when the Ottawa SAH Rule is used in ED diagnostic decision-making.

Background

Headaches represent about 2.8% of emergency department (ED) visits per year.[1] Most headaches are self-limited, but subarachnoid hemorrhage (SAH) is life threatening and is classically described as a sudden onset "thunderclap headache" reaching maximal severity within seconds. The differential diagnosis of acute onset headaches also includes cerebral vasospasm, hypophyseal apoplexy, venous sinus thrombosis, vascular dissection, cough, exertional and postcoital headache, and migraine.[2-6] Migraine-like headaches are at least 50 times more common than SAH among ED headache patients.[7]

Evidence-Based Emergency Care: Diagnostic Testing and Clinical Decision Rules, Third Edition.
Edited by Jesse M. Pines, Fernanda Bellolio, Christopher R. Carpenter, and Ali S. Raja.
© 2023 John Wiley & Sons Ltd. Published 2023 by John Wiley & Sons Ltd.

A meta-analysis of ED-based studies provided a pooled point estimate of 7.5% SAH incidence when emergency physicians were concerned about SAH.[8] Missed SAH are a substantial medical malpractice risk,[9,10] so the evidence-based diagnostic approach to headache epitomizes emergency medicine via a highly lethal condition without a pathognomonic presentation nested within a high-volume complaint for which the vast majority do not have a life-threatening etiology.

Approximately 85% of SAH are caused by ruptured aneurysms. Box 46.1 provides the differential diagnosis of nontraumatic SAH. Perimesencephalic bleeds are the second most common etiology. Usually, SAH is diagnosed by noncontrast head computed tomography (CT) (Figure 46.1). The diagnostic accuracy of head CT can be improved by incorporating the suggestions noted in Box 46.2.[11]

Because early generation CTs missed up to 5% of SAH, classic teaching emphasized the need to proceed to lumbar puncture (LP) to exclude SAH. However, LP infrequently identifies SAH after a negative head CT: the number of LPs required to identify one aneurysmal SAH amenable to surgical intervention after a negative CT performed within 6 hours of symptom onset ranges from 91 to 15,200 LPs.[12-14] Test-treatment threshold analyses provide another way to quantify risks and benefits of a diagnostic test. Two separate test-treatment analyses for LP when diagnosing SAH provide similar results: only patients with post-CT SAH probability between 2% and 9% have benefits outweighing risk associated with LP if imaged within 6 hours and

---

Box 46.1   Differential diagnosis of spontaneous SAH

Cerebral aneurysm

Perimesencephalic

Isolated convexity

Vascular malformations (arteriovenous malformations)

Arterial dissection

Cerebral amyloid angiopathy

Moyamoya

Vasculitis (posterior reversible encephalopathy syndrome, reversible cerebral vasoconstriction syndrome, lupus)

Coagulopathy (thrombocytopenia, anticoagulation)

Sickle cell disease

Hypertension

Sympathomimetic drugs

Source: Carpenter *et al.* [8]/John Wiley & Sons.

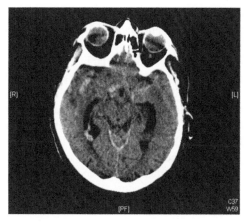

Figure 46.1 Noncontrast head computed tomography (CT) showing an acute subarachnoid hemorrhage.

Box 46.2   Factors to reduced post-CT missed SAH

Patient Factors
- Time of headache onset defined unambiguously
- CT performed within 6 hours of headache onset

Radiological Factors
- Third generation or newer CT scanner
- Technically adequate CT without motion artifact
- Thin cuts less than or equal to 5 mm through the base of the brain
- Hematocrit > 30%
- Radiologist interpreting the scan is attending level or with equivalent experience reading brain scans
- Radiologist specifically examines CT for subtle hydrocephalus, small quantity of blood in dependent portions of ventricles, and isodense or hyperdense material in the basal cisterns

Communication Factors
- Emergency clinician communicates specific concern of "severe acute headache, evaluate for SAH" to the radiologist
- Adequate and accurate discussion of post-CT risk of SAH with patients

Source: Adapted from [11].

lacking any CT evidence of SAH.[8,15] Based upon the diagnostic accuracy of CT described below, the *pretest probability* of SAH would need to exceed 70% for a CT obtained within 6 hours for the posttest probability to fall within the 2–9% range. The 70% pretest probability is far higher than any ED SAH prevalence reported. In addition, LP is not a harmless procedure. Post-LP headache rates are 6–30%,[16] many patients are reluctant to undergo LP,[17] and clinicians often do not obtain LPs due to time constraints and low diagnostic yield.[18,19] LPs are also often inconclusive. "Traumatic taps" (cerebrospinal fluid [CSF] red blood cells [RBC] secondary to the invasive procedure rather than SAH) occur in about one in six LPs with no universally accepted methods to differentiate SAH CSF RBCs from procedural blood.[20]

Clinical question

Can history, physical exam, and/or decision aids accurately and reliably distinguish patients at increased or decreased risk of nontraumatic SAH?
The American College of Emergency Physician's (ACEP) 2019 Clinical Policy on "Acute Headache" and a 2016 diagnostic meta-analysis both emphasize that no element of history or physical exam alone accurately rule in or rule out SAH.[8,21] Objective neck stiffness (pooled positive likelihood ratio [LR+] 6.6) and self-reported stiff neck (pooled LR+ 4.1) most accurately rule in SAH, while the absence of "worst headache of life" (pooled negative likelihood ratio [LR−] 0.24) most accurately rule out SAH. The diagnostic accuracy of history and physical exam are summarized in Tables 46.1 and 46.2, respectively.[8]

The ACEP Clinical Policy provides a Level B recommendation in favor of the Ottawa SAH Rule to rule out SAH safely without a CT or LP. The Ottawa SAH decision aid (Figure 46.2) identifies patients *with suspicion for SAH* (which does not mean every ED headache patient) as low-risk if none of the following features is present: age ≥40, neck pain or stiffness, witnessed loss of consciousness, headache onset with exertion, thunderclap description, or limited neck flexion on examination. The initial validation of the Ottawa SAH decision aid demonstrated a LR− = 0.02 (CI 0.00–0.39).[22] Subsequent multisite validation in Canada demonstrated 100% sensitivity and LR− = 0.[23] Researchers continue attempts to improve the diagnostic performance of the Ottawa SAH Rule[24] or derive new decision aids.[25] Theoretically, using the Ottawa SAH would safely decrease CT rates, but prospective implementation studies demonstrate no decrease in CT ordering, although a 14% reduction in LPs and 2.5% lower admission rate has been observed.[26]

Table 46.1 Predictors of SAH from history

Risk factor (number of studies)	Sensitivity, % (95% CI)	Specificity, % (95% CI)	Positive LR (95% CI)	Negative LR (95% CI)
Arrival by ambulance				
Pooled accuracy (2)	59 (53–65)	80 (78–81)	2.95 (2.23–3.89)	0.51 (0.44–0.63)
Awoke from sleep				
Pooled accuracy (2)	11 (8–16)	82 (80–83)	0.63 (0.45–0.89)	1.09 (1.04–1.14)
Blurred vision				
Pooled accuracy (2)	11 (2–28)	95 (92–98)	3.14 (0.31–31.43)	0.85 (0.44–1.63)
Burst or explosion onset				
Pooled accuracy (5)	58 (52–64)	47 (45–49)	1.10 (0.75–1.60)	0.88 (0.56–1.38)
Diplopia (1)	0 (0–15)	98 (94–100)	0.96 (0.05–19.33)	1.00 (0.94–1.07)
ED transfer				
Pooled accuracy (2)	18 (13–23)	92 (91–93)	2.20 (1.65–2.91)	0.90 (0.85–0.95)
Exertion at onset				
Pooled accuracy (5)	29 (24–34)	83 (82–84)	1.46 (1.16–1.83)	1.20 (0.80–1.79)
Family history cerebral aneurysm (1)	0 (0–13)	92 (87–95)	0.22 (0.01–3.54)	1.07 (1.00–1.15)
Female sex				
Pooled accuracy (6)	58 (53–62)	41 (39–42)	1.10 (0.93–1.31)	0.93 (0.73–1.12)
Intercourse at onset				
Pooled accuracy (4)	7 (4–10)	94 (93–95)	1.20 (0.79–1.82)	1.00 (0.97–1.03)
Loss of consciousness				
Pooled accuracy (4)	16 (12–20)	95 (94–96)	1.87 (0.72–4.86)	0.91 (0.83–1.00)
Male				
Pooled accuracy (3)	42 (32–53)	54 (50–58)	0.90 (0.68–1.18)	1.23 (0.88–1.72)
Nausea				

(Continued)

Table 46.1 (*Continued*)

Risk factor (number of studies)	Sensitivity, % (95% CI)	Specificity, % (95% CI)	Positive LR (95% CI)	Negative LR (95% CI)
Pooled accuracy (5)	77 (70–84)	34 (30–37)	1.15 (0.92–1.44)	0.74 (0.34–1.61)
Neck stiffness, subjective				
Pooled accuracy (5)	33 (28–38)	95 (94–95)	4.12 (2.24–7.59)	0.73 (0.66–0.80)
Onset <1 minute (1)	50 (34–66)	45 (32–58)	0.91 (0.62–1.33)	1.11 (0.74–1.68)
Onset 1–5 minutes (1)	24 (12–39)	87 (75–94)	1.79 (0.77–4.14)	0.88 (0.72–1.07)
Onset <1 hour (1)	100 (95–100)	12 (9–16)	1.13 (1.09–1.19)	0.06 (0–0.95)
Photophobia				
Pooled accuracy (4)	38 (29–47)	58 (54–62)	1.07 (0.67–1.71)	1.05 (0.87–1.40)
PMH chronic headache (1)	19 (7–39)	79 (73–85)	0.93 (0.40–2.91)	1.02 (0.83–1.24)
PMH of hypertension (1)	31 (14–52)	80 (74–85)	1.53 (0.81–2.91)	0.87 (0.66–1.13)
Scotomata (1)	0 (0–15)	93 (87–97)	0.28 (0.02–4.72)	1.06 (0.98–1.14)
Similar headache in past (1)	19 (9–34)	90 (79–96)	1.90 (0.71–5.09)	0.90 (0.76–1.07)
Vomiting				
Pooled accuracy (4)	65 (59–69)	72 (71–74)	1.92 (1.48–2.48)	0.52 (0.45–0.61)
Worst headache of life				
Pooled accuracy (3)	89 (85–93)	23 (22–25)	1.09 (0.85–1.41)	0.36 (0.01–14.22)

Source: Data from [8].

Table 46.2 Predictors of SAH from physical exam

Risk factor (number of studies)	Sensitivity, % (95% CI)	Specificity, % (95% CI)	Positive LR (95% CI)	Negative LR (95% CI)
Altered mental status				
Pooled accuracy (4)	31 (21–41)	93 (90–95)	3.26 (1.93–5.52)	0.87 (0.78–0.98)
Focal neuro deficit				
Pooled accuracy (4)	31 (21–41)	93 (90–95)	3.26 (1.93–5.52)	0.81 (0.67–0.97)
Lethargy (1)	39 (17–64)	82 (72–90)	2.19 (1.04–4.64)	0.74 (0.51–1.09)
Neck stiffness, objective				
Pooled accuracy (3)	29 (24–35)	96 (95–96)	6.59 (3.95–11.00)	0.78 (0.68–0.90)

Source: Data from [8].

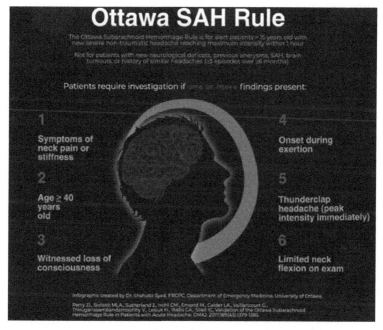

Figure 46.2 The components of the Ottawa SAH Rule. (Infographic Created by Dr. Shahabz Syed, FRCPC, Department of Emergency Medicine, University of Ottawa.)

Clinical question

Can noncontrast CT within 6 hours accurately identify headache patients at low risk of SAH?

One of the first diagnostic studies of nontraumatic SAH investigated the need for LP in patients who presented within the first 12 hours of headache onset with normal neurological examinations. All patients had a noncontrast head CT followed by a LP (at 12 or more hours from the headache onset) if the head CT was negative. CT identified SAH in 117 patients, but CSF analysis showed SAH in two additional patients. Therefore, in two out of 119 patients with SAH, the head CT was negative, which is a sensitivity of 98% (CI 92–100).[27]

Another group studied 6 years of data of patients with SAH from 1988 to 1994.[5] They excluded patients younger than 2 years or who had a history of head trauma within 24 hours of onset of symptoms and stratified patients into two groups based on symptom duration (<24 hours and >24 hours). All patients with negative head CTs received a diagnostic LP. In 181 patients, the sensitivity of CT was 93% for patients whose head CT was performed within 24 hours of symptom onset as opposed to 84% for patients whose head CT was performed after 24 hours for an overall sensitivity of 92% indicating that, as time goes by, the sensitivity of CT for the detection of SAH decreases.

CT accuracy was evaluated in a prospective study across 11 tertiary care EDs in Canada from 2000 to 2009.[9] They enrolled neurologically intact adults with a new headache peaking in intensity within 1 hour of onset where the patient had a CT to rule out SAH. In 3132 patients (of which 82% had their worst headache ever), 240 (8%) had SAH. The LR+ of CT for SAH was 5366 (CI 335–85,786) and the LR– was 0.07 (CI 0.05–0.11). In a subgroup analysis of 953 patients who were scanned within 6 hours of symptoms, all 121 patients with SAH were detected on CT representing a LR+ 1659 (CI 104–26,504) and a LR– of 0 (CI 0–0.07).[18]

Two subsequent meta-analyses provide a pooled LR– 0.01 (0.00–0.04) for CT within 6 hours of headache onset with minimal statistical heterogeneity,[8,11] although only based on two studies.[18,28] Based on the same two studies CT beyond 6 hours is less accurate and less precise with LR– 0.07 (95% CI 0.01–0.61). Table 46.3 provides the diagnostic accuracy of CT across all prospective and retrospective studies over the last 25 years.

Clinical question

Can CT angiogram accurately identify headache patients with aneurysmal SAH?

Based on two Level III studies,[31,32] the ACEP Clinical Policy provides a Level C recommendation (consensus only) to "perform LP or CT angiography (CTA)

Table 46.3 CT accuracy at any interval since headache

Risk factor	Sensitivity, % (95% CI)	Specificity, % (95% CI)	Positive LR (95% CI)	Negative LR (95% CI)
Altered mental status				
van der Wee et al.[27]	98	100	111.63	0.02
	(94–100)	(94–100)	(7.07–1763.23)	(0.01–0.07)
Boesiger and	100	99	106.48	0.07
Shiber[29]	(54–100)	(97–100)	(21.36–530.82)	(0.00–1.04)
O'Neill et al.[30]	76 (55–91)	100	138.00	0.25
		(96–100)	(8.62–2209.28)	(0.13–0.49)
Perry et al.[18]	93 (89–96)	100	5365.85	0.07
		(100–100)	(335.63–85,786.14)	(0.05–0.11)
Backes et al.[28]	95 (89–95)	100	276.85	0.05
		(97–100)	(17.39–4406.77)	(0.02–0.12)
Pooled accuracy	**94**	**100**	**267.26**	**0.07**
	(91–96)	**(100–100)**	**(57.67–1238.49)**	**(0.03–0.17)**

Source: Data from [8].

to safely rule out SAH in the adult ED patient who is still considered to be at risk for SAH after a negative noncontrast head CT."[21] In SAH patients, CTA sensitivity for detecting aneurysms ranged from 86% to 100% with a pooled sensitivity of 98% (97–99) with a specificity of 100% (7–100).[8] Paradoxically, CTA may have problems with false positives and false negatives. False-negative aneurysms occur in the internal carotid/posterior communicating artery near the skull base due to poor visualization in these areas. False-positive CTA can lead to over-diagnosis and over-testing.[33] Up to 2% of the general population live with asymptomatic cerebral aneurysms.[34] CTA may also identify aneurysms that were not the cause of the presenting symptoms and are unlikely to ever rupture, but once identified create patient anxiety and increased medical expenses.[35,36] One diagnostic approach to differentiate false-positive cerebral aneurysms from true positives likely to benefit from interventions would be to obtain LP post-CT to evaluate for CSF RBCs if there is a clinical question whether the aneurysm is incidental.[37]

Comment

ED SAH diagnosis research consists largely of studies with major limitations. Most of the studies presented are retrospective and did not follow up on patients who were discharged home without any testing or just a negative head CT. This is important because there may have been cases of SAH that were missed, either because no testing was performed or because no LP was performed.[38] As discussed in Chapter 6, the name for this phenomenon is *partial verification bias* and the consequences include artificially elevated sensitivity and lowered specificity compared with their true values where this bias is removed.[39] Lingering uncertainty around these studies result in some physicians continuing to advocate for the historical post-CT LP every time.[40]

Considerable between-study differences exist in the prevalence of SAH, ranging from 8% to 67%. *Spectrum bias* (see Chapter 6) may skew observed sensitivity and specificity. In populations with higher rates of SAH (neurosurgical studies representing the sickest of the sick), observed sensitivity in the study may be higher than true values were this bias eliminated. On the other hand, in populations with lower rates of SAH (ED headache populations representing the most well of the well), specificity may be higher than true values where spectrum bias is eliminated.[39]

However, what is clear from these studies is that test sensitivity decreases as time passes from the onset of the acute headache. There were also variable definitions for a positive LP. Because there are no widely accepted, validated criteria for a positive LP, it can be difficult to distinguish a traumatic LP (in which RBCs from the mechanical process of performing the procedure get into the CSF specimen) from a true positive LP. In addition, most SAH studies had small sample sizes from one hospital, which limits the precision and generalizability of conclusions.

The most common root cause for missed SAH is failure to obtain a CT.[9] In patients presenting with a "worst headache," or a severe headache in patients who do not usually get headaches, or chronic headaches with a change in their headache symptoms, noncontrast head CT is useful to rule out the diagnosis of SAH. If the CT is nondiagnostic, the decision threshold to perform LP or obtain CTA on patients is dependent on the pretest probability for disease and merits shared decision-making with patients.[41] Given the small risk of LP complications including postdural headache and lower back pain, it is a reasonable practice to rule out SAH without an LP or CTA, after a negative CT if the clinician has a low pretest probability and the headache began within 6 hours. Clinicians should be cautious in patients with headaches that began greater than 6 hours prior to arrival, and particularly beyond 24 hours. In such delayed presentations, LP is important to rule out SAH even after a negative CT.

References

1. Centers for Disease Control and Prevention. National Hospital Ambulatory Medical Care Survey: 2015 Emergency Department Summary Tables. https://www.cdc.gov/nchs/data/nhamcs/web_tables/2015_ed_web_tables.pdf. Accessed October 8, 2021.

2. Landtblom AM, Fridriksson S, Boivie J, Hillman J, Johansson G, Johansson I. Sudden onset headache: A prospective study of features, incidence and causes. *Cephalalgia.* 2002; 22: 354–60.

3. Dodick DW, Wijdicks EF. Pituitary apoplexy presenting as a thunderclap headache. *Neurology.* 1998; 50: 1510–1.

4. de Bruijn SF, Stam J, Kappelle LJ. Thunderclap headache as first symptom of cerebral venous sinus thrombosis. CVST Study Group. *Lancet.* 1996; 348: 1623–5.

5. Cordenier A, De Hertogh W, De Keyser J, Versijpt J. Headache associated with cough: A review. *The Journal of Headache and Pain.* 2013; 14: 42.

6. Pascual J, Iglesias F, Oterino A, Vasquez-Barquero A, Berciano J. Cough, exertional, and sexual headaches: An analysis of 72 benign and symptomatic cases. *Neurology.* 1996; 46: 1520–4.

7. Edlow JA. Diagnosis of subarachnoid hemorrhage in the emergency department. *Emergency Medicine Clinics of North America.* 2003; 21: 73–87.

8. Carpenter CR, Hussain AM, Ward MJ et al. Spontaneous subarachnoid hemorrhage: A systematic review and meta-analysis describing the diagnostic accuracy of history, physical examination, imaging, and lumbar puncture with an exploration of test thresholds. *Academic Emergency Medicine.* 2016; 23: 963–1003.

9. McNeill A. Neurological negligence claims in the NHS from 1995 to 2005. *European Journal of Neurology.* 2007; 14: 399–402.

10. Coysh T, Breen DP. A nationwide analysis of successful litigation claims in neurological practice. *JRSM Open.* 2014; 5: 2042533313518914.

11. Dubosh NM, Bellolio MF, Rabinstein AA, Edlow JA. Sensitivity of early brain computed tomography to exclude aneurysmal subarachnoid hemorrhage: A systematic review and meta-analysis. *Stroke.* 2016; 47: 750–5.

12. Brunell A, Ridefelt P, Zelano J. Differential diagnostic yield of lumbar puncture in investigation of suspected subarachnoid haemorrhage: A retrospective study. *Journal of Neurology.* 2013; 260: 1631–6.

13. Sayer D, Bloom B, Fernando K et al. An observational study of 2,248 patients presenting with headache, suggestive of subarachnoid hemorrhage, who received lumbar punctures following normal computed tomography of the head. *Academic Emergency Medicine.* 2015; 22: 1267–73.

14. Blok KM, Rinkel GJ, Majoie CB et al. CT within 6 hours of headache onset to rule out subarachnoid hemorrhage in nonacademic hospitals. *Neurology.* 2015; 84: 1927–32.

15. Taylor RA, Singh GH, Marcolini EG, Meyers HP, Faust JS, Newman DH. Determination of a testing threshold for lumbar puncture in the diagnosis of subarachnoid hemorrhage after a negative head computed tomography: A decision analysis. *Academic Emergency Medicine.* 2016; 23: 1119–27.

16. Seupaul RA, Somerville GG, Viscusi C, Shepard AJ, Hauter WE. Prevalence of postdural puncture headache after ED performed lumbar puncture. *The American Journal of Emergency Medicine.* 2005; 23: 913–5.

17. Czuczman AD, Thomas LE, Boulanger AB et al. Interpreting red blood cells in lumbar puncture: Distinguishing true subarachnoid hemorrhage from traumatic tap. *Academic Emergency Medicine.* 2013; 20: 247–56.

18. Perry JJ, Stiell IG, Sivilotti ML *et al.* Sensitivity of computed tomography performed within six hours of onset of headache for diagnosis of subarachnoid haemorrhage: prospective cohort study. *BMJ.* 2011; 343: d4277.

19. Kumar A, Niknam K, Lumba-Brown A *et al.* Practice variation in the diagnosis of aneurysmal subarachnoid hemorrhage: A survey of US and Canadian emergency medicine physicians. *Neurocritical Care.* 2019; 31: 321–8.

20. Shah KH, Richard KM, Nicholas S, Edlow JA. Incidence of traumatic lumbar puncture. *Academic Emergency Medicine.* 2003; 10: 151–4.

21. Godwin SA, Cherkas DS, Panagos PD, Shih RD, Byyny R, Wolf SJ. Clinical policy: Critical issues in the evaluation and management of adult patients presenting to the emergency department with acute headache. *Annals of Emergency Medicine.* 2019; 74: e41–74.

22. Perry JJ, Stiell IG, Sivilotti ML *et al.* Clinical decision rules to rule out subarachnoid hemorrhage for acute headache. *JAMA.* 2013; 310: 1248–55.

23. Perry JJ, Sivilotti MLA, Sutherland J *et al.* Validation of the Ottawa subarachnoid hemorrhage rule in patients with acute headache. *CMAJ.* 2017; 189: E1379–85.

24. Cheung HY, Lui CT, Tsui KL. Validation and modification of the Ottawa subarachnoid haemorrhage rule in risk stratification of Asian Chinese patients with acute headache. *Hong Kong Medical Journal.* 2018; 24: 584–92.

25. Kimura A, Kobayashi K, Yamaguchi H *et al.* New clinical decision rule to exclude subarachnoid haemorrhage for acute headache: A prospective multicentre observational study. *BMJ Open.* 2016; 6: e010999.

26. Perry JJ, Sivilotti MLA, Émond M *et al.* Prospective implementation of the Ottawa subarachnoid hemorrhage rule and 6-hour computed tomography rule. *Stroke.* 2020; 51: 424–30.

27. van der Wee N, Rinkel GJ, Hasan D, van Gijn J. Detection of subarachnoid haemorrhage on early CT: Is lumbar puncture still needed after a negative scan? *Journal of Neurology, Neurosurgery, and Psychiatry.* 1995; 58: 357–9.

28. Backes D, Rinkel GJ, Kemperman H, Linn FH, Vergouwen MD. Time-dependent test characteristics of head computed tomography in patients suspected of nontraumatic subarachnoid hemorrhage. *Stroke.* 2012; 43: 2115–9.

29. Boesiger BM, Shiber JR. Subarachnoid hemorrhage diagnosis by computed tomography and lumbar puncture: are fifth generation CT scanners better at identifying subarachnoid hemorrhage? *Journal of Emergency Medicine.* 2005; 29: 23–7.

30. O'Neill J, McLaggan S, Gibson R. Acute headache and subarachnoid haemorrhage: a retrospective review of CT and lumbar puncture findings. *Scottish Medical Journal.* 2005; 50: 151–3.

31. Menke J, Larsen J, Kallenberg K. Diagnosing cerebral aneurysms by computed tomographic angiography: Meta-analysis. *Annals of Neurology.* 2011; 69: 646–54.

32. El Khaldi M, Pernter P, Ferro F *et al.* Detection of cerebral aneurysms in nontraumatic subarachnoid haemorrhage: Role of multislice CT angiography in 130 consecutive patients. *La Radiologia Medica.* 2007; 112: 123–37.

33. Carpenter CR, Raja AS, Brown MD. Overtesting and the downstream consequences of overtreatment: Implications of "preventing overdiagnosis" for emergency medicine. *Academic Emergency Medicine.* 2015; 22: 1484–92.

34. Edlow JA. What are the unintended consequences of changing the diagnostic paradigm for subarachnoid hemorrhage after brain computed tomography to computed tomographic angiography in place of lumbar puncture? *Academic Emergency Medicine.* 2010; 17: 991–5.

35. Otawara Y, Ogasawara K, Kubo Y *et al.* Anxiety before and after surgical repair in patients with asymptomatic unruptured intracranial aneurysm. *Surgical Neurology.* 2004; 62: 28–31.

36. Scharf E, Pelkowski S, Sahin B. Unruptured intracranial aneurysms and life insurance underwriting. *Neurology: Clinical Practice.* 2017; 7: 274–7.

37. Probst MA, Hoffman JR. Computed tomography angiography of the head is a reasonable next test after a negative noncontrast head computed tomography result in the emergency department evaluation of subarachnoid hemorrhage. *Annals of Emergency Medicine.* 2016; 67: 773–4.

38. Hoffman JR. Computed tomography for subarachnoid hemorrhage: What should we make of the "evidence". *Annals of Emergency Medicine.* 2001; 37: 345–9.

39. Kohn MA, Carpenter CR, Newman TB. Understanding the direction of bias in studies of diagnostic test accuracy. *Academic Emergency Medicine.* 2013; 20: 1194–206.

40. Chin N, Sarko J. Tried and true and still the best: Lumbar puncture, not computed tomography angiogram, for the diagnosis of subarachnoid hemorrhage. *Annals of Emergency Medicine.* 2016; 67: 774–5.

41. Hess EP, Grudzen CR, Thomson R, Raja AS, Carpenter CR. Shared decision-making in the emergency department: Respecting patient autonomy when seconds count. *Academic Emergency Medicine.* 2015; 22: 856–64.

Chapter 47 **Acute Stroke**

John Bedolla[1] and Jesse M. Pines[2,3]

[1] Department of Surgery and Perioperative Care, Dell Medical School, University of Texas at Austin, Austin, TX, USA
[2] US Acute Care Solutions, Canton, OH, USA
[3] Department of Emergency Medicine, Drexel University, Philadelphia, PA, USA

Highlights

- Rapid evaluation of patients with acute stroke by noncontrast head CT (NCHCT) rules out intracranial hemorrhage in patients who may be candidates for intravenous thrombolysis (≤4.5 hours from symptom onset).
- NCHCT has poor sensitivity for ischemic stroke at about 30%. Positive findings for acute ischemic stroke on NCHCT indicate completed stroke and represent a contraindication to intravenous thrombolytics.
- When large vessel occlusion is suspected clinically by a high National Institutes of Health Stroke Scale (NIHSS), computed tomography (CT) angiogram of the head and neck is warranted to demonstrate clot treatable with intra-arterial thrombolysis and/or clot retrieval.
- Diffusion-weighted magnetic resonance imaging (dwMRI) is highly sensitive for ischemic stroke overall (~97%) but has a 10% false negative rate for posterior circulation strokes. The most important uses for dwMRI are to evaluate for noncompleted stroke in the setting of uncertainty of time of onset, and when deficits are equivocal or subtle.
- The use of CT perfusion or diffusion/perfusion MRI can help identify patients with wake-up strokes and those presenting in the late window (after 6 hours), that have large areas of ischemic penumbra and might benefit from acute interventions.

Evidence-Based Emergency Care: Diagnostic Testing and Clinical Decision Rules, Third Edition.
Edited by Jesse M. Pines, Fernanda Bellolio, Christopher R. Carpenter, and Ali S. Raja.
© 2023 John Wiley & Sons Ltd. Published 2023 by John Wiley & Sons Ltd.

- The recognition of stroke in the emergency room (ROSIER) scale is a useful way to discriminate stroke mimics in the ED using clinical criteria.
- Because NIHSS of zero is very rare (<1%) in patients diagnosed with stroke, it can be a useful way to help exclude in the diagnosis of stroke in the ED.

Background

Stroke is the leading cause of disability and the third-leading cause of death in the United States. Rapid bedside and radiological evaluation of cases of suspected acute stroke within 4.5–6 hours of symptom onset are critical in the assessment of patients potentially eligible for intravenous (IV) and intra-arterial thrombolysis. In acute ischemic stroke (Figure 47.1), the central event is an acute vascular occlusion; however, 15% of strokes are hemorrhagic (Figure 47.2). Hemorrhagic strokes do not benefit from thrombolysis, as it can worsen bleeding and increase mortality. While this chapter focuses on the diagnosis of stroke, it is important to consider why the diagnosis of stroke is clinically important. Importantly, when the correct diagnosis of stroke is made in a timely way, early interventions such as tissue plasminogen activator (tPA) and endovascular treatment (i.e., mechanical thrombectomy) have been shown to improve outcomes.[1]

The approach to diagnostic imaging depends on patient characteristics, time since symptoms onset, and local availability of imaging and stroke expertise. Traditionally, noncontrast head computed tomography (NCHCT) has been the first imaging modality in acute stroke in the emergency department (ED) (Figure 47.1). NCHCT can rule out hemorrhagic stroke,

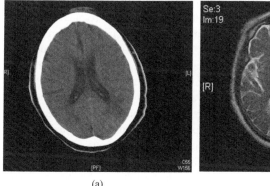
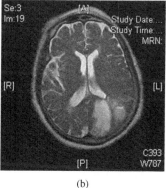

(a)   (b)

Figure 47.1 Noncontrast head CT showing ischemic stroke in the left posterior cerebral artery region (a), confirmed on MRI (b).

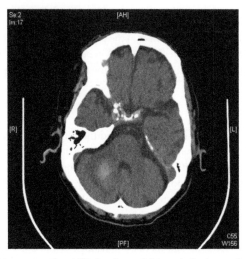

Figure 47.2 Noncontrast head CT showing a right cerebellar hemorrhage.

completed stroke, and also exclude other potential causes of acute neurological symptoms. NCHCT is widely available, easier, and faster to perform with
shorter scan times and fewer patient exclusions/contraindications, has lower
cost compared to MRI, and is a cost-effective strategy.[2] In cases where a large
vessel occlusion (LVO) is suggested on exam, computed tomography angiogram (CTA) head and neck can also be performed to demonstrate large clots
that are best treated with IV or arterial tPA or mechanical clot retrieval.
A LVO is defined as the occlusion of the internal carotid artery and of the
proximal segments (M1, M2) of the middle cerebral artery. In cases where
the deficit is equivocal or the timing of last known normal is uncertain more
advanced imaging technique, multimodal magnetic resonance imaging
(MRI) with diffusion-weighted imaging (dwMRI) and perfusion MRI, or
computed tomography perfusion (CTP) can be performed after computed
tomography (CT) because these advanced imaging methods are considered a
more accurate diagnostic test for demonstrating acute ischemia. CTP is particularly useful in selecting patients amenable to mechanical thrombectomy,
particularly those within 24 hours of symptoms including those with
unknown symptoms onset (wake-up strokes). Diffusion-weighted magnetic
resonance imaging (dwMRI) is sensitive for acute ischemia, however the primary clinical concerns regarding the use of dwMRI as a solitary test are
(i) reduced ability to detect intracranial hemorrhage in the setting of acute
stroke, (ii) less clinical access to potentially unstable patients, (iii) longer testing times, and (iv) poor availability of rapid MRI.

Clinical question

What is the sensitivity of diagnostic modalities (head CT and MRI) in acute stroke, and does MRI miss acute intracranial hemorrhages?

A study comparing NCHCT to dwMRI included articles in which both head CT and dwMRI were performed within 6–7 hours of the onset of clinical symptoms.[3] A total of eight studies and 909 patients were included. The largest included study was a retrospective review of patients seen in the ED for signs and symptoms of acute stroke.[4] Of 691 patients, 509 had a NCHCT and 122 had dwMRI within 6 hours of ED arrival. They used a primary discharge diagnosis of stroke as the criterion standard. The study reported a sensitivity of NCHCT of 40% and of dwMRI of 97%; the specificity was 92% for both modalities. The positive predictive value (PPV) of head CT and dwMRI were each 96%. The negative predictive value (NPV) were 23% for head CT and 77% for dwMRI.

The authors went on to review seven smaller studies (ranging in sample size from 17 to 54), most with considerable methodological issues including variable inclusion criteria, variable criterion standards for stroke, delays between head CT and dwMRI, and variable blinding of reviewers.[5-11] They then combined data from all eight studies (despite variable inclusion criteria and heterogeneity of the studies) to calculate a sensitivity, specificity, PPV, and NPV for each modality. For dwMRI, their calculated sensitivity was 97% (confidence interval [CI] 94–98%) and their specificity was 100% (CI 88–100%), with a PPV of 100% (CI 98–100%) and a NPV of 91% (CI 75–98%). The sensitivity of head CT was 47 % (CI 43–51%), specificity was 93% (CI 85–97%), the PPV was 97% (CI 94–99%), and the NPV was 23% (CI 19–28%). In this systematic review the authors excluded four studies from the pooled diagnostic test accuracy calculations because these studies did not have patients without a stroke or required a negative CT as part of the original studies, limiting the calculations.

A single center prospective study compared dwMRI to NCHCT in the ED in patients with suspected stroke.[12] MRI detected acute ischemic stroke in 164/356 patients (46%, CI 41–51%) compared with CT in 35/356 patients (10%, CI 7–14%), $p < 0.001$. A subset analysis was performed on patients who were scanned within 3 hours of symptom onset. In those patients, MRI detected acute ischemic stroke in 41/90 (46%, CI 35–56%) and CT detected acute ischemic stroke in 6/90 (7%, CI 3–14%). Using final clinical diagnosis as the criterion standard, they reported a sensitivity of 83% (CI 78–88%) for MRI and 26% (CI 20–32%) for CT. The authors concluded that MRI was better than CT in terms of detecting of acute ischemia. It was also no different in the detection of acute hemorrhage (6% MRI versus 7% CT).

Other studies have confirmed that dwMRI is as sensitive as CT for the detection of acute intracranial hemorrhage. Fiebach *et al.*[13] performed a multicenter study to test the accuracy of MRI for the detection of acute intracranial hemorrhage in patients with suspected stroke. They compared MRI images from 62 patients with intracranial hemorrhages and 62 without intracranial hemorrhages, all of whom were imaged within 6 hours of symptom onset. They used CT as the criterion standard for the diagnosis of intracranial hemorrhage. Experienced readers of MRI were able to detect intracranial hemorrhage on all cases (100% sensitivity; CI 97–100%).

Kidwell *et al.*[14] also compared the accuracy of MRI and CT in the detection of intracranial hemorrhage in patients within 6 hours of acute focal symptoms of stroke in two centers. MRI and CT were equivalent in diagnosing acute hemorrhage, as acute hemorrhage was detected in 25 patients on both MRI and CT. However, in four other patients, acute hemorrhage was detected on MRI but not CT and, in three additional patients, regions that were interpreted as acute hemorrhage on CT were read as chronic hemorrhage on MRI. There was one patient for whom subarachnoid hemorrhage was seen on CT but not on MRI, and chronic hemorrhages (microbleeds) were visualized on MRI in 49 patients that were not seen on CT. The authors concluded that MRI is as accurate as CT in detecting acute hemorrhage in patients with acute focal symptoms of stroke and is more accurate than CT in detecting chronic intracranial hemorrhage.

Two studies have used MRI as the only imaging prior to IV tPA.[15,16] In one study 135 patients had MRI and received tPA as part as a quality improvement study to reduce door to tPA times. However, there is no evidence that MRI is superior to CT for most patients who could be treated with IV thrombolysis.

Clinical question

What findings suggest increased risk of LVO?

LVO in the setting of stroke is important because it can be treated endovascularly with mechanical thrombectomy (Figure 47.3). There are multiple screening scores for LVO, and to date none has emerged as both highly sensitive and highly specific. In a 2018 systematic review of prediction rules for LVO, there were 36 studies that presented information on 34 different LVO prediction instruments.[17] Most of the prediction instruments were derived from elements of the National Institutes of Health Stroke Scale (NIHSS). Many studies included in the review had high risk or unclear risk for bias. Higher NIHSS increased the risk of LVO. In patients with suspected stroke, NIHSS stroke scale of ≥6 has a sensitivity of 80% (CI 75–85%), and a

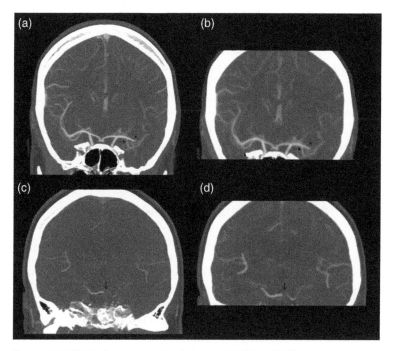

Figure 47.3 CTA brain demonstrating large vessel occlusion (LVO).

specificity of 72% (CI 70–74%), while a NIHSS ≥10 has a sensitivity of 64% (CI 57–70%) and a specificity of 84% (CI 81–87%). Some groups use an NIHSS ≥7 as protocols to denote higher risk of LVO for which CTA of the neck is a useful adjunct. However, no NIHSS cutoff excludes LVO in all cases, making early imaging an important component of stroke evaluation, which includes a CTA of the head and neck along with the NCHCT.

Clinical question

Can dwMRI and CTP predict which stroke patients may benefit from IV tPA when time of stroke onset is unknown?

dwMRI is sensitive and specific within 6 hours and can detect abnormalities within 30 minutes of symptoms onset.[18] In one retrospective study of 569 consecutive patients that received tPA, dwMRI was positive in 91% (n = 518/569) and negative in 8%. One of four patients with stroke mimics had a positive dwMRI. The use of perfusion MRI helped identify 33 of 47 patients with acute stroke that were dwMRI negative. Patients with negative dwMRI had less severe strokes, were more likely to be in the posterior circulation, and had longer time from symptom onset to imaging.[19]

In a large, randomized trial called WAKE-UP which was focused on assessing the efficacy and safety of using thrombolysis based on MRI findings in "wake-up" stroke, specifically where the time of onset is unknown, there were findings of diffusion-weighted imaging (DWI) and fluid-attenuated inversion recovery (FLAIR) mismatch in 479 patients, or approximately half the sample (48.0%) (Figure 47.4).[20] This suggests that patients with wake-up stroke are eligible half the time for safe thrombolysis, meaning that dwMRI can help identify clinically important vascular occlusion in this population. Notably, this strategy also was associated with improved outcomes.[21] The DWI-FLAIR mismatch indicates that there is no vasogenic edema, thus the stroke is relatively acute and potentially eligible for IV thrombolysis. Similarly, CTP estimates the cerebral blood flow and volume, and transit time of contrast through the brain. This estimates the size of the core ischemic area and the penumbra or area of low perfusion. Patients with small ischemic cores and large penumbra are identified by dwMRI or CTP and are the most likely to benefit from acute therapy.

The DEFUSE-3 was a randomized controlled trial (RCT) that included patients with acute strokes in the 6–16 hour window.[22] CTP or dwMRI with

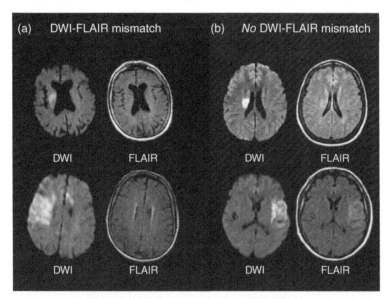

Figure 47.4 dwMRI with FLAIR showing mismatch (a) indicating stroke onset <4.5 hours and match (b), meaning stroke onset 4.5 hours or greater.

MRI perfusion imaging were used to select patients for mechanical thrombectomy. The study demonstrated a benefit of endovascular thrombectomy regardless of whether CT or MRI was used for patient selection, and 75% of the patients were selected with CTP. This study was terminated early for efficacy bringing concerns about the real magnitude of benefit of the intervention (see comment below).

Clinical question

What scales are useful to differentiate stroke from stroke mimics in the ED?

In the ED, it is important to differentiate stroke from stroke mimics.[23] Differentiating stroke mimics from genuine cases of acute stroke is challenging, particularly given the narrow time window to administration of IV thrombolysis or make decisions about other time sensitive stroke treatments. Studies have determined that the prevalence of stroke mimics is approximately 30%.[24] There have been several scales that have been developed to differentiate stroke from stroke mimics. The recognition of stroke in the emergency room (ROSIER) scale (Table 47.1) was developed and validated in 2005 in a combination derivation and validation study.

In development, 343 suspected stroke patients were assessed where 159 were diagnosed with stroke, 167 with nonstroke, 32 with transient ischemic attack (TIA). The common stroke mimic final diagnoses included seizures (23%), syncope (23%), and sepsis (10%). Using a cutoff of 0 on the seven-item ROSIER scale (with a score range from −2 to +5), the sensitivity was 92%, specificity 86%, PPV 88%, and NPV 91%. In a prospective validation of 173 consecutive suspected strokes, the sensitivity was 93%, specificity 83%, PPV 90%, and NPV 88%.

Table 47.1 Elements of the recognition of stroke in the emergency room (ROSIER) scale

Loss of consciousness/syncope (−1)
Seizure (−1)
Asymmetric facial weakness (+1)
Asymmetric arm weakness (+1)
Asymmetric leg weakness (+1)
Speech disturbance (+1)
Visual field deficit (+1)

Note: The ROSIER score varies from −2 to +5. A score of 0 or less is associated with a low likelihood of stroke.

Clinical question

What percentage of patients diagnosed with stroke have an NIHSS of zero?
In a large single-center cohort study, from 2004 to 2008, a total of 2618 strokes were evaluated by the stroke service.[25] Of those only 20 or 0.73% had an NIHSS of zero. While this is limited by the fact that patients without stroke were not included in this study, this suggests that NIHSS may be good discriminator of acute stroke symptoms. In particular, using NIHSS as an approach for a detailed neurological examination in the ED should be considered to detect patients with symptoms of stroke. When patients have an NIHSS of zero, patients can be considered low risk for stroke.

Comment

In emergency care, the current standard in cases of acute stroke is NCHCT to determine the presence of intracranial hemorrhage, detect large strokes, and potentially exclude other neurological causes for stroke symptoms. NCHCT and clinical evaluation are the standards by which the decision to use thrombolysis is typically made. However, head CT has limited sensitivity and thrombolytics are used in cases of stroke mimics. Detecting stroke mimics can be done with good sensitivity using the ROSIER scale. dwMRI is a more sensitive for acute stroke; however, this modality has limited availability, costs more, takes longer to perform, and requires a higher degree of patient participation. dwMRI is also more sensitive than head CT in identifying large-volume strokes that are at increased risk for hemorrhagic transformation and is also more sensitive in detecting chronic intracranial hemorrhage.

A primary historical concern with use of only dwMRI in acute stroke is that head CT is more sensitive in detecting acute intracranial hemorrhage. However, recent studies with newer MRI technology have mostly disproved this issue. Obtaining dwMRI and FLAIR imaging requires additional equipment, software and training and does not come automatically with MRI. Managing wake up stroke, or stroke of uncertain onset is institution dependent, however, the use of dwMRI or CTP can be useful in wake-up stroke to rule out completed infarction. FLAIR or fluid attenuated inversion detects parenchymal hyperdensity, which begins occurring at 4.5 hours after stroke onset. Thus, the combination of ischemia seen on dwMRI with FLAIR imaging showing no hyperdensity (called a "quantitative mismatch") indicates that the stroke is less than 4.5 hours and therefore potentially treatable with thrombolytics.

Care for LVO is a rapidly changing area and best practice is to perform your NIHSS on any patient suspected stroke, simultaneously order a NCHCT with CT angiogram and consult with neurology. Consider adding a CTA of the neck in NIHSS is ≥ 7 along with the NCHCT. However, be willing to order CTA in any case where it's recommended by the neurologist. Finally, NIHSS is an important adjunct to the physical examination in the ED, in particular because patients with acute stroke are very unlikely to have a NIHSS of zero.

References

1. Endovascular treatment versus medical care alone for ischaemic stroke: systematic review and meta-analysis. *BMJ*. 2019; 11(365): l1658.
2. Wardlaw JM, Seymour J, Cairns J, Keir S, Lewis S, Sandercock P. Immediate computed tomography scanning of acute stroke is cost-effective and improves quality of life. *Stroke*. 2004; 35(11): 2477–83.
3. Davis DP, Robertson T, Imbesi SG. Diffusion-weighted magnetic resonance imaging versus computed tomography in the diagnosis of acute ischemic stroke. *Journal of Emergency Medicine*. 2006; 31: 269–77.
4. Mullins ME, Schaefer PW, Sorensen AG *et al*. CT and conventional and diffusion-weighted MR imaging in acute stroke: Study in 691 patients at presentation to the emergency department. *Radiology*. 2002; 224: 353–9.
5. Fiebach J, Jansen O, Schellinger P *et al*. Comparison of CT with diffusion-weighted MRI in patients with hyperacute stroke. *Neuroradiology*. 2001; 43: 628–32.
6. Fiebach JB, Schellinger PD, Jansen O *et al*. CT and diffusion-weighted MR imaging in randomized order. *Stroke*. 2002; 33: 2206–10.
7. Urbach H, Flacke S, Keller E *et al*. Detectability and detection rate of acute cerebral hemisphere infarcts on CT and diffusion-weighted MRI. *Neuroradiology*. 2000; 42: 722–7.
8. Lansberg MG, Albers GW, Beaulieu C, Marks MP. Comparison of diffusion-weighted MRI and CT in acute stroke. *Neurology*. 2000; 54: 1557–61.
9. Gonzales RG, Schaefer PW, Buonanno FS *et al*. Diffusion-weighted MR imaging: Diagnostic accuracy in patients imaged within 6 hours of stroke symptom onset. *Radiology*. 1999; 210: 155–6.
10. Barber PA, Darby DG, Desmond PM *et al*. Identification of major ischemic change, diffusion-weighted imaging versus computed tomography. *Stroke*. 1999; 30: 2059–65.
11. Saur D, Kucinski T, Grzyska U *et al*. Sensitivity and interrater agreement of CT and diffusion-weighted MR imaging in hyperacute stroke. *American Journal of Neuroradiology*. 2003; 24: 878–85.
12. Chalela JA, Kidwell CS, Nentwich LM *et al*. Magnetic resonance imaging and computed tomography in emergency assessment of patients with suspected acute stroke: A prospective comparison. *Lancet*. 2007; 369: 293–8.
13. Fiebach JB, Schellinger PD, Gass A *et al*. Stroke magnetic resonance imaging is accurate in hyperacute intracerebral hemorrhage: A multicenter study on the validity of stroke imaging. *Stroke*. 2004; 35: 502–6.

14. Kidwell CS, Chalela JA, Saver JL *et al.* Comparison of MRI and CT for detection of acute intracerebral hemorrhage. *Journal of the American Medical Association.* 2004; 292(15): 1823–30.

15. Shah S, Luby M, Poole K *et al.* Screening with MRI for accurate and rapid stroke treatment: SMART. *Neurology.* 2015; 84(24): 2438–44.

16. Sølling C, Ashkanian M, Hjort N, Gyldensted C, Andersen G, Østergaard L. Feasibility and logistics of MRI before thrombolytic treatment. *Acta Neurologica Scandinavica.* 2009; 120(3): 143–9.

17. Smith EE, Kent DM, Bulsara KR *et al.* Accuracy of prediction instruments for diagnosing large vessel occlusion in individuals with suspected stroke: A systematic review for the 2018 guidelines for the early management of patients with acute ischemic stroke. *Stroke.* 2018; 49(3): e111–22.

18. Sorensen AG, Buonanno FS, Gonzalez RG *et al.* Hyperacute stroke: Evaluation with combined multisection diffusion-weighted and hemodynamically weighted echo-planar MR imaging. *Radiology.* 1996; 199(2): 391–401.

19. Simonsen CZ, Madsen MH, Schmitz ML, Mikkelsen IK, Fisher M, Andersen G. Sensitivity of diffusion- and perfusion-weighted imaging for diagnosing acute ischemic stroke is 97.5%. *Stroke.* 2015; 46(1): 98–101.

20. Thomalla G, Boutitie F, Fiebach JB *et al.* Stroke with unknown time of symptom onset: Baseline clinical and magnetic resonance imaging data of the first thousand patients in WAKE-UP (efficacy and safety of MRI-based thrombolysis in wake-up stroke: A randomized, doubleblind, placebo-controlled trial). *Stroke.* 2017; 48(3): 770–3.

21. Thomalla G, Simonsen CZ, Boutitie F *et al.* MRI-guided thrombolysis for stroke with unknown time of onset. *The New England Journal of Medicine.* 2018; 379(7): 611–22.

22. Albers GW, Marks MP, Kemp S *et al.* Thrombectomy for stroke at 6 to 16 hours with selection by perfusion imaging. *The New England Journal of Medicine.* 2018; 378(8): 708–18.

23. Hand PJ, Kwan J, Lindley RI, Dennis MS, Wardlaw JM. Distinguishing between stroke and mimic at the bedside: The brain attack study. *Stroke.* 2006; 37: 769–75.

24. Tsivgoulis G, Alexandrov AV, Chang J *et al.* Safety and outcomes of intravenous thrombolysis in stroke mimics: A 6-year, single-care center study and a pooled analysis of reported series. *Stroke.* 2011; 42(6): 1771–4.

25. Martin-Schild S, Albright KC, Tanksley J *et al.* Zero on the NIHSS does not equal the absence of stroke. *Annals of Emergency Medicine.* 2011; 57(1): 42–5.

Chapter 48 **Transient Ischemic Attack**

Ian T. Ferguson and Christopher R. Carpenter

Department of Emergency Medicine, Washington University School of Medicine, St. Louis, MO, USA

Highlights

- Transient ischemic attack (TIA) precedes 23% of strokes; among emergency department (ED) patients, the post-TIA stroke rates are 3% at 2 days and 6% at 7 days.
- Early registry-based validations of the ABCD^2 post-TIA clinical decision rules were promising, but methodologically rigorous clinical decision rule research has demonstrated that the ABCD^2 is nonspecific at recommended thresholds and that different cutoff values do not improve the ABCD^2 prognostic accuracy.
- There are no current validated and acceptably accurate TIA prognostic decision aids for the ED population.
- Clinical-plus scores incorporate imaging into the risk stratification, although these scores require further validation for ED use.
- Rapid ED-based diagnostic protocols may be a safe and cost-effective way to manage patients with suspected TIA.

Background

Historically, the definition of a transient ischemic attack (TIA) included a symptom resolution timeframe of less than 24 hours.[1] This symptom-based definition has been challenged in favor of a tissue-based definition with the advent of higher resolution imaging such as magnetic resonance imaging (MRI) with diffusion-weighted imaging (DWI). TIA is now defined by the American Heart Association (AHA) as "a transient episode of neurological

---

Evidence-Based Emergency Care: Diagnostic Testing and Clinical Decision Rules, Third Edition.
Edited by Jesse M. Pines, Fernanda Bellolio, Christopher R. Carpenter, and Ali S. Raja.
© 2023 John Wiley & Sons Ltd. Published 2023 by John Wiley & Sons Ltd.

dysfunction caused by focal brain, spinal cord, or retinal ischemia, without acute infarction."[1,2] This new definition has no time restriction for symptoms, although 70% of all TIAs resolve within 2 hours of onset.[3] TIA precedes 23% of strokes, and 200,000–500,000 strokes occur annually.[4,5] The diagnostic and therapeutic management of TIA as a medical emergency is a new concept because TIAs were traditionally not linked to strokes. On average, the annual risk of post-TIA stroke is 3–4%,[6] though this is probably a conservative estimate. Johnston *et al.*[7] reported a 3-month risk of 10.5% with half of those occurring within the first 2 days. Emergency department (ED) patients have higher post-TIA stroke rates than other populations: 3.1% at 2 days and 5.8% at 7 days.[8] Thus post-TIA stroke risk stratification models have become a priority amongst neurovascular emergency specialists, and rapid test–treat models are now being evaluated in a variety of healthcare settings.

The symptoms of TIA relate to the brain region suffering ischemia rather than the hemorrhagic, embolic, or atherosclerotic etiology of the low flow state, so causative inferences are not possible at the bedside. Potential etiologies of cerebral ischemia include cardiac emboli from valvular disease or atrial fibrillation (10–15%), large vessel extracranial arterial disease (20–25%), and small vessel intracranial atherosclerosis (10–15%).[6] The first two etiologies can be identified by echocardiography, telemetry, and carotid Doppler. Unfortunately, in 50% of cases, the cause of TIA remains undefined after diagnostic evaluation.[7] Observational studies and randomized trials suggest that stroke specialist care, rapid administration of antiplatelet and lipid-lowering agents, and ED-initiated diagnostic testing within 24 hours reduce 1-year post-TIA stroke rates.[5,8–12] One potential benefit of admitting TIA patients is that in-hospital thrombolysis using the National Institute of Neurological Disorders and Stroke (NINDS) or European Cooperative Acute Stroke Study III (ECASS-III) protocols is more likely in the inpatient setting.[13–15] However, debate continues regarding the cost-effectiveness of hospitalizing TIA patients as opposed to evaluating them in same-day clinics.[16,17]

If TIA patients at increased risk for short-term stroke could be rapidly and accurately identified in ED settings, cost-effectiveness might be less controversial, but simply diagnosing TIA remains challenging. One prospective series found that 20% of all suspected TIAs in the ED were TIA mimics, with the two most common being seizures and migraine.[9] Less frequent causes included hypoglycemia, psychogenic hyperventilation, sepsis, and transient global amnesia.[9] Consequently, TIAs are frequently misdiagnosed in the ED by neurologists and emergency physicians.[18–20] Features associated with a discordant diagnosis of TIA between neurologists and emergency physicians include headache, involuntary movement, and dizziness, while a high ABCD^2 score increases the odds of concordance.[21] MRI with DWI identifies ischemic lesions in one-third of patients even with symptom resolution <1 hour and increases the risk of future stroke, although this imaging modality is not always readily available.[1,2] In addition, practice variability and resource constraints limit the uniform application of rapid diagnostic and therapeutic pathways on all TIA patients.[22,23]

Clinical question

In suspected TIA, can decision aids identify patients at low- or high risk of subsequent stroke within 2 or 7-days?

The American College of Emergency Physicians (ACEP) latest TIA Clinical Policy provides no Level A recommendations for the use of decision aids to identify low-risk patients with suspected TIA who can safely be discharged from the ED. A Level B recommendation is to *not* rely on current risk stratification tools such as the ABCD^2 score for ruling out high-risk patients with suspected TIA.[24]

As of this 2016 ACEP policy, six clinical decision instruments aimed at stratifying the risk of patients with TIA for the development of future stroke had been identified. These are the ABCD, ABCD^2, ABCD^3, California Rule, and the Canadian TIA Score.[7,10–13] Registry data were used to derive and validate the California Rule and the original ABCD Rule. The ABCD^2 rule was derived using components of both the California and original ABCD rules and validated in four different registry-based cohorts (Table 48.1).[11,14,15]. A systematic review of early validation trials for the ABCD^2 observed negative likelihood ratios (LRs) of 0.24 and 0.35 for risk of stroke in 7 and 90 days respectively using the recommended cut-off of <3.[16] However, the only trial to follow established methodological rigor for validating a decision instrument prospectively yielded a negative LR of 0.42 for stroke risk in 7 days using the same cut-off of <3 (Table 48.2)[17,18] Although sensitive, the poor specificity observed for a cut-off of >2 would mean that 87.6% of all patients evaluated for TIA would require emergent investigations from the ED.[17] Therefore, the ABCD^2 should not be used to stratify TIA patients as either high or low risk for stroke within 7 days.

Further modification of the ABCD^2 score using clinical features alone has not improved accuracy,[19] prompting efforts to develop clinical-plus tools which aim to combine clinical features and imaging findings. A number of these scores have been published, including the clinical- and imaging-based prediction (CIP) model, recurrent risk estimator (RRE), ABCD^2-I, ABCD^3-I, and Canadian TIA score.[12,20–23] The ABCD^3-I requires external validation but showed increased discrimination over the ABCD^2 score in the initial derivation sample (*C* statistic 0.92 versus 0.71).[12] The Canadian TIA score incorporates noncontrast computed tomography (CT) and may also be more discriminatory

Table 48.1 Transient ischemic attack (TIA) risk stratification instruments

California rule	
Age >60 years	1 point
Diabetes mellitus	1 point
Symptoms >10 minutes	1 point
Weakness	1 point
Speech deficit	1 point
ABCD rule	
Age >60 years	1 point
Blood pressure >140/90	1 point
Unilateral weakness	2 points
Language disturbance	1 point
Without weakness duration	
>60 minutes	2 points
10–59 minutes	1 point
ABCD^2 rule	
Age >60 years	
Blood pressure >140/90	1 point
Diabetes	2 points
Unilateral weakness	2 points
Language disturbance	1 point
Without weakness duration	
>60 minutes	2 points
10–59 minutes	1 point

Source: Data from [14].

Table 48.2 ABCD^2 likelihood ratio diagnostic accuracy for stroke at 7 and 90 days

ABCD^2 score	Stroke at 7 days (95% confidence interval)	Stroke at 90 days (95% confidence interval)
0	0	0
1	0	0
2	0.61 (0.12–2.38)	0.36 (0.09–1.42)
3	0.13 (0.02–0.91)	0.23 (0.08–0.70)
4	1.07 (0.63–1.84)	1.22 (0.83–1.79)
5	1.53 (0.97–2.39)	1.47 (1.03–2.11)
6	1.19 (0.64–2.22)	1.06 (0.63–1.77)
7	3.89 (1.48–10.19)	4.22 (1.99–8.92)

Source: Data from [17].

than the ABCD^2 score, although it also requires external validation. This score has a total score of −3 to 23 and a negative LR of 0.08 with a score of 6 or less.[13] At this time, neither current risk-stratification instruments nor noncontrast head CT should be used alone to identify ED patients with TIA at low-risk or high risk for stroke at either 2 or 7 days.[24]

Clinical question

In suspected TIA, can carotid ultrasonography and echocardiogram be safely deferred to the post-ED outpatient setting?

There are no Level A or B recommendations from the 2016 ACEP guidelines regarding the safety of deferring ultrasound (US) or echocardiogram in the post-ED outpatient setting.[24] Level C recommendations include obtaining vascular imaging when feasible to identify patients at short-term risk for stroke, including as appropriate carotid US, computed tomography angiography (CTA), or magnetic resonance angiography (MRA). The Clinical Policy does not specify the superiority of one vascular modality over another in the ED setting. In one study, carotid US had the same reported negative LR as MRA to exclude significant carotid stenosis (0.07 with confidence interval [CI] 0.01–0.47).[25] Another study with imaging performed within 15 days of patient enrollment found that the negative LR US was inferior to MRA (0.19 [CI 0.09–0.40] versus 0.07 [CI 0.02–0.27]) for the diagnosis of carotid stenosis.[26] One example of an ED-based diagnostic algorithm for TIA is shown in Figure 48.1.[24] This pathway suggests admission may be not be required in all TIA evaluations if no high-risk criteria are present on initial evaluation, appropriate neurovascular imaging can be obtained in the ED, and patients do not meet any admission criteria as outlined in the figure.[24]

Clinical question

In suspected TIA, can CTA or MRA cerebral circulation imaging accurately identify patients at high risk of stroke within 7-days?

Unremarkable or nondiagnostic DWI imaging does not reduce the need for carotid imaging to evaluate the risk for future stroke.[2] Carotid endarterectomy for symptomatic severe (70–99%) carotid stenosis within 2 weeks of TIA significantly reduces the risk of stroke (Number Needed to Treat = 6 to prevent one death or stroke).[24,27] Therefore, identifying and treating severe carotid stenosis is a surrogate for preventing strokes. Unfortunately, auscultation of carotid bruit is specific but not sensitive to detect severe stenosis so not an adequate screening test to guide imaging decisions in TIA.[28] CTA and MRA have replaced traditional catheter-based angiography to evaluate carotid stenosis.

Imaging used to evaluate for carotid stenosis varies depending on local practice and availability and ACEP Clinical Policy provides a Level C recommendation that carotid US is acceptable with accuracy similar to MRA and CTA. D'Onofrio *et al.*[25] compared carotid Doppler (LR+ 3.2 [CI 1.6–6.2], LR– 0.07 [CI 0.01–0.47]) to MRA (LR+ 3.2 [CI 1.6–6.2] and LR– 0.07 [CI 0.01–0.47]), demonstrating similar diagnostic accuracy identifying carotid

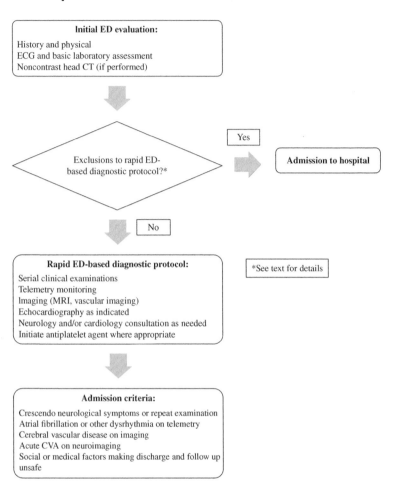

Figure 48.1 Rapid ED-based diagnostic algorithm for TIA. High-risk conditions that preclude assessment in this algorithm include abnormal findings on initial head CT, suspected embolic source (presence of atrial fibrillation, cardiomyopathy, or valvulopathy), known carotid stenosis, previous large stroke, and crescendo TIA. (Lo *et al.* [24]/ With permission of Elsevier.)

stenosis >60%.[25] Another Health Technology Assessment meta-analysis in 2006 demonstrated superior LR+ for CTA and LR– for MRA[29] (Table 48.3). Diagnostic meta-analysis of 23 studies demonstrated carotid US LR+ 115 (CI 59–224) and LR– 0.03 (CI 0.01–0.06), suggesting improved accuracy over time when compared with earlier research.[30] The specificity of MRA is improved with use of three-dimensional imaging.[31]

Table 48.3 Diagnostic accuracy of severe carotid stenosis

Imaging	Positive likelihood ratio	Negative likelihood ratio
CTA	15.4	0.24
Doppler ultrasound	5.6	0.13
MRA	13.4	0.06

Source: Data from [29].

CTA is comparable to DWI for predicting recurrent stroke within 90 days: LR+ of 2.1 for CTA and 1.32 for DWI.[32] MRA is similar in image quality to CTA, although takes longer for safety screening and data acquisition, and is not consistently available, which potentially limits the feasibility and cost-effectiveness of ED MRA.[33]

Clinical question

In suspected TIA, is a rapid ED-based protocol of vascular imaging and echocardiography accurate, safe, and cost-effective?
Early studies evaluating rapid treatment approaches include the early use of existing preventative strategies for stroke (EXPRESS) and the SOS-TIA study. EXPRESS reported an 80% reduction in stroke over a 90-day period after implementation of a rapid referral program to a TIA clinic (median delay from ED presentation to TIA clinic less than 1 day with interquartile range of 0–3).[34] The authors note that the majority of benefit was likely associated with aspirin administered early after ED arrival. In SOS-TIA, patients were referred to the follow-up clinic from outpatient clinics and the ED, with follow-up imaging dictated by assessment from a neurologist in the clinic. There was a decrease in 90-day stroke rates to 1.63% (CI 0.85–3.12) from 6.49% when expected risk was calculated using ABCD².[35] The transient ischemic attack work-up as outpatient assessment of clinical evaluation and safety (TWO ACES) study triaged ED patients with suspected TIA using ABCD² scores < 4 to outpatient follow-up with either MRI and MRA (or CTA), ED vascular imaging (scores 4–5), or inpatient hospitalization (scores > 5). Median follow-up to clinic was 3 days and 76% had an MRI performed before the clinic visit. Thirty-two percent of the outpatient patient cohort had a final diagnosis of TIA or stroke, and of those with an MRI, 9% showed an acute DWI lesion.[36] The Monash transient ischemic attack triaging treatment (M3T) model does not incorporate a clinical risk stratification tool, instead using carotid US and CT to triage patients to urgent (<24 hours) versus less urgent (4–6 week) follow-up. Patients with ≥50% ipsilateral

carotid artery stenosis identified on carotid US were referred for CTA or MRA within 24 hours (>70% lesions were referred immediately to vascular surgery).[37] This model observed a 90-day stroke risk of 1.5% (CI 0.73–3.05) and observed a nonsignificant difference between admitted and nonadmitted patients with regard to stroke outcome.[37]

Cheong et al.[38] evaluated another CTA-based protocol. ED patients with suspected TIA were evaluated with noncontrast CT and CTA in the ED. Patients with a >50% arterial stenosis were admitted to the stroke unit, as were patients with high-risk features, including those with atrial fibrillation not on anticoagulation or sub-therapeutic and those with mechanical valve replacements. Other patients received antiplatelet therapy, were referred to an outpatient TIA clinic, and further imaged via MRI within a median duration of 4 days postevent. Unlike prior similar studies, this algorithm did not utilize carotid US, neurologist review, or ABCD² scores, while still achieving a 2.0% stroke rate at 90 days. However, the pragmatic utility and cost-efficiency of this algorithm are unclear, as the authors do not clearly delineate how they identified those at high risk for TIA.

Two physical exam findings predictive of an ischemic event are unilateral weakness or speech disturbances (dysarthria or dysphasia).[11] If clinical findings associated with high risk for post-TIA stroke are noted in the ED, some advocate for rapid CTA and urgent follow-up within 24 hours for all patients, although the utility of urgent follow-up following negative vascular imaging is debateable.[39]

Comment

One-year follow-up data from the TIAregistry.org project with a cohort of 4789 patients from 21 countries suggest that recurrent risk following a TIA is much lower than previously reported. Prior 90-day risk of stroke or vascular events ranged from 12% to 20% while the TIAregistry risk was 3.7%.[40] This marked reduction may reflect a paradigm shift of TIA viewed as a precursor of stroke with patients receiving more comprehensive secondary stroke prevention. Interventions to reduce post-TIA stroke include early initiation of antiplatelet agents, faster revascularization in those with significant carotid stenosis, and other pharmacological therapies like statins. Incorporating the ABCD² score in the TIAregistry cohort would miss 20% of strokes if urgent treatment was only provided to those with a score of ≥4 so the current ACEP Clinical Policy discourages relying solely on currently available scores[24,40] Although a number of early decision pathways exist, no pathway is superior to reduce post-TIA stroke. Nonetheless, as discussed in Chapter 5, emergency medicine clinicians are stewards of the healthcare system as well as advocates for delivering the appropriate care to patients most likely to benefit at the point in time when the patient requires that care. Every patient with suspected TIA is not a TIA patient or at risk for subsequent stroke – and therefore will not benefit from extensive diagnostic evaluation or referrals. In fact, inappropriate diagnostic testing is sometimes associated with the harms of over-diagnosis and over-treatment.[41] Rapid ED protocols are appropriate in adult patients with suspected TIA without high-risk features.[24] High-risk features include an abnormal initial head CT, suspected embolic source (history of atrial fibrillation, cardiomyopathy, or known valvuloplasty), known carotid stenosis, pervious large stroke, or crescendo TIA.[24]

Early vascular imaging in suspected TIA with high-risk clinical features, whether carotid US, CTA, or MRA, is beneficial. Noncontrast CT is less sensitive than MRI with DWI for ischemic events but should also be performed in suspected TIA given the probability of nonischemic causes for the patient's symptoms.[24] Future ED protocols may better clarify those patients at high-risk requiring advanced vascular imaging in the ED prior to discharge and specify an optimal time for a TIA clinic or neurology follow-up. The role for TIA clinical decision aids within ED care pathways remains uncertain. Future tools and diagnostic algorithms in the ED setting must successfully engage patients in management options and align with their goals of care, in addition to confirming that prognostic accuracy is associated with improved patient-centered outcomes.[42–44]

References

1. Easton JD, Saver JL, Albers GW *et al.* Definition and evaluation of transient ischemic attack: A scientific statement for healthcare professionals from the American Heart Association/American Stroke Association Stroke Council; Council on Cardiovascular Surgery and Anesthesia; Council on Cardiovascular Radiology and Intervention; Council on Cardiovascular Nursing; and the Interdisciplinary Council on Peripheral Vascular Disease. The American Academy of Neurology affirms the value of this statement as an educational tool for neurologists. *Stroke.* 2009; 40(6): 2276–93.
2. Brazzelli M, Chappell FM, Miranda H *et al.* Diffusion-weighted imaging and diagnosis of transient ischemic attack. *Annals of Neurology.* 2014; 75(1): 67–76.
3. Long B, Koyfman A. Best clinical practice: Controversies in transient ischemic attack evaluation and disposition in the emergency department. *The Journal of Emergency Medicine.* 2017; 52(3): 299–310.
4. Kleindorfer D, Panagos P, Pancioli A *et al.* Incidence and short-term prognosis of transient ischemic attack in a population-based study. *Stroke.* 2005; 36(4): 720–3.
5. Rothwell PM, Warlow CP. Timing of TIAs preceding stroke: Time window for prevention is very short. *Neurology.* 2005; 64(5): 817–20.

6. Dhamoon MS, Sciacca RR, Rundek T, Sacco RL, Elkind MS. Recurrent stroke and cardiac risks after first ischemic stroke: The Northern Manhattan Study. *Neurology.* 2006; 66(5): 641–6.

7. Johnston SC, Gress DR, Browner WS, Sidney S. Short-term prognosis after emergency department diagnosis of TIA. *JAMA.* 2000; 284(22): 2901–6.

8. Giles MF, Rothwell PM. Risk of stroke early after transient ischaemic attack: A systematic review and meta-analysis. *Lancet Neurology.* 2007; 6(12): 1063–72.

9. Amort M, Fluri F, Schafer J *et al.* Transient ischemic attack versus transient ischemic attack mimics: Frequency, clinical characteristics and outcome. *Cerebrovascular Diseases.* 2011; 32(1): 57–64.

10. Rothwell PM, Giles MF, Flossmann E *et al.* A simple score (ABCD) to identify individuals at high early risk of stroke after transient ischaemic attack. *Lancet.* 2005; 366(9479): 29–36.

11. Johnston SC, Rothwell PM, Nguyen-Huynh MN *et al.* Validation and refinement of scores to predict very early stroke risk after transient ischaemic attack. *Lancet.* 2007; 369(9558): 283–92.

12. Merwick A, Albers GW, Amarenco P *et al.* Addition of brain and carotid imaging to the ABCD(2) score to identify patients at early risk of stroke after transient ischaemic attack: A multicentre observational study. *Lancet Neurology.* 2010; 9(11): 1060–9.

13. Perry JJ, Sharma M, Sivilotti ML *et al.* A prospective cohort study of patients with transient ischemic attack to identify high-risk clinical characteristics. *Stroke.* 2014; 45(1): 92–100.

14. Carpenter CR, Keim SM, Crossley J, Perry JJ, Best Evidence in Emergency Medicine Investigator Group. Post-transient ischemic attack early stroke stratification: The ABCD(2) prognostic aid. *The Journal of Emergency Medicine.* 2009; 36(2): 194–8; discussion 8–200.

15. Shah KH, Metz HA, Edlow JA. Clinical prediction rules to stratify short-term risk of stroke among patients diagnosed in the emergency department with a transient ischemic attack. *Annals of Emergency Medicine.* 2009; 53(5): 662–73.

16. Galvin R, Geraghty C, Motterlini N, Dimitrov BD, Fahey T. Prognostic value of the ABCD(2) clinical prediction rule: A systematic review and meta-analysis. *Family Practice.* 2011; 28(4): 366–76.

17. Perry JJ, Sharma M, Sivilotti ML *et al.* Prospective validation of the ABCD^2 score for patients in the emergency department with transient ischemic attack. *CMAJ.* 2011; 183(10): 1137–45.

18. Stiell IG, Wells GA. Methodologic standards for the development of clinical decision rules in emergency medicine. *Annals of Emergency Medicine.* 1999; 33(4): 437–47.

19. Raser JM, Cucchiara BL. Modifications of the ABCD^2 score do not improve the risk stratification of transient ischemic attack patients. *Journal of Stroke and Cerebrovascular Diseases.* 2012; 21(6): 467–70.

20. Ay H, Arsava EM, Johnston SC *et al.* Clinical- and imaging-based prediction of stroke risk after transient ischemic attack: The CIP model. *Stroke.* 2009; 40(1): 181–6.

21. Schrock JW, Glasenapp M, Victor A *et al.* Variables associated with discordance between emergency physician and neurologist diagnoses of transient ischemic attacks in the emergency department. *Annals of Emergency Medicine.* 2012; 59: 19–26.
22. Arsava EM, Furie KL, Schwamm LH, Sorensen AG, Ay H. Prediction of early stroke risk in transient symptoms with infarction: Relevance to the new tissue-based definition. *Stroke.* 2011; 42(8): 2186–90.
23. Giles MF, Albers GW, Amarenco P *et al.* Addition of brain infarction to the ABCD² score (ABCD2I): A collaborative analysis of unpublished data on 4574 patients. *Stroke.* 2010; 41(9): 1907–13.
24. Lo BM, Carpenter CR, Hatten BW, Wright BJ, Brown MD. Clinical policy: Critical issues in the evaluation of adult patients with suspected transient ischemic attack in the emergency department. *Annals of Emergency Medicine.* 2016; 68(3): 354–70.e29.
25. D'Onofrio M, Mansueto G, Faccioli N *et al.* Doppler ultrasound and contrast-enhanced magnetic resonance angiography in assessing carotid artery stenosis. *La Radiologia Medica.* 2006; 111(1): 93–103.
26. Nonent M, Ben Salem D, Serfaty JM *et al.* Overestimation of moderate carotid stenosis assessed by both Doppler US and contrast enhanced 3D-MR angiography in the CARMEDAS study. *Journal of Neuroradiology.* 2011; 38(3): 148–55.
27. Rerkasem A, Orrapin S, Howard DP, Rerkasem K. Carotid endarterectomy for symptomatic carotid stenosis. *Cochrane Database of Systematic Reviews.* 2020; 9: CD001081.
28. McColgan P, Bentley P, McCarron M, Sharma P. Evaluation of the clinical utility of a carotid bruit. *QJM.* 2012; 105(12): 1171–7.
29. Wardlaw JM, Chappell FM, Best JJ *et al.* Non-invasive imaging compared with intra-arterial angiography in the diagnosis of symptomatic carotid stenosis: A meta-analysis. *Lancet.* 2006; 367(9521): 1503–12.
30. Rojoa DM, Lodhi AQD, Kontopodis N, Ioannou CV, Labropoulos N, Antoniou GA. Ultrasonography for the diagnosis of extra-cranial carotid occlusion - diagnostic test accuracy meta-analysis. *VASA.* 2020; 49(3): 195–204.
31. Menke J. Diagnostic accuracy of contrast-enhanced MR angiography in severe carotid stenosis: Meta-analysis with metaregression of different techniques. *European Radiology.* 2009; 19(9): 2204–16.
32. Coutts SB, Modi J, Patel SK, Demchuk AM, Goyal M, Hill MD. CT/CT angiography and MRI findings predict recurrent stroke after transient ischemic attack and minor stroke: Results of the prospective CATCH study. *Stroke.* 2012; 43(4): 1013–7.
33. Graham BR, Menon BK, Coutts SB, Goyal M, Demchuk AM. Computed tomographic angiography in stroke and high-risk transient ischemic attack: Do not leave the emergency department without it! *International Journal of Stroke.* 2018; 13(7): 673–86.
34. Rothwell PM, Giles MF, Chandratheva A *et al.* Effect of urgent treatment of transient ischaemic attack and minor stroke on early recurrent stroke (EXPRESS study): A prospective population-based sequential comparison. *Lancet.* 2007; 370(9596): 1432–42.

35. Lavallee PC, Meseguer E, Abboud H *et al.* A transient ischaemic attack clinic with round-the-clock access (SOS-TIA): Feasibility and effects. *Lancet Neurology.* 2007; 6(11): 953–60.
36. Olivot JM, Wolford C, Castle J *et al.* Two aces: Transient ischemic attack work-up as outpatient assessment of clinical evaluation and safety. *Stroke.* 2011; 42(7): 1839–43.
37. Sanders LM, Srikanth VK, Jolley DJ *et al.* Monash transient ischemic attack triaging treatment: Safety of a transient ischemic attack mechanism-based outpatient model of care. *Stroke.* 2012; 43(11): 2936–41.
38. Cheong E, Toner P, Dowie G, Jannes J, Kleinig T. Evaluation of a CTA-triage based transient ischemic attack service: A retrospective single center cohort study. *Journal of Stroke and Cerebrovascular Diseases.* 2018; 27(12): 3436–42.
39. Kamal N, Hill MD, Blacquiere DP *et al.* Rapid assessment and treatment of transient ischemic attacks and minor stroke in canadian emergency departments: Time for a paradigm shift. *Stroke.* 2015; 46(10): 2987–90.
40. Amarenco P, Lavallee PC, Labreuche J *et al.* One-year risk of stroke after transient ischemic attack or minor stroke. *The New England Journal of Medicine.* 2016; 374(16): 1533–42.
41. Carpenter CR, Raja AS, Brown MD. Overtesting and the downstream consequences of overtreatment: implications of "preventing overdiagnosis" for emergency medicine. *Academic Emergency Medicine.* 2015; 22(12): 1484–92.
42. Finnerty NM, Rodriguez RM, Carpenter CR *et al.* Clinical decision rules for diagnostic imaging in the emergency department: A research agenda. *Academic Emergency Medicine.* 2015; 22(12): 1406–16.
43. Kanzaria HK, McCabe AM, Meisel ZM *et al.* Advancing patient-centered outcomes in emergency diagnostic imaging: A research agenda. *Academic Emergency Medicine.* 2015; 22(12): 1435–46.
44. Kanzaria HK, Booker-Vaughns J, Itakura K *et al.* Dissemination and implementation of shared decision making into clinical practice: A research agenda. *Academic Emergency Medicine.* 2016; 23(12): 1368–79.

Chapter 49 **First-Episode Seizure**

Jesse M. Pines[1,2] and Christopher R. Carpenter[3]

[1] US Acute Care Solutions, Canton, OH, USA
[2] Department of Emergency Medicine, Drexel University, Philadelphia, PA, USA
[3] Department of Emergency Medicine, Washington University School of Medicine, St. Louis, MO, USA

Highlights

- The majority of seizures in the ED will not have a clear diagnosis established.
- Routine imaging and laboratory testing can be safely deferred in most children with febrile seizures.
- Withdrawal seizures represent the minority of alcohol-related seizures.
- All reproductive-aged females with a new-onset seizure should have a pregnancy test and careful consideration for eclampsia.
- In adults with first seizure, assessment of sodium and glucose is indicated.
- Brain CT is indicated in adults after a first unprovoked seizure but may be deferred to the outpatient setting in some patients.
- All patients do not need to be admitted to the hospital following the first unprovoked seizure to reduce adverse events.
- To diagnose aid in the diagnosis of seizures, several lab tests can differentiate seizures versus nonseizure disorders including creatine kinase, prolactin, and lactic acid.

Background

There are nearly 1 million emergency department (ED) visits per year for seizures, with a prevalence rate of 346 per 100,000 US adults.[1] The prevalence is highest in 18–44 year age group with a rate of 402/100,000. The vast majority of patients less than 65 years are ultimately discharged from the ED (88%), as

---

Evidence-Based Emergency Care: Diagnostic Testing and Clinical Decision Rules, Third Edition.
Edited by Jesse M. Pines, Fernanda Bellolio, Christopher R. Carpenter, and Ali S. Raja.
© 2023 John Wiley & Sons Ltd. Published 2023 by John Wiley & Sons Ltd.

compared to the 65–84 age group where 50% are discharged, and 40% in the age 85+ group. The total costs of ED visits related to seizures are estimated at more than $1.15 billion U.S. dollars. The time-to-diagnosis of ED seizure is a source of healthcare disparities.[2] The initial impression of seizure changes in up to 25% of ED cases within a short period of time with additional information.[3]

Patients with known seizure disorder should be evaluated distinctly from first-episode seizure patients presenting to the ED. This chapter will focus on the diagnostic approach to the first-episode seizure patients. One-fifth of first-episode seizure patients are not recognized during their first ED evaluation.[4] In particular, migraine headaches and syncope are frequently misdiagnosed as seizure, and sometimes stroke.[5] After a first seizure, up to 40–50% of patients will have a recurrence within 2 years.[6] This makes it vitally important to ensure that patients who have seizures have clear follow-up instructions and are educated about the potential for seizure recurrence.

The top three etiologies of seizures in ED patients older than 5 years are toxins (19%), head injury (8%), and epilepsy (7%).[7] Toxins include ethanol, but only 22% of seizures attributed to alcohol abuse can be explained by withdrawal.[8] Therefore, the diagnosis of an alcohol withdrawal seizure should be one of exclusion. Other toxins associated with seizures include cocaine, lidocaine, meperidine, bupropion, carbon monoxide, tramadol, fentanyl, synthetic cannabinoids, organophosphates, and nerve agents.[9–11] Unrecognized dysrhythmia can mimic seizures.[12,13] Less common diagnoses like cerebral vein thrombosis can also present with seizures.[14]

Status epilepticus is defined as seizures persisting for over 30 minutes or multiple seizures without a return to normal consciousness in between. In the ED, status epilepticus represents 7% of seizures.[15] Mortality for status epilepticus is 3% in children and increases to 38% in older adults.[16] One-quarter of status epilepticus cases are nonconvulsive, which can be a challenging diagnosis, as the patient may present with altered mental statuses such as lethargy or coma.[17] Additionally, when seizures are not witnessed by bystanders, emergency physicians must differentiate syncope from seizure. Elevated serum creatine kinase measured 4 hours after loss of consciousness can distinguish syncope from tonic-clonic seizure.[18,19]

In children, febrile seizures represent one-third of seizures presenting to the ED.[8] In order to establish the diagnosis of simple febrile seizure, all criteria in Table 49.1 must be met.[20] Complex febrile seizures are less well defined and represent a heterogeneous mixture of etiologies. Children with a simple febrile seizure are not at increased risk to develop adult epilepsy compared with those who never had a febrile seizure. However, the risk of recurrent febrile seizure is high, ranging from 12% to 50% depending upon whether

Table 49.1 Essential criteria to define *simple* febrile seizure

Age 6 months–5 years
Tonic-clonic seizure
Resolution of convulsions within 15 minutes
Normal mental status after convulsion
Documentation of fever >38.0 °C
Only one seizure in 24-hour period
Absence of preceding neurological abnormality

Source: Data from [20].

the seizure occurred in an infant or toddler. This is a key message that should be explained to parents when discharging a child with a febrile seizure.

Pregnant women without preexisting epilepsy can develop a gestational seizure disorder called *eclampsia*. Preeclampsia usually precedes the development of seizures with hypertension, edema, and +/– proteinuria beginning after the 20th week of pregnancy.[21] One-quarter of eclampsia seizures occur before labor, one-half during labor, and the rest occur up to 10 days postpartum.[22,23] Maternal risk factors for preeclampsia include a family history of preeclampsia, multiple gestations, renal disease, diabetes preceding the pregnancy, nulliparity, and extremes of age.[24]

Psychogenic seizures, formerly referred to as *pseudoseizures*, are a diagnosis of exclusion in the ED with a general population prevalence of 0.002–0.33%.[25] Psychogenic seizures are sometimes difficult to distinguish from other seizures and are a source of significant healthcare expense.[26,27] Psychogenic seizures can also stigmatize patients.[28] About one in three patients receive an antiepileptic medication for psychogenic seizures which are not effective in preventing them.[29] In addition, the mean delay between seizure onset and psychogenic seizure diagnosis is 7 years.[30] Among patients referred to definitive epilepsy diagnostic centers, 30% are ultimately diagnosed with psychogenic seizures.[31] To further complicate the issue, epilepsy can coexist with psychogenic seizures in 5–40% of cases.[32] Psychogenic seizures may be distinguished from neurogenic seizures by duration (often >90 seconds), presence of corneal reflex, prevention of hand falling on the face, being awake or conversant during the attack, and the absence of a postictal phase or event-related amnesia.[33,34]

Clinical question

What diagnostic tests should be performed in well-appearing children following a febrile seizure?

In well-appearing children with first complex seizure associated with fever, the incidence of significant intracranial pathology is rare (0%, CI 0–4%) and central nervous system (CNS) imaging can often be safely deferred. However, this has several important exclusions including those with prior neurosurgery, significant neurological disorder, or chronic medical illness.[35-37] Similarly, studies have not demonstrated any role in routinely evaluating electrolytes or glucose in first-episode febrile or afebrile pediatric seizure patients.[14,38-40] However, laboratory testing is indicated in the ill-appearing child with vomiting, diarrhea, dehydration, or failure to return to his or her baseline mental status.

Clinical question

Which diagnostic tests should be performed in well-appearing adults presenting to the ED following a first-episode unprovoked seizure?

The American College of Emergency Physicians has provided two Clinical Policies upon which to base diagnostic decision making.[41,42] Some of these recommendations are summarized in Figure 49.1. No Level A recommendations were published. The 2004 American College of Emergency Physicians (ACEP) Clinical Policy provides Level B evidence for the following ED diagnostic studies following a first-episode unproved seizure.

- Electroencephalogram (EEG)
- Computed tomography (CT) or magnetic resonance imaging (MRI) neuroimaging
- Serum glucose
- Serum sodium
- Pregnancy test in reproductive-aged females

   The 2004 Clinical Policy authors found insufficient evidence to support or refute routine toxicology screening or lumbar puncture and did not address the role of lactate to prolactin to distinguish seizure from other forms of transient alterations of consciousness.[43,44] Furthermore, when the new-onset seizure patient has returned to a normal baseline, deferred outpatient neuroimaging is sufficient when reliable follow-up is available (e.g., MRI and EEG). The indications for consulting neurology and/or obtaining an EEG in the ED (versus in outpatient follow-up) are not defined by the Clinical Policy. However, the sensitivity of EEG to detect a specific seizure focus decreases with increased time from the event, so ensuring prompt neurology referral who can schedule an urgent outpatient EEG is useful.

   Although many electrolyte abnormalities will be suspected on history and physical exam in such patients, unexpected hypoglycemia or hyponatremia will sometimes be identified by laboratory evaluation.[45-47] The same is true for CNS imaging. In one study of 259 patients with clinically suspected alcohol withdrawal seizures, 16 (6%) had an intracranial lesion on head CT, 10 of

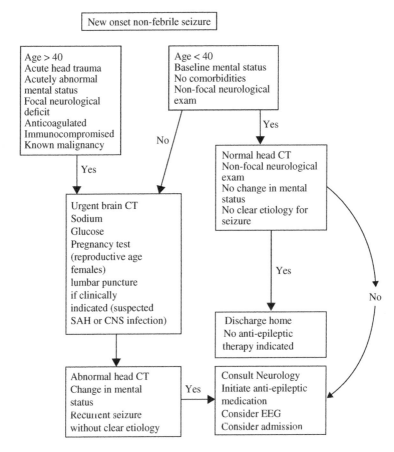

Figure 49.1 Diagnostic evaluation of first-time seizure.

which altered subsequent clinical management.[48] A multidisciplinary clinical policy on neuroimaging for such patients recommended that a head CT be obtained in the ED whenever an acute intracranial process is suspected, in the presence of a focal neurological deficit, after acute head trauma, for patients older than 40 years, if focal onset before generalized seizure ensued, or if a history of malignancy, immunocompromising illness, fever, persistent headache, or anticoagulation exists.[49] More recently, another study demonstrated abnormal findings in 5% of CTs and 19% or MRIs after a first seizure.[44] The frequency of abnormal CT findings increases with age.

Lower quality evidence suggests that serum prolactin levels measured 10–20 minutes after a suspected psychogenic seizure may be useful to distinguish them from tonic-clonic seizures. A recent systematic review on the topic examined 16 studies. All found that prolactin levels increase after epileptic seizures, especially in the first 10–20 minutes after the seizure occurs.[50] Among studies where capillary prolactin level measurements were included, test sensitivity for the diagnosis of seizures (all epileptic seizure types), generalized tonic-clonic seizures, focal impaired awareness seizures, and focal aware seizures (FAS) was 67%, 67%, 34%, and 11%, respectively. By comparison, the specificity was 99 %.

This means that an elevated prolactin level supports the diagnosis of generalized tonic-clonic seizure, but a normal prolactin level does not sufficiently diagnose psychogenic seizures. Transient lactic acidosis is also common following a generalized tonic-clonic seizure.[44,51] In a retrospective study of 270 patients with generalized tonic-clonic seizures, psychogenic seizures, or syncope, a serum lactate above 2.4 mmol/L was 85% sensitive and 88% specific to differentiate tonic-clonic seizures from other events in males. The sensitivity and specificity dropped to 64% and 85%, respectively.

Clinical question

Following a normal first unprovoked seizure evaluation in adults, should patients be admitted to the hospital?

There is limited evidence on the incidence of mortality and recurrent seizures following an ED evaluation of seizures. One study did examine the rate of recurrent seizures within 6–24 hours in two EDs which included both provoked and unprovoked seizures in 1025 patients.[52] The average time to early seizure recurrence was 2 hours, and more than 85% of seizures recurred within 3 hours. Patients with nonalcoholic seizures had the lowest rate of early seizure current (at 9%), while in alcoholics the rate was 25%.

With regard to the longer-term risk of a seizures, a study of 232 patients assessed patients who were referred to a clinic after a first-time seizure.[53] More than half of the sample was referred from the ED, and 1 in 5 had been admitted to the hospital. Overall, 9% experienced a repeat seizure while waiting for a 6-week seizure clinic appointment. No data were provided in the study assessing whether a specific cause for seizures was detected among patients admitted to the hospital. While there is limited evidence on whether hospital admission is necessary to reduce adverse events, a 2014 guideline from the American College of Emergency Physicians did not recommend admitting all patients to the hospital following a first unprovoked seizure, with a Level 3 of evidence (i.e., expert opinion).[42]

Comment

Seizures are a common presentation to the ED with significant variability in care.[54] A primary role of the ED is to differentiate seizures versus nonseizure conditions, to offer treatment for specific types of seizures (e.g., alcohol withdrawal, status epilepticus, and eclampsia), and to perform the correct diagnostic testing to identify the underlying seizure causes. In our review, no trials exist defining the diagnostic accuracy of tests in seizure patients. Additionally, no outcomes-based studies have been published to assess the utility of laboratory or CNS imaging in first-time seizure patients. Figure 49.1 provides an algorithmic approach to the management of seizure patients in the ED that is based upon available guidelines and provides opportunities to improve local seizure pathways.[55] Future research is needed to explore the subset of patients most likely to benefit from early (versus delayed) CT and EEG, as well as the diagnostic accuracy of history and physical exam to distinguish psychogenic seizures from neurogenic seizures. Clinicians need to approach each seizure patient as a neurogenic seizure until proven otherwise.

References

1. Martindale JL, Goldstein JN, Pallin DJ. Emergency department seizure epidemiology. *Emergency Medicine Clinics of North America*. 2011; 29(1): 15–27.
2. Bensken WP, Navale SM, Andrew AS, Jobst BC, Sajatovic M, Koroukian SM. Delays and disparities in diagnosis for adults with epilepsy: Findings from U.S. Medicaid data. *Epilepsy Research*. 2020; 166: 106406. doi: 10.1016/j.eplepsyres.2020.106406.
3. Fonseca Hernández E, Olivé Gadea M, Requena Ruiz M et al. Reliability of the early syndromic diagnosis in adults with new-onset epileptic seizures: A retrospective study of 116 patients attended in the emergency room. *Seizure*. 2018; 61: 158–63.
4. Leung H, Man CY, Hui ACF, Wong KS, Kwan P. Agreement between initial and final diagnosis of first seizures, epilepsy and non-epileptic events: A prospective study. *Journal of Neurology, Neurosurgery and Psychiatry*. 2008; 79(10): 1144–7.
5. Moeller JJ, Kurniawan J, Gubitz GJ, Ross A, Bhan V. Diagnostic accuracy of neurological problems in the emergency department. *Canadian Journal of Neurological Sciences*. 2008; 35(3): 335–41.
6. Berg AT, Shinnar S. The risk of seizure recurrence following a first unprovoked seizure: A quantitative review. *Neurology*. 1991; 71(7): 965–72.
7. Beghi E. The epidemiology of epilepsy. *Neuroepidemiology*. 2020; 54(2): 185–91.
8. Krumholz A, Grufferman S, Orr ST, Stern BJ. Seizures and seizure care in an emergency department. *Epilepsia*. 1989; 30(2): 175–81.

9. Holland RW, Marx JA, Earnest MP, Ranniger S. Grand mal seizures temporally related to cocaine use: Clinical and diagnostic features. *Annals of Emergency Medicine*. 1992; 21(7): 772–6.

10. Sharma S, Riviello JJ, Harper MB, Baskin MN. The role of emergent neuroimaging in children with new-onset afebrile seizures. *Pediatrics*. 2003; 111(1): 1–5.

11. Wolfe CE, Wood DM, Dines A et al. Seizures as a complication of recreational drug use: Analysis of the Euro-DEN Plus data-set. *Neurotoxicology*. 2019; 73: 183–7.

12. González A, Aurlien D, Larsson PG et al. Seizure-like episodes and EEG abnormalities in patients with long QT syndrome. *Seizure*. 2018; 61: 214–20. doi: 10.1016/j.seizure.2018.08.020.

13. Schwarzkoph M, Yin L, Hergert L, Drucker C, Counts CR, Eisenberg M. Seizure-like presentation in OHCA creates barriers to dispatch recognition of cardiac arrest. *Resuscitation*. 2020; 156: 230–6.

14. Liberman AL, Gialdini G, Bakradze E, Chatterjee A, Kamel H, Merkler AE. Misdiagnosis of cerebral vein thrombosis in the emergency department. *Stroke*. 2018; 49(6): 1504–6.

15. Huff JS, Morris DL, Kothari RU, Gibbs MA. Emergency department management of patients with seizures: A multicenter study. *Academic Emergency Medicine*. 2001; 8(6): 622–8.

16. Delorenzo RJ, Hauser WA, Towne AR et al. A prospective, population-based epidemiologic study of status epilepticus in Richmond, Virginia. *Neurology*. 1996; 46(4): 1029–35.

17. Drislane FW. Presentation, evaluation, and treatment of nonconvulsive status epilepticus. *Epilepsy & Behavior*. 2000; 1(5): 301–14.

18. Libman MD, Potvin L, Coupal L, Grover SA. Seizure vs. syncope: Measuring serum creatine kinase in the emergency department. *Journal of General Internal Medicine*. 1991; 6(5): 408–12.

19. Goksu E, Oktay C, Kilicaslan I, Kartal M. Seizure or syncope: The diagnostic value of serum creatine kinase and myoglobin levels. *European Journal of Emergency Medicine*. 2009; 16(2): 84–6.

20. Hampers LC, Spina LA. Evaluation and management of pediatric febrile seizures in the emergency department. *Emergency Medicine Clinics of North America*. 2011; 29(1): 83–93.

21. Gestational hypertension and preeclampsia: ACOG Practice Bulletin, number 222. *Obstetrics and Gynecology*. 2020; 135(6): e237–60.

22. Sibai BM. Diagnosis, prevention, and management of eclampsia. *Obstetrics and Gynecology*. 2005; 105(2): 402–10.

23. Yancey LM, Withers E, Bakes K, Abbott J. Postpartum preeclampsia: Emergency department presentation and management. *The Journal of Emergency Medicine*. 2011; 40(4): 380–4.

24. Stead LG. Seizures in pregnancy/eclampsia. *Emergency Medicine Clinics of North America*. 2011; 29(1): 109–16.

25. Benbadis SR, Allen-Hauser W. An estimate of the prevalence of psychogenic non-epileptic seizures. *Seizure.* 2000; 9(4): 280–1.
26. Wasserman D, Herskovitz M. Epileptic vs psychogenic nonepileptic seizures: A video-based survey. *Epilepsy & Behavior.* 2017; 73: 42–5.
27. Seneviratne U, Low ZM, Low ZX et al. Medical health care utilization cost of patients presenting with psychogenic nonepileptic seizures. *Epilepsia.* 2019; 60(2): 349–57.
28. Karakis I, Janocko NJ, Morton ML et al. Stigma in psychogenic nonepileptic seizures. *Epilepsy & Behavior.* 2020; 111: 107269.
29. Benbadis SR. How many patients with pseudoseizures receive antiepileptic drugs prior to diagnosis? *European Neurology.* 1999; 41(2): 114–5.
30. Reuber M, Fernandez G, Bauer J, Helmstaedter C, Elger CE. Diagnostic delay in psychogenic nonepileptic seizures. *Neurology.* 2002; 58(3): 493–5.
31. Friedman JH, Lafrance WC. Psychogenic disorders: The need to speak plainly. *Archives of Neurology.* 2010; 67(6): 753–5.
32. Bodde NM, Brooks JL, Baker GA et al. Psychogenic non-epileptic seizures: Definition, etiology, treatment, and prognostic issues: A critical review. *Seizure.* 2009; 18(8): 543–53.
33. Leis AA, Ross MA, Summers AK. Psychogenic seizures: Ictal characteristics and diagnostic pitfalls. *Neurology.* 1992; 42(1): 95–9.
34. Jagoda A, Riggio S. Psychogenic convulsive seizures. *American Journal of Emergency Medicine.* 1993; 11(6): 626–32.
35. Garvey MA, Gaillard WD, Rusin JA et al. Emergency brain computed tomography in children with seizures: Who is most likely to benefit? *Journal of Pediatrics.* 1998; 133(5): 664–9.
36. Maytal J, Krauss JM, Novak G, Nagelberg J, Patel M. The role of brain computed tomography in evaluating children with new onset seizures in the emergency department. *Epilepsia.* 2000; 41(8): 950–4.
37. Teng D, Dayan P, Tyler S et al. Risk of intracranial pathologic conditions requring emergency intervention after a first complex febrile seizure episode among children. *Pediatrics.* 2006; 117(2): 304–8.
38. Gerber MA, Berliner BC. The child with a "simple" febrile seizure: Appropriate diagnostic evaluation. *American Journal of Diseases in Children.* 1981; 135(5): 431–3.
39. Nypaver MM, Reynolds SL, Tanz RR, Davis AT. Emergency department laboratory evaluation of children with seizures: Dogma or dilemma? *Pediatric Emergency Care.* 1992; 8(1): 13–6.
40. Sharieff GQ, Hendry PL. Afebrile pediatric seizures. *Emergency Medicine Clinics of North America.* 2011; 29(1): 95–108.
41. ACEP Clinical Policies Subcommittee. Critical issues in the evaluation and management of adult patients presenting to the emergency department with seizures. *Annals of Emergency Medicine.* 2004; 43(5): 605–25.
42. Huff JS, Melnick ER, Tomaszewski CA et al. Clinical policy: Critical issues in the evaluation and management of adult patients presenting to the emergency department with seizures. *Annals of Emergency Medicine.* 2014; 63(4): 437–47.e15.

43. Magnusson C, Herlitz J, Höglind R *et al.* Prehospital lactate levels in blood as a seizure biomarker: A multi-center observational study. *Epilepsia.* 2021; 62(2): 408–15.

44. Doğan EA, Ünal A, Ünal A, Erdoğan Ç. Clinical utility of serum lactate levels for differential diagnosis of generalized tonic-clonic seizures from psychogenic non-epileptic seizures and syncope. *Epilepsy & Behavior.* 2017; 75: 13–7.

45. Turnbull TL, Vanden Hoek TL, Howes DS, Eisner RF. Utility of laboratory studies in the emergency department patient with a new-onset seizure. *Annals of Emergency Medicine.* 1990; 19(4): 373–7.

46. Tardy B, Lafond P, Convers P *et al.* Adult first generalized seizure: Etiology, biological tests, EEG, CT scan, in an ED. *American Journal of Emergency Medicine.* 1995; 13(1): 1–5.

47. Bradford JC, Kyriakedes CG. Evaluation of the patient with seizures: An evidence based approach. *Emergency Medicine Clinics of North America.* 1999; 17(1): 203–20.

48. Earnest MP, Feldman H, Marx JA, Harris JA, Biletch M, Sullivan LP. Intracranial lesions shown by CT scans in 259 cases of first alcohol-related seizures. *Neurology.* 1988; 38(10): 1561–5.

49. American College of Emergency Physicians, American Academy of Neurology, American Association of Neurological Surgeons, and American Society of Neuroradiology. Practice parameter: Neuroimaging in the emergency patient presenting with seizure (summary statement). *Annals of Emergency Medicine.* 1996; 28(1): 114–8.

50. Wang YQ, Wen Y, Wang MM, Zhang YW, Fang ZX. Prolactin levels as a criterion to differentiate between psychogenic non-epileptic seizures and epileptic seizures: A systematic review. *Epilepsy Research.* 2021; 169: 106508.

51. Lipka K, Bülow HH. Lactic acidosis following convulsions. *Acta Anaesthesiologica Scandinavica.* 2003; 47(5): 616–8.

52. Choquet C, Depret-Vassal J, Doumenc B *et al.* Predictors of early seizure recurrence in patients admitted for seizures in the emergency department. *European Journal of Emergency Medicine.* 2008; 15: 261–7.

53. Breen DP, Dunn MJ, Davenport RJ *et al.* Epidemiology, clinical characteristics, and management of adults referred to a teaching hospital first seizure clinic. *Postgraduate Medical Journal.* 2005; 81: 715–8.

54. Williams J, Doherty J, Di Blasi C, Mabarak D, Kennedy U, Doherty CP. Seizure care in the emergency department. Identifying and bridging the gaps. A study of care and outcomes from 644 seizure presentations. *Epilepsy & Behavior.* 2018; 78: 226–31.

55. Male LR, Noble A, Snape DA, Dixon P, Marson T. Perceptions of emergency care using a seizure care pathway for patients presenting to emergency departments in the North West of England following a seizure: A qualitative study. *BMJ Open.* 2018; 8(9): e021246.

SECTION 8
Miscellaneous: Hematology Ophthalmology Pulmonology Rheumatology and Geriatrics

Chapter 50 **Pulmonary Embolism**

Lauren Westafer[1] and Ali S. Raja[2]

[1]Department of Emergency Medicine, University of Massachusetts Chan Medical School – Baystate, Springfield, MA, USA
[2]Department of Emergency Medicine, Massachusetts General Hospital, Harvard Medical School, Boston, MA, USA

Highlights

- Pulmonary embolism (PE) is a potentially lethal condition that can present atypically but overtesting is common.
- Scoring systems like the PERC rule, the Wells criteria, the Geneva score, and the YEARS algorithm can guide clinicians about the likelihood of PE.
- Diagnostic evaluation for PE involves risk stratification coupled with D-dimer testing for low-risk to intermediate-risk patients.
- High-risk patients with suspected PE should receive a chest CT pulmonary angiogram (CTPA) to rule out PE.

Background

Diagnosing pulmonary embolism (PE) represents a challenge in emergency care because it can present with nonspecific symptoms and can be potentially, but not commonly, lethal. However, detecting PE should also be balanced with the potential for over-testing, over-diagnosis, and over-treatment of PE, particularly when a diagnosis of PE is sought in very low-risk patients.[1] PEs are commonly encountered in the emergency department (ED), with nearly 200,000 ED patients receiving a diagnosis of PE in 2016.[2] Accurate and timely identification of patients with PE in the ED can minimize complications and morbidity. The challenge in diagnosing PE in the ED is the appropriate selection

Evidence-Based Emergency Care: Diagnostic Testing and Clinical Decision Rules, Third Edition.
Edited by Jesse M. Pines, Fernanda Bellolio, Christopher R. Carpenter, and Ali S. Raja.
© 2023 John Wiley & Sons Ltd. Published 2023 by John Wiley & Sons Ltd.

of patients for diagnostic testing and risk stratification based on clinical findings. The following is not meant to be a comprehensive review of all aspects of the diagnosis of PE in the ED; rather, it is a compilation of clinically relevant questions, and studies providing objective data for specific clinical questions.

There are multiple tests for PE, including D-dimer (enzyme-linked immunosorbent assay [ELISA] or whole-blood assay), computed tomographic pulmonary angiogram (CTPA), ventilation–perfusion (V/Q) scan, and pulmonary angiogram. It is important in the case of suspected PE to choose testing strategies that employ blood tests first such as D-dimer in lower-risk patients rather than starting with high-radiation costly tests such as CTPA or V/Q, when D-dimer is appropriate. Choice of a test traditionally focuses on assessment of pretest probability of the disease based on objective clinical criteria where lower-risk patients can be risk-stratified using D-dimer, or even no testing, to exclude PE and higher risk patients traditionally receive a chest CTPA or V/Q scan. Because pulmonary angiogram, long considered the criterion standard test for PE, has a 1.5% incidence of serious complication just from receiving the test, it is rarely used to make a diagnosis and/or guide patient management.

Clinical question

In patients with suspected acute PE, can a risk stratification tool be used to identify patients who need no further testing for PE?

While D-dimer can be helpful in ruling out PE without imaging if applied to low or intermediate-risk patients, overuse of the D-dimer to screen for possible PE can have negative consequences because of its low specificity. Using D-dimer in high-risk patients should be avoided because it is not sensitive enough to completely rule out PE. As patients with elevated D-dimers commonly undergo CTPA to rule out PE,[3] and the number of negative CTPAs for PE is high (90–95% in the United States), selecting which patients need any testing to rule out PE is clinically helpful.[4,5] Kline et al.[6] aimed to derive and test clinical criteria for patients that did not require D-dimer testing, creating a prediction rule, called the pulmonary embolism rule out criteria (PERC). The authors sought to find variables that were associated with the absence of PE. In the derivation study, the prevalence of PE was 11%. The final model that was derived consisted of eight criteria (Table 50.1). If all are negative, the patient does not require any testing for PE and PE can be ruled out on clinical grounds. In other words, a patient lacking any of the PERC criteria is so low-risk for PE that they do not require a D-dimer or further imaging to reduce the risk further and to continue to evaluate these very low-risk patients further will ultimately harm more patients than will be helped by over-testing as explained in Chapter 1 with test-treatment thresholds.

Table 50.1 The Pulmonary Embolism Research Consortium (PERC) criteria for suspected pulmonary embolism

---

Age <50 years
Pulse <100 beats per minute
Oxygen saturation >94%
Absence of unilateral leg swelling
No hemoptysis
No recent trauma or surgery
No history of deep vein thrombosis or pulmonary embolus
No hormone use

Source: Data from [2].

A validation set included 1427 low-risk patients, 8% of whom had PE. The rule was negative (did not meet any criteria) in 25% of them. Among those who were PERC rule negative, the proportion with PE was only 1.4% (confidence interval [CI] 0.4–3.2%). The authors concluded that these low-risk patients did not need a test for PE. The PERC criteria have been validated in a prospective study of patients with suspected PE in 13 EDs, who had a gestalt pretest probability <15%. The main study outcome was any image-proven venous thromboembolism (VTE) or all-cause death within 45 days of presentation.[7] In 8138 patients, they reported a low suspicion for PE and all PERC criteria being negative in 1666 patients (20% of the sample). Within 45 days, 561 patients (7%) had been diagnosed with any VTE and 56 had died. For the 1666 with low suspicion and PERC-negative patients, 15 had VTE and one patient died. Low suspicion and being PERC negative yielded a sensitivity of 97% (CI 96–99%) and a specificity of 22% (CI 21–23%). A cluster-randomized validation study of PERC in 1916 patients who were evaluated for possible PE found 0.1% of patients in the PERC group had a PE at 3 months and met noninferiority for incidence of PE at follow-up. Ten percent fewer patients in PERC group underwent imaging for PE.[8]

In 2018, the American College of Emergency Physicians Clinical Policy on Adult Venous Thromboembolic Disease gave a Level B recommendation to the following statement, "For patients who are at low risk for acute PE, use the Pulmonary Embolism Rule out Criteria (PERC) to exclude the diagnosis without further diagnostic testing."[9]

Clinical question

What is the Wells criteria for pretest probability of PE?
The initial derivation of the Wells criteria for PE involved the development of a scoring system to calculate pretest probability in patients with suspected PE.[10]

Table 50.2 The Wells criteria to assess pretest probability for suspected pulmonary embolism

Clinical factor	Point score*
Clinical deep vein thrombosis (DVT) (objective leg swelling, tenderness)	3
Heart rate ≥100 beats/minute	1.5
Immobilization >3 days or surgery in previous 4 weeks	1.5
Previous DVT or pulmonary embolus (PE)	1.5
Hemoptysis	1
Malignancy	1
PE as likely as, or more likely than, alternative diagnosis	3

*Interpretation of point total: <2 points: low risk (mean probability = 3.6%); 2–6 points: moderate risk (mean probability = 20.5%); and ≥6 points: high risk (mean probability = 66.7%).
Source: Data from [5].

The authors used a randomly selected sample of 80% of the patients who had participated in a prospective cohort study of patients with suspected PE who also received D-dimer testing (SimpliRED), and performed logistic regression analysis using 40 clinical variables to create a clinical prediction rule. Seven variables ended up being predictive of PE and were termed the Wells criteria for PE (Table 50.2). They created cut points for the new rule and two separate scoring systems; one that classifies patients as having low, intermediate, or high probability of PE, and a second that dichotomizes the Wells criteria into *PE likely* and *PE unlikely*. The goal of the dichotomous scoring was to simplify the risk stratification process and include a subgroup of patients who were PE unlikely and had a negative D-dimer, and therefore would have a PE prevalence of less than 2%. Notably, studies have determined that the testing threshold for PE is in the approximately 1–2% prevalence range.[11,12] For more information on test-treatment thresholds, see Chapter 1. The authors then applied these probabilities to the remaining 20% of the sample (to validate the scoring system).

A validation study of the dichotomized Wells score in 3306 patients found that when a normal quantitative D-dimer (VIDAS or Tinaquant) was combined with a PE unlikely probability, the 3-month incidence of VTE was 0.5% (95% CI 0.2–1.1). The authors concluded that a combination of a score ≤4 and a negative D-dimer may have a negative predictive value where safe discharge is possible in patients with suspected PE.[13] While a negative D-dimer combined with low pretest probability or *PE Unlikely* Wells score has been demonstrated to be safe, Warren *et al.* examined the utility of the D-dimer in the intermediate risk Wells group in a study with an overall PE prevalence of 22.7%. In 2531 patients evaluated for possible PE, 1679 (66.3%) patients had an intermediate Wells score (2–6). When combined with a negative D-dimer (IL-test or Bio-Pool), this resulted in a sensitivity of 99.5% (95% CI 98.1–99.9). When this same population was dichotomized, only 946 (37.3%) patients had a score of *PE Unlikely* and would have been eligible for D-dimer testing.[14]

Clinical question

What is the Geneva score for PE, and how does this compare to the Wells score?
The Geneva score is another risk stratification tool for patients with potential PE. The original scoring system required arterial blood gas analysis, which is painful and is unnecessary in low-risk patients.[8] The revised Geneva score, however, does not include arterial blood gas analysis. The scoring system differs from Wells in that it does not require an assessment by the physician about whether PE is the leading diagnosis. The revised Geneva score was derived in 965 consecutive patients who were evaluated for PE according to a standardized protocol. A total of 23% in the derivation cohort and 26% in the validation cohort had PE. The area under the receiver operating curve (ROC) was 0.74 (CI 0.70–0.78) in both the derivation and validation datasets. The revised Geneva score (see Table 50.3) also performed well in an external validation cohort of 756 patients.

Clinical question

How can age-adjusted D-dimer be incorporated into the evaluation of PE?
Historically, a dichotomous D-dimer threshold has been used. However, D-dimer concentrations increase with age, resulting in a lower specificity of D-dimer testing in patients with suspected PE. Douma *et al.* aimed to retrospectively derive and validate an age-dependent D-dimer cut-off value. The derivation cohort included 1721 outpatients who underwent evaluation for possible PE using the VIDAS D-dimer assay. The authors plotted the D-dimer cut-off against 10-year age groups (for those >50 years old) and used linear regression to find an age-adjusted value. They found that a D-dimer cut-off of a 10 µg/L increase per patient year after age 50 to have a failure rate of 0.2% (95% CI 0–1.0) in the derivation cohort. They then assessed the cut-off in two retrospective validation cohorts and the age-adjusted D-dimer cut-off had failure rates of 0.6% (95% CI 0.3–1.3) and 0.3% (0.1–1.1).[15] In a prospective study of 3324 ED patients with an overall prevalence of PE of 19%, the 3-month risk of missed PE using the age-adjusted D-dimer cut-off (VIDAS, Tina-quant, Cobas h 232,

Table 50.3 The revised Geneva score

Risk factors		Points
Age >65 years		1
Previous deep venous thrombosis or pulmonary embolus		3
Surgery or fracture within 1 month		2
Active malignancy		2
Symptoms		
Unilateral lower limb pain		3
Hemoptysis		2
Clinical signs		
Heart rate 75–94 beats/minute		3
Heart rate ≥95 beats/minute		5
Pain on lower limb deep vein palpation and unilateral edema		4

Total score		Prevalence of PE (%)*
0–3	Low risk	7.9
4–10	Intermediate risk	28
≥11	High risk	74

* In the validation cohort.
Source: Data from [8].

STA-Liatest, D-dimer HS500, and Innovance) was 0.3% (95% CI 0.1–1.7). Using this cut-off, which is practically obtained by multiplying the age by 10 μg/L, PE could be excluded on the basis of a D-dimer in an additional 11.6% of patients.[16] In 2018, the American College of Emergency Physicians Clinical Policy on Adult Venous Thromboembolic Disease gave a Level B recommendation to the following statement, "In patients older than 50 years deemed to be low or intermediate risk for acute PE, clinicians may use a negative age-adjusted D-dimer* result to exclude the diagnosis of PE. *For highly sensitive D-dimer assays using fibrin equivalent units (FEU) use a cutoff of age × 10 μg/L; for highly sensitive D-dimer assays using D-dimer units (DDU), use a cutoff of age × 5 μg/L."[9]

Clinical question

Can a higher D-dimer threshold (1000 μg/L DDU) be used to exclude PE in patients with a low pretest probability of PE?

The D-dimer test is historically dichotomized, with most assays using a threshold of <500 μg/L as negative. However, this cut-off has poor specificity for PE. Two algorithms have evaluated the use of a higher D-dimer threshold of 1000 μg/L in patients with low pretest probability for PE: the YEARS algorithm

Table 50.4 The YEARS algorithm components

Hemoptysis
Clinical signs of DVT
PE is the most likely diagnosis

Source: Data from [9].

and the Pulmonary Embolism Graduated d-Dimer (PEGeD) algorithm. Van der Hulle *et al.* proposed the YEARS algorithm, which uses a simplified Wells score (Table 50.4). If a patient satisfies 0 YEARS items, a D-dimer threshold <1000 µg/L is deemed "negative" whereas if a patient satisfies >1 YEARS items, the D-dimer threshold is set at <500 µg/L. They prospectively evaluated this algorithm in 3616 patients with possible PE using several D-dimer assays (VIDAS, Tinaquant, STA-LIA, Innovance) and following patients for 3 months. At 3 months, the conservative estimate of incidence of symptomatic VTE was 0.78% (95% CI 0.49–1.2), assuming all five patients lost to follow-up had VTE.[17] A multicenter evaluation of the YEARS algorithm in 1789 ED patients in the United States found that this algorithm would have resulted in missed PEs in 0.5% of cases (95% CI 0.18–1.1), and using this algorithm would have resulted in 14% fewer imaging studies.[18]

The PEGeD study combined a D-dimer (adjusted for clinical probability) with the Wells score. In this prospective study of 2017 patients undergoing evaluation for PE, the D-dimer threshold for patients who had a Wells score ≤4 (*PE Unlikely*) was set at <1000 µg/L.[19] However, in patients who had an intermediate probability of PE (4.5–6), the D-dimer threshold remained the traditional <500 µg/L. At 90 days, the incidence of VTE was 0% (95% CI 0–0.29). However, 9 of the 1285 patients with a Wells score ≤4 and a D-dimer <1000 µg/L were lost to follow up. A conservative estimate assuming all nine patients had VTE would result in a 90-day VTE incidence of 0.7% (95% CI 0.32–1.33). The PEGeD algorithm resulted in 17.6% fewer imaging studies compared with the traditional Wells score and D-dimer thresholds. This algorithm has not been validated to date.

Clinical question

Can computed tomography (CT) of the chest be used as a diagnostic endpoint in patients at high risk for PE?

Early generation CT scanners initially showed poor sensitivity (70%) for demonstrating PE on chest CT.[20] However, in a prospective study of 756 patients who were referred to the ED with a suspicion of PE (prevalence of 26%), 524 patients with either a high clinical probability or low-or-intermediate probability and a positive D-dimer (ELISA) had both lower

extremity ultrasound and chest CT. At 3-month follow-up, the overall risk of
deep vein thrombosis (DVT) and PE was estimated at 1.5% (95% CI 0.8–
3.0%) if the D-dimer and CTPA had been the only tests to rule out PE.[21] In a
study of 3306 patients that included mostly outpatients with suspected PE,
patients with a Wells score >4 had a CTPA. Patients with elevated D-dimers
underwent CTPA.[22] The 3-month DVT and PE risk in patients who were not
treated on the basis of a negative chest CT was 1.1% (CI 0.6–1.9%). This was
independent of the pretest probability for PE. Van der Hulle *et al.* conducted
a patient-level meta-analysis using data from four prospective studies using
Wells criteria, D-dimer, and CTPA, with an overall prevalence of 24%. At
3 months, the incidence of VTE in those in whom PE was excluded was 1.2%
(95% CI 0.48–2.6%) and the risk of fatal PE was 0.11% (95% CI 0.02–0.70).
However, in the subgroup of patients with a Wells score >6, the 3-month
incidence of VTE was 6.3% (95% CI 3.0–12%).[4,23,24] It is important to note
that the prevalence of PE was much higher in these studies compared with
those conducted solely in the United States (24% versus 4–11%). Additionally,
higher resolution CT scanners (≥64 row) are commonly used and available
in the United States. Thus, the ability of a CTPA to exclude PE in patients
with a high probability of PE and a negative CTPA depends on the local prevalence of PE and type of scanner used.

Clinical question

Which, if any, risk stratification tools can be used in pregnancy to exclude PE?
Pregnancy and the postpartum period carry an elevated risk of VTE. Yet historically, the evaluation of pregnant patients for PE has been complicated due
to the lack of risk stratification tools that include pregnant patients. For
example, Wells did not include pregnant patients and while the PERC derivation cohort included some pregnant patients, pregnancy has been identified
as one of the more common instances in which PERC misses PEs.[25]
Additionally, the D-dimer is known to increase throughout pregnancy, limiting the utility of traditional cut-offs.[26,27] Recently, however, pregnancy-
adapted versions of the Revised Geneva score and YEARS algorithm have
been examined in pregnant patients.

Righini *et al.* evaluated an algorithm comprising the Revised Geneva
score, leg ultrasound, CTPA and/or V/Q scan, and D-dimer in 367 pregnant
patients. None of the 367 patients in whom PE was excluded had symptomatic VTE during the 3-month follow-up period, and PE was excluded in
11.6% of patients without imaging – all of whom would presumably have
received imaging otherwise.[28] The Artemis study evaluated the use of the
YEARS algorithm and leg ultrasound in 498 pregnant patients with suspected

PE.[29] In this cohort, only one patient in whom PE was excluded was diagnosed with DVT at 3-month follow-up and no patients were diagnosed with PE during this period. The YEARS algorithm was more efficient than the combination of the Revised Geneva score, ultrasound, and the standard D-dimer threshold, and imaging was avoided in 65% of patients enrolled in the first trimester, 46% in the second trimester, and 32% in the third trimester. Langlois et al.[29] retrospectively evaluated the YEARS algorithm in the Righini et al. cohort and found that it was safe and would have resulted in fewer imaging studies than the pregnancy-adapted Revised Geneva score. It is important to note, however, that the overall prevalence of PE in these cohorts was approximately 6% and the tools may perform differently in higher prevalence populations. Goodacre et al. retrospectively assessed the performance of both the Revised Geneva and the YEARS algorithm (without the leg ultrasound component) in 219 pregnant patients who were imaged for PE and found that the YEARS strategy would have missed 41.6% of PEs and the Revised Geneva score strategy would have missed 25% of PEs. However, most patients in this study received empiric anticoagulation, which may falsely lower the D-dimer.[30] This is likely indicative of a very different patient population, as empiric anticoagulation for presumptive PE is at odds with not satisfying the criteria "PE is the most likely diagnosis."

Comment

Over the past 20 years, the assessment of ED patients for possible PE has changed considerably. There is considerable information available on test characteristics of risk stratification tools, laboratory tests, and imaging studies, making the application of evidence-based medicine at the bedside a practicable reality. There is good evidence that a D-dimer can be used safely in patients who are at low to intermediate risk of PE and that in certain populations, such as older adults or those with low pretest probability of PE, a higher D-dimer threshold can be used. Further evidence demonstrates that multidetector CTPA is a safe way to evaluate patients for PE in higher-risk presentations.

Deciding which patients to not test for PE is challenging, because a high negative predictive value requires a very low-risk population. Patient selection for any diagnostic testing for PE is highly applicable in the ED because the choice of whether or not to consider a patient at any risk for PE occurs much more frequently than discriminating between intermediate- and high-risk patients. The PERC rule has performed well in validation studies, and it is useful in identifying patients at low risk of PE who need no further testing. The PERC rule should not be applied to a higher risk group, however, because it does not include all risk factors for VTE and the number of false negatives would be too high for safe use.

Finally, all reviewed studies appear to agree that when the criterion standard test (pulmonary angiogram) is not undertaken, or D-dimer is used for low-and intermediate-risk patients, there is always a small chance that a patient will be sent home with PE. Where we draw the line – that is, where we set our standard for risk tolerance with our patients – is very physician- and practice-specific. Emergency physicians should make sure to thoroughly explain the risks and benefits of diagnostic strategies to their patients and involve them in the decision-making process for this highly challenging disease.

References

1. Geersing G-J, Takada T, Klok FA *et al*. Ruling out pulmonary embolism across different healthcare settings: A systematic review and individual patient data meta-analysis. *PLoS Medicine*. 2022; 19(1): e1003905.
2. HCUPnet. *Healthcare cost and utilization project*. Rockville (MD): Agency for Healthcare Research and Quality; 2018.
3. Feng LB, Pines JM, Yusuf HR, Grosse SD. U.S. Trends in computed tomography use and diagnoses in emergency department visits by patients with symptoms suggestive of pulmonary embolism, 2001-2009. *Academic Emergency Medicine*. 2013; 20(10): 1033–40.
4. Venkatesh AK, Agha L, Abaluck J, Rothenberg C, Kabrhel C, Raja AS. Trends and variation in the utilization and diagnostic yield of chest imaging for medicare patients with suspected pulmonary embolism in the emergency department. *American Journal of Roentgenology*. 2018; 210(3): 572–7.
5. Kindermann DR, McCarthy ML, Ding R *et al*. Emergency department variation in utilization and diagnostic yield of advanced radiography in diagnosis of pulmonary embolus. *The Journal of Emergency Medicine*. 2014; 46(6): 791–9.
6. Kline JA, Mitchell AM, Kabrhel C, Richman PB, Courtney DM. Clinical criteria to prevent unnecessary diagnostic testing in emergency department patients with suspected pulmonary embolism. *Journal of Thrombosis and Haemostasis: JTH*. 2004; 2(8): 1247–55.
7. Kline JA, Courtney DM, Kabrhel C *et al*. Prospective multicenter evaluation of the pulmonary embolism rule-out criteria. *Journal of Thrombosis and Haemostasis: JTH*. 2008; 6(5): 772–80.
8. Freund Y, Cachanado M, Aubry A *et al*. Effect of the pulmonary embolism rule-out criteria on subsequent thromboembolic events among low-risk emergency department patients. *Journal of the American Medical Association*. 2018; 319(6): 559.
9. American College of Emergency Physicians Clinical Policies Subcommittee (Writing Committee) on Thromboembolic Disease, Wolf SJ, Hahn SA *et al*. Clinical policy: Critical issues in the evaluation and management of adult patients presenting to the emergency department with suspected acute venous thromboembolic disease. *Annals of Emergency Medicine*. 2018; 71(5): e59–109.

10. Wells P, Anderson D, Rodger M *et al*. Derivation of a simple clinical model to cate-gorize patients probability of pulmonary embolism: Increasing the models utility with the SimpliRED D-dimer. *Thrombosis and Haemostasis*. 2000; 83(03): 416–20.

11. Pines JM, Lessler AL, Ward MJ, Mark Courtney D. The mortality benefit threshold for patients with suspected pulmonary embolism. *Academic Emergency Medicine*. 2012; 19(9): E1109–13.

12. Lessler AL, Isserman JA, Agarwal R, Palevsky HI, Pines JM. Testing low-risk patients for suspected pulmonary embolism: A decision analysis. *Annals of Emergency Medicine*. 2010; 55(4): 316–26.e1.

13. Huisman MV. Effectiveness of managing suspected pulmonary embolism using an algorithm combining clinical probability, D-dimer testing, and computed tomography. *Journal of the American Medical Association*. 2006; 295(2): 172.

14. Warren D, Matthews S. Pulmonary embolism: Investigation of the clinically assessed intermediate risk subgroup. *British Journal of Radiology*. 2012; 85(1009): 37–43.

15. Douma RA, Le Gal G, Söhne M *et al*. Potential of an age adjusted D-dimer cut-off value to improve the exclusion of pulmonary embolism in older patients: A retrospective analysis of three large cohorts. *BMJ*. 2010; 340(7753): 962.

16. Righini M, Van Es J, Den Exter PL *et al*. Age-adjusted D-dimer cutoff levels to rule out pulmonary embolism: The ADJUST-PE study. *Journal of the American Medical Association*. 2014; 311(11): 1117–24.

17. van der Hulle T, Cheung WY, Kooij S *et al*. Simplified diagnostic management of suspected pulmonary embolism (the YEARS study): A prospective, multicentre, cohort study. *The Lancet*. 2017; 390(10091): 289–97.

18. Kabrhel C, Van Hylckama Vlieg A, Muzikanski A *et al*. Multicenter evaluation of the YEARS criteria in emergency department patients evaluated for pulmonary embolism. *Academic Emergency Medicine : Official Journal of the Society for Academic Emergency Medicine*. 2018; 25(9): 987–94.

19. Kearon C, de Wit K, Parpia S *et al*. Diagnosis of pulmonary embolism with D-dimer adjusted to clinical probability. *New England Journal of Medicine*. 2019; 381(22): 2125–34.

20. Yazdani M, Lau CT, Lempel JK *et al*. Historical evolution of imaging techniques for the evaluation of pulmonary embolism: RSNA centennial article. *Radiographics*. 2015; 35(4): 1245–62.

21. Perrier A, Roy P-M, Sanchez O *et al*. Multidetector-row computed tomography in suspected pulmonary embolism. *New England Journal of Medicine*. 2005; 352(17): 1760–8.

22. Van Belle A, Büller H, Huisman M, Huisman P, Kaasjaer K, Kamphuisen P. Effectiveness of managing suspected pulmonary embolism using an algorithm. *Journal of the American Medical Association*. 2006; 295(2): 172–9.

23. van der Hulle T, Douma R, Klok F *et al*. Is a normal computed tomography pulmonary angiography safe to rule out acute pulmonary embolism in patients with a likely clinical probability? *Thrombosis and Haemostasis*. 2017; 117(08): 1622–9.

24. Kline JA, Garrett JS, Sarmiento EJ, Strachan CC, Courtney DM. Over-testing for suspected pulmonary embolism in american emergency departments. *Circulation. Cardiovascular Quality and Outcomes.* 2020; 13(1): 1–10.
25. Kline JA, Slattery D, O'Neil BJ *et al.* Clinical features of patients with pulmonary embolism and a negative PERC rule result. *Annals of Emergency Medicine.* 2013; 61(1): 122–4.
26. Murphy N, Broadhurst D, Khashan A, Gilligan O, Kenny L, O'donoghue K. Gestation-specific D-dimer reference ranges: A cross-sectional study. *BJOG: An International Journal of Obstetrics and Gynaecology.* 2015; 122: 395–400.
27. Kline JA, Williams GW, Hernandez-Nino J. D-Dimer concentrations in normal pregnancy: New dignostic threshold are need. *Clinical Chemistry.* 2005; 51(5): 825–9.
28. Righini M, Robert-Ebadi H, Elias A *et al.* Diagnosis of pulmonary embolism during pregnancy. *Annals of Internal Medicine.* 2018; 169(11): 766–73.
29. Langlois E, Cusson-Dufour C, Moumneh T *et al.* Could the YEARS algorithm be used to exclude PE during pregnancy? Data from the CT - PE - pregnancy study. *Journal of Thrombosis and Haemostasis.* 2019; 17(8): 1329–34.
30. Goodacre S, Nelson-Piercy C, Hunt BJ, Fuller G. Accuracy of PE rule-out strategies in pregnancy: Secondary analysis of the DiPEP study prospective cohort. *Emergency Medicine Journal.* 2020; 37(7): 423–8.

Chapter 51 **Deep Vein Thrombosis**

Ali S. Raja[1] and Jesse M. Pines[2,3]

[1] Department of Emergency Medicine, Massachusetts General Hospital, Harvard Medical School, Boston, MA, USA
[2] US Acute Care Solutions, Canton, OH, USA
[3] Department of Emergency Medicine, Drexel University, Philadelphia, PA, USA

Highlights

- In evaluating patients with suspected DVT, two-point ultrasound (femoral vein at the groin + popliteal fossa) are similar to whole-leg ultrasound, which includes the calf, and serial ultrasound.
- Compared to radiologist-performed ultrasound, emergency physician-performed ultrasound is highly sensitive and specific; however, methodological concerns in studies may overestimate the sensitivity.
- The Wells criteria can guide clinicians about the likelihood of VTE.
- D-Dimer is highly sensitive in detecting DVT but poorly specific. D-Dimer sensitivity is similarly high in cancer patients, but even less specific than in undifferentiated populations. Diagnostic evaluation for DVT can involve risk assessment coupled with D-dimer testing for low-risk to very-low-risk patients.

Background

Deep-vein thrombosis (DVT) is a blood clot within the deep veins. It commonly occurs in the legs but can also form in the upper extremity, mesenteric, and cerebral veins. Similar to pulmonary embolism (PE), DVT is part of the venous thromboembolism (VTE) disorders.[1] Mortality from

---

Evidence-Based Emergency Care: Diagnostic Testing and Clinical Decision Rules, Third Edition.
Edited by Jesse M. Pines, Fernanda Bellolio, Christopher R. Carpenter, and Ali S. Raja.
© 2023 John Wiley & Sons Ltd. Published 2023 by John Wiley & Sons Ltd.

upper and lower extremity DVT occurs when a DVT breaks free and causes PE, which can lead to sudden cardiovascular collapse and other morbidity.

While a diagnosis of DVT is commonly considered in the ED when patients have leg swelling, calf pain, or other symptoms, they are often "silent" and are often diagnosed at autopsy. This makes the incidence of DVT difficult to estimate. The annual incidence of DVT has been estimated at 80 in 100,000 with a prevalence of leg DVT being significantly higher at 1 in 1000.[2,3] In the United States, greater than 200,000 people develop DVTs every year, with 1 in 4 cases also causing PE.[4]

Both DVT as well as PE are common and often "silent" and thus go undiagnosed or are only picked up at autopsy. Therefore, the incidence and prevalence are often underestimated. It is thought the annual incidence of DVT is 80 cases per 100,000, with a prevalence of lower limb DVT of 1 case per 1000 population. Annually in the United States, more than 200,000 people develop venous thrombosis; of those, 50,000 cases are complicated by PE. DVT is relatively rare in children and young adults; at the age of 40, the risk of DVT increases with age. Common conditions associated with DVT include cancer, heart failure, chronic obstructive pulmonary disease, and postsurgical patients.[5]

Accurate and timely identification of patients with DVT can minimize complications and morbidity. However, like PE, DVT is a relatively rare disease, which is often suspected but infrequently diagnosed. In the United States, approximately 1 in every 1000 ED visits results in the diagnosis of DVT.[6] As with PE, the challenge in diagnosing DVT in the ED is the appropriate selection of patients for diagnostic testing and risk stratification based on clinical findings.

Venous noncompressibility on ultrasound is the major diagnostic criterion for DVT. Compression ultrasound, however, is not specific or sensitive for detecting DVT in patients with asymptomatic proximal DVT or in patients with DVT in the calf.[7] It also demonstrates limited accuracy in cases of chronic DVT. The use of ultrasound is further limited in patients who are obese or who have edema.[8,9] However, despite these limitations, leg compression ultrasound is often used to detect DVT in the ED. Traditionally, only the proximal veins (from the femoral veins down to the calf, where they join the popliteal veins) are studied. While approximately 50% of DVTs begin in the calf,[10] more than 70% of symptomatic DVTs involve the popliteal vein and more proximal leg veins.[11] In patients with calf DVTs that may not be detected on the first ED ultrasound, about 20% will extend more proximally within about a week. As DVTs that do not extend above the calf very rarely cause PE, proximal DVTs are at much higher risk for propagation and for causing PE.

Clinical question

How sensitive is ultrasound for the detection of DVT?

A recent systematic review and meta-analysis by Bhatt *et al.* reviewed the accuracy of several diagnostic tests for the diagnosis of DVT. A total of 43 studies met inclusion criteria and were reviewed by the authors, and included analyses of proximal compression ultrasound (Figure 51.1), whole leg ultrasound and serial ultrasound (defined as a diagnostic strategy involving a repeat ultrasound for patients with initial negative ultrasound).[12] Either venography or clinical follow-up were acceptable as reference standards, and studies of both inpatients and outpatients were included.

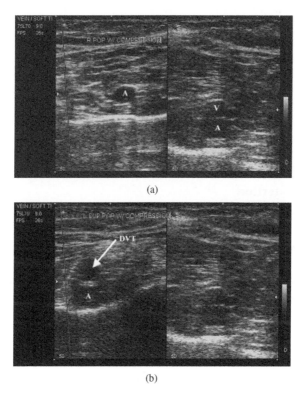

(a)

(b)

Figure 51.1 Compression ultrasound of the right and left popliteal vessels. (a) The screen is split to show the noncompressed normal anatomy on the right-hand side and the compressed anatomy of the left-hand side. (b) The left popliteal vein is noncompressible and represents a deep vein thrombosis. Note: A = artery; and V = vein. (Courtesy of Anthony J. Dean, MD.)

Proximal compression ultrasound, which is the test most commonly used in the ED, typically involves evaluation of the trifurcation of the popliteal vein and more proximal veins. It was evaluated in 13 studies that included a total of 4036 patients. Overall, it had a pooled sensitivity of 90.1% (CI 86.5–92.8%) and a specificity of 98.5% (CI 97.6–99.1%) for the diagnosis of DVT.[12]

In contrast to proximal compression ultrasound, whole-leg ultrasound evaluates the entire length of the leg veins, including the calf. There were fewer studies that included data on whole-leg ultrasound; a total of 10 studies included 1725 patients. The pooled sensitivity for whole-leg ultrasound was 94.0% (CI 91.3–95.9%), with a pooled specificity of 97.3% (CI 94.8–98.6%).

Finally, serial ultrasound had, predictably, the best test characteristics of the ultrasound strategies. Six studies, with 2415 patients, evaluated serial ultrasound, with a pooled sensitivity of 97.9% (CI 96.0–98.9) and specificity of 99.8 (CI 99.3–99.9).

Another systematic review examined emergency physician-performed ultrasound to rule out DVT compared to radiologist-performed US.[13] A total of four studies were included, and there were some methodologic flaws noted. Nevertheless, there was a pooled sensitivity of 95% (95 CI 87–99%), and a specificity of 96% (95% CI 87–99%). The authors concluded that emergency physician-performed US was shown to be accurate; however, they also noted that, given the variation in the studies, the estimates may be overly optimistic.[13]

Clinical question

What are the Wells criteria for pretest probability of DVT?
In addition to the Wells criteria for PE discussed in Chapter 50, Wells *et al.*[14–16] also derived and validated a similar rule for DVT (Table 51.1). In the validation study, all patients had ultrasonography and venography. In 529 patients, the Wells criteria for DVT predicted the prevalence of DVT in high-risk (85%), medium-risk (33%), and low-risk (5%) cases.[14]

Clinical question

What are the test characteristics of D-dimer testing in the diagnosis of DVT?
The test characteristics of a negative D-dimer to exclude DVT are dependent on the type of assay. Assays are either high sensitivity or moderate sensitivity. As the sensitivity of the assay drops, so too does the ability to use a negative test to rule out DVT. While there are many commercially available D-dimer assays, there are two specific methods that have been studied extensively: enzyme-linked immunosorbent assay (ELISA) and whole-blood assays.

Table 51.1 The Wells criteria for deep vein thrombosis (DVT)

Clinical feature	Score
Active cancer (current treatment or within 6 months or palliative)	1
Paralysis, paresis, or recent immobilization	1
Recently bedridden for > than 3 days or major surgery, within 4 weeks	1
Localized calf tenderness	1
Entire leg swollen	1
Calf swelling >3 cm compared with the asymptomatic leg (10 cm below tibial tuberosity)	1
Pitting edema in the symptomatic leg	1
Collateral superficial veins (nonvaricose)	1
Alternative diagnosis as likely as, or greater than, that of DVT	−2

Note: High risk: ≥3 points; moderate risk: 1–2 points; and low risk: ≤0 points.
Source: Data from [5].

Among the different assays, there is wide variation in the sensitivity, normal reference ranges, and cutoff points. A meta-analysis of different D-dimer assays reported a sensitivity of ≥95% for ELISA and certain immuno-turbidimetric tests but also reported a low specificity (≥40%) at a cutoff of ≥500 ng/dL to exclude DVT.[17] Other D-dimer assays such as whole-blood and quantitative latex agglutination assays are less sensitive with a reported rate of about 85% but more specific at about 65%.[17]

The recent systematic review and meta-analysis by Bhatt et al.[12] also reviewed the test characteristics of D-dimer for the diagnosis of DVT, with 16 studies that included 5253 patients. The D-dimer studies used ultrasound, venography, or clinical follow-up as their reference standards. The pooled sensitivity of D-dimer for DVT was 96.1% (CI 92.6–98.0%) and the pooled specificity was 35.7% (CI 29.5–42.4%).

An earlier systematic review by Wells et al.[18] examined 14 studies on 8000 patients examining this question. In the low-, medium-, and high-risk groups using the Wells criteria, the prevalence of DVT was 5%, 17%, and 53%, respectively. In pooled analysis, the sensitivity and specificity of D-dimer in the low-probability group were 88% (CI 81–92%) and 72% (CI 65–78%), in the medium-probability group were 90% (CI 80–95%) and 58% (CI 49–67%), and in the high-probability group were 92% (CI 85–96%) and 45% (CI 37–52%). Likelihood ratios are calculated in Table 51.2.

Another recent systematic review assessed the sensitivity of D-dimer to detect DVT in cancer patients.[19] This is important because patients with malignancy are at higher risk for VTE. For DVT, D-dimer was 94% (CI 90–98%) sensitive, and 46% (40–53%) specific.

Table 51.2 Test characteristics for D-dimer testing in Wells-stratified patients

	Pretest probability		
Specific measure	Low	Moderate	High
LR+	3.14	2.14	1.67
LR−	0.17	0.17	0.18
Negative predictive value	99%	96%	84%
Positive predictive value	17%	32%	66%

Source: Data from [18].

Clinical question

What is the difference in outcomes for patients who received a whole-leg ultrasound (including the calf) compared to a proximal-leg ultrasound with D-dimer to rule out DVT?

A randomized trial was conducted across 14 Italian universities or community hospitals to answer this question surrounding whole-leg ultrasound, which permits the detection of calf vein thrombosis but typically requires more skilled operators.[20] Patients were included who had their first episode of suspected DVT in the lower extremities, and they were randomized to undergo either two-point ultrasound (where the ultrasound is applied to the common femoral vein at the groin and the popliteal vein at the popliteal fossa) along with a D-dimer test, versus whole-leg ultrasound. In the two-point ultrasound group, patients with a normal ultrasound but a positive D-dimer were scheduled for a follow-up ultrasound at 1 week. The major study outcome was the 3-month incidence of symptomatic VTE in patients with an initially normal evaluation. A total of 2098 patients were randomized (whole-leg ultrasound: 1053; and two-point ultrasound: 1045). Symptomatic VTE was detected in seven out of 801 patients in the two-point ultrasound group versus nine out of 763 patients in the whole-leg ultrasound group. This met the equivalence criterion with an observed difference of 0.3% (CI −1.4% to 0.8%). The authors concluded that the two diagnostic strategies were equivalent in managing patients with suspected DVT.

Comment

Over the past 20 years, the assessment of ED patients for possible DVT has changed considerably.[21] Given the substantial quality and quantity of research available on the accuracy and reliability of decision aids, laboratory tests, and imaging studies, DVT evaluation is a prime example of the applicability of evidence-based practice.

The American College of Physicians and American Academy of Family Physicians summarized the evidence in their Clinical Practice Guideline on the diagnosis of DVT (and PE) in 2007 and these recommendations have not been updated since then[22]. The diagnosis can be ruled out in a low- and moderate-risk patients (as defined by Wells) with a negative D-dimer, obviating the need for ultrasound testing. A positive D-dimer should lead to ultrasound testing.

In contrast, all high-risk patients, particularly those with cancer, should also have an ultrasound test in order to rule out DVT (a negative D-dimer cannot rule out the disease in these patients). Additionally, in moderate- or high-risk patients who have a 2-point compression ultrasound (rather than a whole-leg ultrasound), a serial ultrasound exam in 1 week should be obtained, given the prevalence of DVT in these patients.

References

1. Goldhaber SZ. Risk factors for venous thromboembolism. *Journal of the American College of Cardiology.* 2010; 56(1): 1–7.
2. Hansen AT, Juul S, Knudsen UB, Hvas AM. Low risk of venous thromboembolism following early pregnancy loss in pregnancies conceived by IVF. *Human Reproduction.* 2018; 33(10): 1968–72.
3. Sharif S, Eventov M, Kearon C et al. Comparison of the age-adjusted and clinical probability-adjusted D-dimer to exclude pulmonary embolism in the ED. *The American Journal of Emergency Medicine.* 2019; 37(5): 845–50.
4. Delluc A, Mao RL, Tromeur C et al. Incidence of upper-extremity deep vein thrombosis in western France: A community-based study. *Haematologica.* 2019; 104(1): e29–31.
5. White RH. The epidemiology of venous thromboembolism. *Circulation.* 2003; 107(23_suppl_1): I–4.
6. Singer AJ, Thode HC, Peacock WF. Admission rates for emergency department patients with venous thromboembolism and estimation of the proportion of low risk pulmonary embolism patients: A US perspective. *Clinical and Experimental Emergency Medicine.* 2016; 3(3): 126–31.
7. Zhang Y, Xia H, Wang Y et al. The rate of missed diagnosis of lower-limb DVT by ultrasound amounts to 50% or so in patients without symptoms of DVT: A meta-analysis. *Medicine (Baltimore).* 2019; 98(37): e17103.
8. Saranteas T. Limitations in ultrasound imaging techniques in anesthesia: Obesity and muscle atrophy? *Anesthesia & Analgesia.* 2009; 109(3): 993–4.
9. Saranteas T, Karakitsos D, Alevizou A, Poularas J, Kostopanagiotou G, Karabinis A. Limitations and technical considerations of ultrasound-guided peripheral nerve blocks: Edema and subcutaneous air. *Regional Anesthesia and Pain Medicine.* 2008; 33(4): 353–6.
10. Robert-Ebadi H, Righini M. Management of distal deep vein thrombosis. *Thrombosis Research.* 2017; 149: 48–55.

11. Trinchero A, Scheres LJJ, Prochaska JH *et al.* Sex-specific differences in the distal versus proximal presenting location of acute deep vein thrombosis. *Thrombosis Research.* 2018; 172: 74–9.

12. Bhatt M, Braun C, Patel P *et al.* Diagnosis of deep vein thrombosis of the lower extremity: A systematic review and meta-analysis of test accuracy. *Blood Advances.* 2020; 4(7): 1250–64.

13. Burnside PR, Brown MD, Kline JA. Systematic review of emergency physician-performed ultrasonography for lower-extremity deep vein thrombosis. *Academic Emergency Medicine.* 2008; 15(6): 493–8.

14. Wells PS, Hirsh J, Anderson DR *et al.* Accuracy of clinical assessment of deep-vein thrombosis. *Lancet.* 1995; 345(8961): 1326–30.

15. Wells PS, Anderson DR, Bormanis J *et al.* Value of assessment of pretest probability of deep-vein thrombosis in clinical management. *The Lancet.* 1997; 350(9094): 1795–8.

16. Wells PS, Anderson DR, Rodger M *et al.* Evaluation of D-dimer in the diagnosis of suspected deep-vein thrombosis. *The New England Journal of Medicine.* 2003; 349(13): 1227–35.

17. Stein PD, Hull RD, Patel KC *et al.* D-dimer for the exclusion of acute venous thrombosis and pulmonary embolism: A systematic review. *Annals of Internal Medicine.* 2004; 140(8): 589–602.

18. Wells PS, Owen C, Doucette S, Fergusson D, Tran H. Does this patient have deep vein thrombosis? *Journal of the American Medical Association.* 2006; 295(2): 199–207.

19. De Wit K, Parpia S, Sunavsky A, Ilic A, Germini F, Carney BJ. Diagnostic accuracy of D-dimer for pulmonary embolism and lower limb deep vein thrombosis testing in people with cancer: A meta-analysis. *Blood.* 2021; 138: 3218.

20. Bernardi E, Camporese G, Büller HR *et al.* Serial 2-point ultrasonography plus D-dimer vs whole-leg color-coded Doppler ultrasonography for diagnosing suspected symptomatic deep vein thrombosis: A randomized controlled trial. *Journal of the American Medical Association.* 2008; 300(14): 1653–9.

21. Wells PS, Ihaddadene R, Reilly A, Forgie MA. Diagnosis of venous thromboembolism: 20 years of progress. *Annals of Internal Medicine.* 2018; 168(2): 131–40.

22. Qaseem A, Snow V, Barry P *et al.* Current diagnosis of venous thromboembolism in primary care: A clinical practice guideline from the American Academy of Family Physicians and the American College of Physicians. *Annals of Family Medicine.* 2007; 5(1): 57–62.

Chapter 52 **Temporal Arteritis**

Ali S. Raja[1] and Fernanda Bellolio[2]

[1] Department of Emergency Medicine, Massachusetts General Hospital, Harvard Medical School, Boston, MA, USA
[2] Department of Emergency Medicine, Mayo Clinic, Rochester, MN, USA

Highlights

- Temporal arteritis typically presents as an acute unilateral headache in older adults and can cause permanent visual impairment.
- Definitive diagnosis is achieved with temporal artery biopsies.
- Temporal artery ultrasound is emerging as a noninvasive alternative to diagnosing temporal arteritis.
- Jaw claudication alone (LR+ 4–6) or in combination with scalp tenderness and/or headache (LR+ 15–17) is predictive of temporal arteritis.
- An erythrocyte sedimentation rate (ESR) (LR– 0.2–0.03) is a good screening tool for temporal arteritis.

Background

Temporal arteritis, also known as *giant cell arteritis*, is an inflammatory condition characterized by focal, granulomatous changes of branches of the carotid artery that lead to vessel damage, stenosis, and eventual occlusion. Histopathologic findings from temporal artery biopsies include multinucleated giant cells, necrotic tissue, and lymphocytic infiltration of the inflamed vessel wall. The classic description of the clinical manifestations of temporal arteritis includes a new temporal headache that can wax and wane, jaw claudication (and even trismus-like symptoms), and visual symptoms (from floaters to transient monocular vision loss).

Evidence-Based Emergency Care: Diagnostic Testing and Clinical Decision Rules, Third Edition.
Edited by Jesse M. Pines, Fernanda Bellolio, Christopher R. Carpenter, and Ali S. Raja.
© 2023 John Wiley & Sons Ltd. Published 2023 by John Wiley & Sons Ltd.

Table 52.1 American College of Rheumatology (ACR) diagnostic criteria for temporal arteritis

- Age ≥ 50 years
- New onset of localized headache
- Temporal artery tenderness or decreased pulse
- Elevated erythrocyte sedimentation rate (ESR) (Westergren) ≥ 50 mm/hour
- Positive temporal artery biopsy

Source: Data from [2].

Temporal arteritis is a disease process of older adults and is reported as the most common systemic vasculitis in this age group, estimated to occur in approximately 23 per 100,000 women aged 50 years and older, and approximately one-third as many men. While the mortality associated with temporal arteritis is not different from that for those without the condition, its principal morbidity is the risk for permanent visual impairment, as greater than 20% of patients with temporal arteritis develop permanent visual loss.[1] The American College of Rheumatology (ACR) diagnostic criteria are listed in Table 52.1.[2] Patients with three of the five criteria are considered to have temporal arteritis; however, it is usually a heightened clinical suspicion that prompts a biopsy that leads to the diagnosis.

While treatments are available that markedly decrease the likelihood of developing permanent visual loss, it is sometimes difficult to determine which patients should receive a biopsy in order to make the diagnosis. Thus, research into the diagnosis of temporal arteritis has focused on the historical features, physical exam findings, and laboratory results that may help determine which patients should be treated and subsequently referred for temporal artery biopsy. Newer research has focused on the use of ultrasound as an additional diagnostic adjunct for the diagnosis of the disease.

Clinical question

Which factors in a patient's history, physical exam, and laboratory values are predictive of having temporal arteritis?

Two large studies have examined signs and symptoms associated with temporal arteritis.[3,4] Both studies included only patients who had undergone biopsies of the temporal artery, and thus both used biopsy as their criterion standard. The prevalence of temporal arteritis in patients sent for temporal artery biopsy in these studies ranged from 33% to 39%, but it should be noted that the prevalence of temporal arteritis in all patients older than 50 years has been estimated to be 1 in 500.[5] Neither study was able to assess the interobserver reliability of the clinical findings as they were typically taken from

Table 52.2 Clinical findings and laboratory findings in the diagnosis of temporal arteritis

Variable	Positive likelihood ratio (LR+)	Negative likelihood ratio (LR−)
Jaw claudication[3]	4.2 (2.8–6.2)	0.7 (0.6–0.8)
Diplopia[3]	3.4 (1.3–8.6)	0.95 (0.9–0.99)
Beading of temporal artery[3]	4.6 (1.1–18.4)	0.93 (0.88–0.99)
Prominent or enlarged temporal artery[3]	4.3 (2.1–8.9)	0.6 (0.5–0.9)
Elevated erythrocyte sedimentation rate (ESR)[*] [3]	1.1 (1–1.2)	0.2 (0.08–0.5)
Jaw claudication[4]	6.7 (4.9–9.1)	0.6 (0.5–0.7)
Scalp tenderness[4]	3 (2.3–3.9)	0.75 (0.7–0.81)
Jaw claudication + scalp tenderness[4]	17 (8–36)	0.84 (0.8–0.88)
Headache + jaw claudication + scalp tenderness[4]	15 (7–32)	0.86 (0.82–0.9)
Double vision[4]	3.5 (1.4–8.6)	0.97 (0.95–1)
Elevated ESR[**][4]	1.16 (1.11–1.21)	0.28 (0.17–0.45)
Elevated ESR[***][4]	1.19 (1.15–1.22)	0.03 (0–0.13)

[*] Among all patients (normal range not defined).
[**] Among all patients (normal range 0–22 mm/hour for men and 0–29 mm/hour for women).
[***] Among patients not taking steroids (normal range 0–22 mm/hour for men and 0–29 mm/hour for women).
Source: Data from [3,4] as shown in "Variable" column.

retrospective chart reviews. Table 52.2 shows the clinical variables from each study associated with the diagnosis of temporal arteritis.

Jaw claudication, diplopia, and temporal artery beading or prominence had moderate predictive power; however, when combinations of factors were considered that included jaw claudication, LR+s were highly accurate for predicting a positive temporal arteritis biopsy result. Notably, the combination of jaw claudication, a new headache, and scalp tenderness had a LR+ of 15 (confidence interval [CI] 7–32). Other symptoms commonly assessed that were positively associated with a diagnosis of temporal arteritis included headache of any type, anorexia, fever, weight loss, fatigue, myalgias, vertigo, or polymyalgia rheumatica; however, none of these symptoms individually had a likelihood ratio that was sufficiently greater than 1.0 to be considered useful.

Erythrocyte sedimentation rate (ESR) values were clinically useful when they were normal (LR− of 0.2–0.28). Among the subset of patients not on steroids at the time of ESR testing, a normal ESR made temporal arteritis

```
Score =      - 240
             + 48 (if headache present)
             + 108 (if jaw claudication present)
             + 56 (if scalp tenderness present)
             + 70 (if ischemic optic neuropathy present)
             + ESR (mm/h)
             + Age (years)
Risk assessment:
       Score < -110 = Low risk (probability < 10%)
       Score ≥ 70 = High risk (probability > 80%)
```

Figure 52.1 Temporal artery biopsy formula. (Data from [4].)

very unlikely. Nevertheless, there have been case reports of temporal arteritis despite normal ESR values prior to steroids,[6] so ESR alone should not be used to rule out the disease in patients with otherwise classic symptomatology. Notably, the exact cutoff for an "elevated ESR" was not defined in the meta-analysis by Smetana *et al.*[3] since several studies they pooled did not give exact values, but Younge *et al.*[4] used ESR cutoffs of 22 mm/hour for men and 29 mm/hour for women.

Based on their results given in this section, Younge *et al.*[4] developed a temporal arteritis biopsy formula (Figure 52.1) that estimates the probability of a patient referred for temporal artery biopsy having temporal arteritis. They used logistic regression to identify a model that predicted results of the temporal artery biopsy and then developed an equation with coefficients that maximized the receiver operator characteristic (ROC) of their model. While their formula was developed based on a referral population of patients older than 50 years, it is based on the largest series of temporal arteritis patients in the literature and is likely applicable to patients of similar age in the ED.

Clinical question

What are the diagnostic test characteristics of temporal artery ultrasound for the diagnosis of temporal arteritis?

Although considered generally a safe procedure, temporal artery biopsy has a complication rate of around 0.5%, including infection, hematoma formation, and rare injuries to branches of the facial nerve.[7] It is invasive, and patients often undergo bilateral biopsies of arterial sections several centimeters long. Therefore, ultrasound has been investigated as a way to avoid the need for biopsy. A 2005 meta-analysis examined a number of temporal artery ultrasound studies.[8] Patients were classified as having temporal arteritis from either biopsy confirmation or meeting the ACR criteria (Table 52.1).

Table 52.3 Temporal artery ultrasound findings for temporal arteritis

Variable	Number of patients	Positive likelihood ratio (LR+)	Negative likelihood ratio (LR–)
Any ultrasound abnormality (halo, sign, stenosis, or occlusion) versus biopsy [8]	332	4 (3.1–5.1)	0.15 (0.06–0.39)
Any ultrasound abnormality (halo, sign, stenosis, or occlusion) versus ACR criteria[8]	853	22 (15–31)	0.14 (0.08–0.23)
Halo sign alone versus ACR criteria[9]	525	7.6 (5.3–11)	0.35 (0.28–0.44)
Halo sign alone versus biopsy [10]	357	4.1 (3.2–6)	0.3 (0.22–0.41)

Source: Data from [8].

The study examined 2036 patients and found that any ultrasound-specific findings including a halo sign, stenosis, or occlusion of the temporal artery were highly predictive of temporal arteritis regardless of whether the ultimate diagnosis was confirmed using biopsy or the ACR criteria.

Two additional systematic reviews, both published in 2010, have also addressed ultrasound of the temporal arteries to diagnose temporal arteritis. The halo sign, when seen during temporal artery ultrasound, is described as a hypoechoic (dark) ring around the temporal artery wall representing edema and inflammation. Arida et al.[9] reviewed prospective studies with patients diagnosed with temporal arteritis using the ACR criteria and examined the diagnostic test characteristics of the halo sign. Ball et al.[10] reviewed studies of patients who had undergone temporal arteritis biopsies and reported on the diagnostic test parameters of the halo sign (Table 52.3). Overall, the halo sign had moderate predictive value to be clinically useful, whether compared to biopsy confirmation or the ACR criteria.

Comments

The diagnosis of temporal arteritis can be elusive and should be considered if a patient older than 50 years complains of any number of symptoms including headache, diplopia or visual loss, scalp tenderness, or jaw claudication. Clinicians should maintain a cautious level of concern given the long-term morbidity of permanent visual loss associated with temporal arteritis. Furthermore, temporal arteritis has segmental involvement in the arteries (skipping some areas), and false negatives can occur in temporal artery biopsy. Treatment considerations should be modified on the entirety of the clinicians' suspicion based on the timing of the symptoms and any competing alternative diagnoses.

It should be noted that the studies used to generate the associations noted in this chapter were retrospective in nature, and the reported associations represent findings from a highly selective group of patients: those who actually underwent temporal artery biopsy. This form of verification bias, when only those patients in whom there was a sufficiently high suspicion of the disease underwent the criterion standard procedure, needs to be considered when applying and interpreting the findings to unselected patients in an ED setting. Unfortunately, the low prevalence of temporal arteritis in the general population would require any prospective study examining predictive factors to enroll a prohibitive number of patients, many of whom would not ultimately undergo temporal artery biopsy.

While not highly specific, an elevated ESR is highly sensitive (especially in patients not taking steroids) and is associated with useful negative likelihood ratios for ruling out the disease. Therefore, as an inexpensive, widely available lab test, it is a reasonable test to obtain. Jaw claudication alone is moderately predictive of temporal arteritis but, when combined with a new headache and scalp tenderness, the combination of all three is appropriate for ruling in the disease and initiating treatment in the ED.

Ample prospective evidence indicates that temporal artery ultrasound may be a reasonable noninvasive alternative to artery biopsy for diagnosing temporal arteritis. However, technical competency will likely be limited to centers that perform high volumes of these specialized ultrasound studies, effectively minimizing its widespread usefulness.

References

1. Gonzalez-Gay MA, Martinez-Dubois C, Agudo M et al. Giant cell arteritis: Epidemiology, diagnosis, and management. *Current Rheumatology Reports.* 2010; 12(6): 436–42.
2. Hunder GG, Bloch DA, Michel BA et al. The American College of Rheumatology 1990 criteria for the classification of giant cell arteritis. *Arthritis and Rheumatism.* 1990; 33(8): 1122–8.
3. Smetana GW, Shmerling RH. Does this patient have temporal arteritis? *Journal of the American Medical Association.* 2002; 287(1): 92–101.
4. Younge BR, Cook BE Jr, Bartley GB, Hodge DO, Hunder GG. Initiation of glucocorticoid therapy: Before or after temporal artery biopsy? *Mayo Clinic Proceedings.* 2004; 79(4): 483–91.
5. Lawrence RC, Helmick CG, Arnett FC et al. Estimates of the prevalence of arthritis and selected musculoskeletal disorders in the United States. *Arthritis and Rheumatism.* 1998; 41(5): 778–99.

6. Ciccarelli M, Jeanmonod D, Jeanmonod R. Giant cell temporal arteritis with a normal erythrocyte sedimentation rate: Report of a case. *American Journal of Emergency Medicine.* 2009; 27(2): 255.e1–3.

7. Ikard RW. Clinical efficacy of temporal artery biopsy in Nashville, Tennessee. *Southern Medical Journal.* 1988; 81(10): 1222–4.

8. Karassa FB, Matsagas MI, Schmidt WA, Ioannidis JPA. Meta-analysis: Test performance of ultrasonography for giant-cell arteritis. *Annals of Internal Medicine.* 2005; 142(5): 359–69.

9. Arida A, Kyprianou M, Kanakis M, Sfikakis PP. The diagnostic value of ultrasonography-derived edema of the temporal artery wall in giant cell arteritis: A second meta-analysis. *BMC Musculoskeletal Disorders.* 2010; 11: 44.

10. Ball EL, Walsh SR, Tang TY, Gohil R, Clarke JMF. Role of ultrasonography in the diagnosis of temporal arteritis. *British Journal of Surgery.* 2010; 97(12): 1765–71.

Chapter 53 **Intraocular Pressure**

Ali S. Raja[1] and Jesse M. Pines[2,3]

[1] Department of Emergency Medicine, Massachusetts General Hospital, Harvard Medical School, Boston, MA, USA
[2] US Acute Care Solutions, Canton, OH, USA
[3] Department of Emergency Medicine, Drexel University, Philadelphia, PA, USA

Highlights

- Elevated intraocular pressure (IOP) is associated with glaucoma, the leading cause of blindness and visual impairment worldwide.
- The criterion standard for measuring IOP in most studies is Goldmann applanation tonometry; however, it is not typically available in the emergency department.
- Portable tonometers are good screening tools for the detection of elevated IOP, but they perform with variable accuracy.

Background

Glaucoma is a leading cause of blindness and visual impairment worldwide and occurs as a result of increased intraocular pressure (IOP), which is typically due to either acute narrowing of the anterior chamber angle (angle closure glaucoma) or progressively decreasing aqueous humor outflow and increasing aqueous humor production (open-angle glaucoma). Patients may seek acute care for symptoms related to elevated IOP that include not only eye pain but also visual impairment, nausea, vomiting, and headache. Measuring IOP is an essential component of the evaluation of patients suspected of having glaucoma (of both the acute closed-angle and open-angle types) as well as blunt eye trauma and iritis. Measurements above

---

Evidence-Based Emergency Care: Diagnostic Testing and Clinical Decision Rules, Third Edition.
Edited by Jesse M. Pines, Fernanda Bellolio, Christopher R. Carpenter, and Ali S. Raja.
© 2023 John Wiley & Sons Ltd. Published 2023 by John Wiley & Sons Ltd.

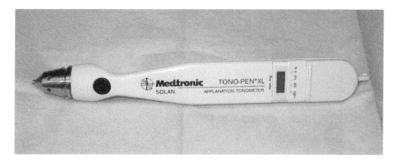

Figure 53.1 The Tono-Pen XL tonometer.

20–22 mmHg are abnormal and should prompt evaluation by an ophthalmologist, either in the acute care setting or through urgent referral.

Different methods of measuring IOP are available and are broadly divided into applanation, indentation, noncontact (air puff), rebound, and transpalpebral techniques. The Goldmann applanation tonometer is mounted on a slit lamp and consists of an applanation prism that comes into contact with the patient's fluorescein-stained cornea using a cobalt-blue light filter, creating lighted semicircles. Correct alignment of the semicircles is translated into a pressure reading. The Goldmann applanation method has been accepted as the criterion standard for most studies. The main limitation of the Goldmann tonometer technique is that accurate readings are not possible with cornea irregularities, scarring, or edema.

The most common indentation method uses the Tono-Pen (Figure 53.1). This is a handheld device that uses gentle manual indentations of the cornea (Figure 53.2) with the tip of the pen-like instrument to produce electronically averaged readings of IOP. The Tono-Pen is portable and utilizes a disposable rubber tip cover, making it ideal for the acute care setting and rapid sequential uses. The Schiotz tonometer is another common indentation tonometry method that uses a small weighted device to indent the cornea in the supine patient (Figure 53.3). The amount of indentation is measured against a calibrated weight, and the IOP is then determined. Noncontact methods that utilize puffs of air to flatten the cornea, and then measure the IOP by correlating it to the time to corneal flattening, are not typically used in the emergency department (ED). Rebound tonometers, such as the Icare Tonometer (Figure 53.4), bounce a small plastic-tipped metal probe on the cornea and calculate the IOP based on the induction current it creates upon its return through an induction coil. The Icare Tonometer has the advantage of not requiring topical anesthetic and has even been

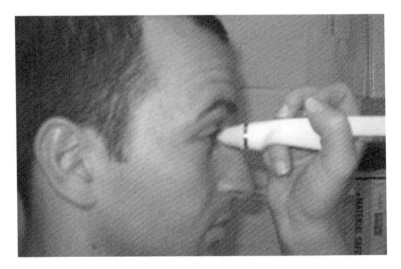

Figure 53.2 Use of the Tono-Pen XL to measure intraocular pressure.

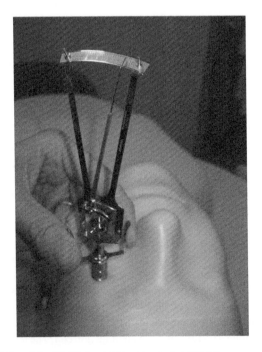

Figure 53.3 Use of the Schiotz tonometer on a supine patient.

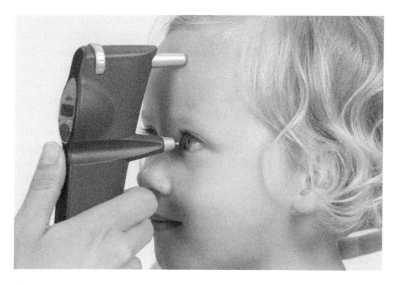

Figure 53.4 Use of the Icare tonometer. (Used with permission of Icare-USA.)

trialed as a device that patients can use at home to monitor IOP.[1] Finally, transpalpebral tonometry using the Diaton tonometer allows for IOP measurement through the upper eyelid, eliminating contact with the cornea completely.

While the Goldmann applanation method has been accepted as the criterion standard for most studies, most emergency physicians are not trained in its use. It is bulky, nonportable, expensive, and not widely available in acute care settings. Similarly, noncontact methods using puffs of air are cost prohibitive. These limitations make the search for suitable alternatives to measure IOP in the acute care setting desirable. While indentation devices (including the Schiotz and Tono-Pen) are currently available in most EDs, newer rebound and transpalpebral tonometers are being marketed and are also within the budgetary constraints of most EDs.

Clinical question

Are IOP measurements using the Schiotz tonometer, Tono-Pen, Icare Tonometer, or Diaton Tonometer reliable and accurate compared to IOP measurements using the criterion standard, Goldmann applanation tonometry?
Several small studies have compared IOP measurements using Goldmann tonometry against a Schiotz, the Tono-Pen, or both. Jackson *et al.*[2] in Australia performed and analyzed serial IOP measurements using the

Tono-Pen and the Schiotz in 72 patients. Patients were recruited from a general practice, were >50 years old, and had no prior history of glaucoma. IOP was first assessed using a Goldmann tonometer by an ophthalmologist, followed by measurement by the Schiotz and the Tono-Pen. An independent observer recorded the pressure reading, and the physicians were blinded to the results. A total of 19 patients (26%) were found to have elevated IOP ($\geq$21 mmHg), of which 18 followed up after the study for specialized eye care. Only five of these had persistently elevated IOPs. The Schiotz was the most reliable with 64–76% of IOP values falling to within ±4 mmHg of the criterion standard measured IOP. The Tono-Pen was extremely variable, with 10–95% of values falling within ±4 mmHg of the Goldmann tonometer. Most measurements using the Tono-Pen tended to underestimate the pressure. This study utilized three examining physicians, and there was measurement variation by physician with each method examined.

A small study out of Missouri examined IOP measurements with several portable tonometers, including the Tono-Pen and the Schiotz, with Goldmann tonometry as the criterion standard.[3] A total of 31 patients (58 eyes) from a glaucoma clinic were enrolled and analyzed in the study. Methods of obtaining IOP were standardized, and the orders of examinations were randomized following initial IOP measurements by Goldmann tonometry. Physicians were not blinded to the individual results from each method. Results are shown in Table 53.1. Both Tono-Pen and Schiotz tonometers underestimated IOP by 2–3 mmHg compared to the Goldmann tonometer.

In another small Australian study, researchers compared IOP measurements with the Tono-Pen and the Goldmann to determine if measurements were similar (to within 2 mmHg).[4] One hundred and thirty-eight patients were recruited from a glaucoma clinic; 22 more patients were enrolled who had known elevated IOPs. Among the 138 patients, IOPs ranged from 3 to 47. Reproducibility of the results was excellent, as reflected in an intraclass

Table 53.1 Results of IOP measurement (n = 58 eyes)

Tonometer	Mean intraocular pressure (mmHg)	95% CI range (mmHg)	Standard error	Mean difference from Goldmann (mmHg)
Goldmann	18.2	Data not shown	0.8	–
Tono-Pen	15.8	7.7	0.6	2.5*
Schiotz	15.3	9.7	0.8	2.9*

*$p<0.05$.
Source: Data from [3].

correlation coefficient (ICC) of 0.97 for the Goldmann tonometer and 0.95 with the Tono-Pen. Analysis of paired IOP readings revealed no statistical differences between methods (mean difference Tono-Pen – Goldmann: right eyes = −0.4 mmHg, confidence interval [CI] −6 to 5 mmHg; left eyes = −0.3 mmHg, CI −5 to 5 mmHg). Examination of three pressure ranges (0–10, 11–20, and 20–30) revealed divergence of agreement at the high pressures. Results of IOP measurements among the 22 patients with known elevated pressures (range 24–58) revealed a significant difference between methods (mean difference −4.2 mmHg, CI −13.0 to 5.0 mmHg), with the Tono-Pen consistently yielding lower values. These researchers concluded that while Tono-Pen measurements are reproducible, the accuracy at higher IOPs may be underestimated.

British researchers compared IOP measurements using both Goldman tonometry and the Tono-Pen in 105 patients from primary eye and glaucoma clinics with standardized methods across all clinics.[5] Mean IOP with the Tono-Pen was 0.6 mmHg lower than the Goldmann measurements, and these differences did not vary depending on ranges of pressures (Table 53.2).

Rebound tonometers, such as the Icare and IOPen (Figure 53.5) tonometers, have been garnering more interest given the fact that they can be used without topical anesthetic. In a study comparing the Icare, IOPen, and Goldman tonometers, Jorge et al.[6] studied the right eyes of 101 consecutive adult patients with good general and ocular health. The measurements for each device were taken by the same investigator for all patients to minimize variation, and the devices were used in random order. The mean (and standard deviation) of the Goldmann applanation tonometer was 15.7 mmHg (4.1), the IOPen was 12.8 mmHg (3.7), and the Icare was 16.0 mmHg (4.6). When compared to the Goldmann IOP measurements, the IOPen measurements were consistently (and significantly) lower, while the Icare measurements were not statistically different (Table 53.3).

Similar results were found by Pakrou et al.[7] who compared Icare and Goldmann tonometry in 292 eyes of 153 subjects. They found significant

Table 53.2 Comparisons of IOP measurements using Goldmann and Tono-Pen tonometry

Tonometer (n = 105)	Mean intraocular pressure (mmHg)	Range (mmHg)	Standard deviation	Mean difference from Goldmann (mmHg)
Goldmann	17.2	9–32	4.3	–
Tono-Pen	16.6	7–29	4.4	0.6*

*p = 0.3.
Source: Data from [5].

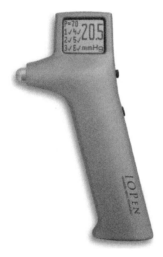

Figure 53.5 The IOPen tonometer. (Used with permission of Medicel AG.)

Table 53.3 Comparisons of IOP measurements using IOPen and Icare tonometers

Comparison (n = 101)	Mean difference (mmHg)	Standard deviation	p-value using Wilcoxon signed rank test
IOPen-Goldmann	−2.94	4.65	<0.001
Icare-Goldman	0.27	3.16	0.310

Note: IOP = intraocular pressure.
Source: Data from [6].

agreement between the two methods (intraclass correlation $r = 0.95$) with mean differences between the two devices of 0.4 mmHg in the right eyes and 0.8 mmHg in the left eyes. Despite the fact that no topical anesthesia was used for the Icare, 74% of patients rated it as more comfortable than the Goldmann applanation tonometer.

Transpalpebral tonometry is the newest noninvasive method for measuring IOP, and the Diaton tonometer is the first commercially available tonometer applying the technique (Figure 53.6). Li *et al.*[8] studied the accuracy of the Diaton tonometer when compared to the Goldmann tonometer in 129 patients. They found that the Diaton results correlated moderately with the Goldmann (criterion standard) results ($r = 0.78$) and were most closely correlated in patients between the ages of 20 and 50 years (mean difference 0.53 ± 3.4 mmHg). However, overall, only 76% of patients had less than

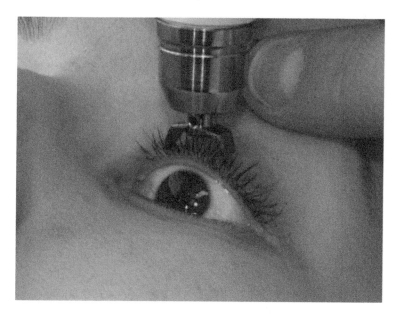

Figure 53.6 The Diaton transpalpebral tonometer. (Used with permission of BiCOM Inc.)

3 mmHg difference between the two readings, leading the investigators to conclude that the Diaton is not yet ready for use in routine clinical practice given the significant proportion of patients with wider variation in IOP as measured by both devices.

Comments

The clinical question of concern is whether portable, smaller, and more widely available instruments can be used to reliably and accurately measure IOP. These studies confirm that the reliability of the Tono-Pen is sound. That is, the results are reproducible across different users with acceptable minimal differences in the absolute pressure measurements. While the data are not overwhelmingly convincing with regard to the reliability of the Schiotz and Icare, it is our opinion that they are likely no worse than the Tono-Pen.

The issue of accuracy is a more technical concern and appears to vary across studies. One study presented measured agreement to within 4 mmHg of the criterion standard, while another study used a 2 mmHg difference as meaningful. Deciding on what constitutes a clinically significant difference from the criterion standard is always a concern. A 2 mmHg difference is seemingly negligible, but a 4 or 5 mmHg difference could significantly affect both the immediate and near-future treatment of a patient. While some early studies of the original Tono-Pen found variable pressure readings, more recent studies using the XL model indicate that measurements are reasonably accurate and do not differ significantly from the Goldmann tonometry measurements. Similar to the discussion of reliability, the accuracy of the Schiotz is not thought to differ greatly from that of the Tono-Pen. While there are fewer studies available for the newer Icare rebound tonometer, it appears to be at least as reliable as the Tono-Pen, while the newest device, the Diaton tonometer, is currently too inaccurate to use in clinical practice.

The Tono-Pen, the Schiotz, or the Icare can serve as screening tools for patients suspected of having abnormal IOPs. Patients should be treated according to the timing, severity, and history of their symptoms in conjunction with the measured IOP values. However, the diagnosis of ocular hypertension or glaucoma should not be excluded solely based on the IOP readings obtained in the ED. An emergent ophthalmology consult should be obtained when there is both sufficient concern by the treating physician and elevated IOP measurements. Borderline or normal IOP measurements should be referred for urgent eye evaluation by a specialist.

References

1. Asrani S, Chatterjee A, Wallace DK, Santiago-Turla C, Stinnett S. Evaluation of the ICare rebound tonometer as a home intraocular pressure monitoring device. *Journal of Glaucoma*. 2011; 20(2): 74–9.
2. Jackson C, Bullock J, Pitt M et al. Screening for glaucoma in a Brisbane general practice: The role of tonometry. *Australian and New Zealand Journal of Ophthalmology*. 1995; 23(3): 173–8.
3. Wingert TA, Bassi CJ, McAlister WH, Galanis JC. Clinical evaluation of five portable tonometers. *Journal of the American Optometric Association*. 1995; 66(11): 670–4.
4. Horowitz GS, Byles J, Lee J, D'Este C. Comparison of the Tono-Pen and Goldmann tonometer for measuring intraocular pressure in patients with glaucoma. *Clinical and Experimental Ophthalmology*. 2004; 32(6): 584–9.
5. Tonnu P-A, Ho T, Sharma K et al. A comparison of four methods of tonometry: Method agreement and interobserver variability. *British Journal of Ophthalmology*. 2005; 89(7): 847–50.
6. Jorge J, Fernandes P, Queirós A et al. Comparison of the IOPen and iCare rebound tonometers with the Goldmann tonometer in a normal population. *Ophthalmic and Physiological Optics*. 2010; 30(1): 108–12.

7. Pakrou N, Gray T, Mills R, Landers J, Craig J. Clinical comparison of the Icare tonometer and Goldmann applanation tonometry. *Journal of Glaucoma.* 2008; 17(1): 43–7.

8. Li Y, Shi J, Duan X, Fan F. Transpalpebral measurement of intraocular pressure using the Diaton tonometer versus standard Goldmann applanation tonometry. *Graefe's Archive for Clinical and Experimental Ophthalmology.* 2010; 248: 1765–70.

Chapter 54 **Asthma**

Jesse M. Pines[1,2] and Fernanda Bellolio[3]

[1] US Acute Care Solutions, Canton, OH, USA
[2] Department of Emergency Medicine, Drexel University, Philadelphia, PA, USA
[3] Department of Emergency Medicine, Mayo Clinic, Rochester, MN, USA

Highlights

- Asthma is common and responsible for many ED visits and hospitalizations every year.
- Hospitalization rates are high for all asthmatics, and relapse following ED visits is frequent among both adults (~15%) and children (~10%).
- Assessment of global function and specific clinical factors are reliable between different providers caring for asthmatics in the ED.
- Numerous asthma scoring systems have been developed, but few have been rigorously validated and replicated.
- The Pediatric Assessment Severity Score (PASS) and the Pediatric Respiratory Assessment Measure (PRAM) both distinguish between patients requiring admission and those stable for discharge, but their practical application has not been demonstrated.
- No uniform set of variables reliably predicts the need for hospitalization or the risk of treatment relapse in adult asthmatics.

Background

Asthma is a chronic disease affecting over 16 million adults and 5 million children in the United States alone, with nearly 20% requiring hospitalization annually. Worldwide estimates place the number of asthmatics at over 300 million.[1] In a recent report from the Centers for Disease Control and Prevention, it was estimated that from 2011 to 2016, among 161 million

---

Evidence-Based Emergency Care: Diagnostic Testing and Clinical Decision Rules, Third Edition.
Edited by Jesse M. Pines, Fernanda Bellolio, Christopher R. Carpenter, and Ali S. Raja.

working adults in the United States, 7% had asthma. Among asthmatic, 45% experienced an asthma attack, and 10% had an asthma-related emergency department (ED) visit in the prior year.[2] Asthma prevalence is highest among workers employed in the health care and social assistance industry (8.8%) and in health care support occupations (8.8%). Efforts to improve outpatient care for asthma have been promoted through the development of treatment guidelines, but many patients remain either undertreated or undiagnosed. Data from 2016 to 2018 demonstrated there were more than 1.6 million ED visits in the United States per year. The rate of ED visits per 10,000 population is considerably higher among children (88) than adults (42).[3] It is also higher among women (50) than men (31). Rates of ED visits in asthma decrease with increasing age. In addition, blacks have significantly higher rates of visits for asthma (164), as compared to Hispanics (60) and whites (31).

While standard ED asthma management is straightforward (including bronchodilators, steroids, and occasionally adjunctive treatments including magnesium), a certain percentage of refractory asthmatics will require hospitalization and monitoring.[4] Since this decision is often the crux of the ED evaluation of a patient with asthma, studies have sought to classify asthma severity and predict which patients will require hospitalization and which, if discharged, will relapse.

Clinical question

Are there scoring systems for ED patients that accurately and reliably predict asthma severity, the need for hospitalization, or relapses after treatment?
Distinct pediatric and adult acute asthma short-term outcome predictors and severity assessment scores exist. Therefore, this section presents pediatric and adult instruments separately.

Reproducibility of the clinical exam

In 2003, Stevens *et al.*[5] examined the interrater reliability of physical exam findings in children with asthma to address the concern that findings from clinical trials may not represent actual clinical practice because specially trained staff are usually involved in the research setting. Reproducibility of key physical findings and an overall global gestalt about the severity of a patient's condition by different people across different levels of training is the first step in establishing that any scoring system can be successfully developed and used clinically. The observers in this study included pediatric emergency physicians ($n = 20$), pediatric ED nurses ($n = 50$), and hospital respiratory therapists (n = 50). The observers received no prior specialized training on physical exam assessment for the study. Patients aged 1–16 years from a large urban children's hospital presenting with acute asthma were the examination subjects. Observers independently and simultaneously rated the following aspects on a standardized form on a scale of one to three or four: work of breathing, wheezing, decreased air entry, increased expiratory time, breathlessness, mental status, and respiratory rate. A global assessment of "overall" severity (options included asymptomatic, mild, moderate, and severe) was also presented, as was a composite total score.

Weighted kappa statistics for each component of the score (used to determine interrater reliability) for 230 pairs of exams ranged from 0.61 to 0.74, while the overall severity (weighted kappa 0.80) and total scores (weighted kappa 0.82) had excellent agreement. Paired observers who were practitioners of the same profession (physicians, nurses, or respiratory therapists) had slightly better interrater reliability for the elements assessed. The authors felt this supported the use of structured and standardized formats to assess pediatric asthmatic patients. More reassuring was that, among a diverse group of care providers, a high level of agreement was found in the clinical assessment of acute asthmatics.

Severity scores in asthmatic children

Numerous pediatric asthma scores have been developed to assess asthma, including discriminative scores (designed to gauge severity at a single point in time), predictive scores (aimed at predicting particular outcomes), and evaluative scores (allowing documentation of changes over time). Many of the early scoring systems were developed using small numbers of select subjects, impacting the generalizability of the results. Of the 16 pediatric asthma scores as of 1994, 11 had sample sizes of <100 study subjects, and only one had >300 study subjects.[6] More concerning and critical is that most were not (and have not been) thoroughly evaluated; none have been validated or assessed in terms of their impact on clinical behavior.[7]

In 2004, Gorelick et al.[8] published a pediatric asthma score, the Pediatric Assessment Severity Score (PASS), that was developed and vigorously validated on a large diverse pediatric asthma population, with no exclusions based on severity or disposition (home or admission). The PASS was validated and tested for reliability and responsiveness on a group of 1221 pediatric asthmatics in two EDs with an enrollment rate of 89% (out of 1379 eligible patients). Forty-one percent (n = 503) were admitted to an inpatient service. Clinical items examined during the study for inclusion in the final score had been included in prior clinical asthma scores and were acceptable to and pertinent by the clinicians at the study sites. The final three-item score included an assessment of wheezing (none or mild, moderate, or severe or absent due to poor air exchange), work of breathing (none or mild, moderate, or severe), and prolongation of expiration (normal or mildly prolonged, moderately prolonged, or severely prolonged). Items assessed but not included in the final score included air entry, tachypnea, and mental status.

The three-item PASS score discriminated admitted versus discharged patients with a high level of confidence: area under the curve (AUC) for the receiver operator characteristic (ROC) curves for each of the two EDs was 0.83 (confidence interval [CI] 0.80–0.86) and 0.85 (CI 0.81–0.89). The new score also was responsive to changes (e.g., improvements) on serial assessment; scores improved by 51–79% among those discharged home, whereas in those asthmatics admitted for inpatient care the scores improved only 25–32%. By comparison, the peak expiratory flow rate (PEFR) also improved by 25–32%, but the change was similar between admitted and discharged patients.

In 2008, Ducharme et al.[9,10] assessed whether their previously published Preschool Respiratory Assessment Measure (which had been developed and internally validated in children aged 3–6 years) could be expanded as the *Pediatric* Respiratory Assessment Measure (PRAM). They examined the validity, responsiveness, and reliability of PRAM in children from 2 to 17 years old, and found that it had predictive validity in that higher values of PRAM were associated with higher rates of admission, both at triage and after initial bronchodilation. PRAM was also responsive to change, as demonstrated by a Guyatt responsiveness coefficient of 0.7 (used to detect the ability of an evaluative instrument to detect change over time; 0.5 and 0.8 are considered moderate to large effect sizes, respectively), which was calculated by determining the ratio of the change in PRAM after initial bronchodilation among discharged patients to the standard deviation of the change in PRAM of the patients who were admitted. Last, the overall score was found to have high interrater reliability when assessed by a physician and a nurse ($\kappa = 0.78$) for 254 children aged 2–17 years. PRAM, which contains more components than PASS, measures scalene muscle contraction, suprasternal retractions, wheezing, air entry, and oxygen saturation (SpO2).

When Gouin et al.[11] performed a prospective external validation of both PRAM and PASS on 283 patients in 2010, they found that both scores had good initial discriminative ability. The scores were measured at triage and again after 90 minutes. Their initial performance as predictors of a length of stay of greater than 6 hours and/or admission was equal (PRAM AUC = 0.69 [CI 0.59–0.79] and PASS AUC = 0.70 [CI 0.60–0.80]) but, at 90 minutes, PRAM improved (AUC = 0.82 [CI 0.73–0.90]) while PASS remained steady

(AUC = 0.72 [CI 0.62–0.82]). Nevertheless, given that this is the only external comparison of both scores, PASS remains a valid prognostic screening instrument.

Predicting hospitalization in asthmatic children

A large prospective multicenter study by the Multicenter Airway Research Collaboration (MARC) investigators examined risk factors and predictors of hospital admission among children aged 2–17 years seen in 44 EDs from 1997 to 1998.[12] Enrolling sites were from 37 general hospitals and 7 children's hospitals across 18 US states and four Canadian provinces. Prospective enrollment occurred 24 hours per day over a median of 2 weeks. Repeat ED visits and patients discharged from the ED against medical advice were excluded.

A total of 1601 eligible children presenting to EDs with acute asthma were identified, and 1178 patients were included in the analysis (74%). The admission rate was 23% (CI 21–26%) with an interquartile range of 11–31% across the 44 EDs. Multivariate logistic regression modeling produced patient variables that were independently predictive of hospital admission (Table 54.1). PEFR was not included in the logistic regression model because it could be measured in only 23% of children. However, in those 23% with PEFR measurements, admitted children had lower initial PEFRs compared to nonadmitted children (percentage predicted 36% versus 50%, mean difference: 14%). Demographic factors were not predictive of admission.

The MARC investigators also examined the initial room air oxygen saturation reading to determine if, as a single variable, it could predict hospital admission in asthmatic children.[13] The study differed from prior studies in

Table 54.1 Independent predictors of hospital admission in children with asthma from multivariate logistic regression

	Odds ratio	Confidence interval (CI)
Oxygen saturation (per decrease of 5%)	2.2	1.6–3.0
Number of inhaled beta-agonist during ED stay	2.1	1.8–2.4
Prior admission for asthma within past year	1.7	1.1–2.8
Pulmonary index score	1.3	1.1–1.4
Not taking corticosteroids at the time of emergency department visit	0.3	0.2–0.6
No comorbidities	0.3	0.1–0.7

Source: Data from [12].

both the number of enrolled patients and the multicenter study design, strengthening its generalizability. Initial oxygen saturation was documented for 1040 children with a mean reading of 95%, and the ROC curve predicting hospitalization in the study cohort had an AUC value of 0.76, demonstrating only moderate discriminatory ability, from which we can conclude that initial oxygen saturation is not useful as a single predictor variable for admission.

In 2015, Arnold et al.[14] developed and internally validated a novel decision tool for asthma admission in children, called the asthma prediction rule (APR) in children aged 5-17. Using data from 2008 to 2013, the authors modeled admission for more than 24 hours as the primary outcome. The decision to admit by the treating team was a secondary outcome. There were 15 demographic characteristics, asthma chronic control measures, and pulmonary examination findings at triage and before treatment used as predictors. In 928 children, several factors were associated with a higher risk for both outcomes. For need for hospitalization, older age (adjusted odds ratio [aOR] 1.5 [CI 1.0–2.2]), female gender (aOR 1.4 [CI 1.0–2.1]), SpO2 (change from 98% to 94%) aOR 2.8 (CI 2.1–3.6), need for albuterol > 2/week 1.3 (CI 0.9–1.9), and Inspiratory to Expiratory ratio (≤1:3 versus 1:1) aOR 4.4 (CI 2.3–8.6), were included in the final rule. To date, the APR has not undergone external validation.

Treatment relapses in asthmatic children

Another large prospective multicenter study by the MARC investigators examined risk factors and predictors of treatment relapses among children aged 2-17 years seen in 44 EDs.[15] Enrolling sites included 37 general hospitals and seven children's hospitals. Only patients discharged from the ED were included. Again, prospective enrollment and data collection occurred 24 hours per day over a median of 2 weeks. Telephone follow-up was 2 weeks after patient discharge to establish relapses. *Relapse* was defined as any urgent visit to an ED for asthma that was unscheduled in the 2 weeks following initial ED discharge.

A total of 1184 patients were enrolled with 303 excluded because they were hospitalized or had severe comorbid conditions. A total of 762 of the remaining 881 (86%) patients had complete follow-up and were included in the analysis. Relapse occurred in 10% (CI 8–13%) of children. There was no difference in relapse rates between general and children's hospitals (12% versus 10%). The four factors independently associated with relapse after multivariate analysis are shown in Table 54.2. The number of ED visits and cigarette smoke exposure variables were no longer significant in a separate analysis

Table 54.2 Independent predictors of treatment relapse in children with asthma from multivariate logistic regression

	Odds ratio	Confidence interval (CI)
Asthma medication other than beta-agonists, steroids, cromolyn, or nedocromil	3.7	2.2–6.3
Age (for every 5-year increase)	1.4	1.0–1.8
Asthma-related emergency department visits in past year (per five visits)	1.2	1.0–1.5
Cigarette smoke exposure	0.5	0.3–0.9

Source: Data from [15].

looking only at relapses occurring within 3 days after ED discharge. There were no differences between relapse and no-relapse patients during the initial ED visit with regard to symptom duration, treatment duration, treatment medications, or steroid prescription for home use.

Predicting hospitalization in asthmatics (children and adults)

Australian researchers asked whether a determination of asthma severity after 1 hour of treatment in the ED is a better predictor of need for admission compared to the initial assessment of asthma severity at ED presentation.[16] This observational cohort analyzed 720 patients presenting to 36 Australian EDs during a 2-week period in 2001. Initial, 1-hour, and postdisposition severity assessments were evaluated. Clinical assessments of adult and pediatric patients followed the National Asthma Guidelines endorsed by the Australian National Asthma Campaign. Assessment had ratings of mild, moderate, and severe or life-threatening (with response meanings for each category) and included the following items: altered consciousness, physical exhaustion, talkativeness, pulsus paradoxus, central cyanosis, wheezing intensity, peak expiratory flow (PEF), forced expiratory volume (FEV_1) (percentage predicted), pulse oximetry on presentation, and need for admission.

Adults comprised 44% of the study cohort, and overall 32% of adult patients required hospital admission. Among patients assessed as having mild asthma either at initial presentation or after 1 hour, over 80% were discharged home. Similarly, over 85% classified as severe at either assessment were admitted. A moderate rating at initial presentation was a poor predictor of need for hospitalization. However, a moderate rating at the 1-hour assessment predicted 84% of individuals who needed admission. The authors concluded that response to therapies after 1 hour for patients presenting to EDs for acute asthma is better than initial severity assessments for predicting hospital admissions.

Predicting hospitalization in asthmatic adults

Investigators used data collected from four prospective cohorts recruited from 64 US and Canadian EDs with 2-week telephone follow-ups in another MARC study that examined patient characteristics associated with hospitalization for acute asthma.[17] The admission rate among the 1805 patients enrolled with complete data was 20% (CI 18–22%). Table 54.3 lists variables that are independently associated with hospitalization. The multivariate model had an AUC value of 0.91, indicating excellent discrimination; however, no external validation of this model has been performed.

Researchers in 88 EDs across the US and Canada collected data during a median 2 weeks from 1999 to 2002 as part of the MARC research alliance to study acute asthma. In an analysis of older versus younger adults presenting with acute asthma, the investigators sought to examine differences in asthma severity, treatments, and outcomes.[18] Ages were divided into three groups: 18–34, 35–54, and ≥55 years old. Patients reporting a history of chronic obstructive pulmonary disease (chronic bronchitis or emphysema) or who had a smoking history of >10 pack-years were excluded. Patient follow-ups were made by telephone interview 2 weeks after the ED visit.

The study enrolled 2064 patients (84% of those eligible), of whom 56% were in the youngest age category and 6% were in the oldest age category.

Table 54.3 Independent predictors of hospitalization in adults with asthma from multivariate logistic regression

	Odds ratio	Confidence interval (CI)
Use of home nebulizers*	2.7	1.6–4.5
Final peak flow (per decrease of 10% predicted)	2.6	2.2–3.1
Female sex	2.1	1.3–3.6
Asthma medications other than beta-agonists or inhaled corticosteroids*	1.9	1.2–3.0
Beta-agonist treatment in the emergency department	1.4	1.3–1.6
Initial peak flow (per increase of 10% predicted)	1.4	1.2–1.7
Initial respiratory rate (per five breaths)	1.3	1.1–1.7

* During the past 4 weeks.
Source: Data from [17].

Table 54.4 Independent predictors of hospitalization in adult asthmatics from multivariate logistic regression

	Odds ratio (CI) of need for hospitalization		
	Age 18–35*	Age 35–54	Age ≥55
Model** excluding peak expiratory flow (PEF) change	1.0	1.2 (0.8–1.7)	2.0 (1.2–3.4)
Model** including PEF change	1.0	1.2 (0.8–2.0)	0.9 (0.4–2.1)

*Reference category.
**Model included variables shown in Table 54.3.
Source: Data from [19].

Overall 348 patients (17%) required hospital admission. Significantly higher admission rates occurred with increasing age categories (13% in the youngest age group, 19% in the middle, and 38% in the oldest). Seriousness of the acute asthma condition at the time of ED presentation based on initial PEF (percentage predicted) was severe for all groups (median 47%). Multivariate modeling revealed that patients aged ≥55 responded the poorest to bronchodilator treatments after controlling for demographic and severity factors. In a logistic regression model that excluded change in PEF, increasing age was an independent predictor of hospital admission. However, age did not predict admission when change in PEF was included in the model (Table 54.4).

Two-week follow-up was available for 64% of all patients. Patients aged ≥55 were hospitalized longer (median stay 2, 3, and 4 days for each progressively older age group) and were more likely to have relapses in the 2 weeks following the initial ED visit (12%, 19%, and 25% for each progressively older age group).

Most recently, Tsai et al.[20] used data from the National Emergency Department Safety Study (NEDSS) and MARC to derive and validate a classification tree designed to risk-stratify patients into groups based on likelihood of admission. They used the NEDSS dataset, which included 1825 patients aged 14–54 years from 63 US EDs for whom eight variables were collected: demographics (age and sex), chronic asthma-related factors (ever hospitalized for asthma), and ED presentation and severity (duration of symptoms, initial oxygen saturation on room air, initial respiratory rate, initial PEF severity, and change in PEF severity). Using recursive partitioning, the authors derived a decision tree based on four clinical variables: change (C) in PEF severity category, any prior hospitalization (H) for asthma, oxygen (O) saturation on room air, and initial PEF (P). This tree was then validated in a cohort of 1335 MARC patients aged 18–54 from 36 EDs across the United States.

The resultant decision tree categorized patients with asthma into seven risk groups based on the four variables noted in this section. Among the seven groups, there was a significant increase in admission risk, from 9% to 48% ($p < 0.001$), between the lowest risk group and the highest risk group, and the tree had satisfactory discriminatory ability, with an AUC of 0.72 in the derivation cohort and 0.65 in the validation cohort. While both these AUCs as well as the fact that no acceptable risk threshold for discharge of asthmatics exists (given the lack of a consensus definition of acceptable risk in this population) currently preclude application of these authors' tree, the methodology used is sound and its application to large datasets of asthmatics is likely to lead to more useful risk stratification tools in the future.

Treatment relapses in asthmatic adults

Using the MARC investigator data collected between 1996 and 1997, Emerman et al.[19] examined factors associated with relapses among adult asthmatics following treatment for acute asthma among 641 patients. A total of 17% reported relapse during the 2 weeks following the initial ED visit. Initial, final, and change in PEFR were not different between patients who did and did not relapse. Multivariate logistic regression modeling found that duration of symptoms lasting from 1 to 7 days (odds ratio [OR] 2.5, CI 1.2–5.2), use of home nebulizers (OR 2.2, CI 1.5–3.9), multiple urgent care visits for asthma (OR 1.4, CI 1.5–3.9), and multiple ED visits for asthma (OR 1.3, CI 1.5–1.5) were all independent predictors associated with relapse after controlling for age, sex, race, primary care provider status, and number of reported asthma triggers.

A systematic review on factors associated with relapse within 4 weeks after and ED visit including 32,923 patients, found an incidence of relapse of 17%. Factors associated with relapse were female gender, prior inhaled steroid use, past healthcare use, and prior intubation. Most relapses occurred within the first week after ED visit, with median relapse rates of 8%, 14%, and 17% at 1, 2, and 4 weeks respectively.[21]

Comments

Asthma is a highly prevalent disease that is responsible for many ED visits and hospitalizations. A number of asthma scoring systems have been developed, primarily for children however, few have been vigorously derived and validated, and none have gained widespread acceptance. While the clinical assessment of acute asthma severity is reproducible, no particular scoring system is more accurate than any other. The PASS and PRAM scores appear to meet the basic criteria for a successful scoring tool: (i) sound derivation and validation on a broad group of unselected study subjects, (ii) using a limited number of clinically relevant items, and (iii) shown to be discriminative and responsive. However, there is not yet a similar tool for use in adult patients, which begs the question: is a separate tool necessary?

Studies have examined sets of predictors of particular outcomes: discharge, hospitalization, and treatment relapse. In children, no set of demographic variables reliably predicts hospital admission. Historical and clinical factors found to be predictive of hospitalization include low initial oxygen saturation, extent of beta-agonist use in the ED (i.e., total number of nebulizer treatments given), prior admissions for asthma in the prior year, and the absence of comorbidities or steroid use at the time of ED visit. Assessment of the need for hospitalization after 1 hour of treatment in the ED appears to be a better predictor of hospitalization compared with the initial assessment because some patients will improve rapidly. For patients treated and discharged, treatment relapse remains high ($\geq 10\%$ in children) and increases with use of asthma medication other than routine medications, as well as annual number of asthma-related ED visits. Among adult asthmatics, several variables appear to predict hospitalization, but none are consistent across studies. Similarly, relapse after treatment in adult asthmatics ($>16\%$ in adults) is associated with duration of symptoms, self-treatment at home, and extent of prior urgent care and ED visits related to asthma.

Overall, no uniform set of predictor variables reliably inform the need for hospitalization or risk of treatment relapse. Some variables such as prior admissions, extent of pharmacologic treatment prior to the ED visit, and evaluation after a period of treatment in the ED are intuitive elements that should influence decisions to admit or discharge a patient. The largest and most diverse collection of studies examining acute asthmatics, from the MARC investigators, as well as the promising development of the PASS, add breadth and depth to the discussion, yet further studies are certainly warranted. Perhaps sets of factors within subgroups of adult asthmatics can be identified that will be predictive as well as responsive indicators for clinical use, much in the same way that pediatric scores have developed separately from adult predictors. Finally, improvements in therapy will necessitate refinements in any prediction tool. We should continue to base patient disposition on the clinical assessment after a short period of intense treatment in the ED. However, additional elements warrant consideration, including issues surrounding access to care, access to appropriate medications, health literacy, and environmental factors, few of which have been incorporated into the clinical studies performed to date.

References

1. Masoli M, Fabian D, Holt S, Beasley R. The global burden of asthma: Executive summary of the GINA Dissemination Committee report. *Allergy.* 2004; 59(5): 469–78.
2. Mazurek JM, Syamlal G. Prevalence of asthma, asthma attacks, and emergency department visits for asthma among working adults - National Health Interview Survey, 2011-2016. *MMWR. Morbidity and Mortality Weekly Report.* 2018; 67(13): 377–86.
3. National Center for Environmental Health. Asthma Emergency Department (ED) Visits 2010–2018. https://www.cdc.gov/asthma/asthma_stats/asthma-ed-visits_2010-2018.html. 2021. Accessed October 22, 2022.
4. Pitts SR, Niska RW, Xu J, Burt CW. National Hospital Ambulatory Medical Care Survey: 2006 emergency department summary. *National Health Statistics Reports.* 2008; 7: 1–38.
5. Stevens MW, Gorelick MH, Schultz T. Interrater agreement in the clinical evaluation of acute pediatric asthma. *Journal of Asthma.* 2003; 40(3): 311–5.
6. van der Windt DA, Nagelkerke AF, Bouter LM, Dankert-Roelse JE, Veerman AJ. Clinical scores for acute asthma in pre-school children: A review of the literature. *Journal of Clinical Epidemiology.* 1994; 47(6): 635–46.
7. McGinn TG, Guyatt GH, Wyer PC *et al.* Users' guides to the medical literature. *Journal of the American Medical Association.* 2000; 284(1): 79–84.
8. Gorelick MH, Stevens MW, Schultz TR, Scribano PV. Performance of a novel clinical score, the Pediatric Asthma Severity Score (PASS), in the evaluation of acute asthma. *Academic Emergency Medicine.* 2004; 11(1): 10–8.
9. Chalut DS, Ducharme FM, Davis GM. The Preschool Respiratory Assessment Measure (PRAM): A responsive index of acute asthma severity. *Journal of Pediatrics.* 2000; 137(6): 762–8.
10. Ducharme FM, Chalut D, Plotnick L *et al.* The Pediatric Respiratory Assessment Measure: A valid clinical score for assessing acute asthma severity from toddlers to teenagers. *Journal of Pediatrics.* 2008; 152(4): 476–80, 480.e1.
11. Gouin S, Robidas I, Gravel J *et al.* Prospective evaluation of two clinical scores for acute asthma in children 18 months to 7 years of age. *Academic Emergency Medicine.* 2010; 17(6): 598–603.
12. Pollack CV, Pollack ES, Baren JM *et al.* A prospective multicenter study of patient factors associated with hospital admission from the emergency department among children with acute asthma. *Archives of Pediatrics and Adolescent Medicine.* 2002; 156(9): 934–40.
13. Keahey L, Bulloch B, Becker AB *et al.* Initial oxygen saturation as a predictor of admission in children presenting to the emergency department with acute asthma. *Annals of Emergency Medicine.* 2002; 40(3): 300–7.

14. Arnold DH, Gebretsadik T, Moons KG, Harrell FE, Hartert TV. Development and internal validation of a pediatric acute asthma prediction rule for hospitalization. *The Journal of Allergy and Clinical Immunology. In Practice.* 2015; 3(2): 228–35.

15. Emerman CL, Cydulka RK, Crain EF *et al.* Prospective multicenter study of relapse after treatment for acute asthma among children presenting to the emergency department. *Journal of Pediatrics.* 2001; 138(3): 318–24.

16. Kelly A-M, Kerr D, Powell C. Is severity assessment after one hour of treatment better for predicting the need for admission in acute asthma? *Respiratory Medicine.* 2004; 98(8): 777–81.

17. Weber EJ, Silverman RA, Callaham ML *et al.* A prospective multicenter study of factors associated with hospital admission among adults with acute asthma. *American Journal of Medicine.* 2002; 113(5): 371–8.

18. Banerji A, Clark S, Afilalo M *et al.* Prospective multicenter study of acute asthma in younger versus older adults presenting to the emergency department. *Journal of American Geriatrics Society.* 2006; 54(1): 48–55.

19. Emerman CL, Woodruff PG, Cydulka RK *et al.* Prospective multicenter study of relapse following treatment for acute asthma among adults presenting to the emergency department. MARC investigators, Multicenter Asthma Research Collaboration. *Chest.* 1999; 115(4): 919–27.

20. Tsai C-L, Clark S, Camargo CA Jr. Risk stratification for hospitalization in acute asthma: The CHOP classification tree. *American Journal of Emergency Medicine.* 2010; 28(7): 803–8.

21. Hill J, Arrotta N, Villa-Roel C, Dennett L, Rowe BH. Factors associated with relapse in adult patients discharged from the emergency department following acute asthma: A systematic review. *BMJ Open Respiratory Research.* 2017; 4(1): e000169.

Chapter 55 **Acute Low Back Pain**

Jesse M. Pines[1,2] and Ali S. Raja[3]

[1] US Acute Care Solutions, Canton, OH, USA
[2] Department of Emergency Medicine, Drexel University, Philadelphia, PA, USA
[3] Department of Emergency Medicine, Massachusetts General Hospital, Harvard Medical School, Boston, MA

Highlights

- Back pain is the leading musculoskeletal complaint in emergency department patients but is usually self-limited.
- To rule out serious causes of low back pain, a detailed history and physical examination should be performed in the ED including a neurological examination.
- The initial diagnostic approach to acute back pain should assess the risk for serious systemic disease through the presence and absence of red flags to guide subsequent imaging decisions.
- Systemic diseases presenting with back pain include aortic aneurysm, cancer, spinal infections, compression fractures, and ankylosing spondylitis.
- In isolation, most elements of history and physical exam are insufficient to rule in or rule out systemic disease etiologies of back pain.

Background

The lifetime incidence of back pain is 90%, and low back pain accounted for 1.5 million emergency department (ED) visits in 2017.[1,2] Only a minority of back pain episodes, approximately 14%, last more than 2 weeks. Low back pain may originate from the lumbar spine, vertebral ligaments, annulus fibrosus, vertebral periosteum, facet joints, paravertebral musculature, blood vessels, or spinal nerve roots. Low back pain may also be a presenting

---

Evidence-Based Emergency Care: Diagnostic Testing and Clinical Decision Rules, Third Edition.
Edited by Jesse M. Pines, Fernanda Bellolio, Christopher R. Carpenter, and Ali S. Raja.
© 2023 John Wiley & Sons Ltd. Published 2023 by John Wiley & Sons Ltd.

Table 55.1 Differential diagnoses of acute back pain

Abdominal aortic aneurysm
Ankylosing spondylosis
Compression fracture
Discitis (or spinal osteomyelitis)
Epidural abscess
Herniated disc
Malignancy
Musculoskeletal inflammation
Occult trauma
Pancreatitis
Pyelonephritis
Reactive or psoriatic spondyloarthritis
Spinal stenosis

symptom for many systemic disease processes (Table 55.1). Clinicians should seek to answer three key questions in the evaluation of acute back pain:[3]
1. Is a serious systemic disease causing the pain?
2. Is there neurological compromise that might require surgical evaluation?
3. Do social or psychological situations exist that could amplify or prolong pain?

Systemic diseases can include vascular disease, cancer, spinal infections, compression fractures, and ankylosing spondylitis. A thorough history is superior to extensive ancillary diagnostic testing to identify these disease processes. For example, abdominal aortic aneurysm is typically found in patients who are older than 60 years, have atherosclerosis, and experience pain at rest.[4]

Cauda equina syndrome is often the result of a massive midline herniated disc, most commonly in the L4–5, L5–S1, or L3–4 disc space.[5] The recognition of cauda equina is most often delayed because the diagnosis was not considered.[6,7] Ankylosing spondylitis typically presents with symptom onset before age 40 years with gradual onset, night pain, morning stiffness, and improvement with exercise.[8] Epidural abscesses progress from back pain with fever to spinal irritation with Lasegue's, Kernig's, and Lhermitte's signs with neck stiffness and sometimes radiation to the arms or legs, to motor-sensory deficits and ultimately paralysis.[9] It is essential that clinicians recognize that the duration of each phase is highly variable and may be extremely short. Risk factors for epidural abscess include intravenous drug abuse, alcohol abuse, obesity, distal bacterial infections, trauma, and invasive procedures.[9–11] ED diagnostic delays in epidural abscesses have occurred in 83.6% of cases, but implementation of a guideline to systematically assess signs and symptoms, erythrocyte sedimentation rate (ESR) and C-reactive protein

(CRP), and then magnetic resonance imaging (MRI), reduced delays to 9.7%.[12] The prevalence of these systemic diseases has not been defined in ED populations. By contrast, in primary care patients with back pain, 4% will have a compression fracture, 3% spondylolisthesis, 0.7% spinal malignancy, 0.3% ankylosing spondylitis, and 0.01% spinal infections.[2]

In a large sample of insurance claims for ED patients with lower back pain aged 18–64 years, imaging was obtained in 34% of visits.[13] However, the study found that between 2011 and 2016, imaging decreased from 35% to 32%. Most patients underwent pain radiography, 3% underwent computed tomography (CT), and 0.8% received an MRI. An earlier study found that in the prior decade, in primary care settings, using MRI as the first-line imaging test for low back pain was not associated with improved functional status, but did result in more surgical interventions and higher costs of care.[14] Similarly, multiple randomized trials have failed to demonstrate any measurable benefit to immediate imaging in the absence of features suggesting serious problems.[15] A recent systematic review examined the impact of imaging (X-ray, CT, and MRI) on costs of care and absence from work.[16] The review found with moderate quality evidence that costs increased among patients receiving X-ray and moderate quality evidence that MRI and CT when performed for back pain increases healthcare utilization.

Emergency physicians are generally more conservative than primary care physicians in the radiographic evaluation of low back pain.[17] Clinical decision support systems have also reduced the inappropriate utilization of lumbar MRI.[18,19] Following back pain diagnostic guidelines reduces costs and improves outcomes, but clinicians rarely follow these recommendations.[20] Although no emergency medicine guidelines exist for the diagnostic evaluation of acute back pain, multiple specialty societies have published guidelines upon which an evidence-based approach can be formulated.[21] In general, the diagnosis being contemplated should guide the initial imaging choice and urgency. "Red flags" generally signal clinicians to expedite advanced imaging considerations, and 22 "red flags" have been identified in various guidelines (Table 55.2).[22] Guidelines for the imaging of suspected spine fractures sometimes diverge because multidetector CT is the method of choice for bony structures (i.e., spinal fracture or bony metastasis), but MRI is the investigation of choice for the spinal cord and ligaments (i.e., cauda equina syndrome or spinal cord infection).[22] The duration of back pain should also be included when deciding whether and when to image patients.

Two key considerations in contemplating test ordering are noteworthy. First, although guidelines are based upon evidence appraisal and expert consensus, they often ignore clinical realities such as malpractice risk and third-party payors' management recommendations.[23] Second, clinicians

Table 55.2 Red flags symptoms for high-risk diagnoses in the ED

Disease	Red flags
Cauda equina syndrome	Fecal incontinence
	Gait abnormality
	Limb weakness
	Saddle numbness
	Urinary retention
	Widespread neuro symptoms
Malignancy	Age > 50
	Cancer history
	Pain at multiple sites
	Pain at rest
	Refractory pain
	Unexplained weight loss
	Urinary retention
Spine fracture	Age ≥ 50 years
	Osteoporosis
	Steroid use
	Structural deformity
Spine infection	Fever
	Immunosuppression
	Intravenous drug abuse
	Systemic illness or toxicity

Source: Data from [21].

mistakenly assume that negative or positive diagnostic test results offer reassurance to anxious patients, while the evidence suggests the opposite.[24] In fact, ordering tests that are unlikely to yield diagnoses for which effective therapies exist (such as back pain) can independently increase the duration of symptoms.[25]

Clinical question

What is the diagnostic accuracy of history and physical exam to identify the various etiologies of acute nontraumatic back pain?

Ankylosing spondylitis patients are usually older than 40 years (Table 55.3). Reduced chest expansion (≤2.5 cm) has a positive likelihood ratio (LR) of 9. None of the other history-related risk factors have a useful positive or negative LR for ankylosing spondylitis.[26] The only clinically significant positive finding for cancer is a past history of cancer. However, the absence of findings does not significantly reduce the probability of malignancy as the etiology of the back pain.[27] Steroid use increases the risk of compression fractures, but

Table 55.3 Diagnostic accuracy of history for systemic disease etiology of back pain

Disease	Element of history	Positive likelihood ratio (LR+)	Negative likelihood ratio (LR−)
Ankylosing spondylitis	4 of 5 calin responses positive*	1.3	0.94
	Age at onset ≤40	1.1	0
	Pain is not relieved when supine	1.6	0.41
	Morning back stiffness	1.6	0.61
	Pain duration >3 months	1.5	0.54
	Reduced chest expansion**	9	0.92
Cancer	Age ≥50	2.7	0.32
	Cancer history	15.5	0.70
	Unexplained weight loss	2.5	0.90
	Failure to improve after 1 month of therapy	3.1	0.77
	No relief with bed rest	1.7	0.22
	Duration of pain >1 month	2.6	0.62
	Age ≥50 or history of cancer or unexplained weight loss or failure of conservative therapy	2.5	0
Compression fracture	Age ≥50 years	2.1	0.26
	Age ≥70 years	5.5	0.81
	Corticosteroid use	12	0.94
	Trauma	2	0.82
Herniated disc	Sciatica	7.9	0.06
Spinal stenosis	Age ≥50 years	3	0.14

*Calin questions were: (i) Onset of back discomfort before age 40 years? (ii) Did the problem begin slowly? (iii) Persistence for at least 3 months? (iv) Morning stiffness? (v) improved by exercise?
** Expansion ≤2.5 cm.
Source: Data from [2].

similar to cancer, the absence of these risk factors does not significantly reduce the posttest probability.[2] The presence of sciatica significantly increases the risk of a disc herniation and the absence reduces the risk significantly.[28,29] The only physical exam finding that increases the risk of a herniated disc is the single-leg sit-to-stand test. This is where the patient attempts to rise from a chair using only one leg. This test differentiates an L3–L4 herniation (if unable to perform) from an L5–S1 herniation and has excellent reliability (kappa = 0.85) (Table 55.4).[30] The ipsilateral straight-leg raise may decrease the probability of a lumbar disc herniation, but the

Table 55.4 Diagnostic accuracy of physical exam for herniation with radiculopathy

Physical exam finding	Positive likelihood ratio (LR+)	Negative likelihood ratio (LR–)
Ankle dorsiflexion weakness	1.2	0.93
Ankle plantar flexion weakness	1.2	0.99
Crossed straight-leg raise	1.6–5.8	0.59–0.90
Great-toe extensor weakness	1.7	0.71
Impaired ankle reflex	1.3	0.83
Ipsilateral straight-leg raise	0.99–2.0	0.04–0.54
Sit-to-stand test	26.0	0.35
Sensory loss	1.0	1.0

Source: Data from [2].

negative LR has a wide range across seven studies extending up to 0.54.[31] No other physical exam finding significantly decreases the probability of a disc herniation.[30-33] No high-quality diagnostic research was identified to describe the diagnostic accuracy of physical exam for spinal stenosis, cancer, compression fractures, or ankylosing spondylitis.[2,34]

Clinical question

What is the diagnostic accuracy of radiologic imaging for acute nontraumatic back pain?

One systematic review has formally assessed the diagnostic accuracy of common imaging modalities.[35] X-rays are useful in the evaluation of cancer and ankylosing spondylitis if positive. However, X-ray lacks the accuracy to reduce posttest probability of disease if negative in cancer, infections, or ankylosing spondylitis (Table 55.5). CT is useful in the evaluation of stenosis whether positive or negative. Yet CT has a wide range of LRs for diagnosing herniated discs. Over half of individuals without back pain have a herniated disc on MRI, and a wide range of likelihoods have been reported.[35] MRI is quite helpful if positive and particularly if negative in cancer and infection. A negative MRI will significantly reduce the posttest probability of stenosis. Radionuclide scanning (single-photon emission computed tomography [SPECT]) can significantly increase or decrease the probability of diagnosing cancer. Nuclear medicine is less useful than MRI for infections and is not useful for ankylosing spondylitis.

Table 55.5 Diagnostic accuracy of imaging for back pain

Imaging choice	Disease	Positive likelihood ratio (LR+)	Negative likelihood ratio (LR−)
X-ray	Cancer	12–120	0.40–0.42
	Infection	1.9	0.32
	Ankylosing spondylitis	*	0.55–0.74
Computed	Herniated disc	2.1–6.9	0.11–0.54
tomography	Stenosis	4.5–22	0.10–0.12
Magnetic resonance	Cancer	8.3–31	0.07–0.19
imaging	Infection	12	0.04
	Herniated disc	1.1–33	0–0.93
	Stenosis	3.2	0.10–0.14
Nuclear medicine	Cancer (SPECT)	9.7	0.14
	Infection	4.1	0.13
	Ankylosing spondylitis	*	0.74

*No value for LR+ has been identified in the existing literature.
Source: Data from [35].

Comment

Back pain is the most common musculoskeletal complaint in ED visits in the United States. Even though back pain has a self-limited natural history in over 90% of patients, clinicians must consider more serious etiologies for each case within the context of the patient's age, comorbid illnesses, psychosocial stressors, potentially occult mechanisms of injury, neurological findings, and symptom duration. To properly exclude serious causes of acute low back pain in the ED, a careful history and physical examination are required including identification of red flag symptoms, and a detailed neurological examination. In cases where red flag symptoms are present or concerning neurological findings, advanced ED imaging should be performed with CT or MRI depending on the diagnostic concern. Emergency medicine clinical decision aids for the more serious causes of back pain have yet to be developed and validated, so costly imaging procedures that delay ED throughput and are most often inconsequential to patient-centric outcomes must be carefully weighed against initial clinical concern and each test's diagnostic accuracy. Guideline-derived algorithms have been shown to increase the efficiency of back pain test ordering in primary care and emergency settings, and currently represent the best approach to reduce variability without compromising patient care.

References

1. National Hospital Ambulatory Medical Care Survey: 2017 Emergency Department Summary Tables. https://www.cdc.gov/nchs/data/nhamcs/web_tables/2017_ed_web_tables-508.pdf. Accessed February 24, 2021.
2. Deyo RA, Rainville J, Kent DL. What can the medical history and physical examination tell us about low back pain? In: Simel DL, Rennie D, editors. *The rational clinical examination: Evidence-based clinical diagnosis.* New York: McGraw-Hill; 2009: 75–86.
3. Deyo RA. Early diagnostic evaluation of low back pain. *Journal of General Internal Medicine.* 1986; 1(5): 328–38.
4. Lederle FA, Simel DL. The rational clinical examination: Does this patient have abdominal aortic aneurysm? *Journal of the American Medical Association.* 1999; 281(1): 77–82.
5. Shapiro S. Medical realities of cauda equina syndrome secondary to lumbar disc herniation. *Spine.* 2000; 25(3): 348–51.
6. Small SA, Perron AD, Brady WJ. Orthopedic pitfalls: Cauda equina syndrome. *American Journal of Emergency Medicine.* 2005; 23(2): 159–63.
7. Jalloh I, Mnihas P. Delays in the treatment of cauda equina syndrome due to its variable clinical features in patients presenting to the emergency department. *Emergency Medicine Journal.* 2007; 24(1): 33–4.
8. Chou R, Qaseem A, Snow V et al. Diagnosis and treatment of low back pain: A joint clinical practice guideline from the American College of Physicians and the American Pain Society. *Annals of Internal Medicine.* 2007; 147(7): 478–91.
9. Reihsaus E, Waldbaur H, Seeling W. Spinal epidural abscess: A meta-analysis of 915 patients. *Neurosurgical Review.* 2000; 23(4): 175–204.
10. Angsuwat M, Kavar B, Lowe AJ. Early detection of spinal sepsis. *Journal of Clinical Neuroscience.* 2009; 17(1): 59–63.
11. Tompkins M, Panuncialman I, Lucas P, Palumbo M. Spinal epidural abscess. *Journal of Emergency Medicine.* 2010; 39(3): 384–90.
12. Davis DP, Salazar A, Chan TC, Vilke GM. Prospective evaluation of a clinical decision guideline to diagnose spinal epidural abscess in patients who present to the emergency department with spine pain. *Journal of Neurosurgery. Spine.* 2011; 14(6): 765–70.
13. Pakpoor J, Raad M, Harris A et al. Use of imaging during emergency department visits for low back pain. *AJR. American Journal of Roentgenology.* 2020; 214(2): 395–9.
14. Jarvik JG, Hollingworth W, Martin B et al. Rapid magnetic resonance imaging vs radiographs for patients with low back pain: A randomized controlled trial. *Journal of the American Medical Association.* 2003; 289(21): 2810–8.
15. Chou R, Fu R, Carrino JA, Deyo RA. Imaging strategies for low-back pain: Systematic review and meta-analysis. *Lancet.* 2009; 373(9662): 463–72.
16. Lemmers GPG, van Lankveld W, Westert GP, van der Wees PJ, Staal JB. Imaging versus no imaging for low back pain: A systematic review, measuring costs, healthcare utilization and absence from work. *European Spine Journal.* 2019; 28(5): 937–50.

17. Webster BS, Courtney TK, Huang YH, Matz S, Christiani DC. Survey of acute low back pain management by specialty group and practice experience. *Journal of Occupational and Environmental Medicine.* 2006; 48(7): 723–32.

18. Gallagher EJ, Trotzky SW. Sustained effect of an intervention to limit ordering of emergency department lumbosacral spine films. *Journal of Emergency Medicine.* 1998; 16(3): 395–401.

19. Blackmore CC, Mecklenburg RS, Kaplan GS. Effectiveness of clinical decision support in controlling inappropriate imaging. *Journal of the American College of Radiology.* 2011; 8(1): 19–25.

20. Becker A, Leonhardt C, Kochen MM *et al.* Effects of two guideline implementation strategies on patient outcomes in primary care: A cluster randomized controlled trial. *Spine.* 2008; 33(5): 473–80.

21. Dagenais S, Tricco AC, Haldeman S. Synthesis of recommendations for the assessment and management of low back pain from recent clinical practice guidelines. *Spine Journal.* 2010; 10(6): 514–29.

22. Roudsari B, Jarvik JG. Lumber spine MRI for low back pain: Indications and yield. *American Journal of Roentgenology.* 2010; 195(3): 550–9.

23. Negrini S, Giovannoni S, Minozzi S *et al.* Diagnostic therapeutic flow-charts for low back pain patients: The Italian clinical guidelines. *Europa Medicophysica.* 2006; 42(2): 151–70.

24. van Ravesteijn H, van Dijk I, Darmon D *et al.* The reassuring value of diagnostic tests: A systematic review. *Patient Education and Counseling.* 2012; 86(1): 3–8.

25. Swedish Council on Technology Assessment in Health Care (SBU). *Back pain, neck pain: An evidence based review.* Report No. 145. Stockholm: Swedish Council on Technology Assessment in Health Care; 2000.

26. Gran JT. An epidemiological survey of the signs and symptoms of ankylosing spondylitis. *Clinical Rheumatology.* 1985; 4(2): 161–9.

27. Deyo RA, Diehl AK. Cancer as a cause of back pain: Frequency, clinical presentation, and diagnostic strategies. *Journal of General Internal Medicine.* 1988; 3(3): 230–8.

28. Deyo RA, Tsui-Wu YJ. Descriptive epidemiology of low-back pain and its related medical care in the United States. *Spine.* 1987; 12(3): 264–8.

29. Spangfort EV. The lumbar disc herniation: A computer-aided analysis of 2,504 operations. *Acta Orthopaedica Scandinavica.* 1972; 142: 1–95.

30. Rainville J, Jouve C, Finno M, Limke J. Comparison of four tests of quadriceps strength in L3 or L4 radiculopathies. *Spine.* 2003; 28(21): 2466–71.

31. van den Hoogen HMM, Koes BW, van Eijk JTM, Bouter LM. On the accuracy of history, physical examination, and erythrocyte sedimentation rate in diagnosing low back pain in general practice: A criteria-based review of the literature. *Spine.* 1995; 20(3): 318–27.

32. Jönsson B, Strömqvist B. Symptoms and signs in degeneration of the lumbar spine: A prospective, consecutive study of 300 operated patients. *The Journal of Bone and Joint Surgery. British Volume.* 1993; 75(3): 381–5.

33. Deville WLJM, van der Windt DAWM, Dzaferagic A, Bezemer PD, Bouter LM. The test of Lasègue: Systematic review of the accuracy in diagnosing herniated discs. *Spine*. 2000; 25(9): 1140–7.

34. Turner JA, Ersek M, Herron L, Deyo R. Surgery for lumbar spinal stenosis: Attempted meta-analysis of the literature. *Spine*. 1992; 17(1): 1–8.

35. Jarvik JG, Deyo RA. Diagnostic evaluation of low back pain with emphasis on imaging. *Annals of Internal Medicine*. 2002; 137(7): 586–97.

Chapter 56 **Intravascular Volume Status**

Ali S. Raja[1] and Christopher R. Carpenter[2]

[1] Department of Emergency Medicine, Massachusetts General Hospital, Harvard Medical School, Boston, MA, USA
[2] Department of Emergency Medicine, Washington University School of Medicine, St. Louis, MO, USA

Highlights

- Accurately assessing volume status in acutely ill ED patients is an important clinical skill and can impact outcomes.
- No studies have assessed the diagnostic accuracy of history for hypovolemia.
- The only useful finding on physical exam to rule in hypovolemia is an abnormal capillary refill, while the most helpful features to rule out hypovolemia are the absence of a dry mouth or tongue furrows.
- The rapid ultrasound for shock and hypotension (RUSH) exam can be used to rule in causes of shock.
- Bedside tests such as the passive leg raise and sonographic inferior vena cava diameter are being evaluated as readily available data to predict fluid responsiveness in critically ill patients.

Background

This chapter focuses on the assessment of volume status in adults because the literature on children is vast and not always applicable to older populations.[1] Volume management decisions are frequently encountered in the emergency department (ED) in patients with trauma or other bleeding states, hot weather, congestive heart failure, sepsis, gastrointestinal, and

---

Evidence-Based Emergency Care: Diagnostic Testing and Clinical Decision Rules, Third Edition.
Edited by Jesse M. Pines, Fernanda Bellolio, Christopher R. Carpenter, and Ali S. Raja.
© 2023 John Wiley & Sons Ltd. Published 2023 by John Wiley & Sons Ltd.

other conditions. The optimal fluid management strategy is not always clear and can carry increased morbidity and mortality with either over- or under-volume resuscitation of patients.[2,3] When encountering a hemodynamically unstable patient, it is not always obvious whether the volume issue is one of preload, afterload, cardiac contractility, or none of these. Consequently, only about one-half of hemodynamically unstable, critically ill patients respond to fluid boluses.[4]

The terminology for volume deficiency conditions can also be confusing. Whereas *volume depletion* refers to extracellular space sodium losses, *dehydration* is the loss of intracellular water that increases plasma sodium levels and osmolality.[5] Clinicians and investigators tend to lump these volume state descriptors together as evidenced by the accepted criterion standard of either an elevated serum urea nitrogen-to-creatinine ratio (which measures volume depletion) or an elevated serum sodium or osmolality (which measures dehydration). Hypernatremia occurs predominantly in geriatric adults with intravascular volume depletion and is associated with a 40% mortality rate. Hypernatremia-related deaths are associated with the type and rate of fluid administration as well as the duration of hypotension.[4,6] In this chapter, we will use the term *hypovolemia* to denote the constellation of dehydration and volume depletion.

Physical exam findings for dehydration or volume depletion include assessing postural vital signs (orthostatics), skin turgor, mucous membrane dryness, capillary refill, urine output, and neurological status. One caveat for orthostatic vital signs is that clinicians should wait at least 2 minutes before measuring supine vital signs, and 1 minute after standing before measuring upright vital signs. Sitting vital signs are far less accurate than standing ones. Also, counting the pulse for 30 seconds is more accurate than for 15 seconds.[7] Capillary refill time is assessed by gently pressing the fingernail of the patient's middle finger while it is positioned at the same level as the heart for 5 seconds before releasing and noting the time required for the nailbed's normal color to return (normally 3 seconds for adults and 4 seconds for the elderly). Skin turgor describes the skin's ability to return to its normal position after being pinched between the examiner's fingers and is a function of elastin-related recoil. No studies on normal recoil times have been identified, but skin turgor decreases (i.e., there is a greater time to return to normal skin position) with age as elastin levels are reduced.

Investigators have evaluated the diagnostic accuracy of postural vital signs following acute blood loss in healthy volunteers following experimental phlebotomy, but with the exception of young otherwise healthy patients with hemorrhage, these lab trials are not applicable to the usual course of events, associated illness or injury, or patient populations routinely evaluated in

ED settings.[5] In summary, these studies suggest that a postural pulse change from lying to standing of ≥30 or severe postural dizziness has 97% sensitivity and 98% specificity for a large blood loss, whereas postural hypotension (>20 mmHg systolic decrease) or supine tachycardia or hypotension are insensitive tests.[5]

Clinical question

In adult patients presenting to the ED with vomiting, diarrhea, or decreased oral intake, what is the diagnostic accuracy of the physical examination for hypovolemia?

Three ED-based studies have reported the diagnostic test characteristics for physical exam (Table 56.1).[8–10] Schriger *et al.* evaluated 32 ED patients with suspected hypovolemia (and frank hypotension or abnormal orthostatic vital signs, mean age 44 years) and 47 volunteer blood donors to assess capillary refill, excluding those on cardiovascular medications. The criterion standard for hypovolemia in the "suspected hypovolemia" subset was not clearly stated in their manuscript. The likelihood ratios for "abnormal capillary refill time" reported in Table 56.1 are in reference to the age- and sex-specific upper limits of normal for capillary refill.[8] Gross *et al.* evaluated 55 patients older than 60 years presenting to one of two academic EDs with suspected dehydration to assess 38 signs and symptoms. As their criterion standard, they used a non-validated Physician Dehydration Rating Scale that relied upon gestalt, vital signs, serum sodium, osmolality, and urea creatinine.[9] Johnson *et al.* assessed 23 pregnant patients in the ED because of hyperemesis gravidarum to assess

Table 56.1 Diagnostic accuracy of physical exam in ED patients to identify hypovolemia not due to blood loss

Finding	Positive likelihood ratio (LR+)	Negative likelihood ratio (LR−)
Orthostatic pulse change >30	1.7	0.8
Orthostatic systolic BP change >20 mmHg	1.5	0.9
Dry axilla	2.8	0.6
Dry mouth	2.0	0.3 (0.1–0.6)
Longitudinal tongue furrows	2.0	0.3 (0.1–0.6)
Sunken eyes	3.4	0.5
Confusion	2.1	0.6
Extremity weakness	2.3	0.7
Speech not clear	3.1	0.5
Abnormal capillary refill time	6.9 (range 3.2–15)	0.7

Source: Data from [8–10].

the diagnostic accuracy of postural vital signs. Their inclusion criteria were a positive β-hCG, ≤16-week gestation by dates, and either a urine-specific gravity ≥1.025 or a urine ketone ≥40 mg/dL. They used percentage dehydration via pre- and posthydration body weight as the criterion standard for hypovolemia.[11] Eaton et al.[12] conducted a fourth non-ED-based study of geriatric adults assessing axillary sweating in 100 consecutive patients admitted to the medicine service (mean age 80 years). Axillary sweating was assessed within 24 hours of admission by applying preweighed tissue paper to the right axilla for 15 minutes with the arm held adducted. The tissue paper was then reweighed. The criterion standard for hypovolemia was a serum urea:creatinine ratio over 1 : 10 and a plasma osmolality above 295 mmol/kg.[10]

Abnormal capillary refill is the only physical exam finding to significantly increase the posttest probability of hypovolemia. The absence of tongue furrows or a dry mouth is the only physical exam findings to significantly decrease the probability of hypovolemia. Combinations of physical exam findings have not been reported, and no high-quality studies have evaluated the accuracy of history in the diagnosis of hypovolemia.

Clinical question

In adult patients presenting to the ED with suspected hypovolemia not caused by blood loss, what is the diagnostic accuracy of lab testing?

Although serum urea nitrogen, sodium, and osmolality have been used as the criterion standard for hypovolemia in the highest quality diagnostic accuracy trials, the accuracy of these labs has not been evaluated in healthy or acutely ill populations. Elevated urine-specific gravity (≥1.020) has also been used as a component of the criterion standard for hypovolemia in several studies. Bartok evaluated the diagnostic accuracy of urine-specific gravity in 25 male collegiate wrestlers using weight-based dehydration as the criterion standard. The laboratory-based urine-specific gravity ≥1.020 had 96% sensitivity and 96% specificity, while the dipstick technique had 87% sensitivity and 91% specificity.[13] The diagnostic accuracy of urine-specific gravity has not been assessed in acutely ill ED patients.

Clinical question

In adult patients with hemodynamic instability and uncertain volume status, what is the diagnostic accuracy of passive leg raising or emergency physician-performed ultrasound to predict volume resuscitation responsiveness?

Passive leg raising has been assessed as a rapid fluid-loading mimic that is simple and reversible. Biais et al.[14] evaluated 34 spontaneously breathing patients with transthoracic echocardiography stroke volume and Vigileo

Table 56.2 Diagnostic accuracy of bedside tests to predict volume responsiveness

Bedside test	Positive likelihood ratio (LR+)	Negative likelihood ratio (LR−)
Passive leg raise echo stroke volume increase ≥13%		
Biais et al.[14]	5.0	0.00
Thiel et al.[11]	11.6	0.20
Passive leg raise Flotrac stroke volume increase ≥16%	8.5	0.17

Source: Data from [11, 14].

(FloTrac) stroke volume measurements after passive leg raising in a semi-recumbent position. Increases of echocardiography stroke volume ≥13% or Flotrac stroke volume ≥16% during passive leg raising were sensitive and specific to predict volume expansion (see Table 56.2). Thiel et al. evaluated the transthoracic ultrasound change in stroke volume following a fluid challenge to assess passive leg raise in intensive care unit patients requiring volume expansion. A change in the passive leg raise stroke volume by ≥15% was predictive of volume responsiveness.[11]

However, while the passive leg raise may be a fluid-loading mimic that temporarily increases stroke volume, its use has not been found to be associated with a mortality benefit. Azadian et al. recently published a systematic review and meta-analysis of five studies that evaluated the passive leg raise as a tool to guide volume resuscitation. They determined that the pooled odds ratio (OR) for mortality with a passive leg raise-guided resuscitation strategy was 0.82 (confidence interval [CI] 0.52–1.30).[15] While the studies could not be blinded and ranged from low to high risk of bias on their evaluation, there is yet no evidence that the use of this tool has a patient-oriented benefit.

The use of emergency physician-performed ultrasound to predict volume resuscitation responsiveness was evaluated by a 2019 systematic review and meta-analysis by Stickles et al.[16] They included four studies in their analysis, with a total of 357 patients. All four studies evaluated the use of protocolized rapid ultrasound for shock and hypotension (RUSH) exams in patients in shock. These RUSH exams are used to evaluate for multiple etiologies of shock, including hypovolemic, cardiogenic, obstructive, and distributive, with imaging performed of the heart, inferior vena cava (IVC), peritoneum, aorta, lungs, and leg veins. In patients with hypovolemic or distributive shock (most relevant to this chapter), a hyperdynamic heart and compressible IVC may be observed on ultrasound. The pooled analysis demonstrated that RUSH exams were not sensitive for either hypovolemic or distributive shock, but were specific for both. Their likelihood ratios are listed in Table 56.3.

Table 56.3 Test characteristics for RUSH exams in hypovolemic and distributive shock

	Shock subtype	
	Hypovolemic	Distributive
LR+	8.25 (3.29–20.69)	17.56 (3.46–89.19)
LR–	0.19 (0.07–0.50)	0.30 (0.11–0.79)

Source: Data from [16].

Comment

Accurate assessment of volume responsiveness in any clinical setting is a challenge, but in the ED, this challenge is magnified by incomplete histories and short evaluation times. Understanding the limitations of history and physical exam is key to safe, efficient volume resuscitation. Unfortunately, the diagnostic accuracy of history has not been studied, and very few elements of the physical exam are helpful to increase or decrease the probability of hypovolemia. High-quality diagnostic trials are needed to determine the accuracy and reliability of history and physical exam in isolation and in various combinations for ED patients with suspected hypovolemia. Additionally, these ED-based diagnostic trials should assess subsets of hypovolemia patients including blood loss hypovolemia, gastrointestinal loss hypovolemia, and critical illness-related hypovolemia to ascertain their reliability, diagnostic accuracy, and volume-responsiveness prognostic potential. To do so, researchers will need to establish a valid criterion standard for hypovolemia and assess the accuracy of clinical gestalt. No clinical decision rule for hypovolemia risk currently exists, but such an aid would be particularly useful in ED subsets at increased risk for adverse outcomes if the assessment of volume status results in the wrong therapy (fluids for the volume-overloaded patient or fluid restriction for the hypovolemia patient). The most helpful elements of physical exam to rule in hypovolemia include an abnormal capillary refill time, sunken eyes, and a dry axilla, while the absence of a dry mouth is the most useful finding to exclude hypovolemia.

References

1. Steiner MJ, DeWalt DA, Byerley JS. Is this child dehydrated? *Journal of the American Medical Association*. 2004; 291(22): 2746–54.
2. Silversides JA, Fitzgerald E, Manickavasagam US *et al.* Deresuscitation of patients with iatrogenic fluid overload is associated with reduced mortality in critical illness*. *Critical Care Medicine*. 2018; 46(10): 1600–7.

3. Jones DG, Nantais J, Rezende-Neto JB, Yazdani S, Vegas P, Rizoli S. Crystalloid resuscitation in trauma patients: Deleterious effect of 5L or more in the first 24h. *BMC Surgery.* 2018; 18(1): 93.

4. Mandal AK, Saklayen MG, Hillman NM, Markert RJ. Predictive factors for high mortality in hypernatremic patients. *The American Journal of Emergency Medicine.* 1997; 15(2): 130–2.

5. McGee S, Abernethy WB, Simel DL. The rational clinical examination. Is this patient hypovolemic? *Journal of the American Medical Association.* 1999; 281(11): 1022–9.

6. Snyder NA, Feigal DW, Arieff AI. Hypernatremia in elderly patients. A heterogeneous, morbid, and iatrogenic entity. *Annals of Internal Medicine.* 1987; 107(3): 309–19.

7. Hollerbach AD, Sneed NV. Accuracy of radial pulse assessment by length of counting interval. *Heart & Lung.* 1990; 19(3): 258–64.

8. Schriger DL, Baraff LJ. Capillary refill – is it a useful predictor of hypovolemic states? *Annals of Emergency Medicine.* 1991; 20(6): 601–5.

9. Gross CR, Lindquist RD, Woolley AC, Granieri R, Allard K, Webster B. Clinical indicators of dehydration severity in elderly patients. *The Journal of Emergency Medicine.* 1992; 10(3): 267–74.

10. Johnson DR, Douglas D, Hauswald M, Tandberg D. Dehydration and orthostatic vital signs in women with hyperemesis gravidarum. *Academic Emergency Medicine.* 1995; 2(8): 692–7.

11. Thiel SW, Kollef MH, Isakow W. Non-invasive stroke volume measurement and passive leg raising predict volume responsiveness in medical ICU patients: An observational cohort study. *Critical Care.* 2009; 13(4): R111.

12. Eaton D, Bannister P, Mulley GP, Connolly MJ. Axillary sweating in clinical assessment of dehydration in ill elderly patients. *BMJ;* 308(6939): 1271.

13. Bartok C, Schoeller DA, Sullivan JC, Clark RR, Landry GL. Hydration testing in collegiate wrestlers undergoing hypertonic dehydration. *Medicine and Science in Sports and Exercise.* 2004; 36(3): 510–7.

14. Biais M, Vidil L, Sarrabay P, Cottenceau V, Revel P, Sztark F. Changes in stroke volume induced by passive leg raising in spontaneously breathing patients: Comparison between echocardiography and Vigileo/FloTrac device. *Critical Care.* 2009; 13(6): R195.

15. Azadian M, Win S, Abdipour A, Kim CK, Nguyen HB. Mortality benefit from the passive leg raise maneuver in guiding resuscitation of septic shock patients: A systematic review and meta-analysis of randomized trials. *Journal of Intensive Care Medicine.* 2022; 37(5): 611–7.

16. Stickles SP, Carpenter CR, Gekle R *et al.* The diagnostic accuracy of a point-of-care ultrasound protocol for shock etiology: A systematic review and meta-analysis. *CJEM.* 2019; 21(3): 406–17.

Chapter 57 **Geriatric Screening**

Christopher R. Carpenter[1] and Fernanda Bellolio[2]

[1] Department of Emergency Medicine, Washington University School of Medicine, St. Louis, MO, USA
[2] Department of Emergency Medicine, Mayo Clinic, Rochester, MN, USA

Highlights

- Cognitive dysfunction is present in approximately 30% of community-dwelling geriatric patients in the emergency department (ED) but is usually not detected by clinicians without focused screening.
- An abnormal Abbreviated Mental Test (AMT-4) increases the probability of dementia, while the Brief Alzheimer's Screen most significantly decreases it.
- The Ottawa 3DY balances brevity and accuracy as an ED dementia screener.
- To rule in or rule out delirium the 4AT is superior to other instruments such as the Brief Confusion Assessment Method or the Delirium Triage Screen.
- Fall studies have not reported the diagnostic accuracy of individual or aggregate risk factors in ED populations, but past falls and cognitive dysfunction appear to be strongly associated with future falls.
- Vulnerability screening instruments (Identification of Seniors at Risk, Triage Risk Screening Tool) do not identify patients at low- or high risk for post-ED adverse outcomes like functional decline, return visits, or death.

Background

The "baby boomers" are individuals born in the United States between 1946 and 1964, marked by a substantial rise in birth rates post-World War II.[1] Baby boomers started turning 65 in 2011, and there were 77 million people older than 65 in 2011, and by 2030, there will be 60 million.[1] Longevity is the result

---

Evidence-Based Emergency Care: Diagnostic Testing and Clinical Decision Rules, Third Edition.
Edited by Jesse M. Pines, Fernanda Bellolio, Christopher R. Carpenter, and Ali S. Raja.
© 2023 John Wiley & Sons Ltd. Published 2023 by John Wiley & Sons Ltd.

of higher income and education, so it comes as no surprise that socioeconomic inequalities widen the gap of life expectancy.[2,3] Terms such as "elderly" are offensive for some of society with alternative terminology like "older adult" or "geriatric" deemed more acceptable.[4] Defining the threshold for "older adults" in the late twentieth century often used aged 65 years or older but may vary across regions depending on populations and resources. Multiorganizational guidelines exist to standardize the "geriatricization" of care in the adult emergency department (ED), though these recommendations are primarily consensus-based rather than research-based.[5] Despite the lack of high-quality supporting evidence, the American College of Emergency Physicians has created Geriatric Emergency Department Guidelines aiming to improve the care seniors receive in the ED. There have been several articles trying to demonstrate the cost-effectiveness for these efforts.[6–8] Most recently, a study by Hwang et al.[9] found that patients cared for in a geriatric ED by a transitional care nurse or social work had lower Medicare expenditures at 30 and 60 days after an ED visit.

Older adults often present to the ED with atypical disease manifestations, including pyuria that is usually not a urinary tract infection[10,11] or minor trauma that is potentially life threatening.[12] In addition, unrecognized co-morbidities like dementia or acute illness like delirium frequently exist, either of which can prolong ED length of stay, admission rates, and preventable readmissions.[13,14] "Geriatric syndromes" include falls,[15] delirium,[16] dementia,[17] frailty,[18] functional decline,[19] and polypharmacy.[20] With aging populations and established guidelines, ED physicians will be increasingly expected to identify and initiate management of prevalent geriatric syndromes in coming decades.[21,22]

Clinical question

In older ED patients at risk for cognitive dysfunction, what are the diagnostic test characteristics of brief dementia screening tests?

Cognitive dysfunction includes mild cognitive impairment, delirium, and dementia. Approximately 30% of older adult ED patients have an abnormal dementia screening test with a range from 12% to 43%.[23] Emergency physicians miss the majority of dementia (and delirium) presenting to the ED.[24,25] Cognitive dysfunction in older ED patients is associated with accelerated functional decline or short-term readmissions,[14] falls,[26] impaired driving safety,[27] lower patient satisfaction,[28] and lower caregiver quality of life.[29] Alzheimer's disease is the most common dementia subtype, afflicts 5 million Americans in 2020 and is projected to increase to 14 million by 2050 with an increase in dementia-related healthcare costs from $305 billion to

$1.1 trillion over that period.[30] Historically, the Mini–Mental State Examination (MMSE) was used to assess for dementia in research settings, but this instrument is not sufficiently brief for practical use clinically, was not originally derived to diagnose dementia, and has not been formally validated in the ED.[23,31,32] The MMSE is particularly inaccurate in identifying mild cognitive impairment with a sensitivity as low as 18%.[33] In addition, the MMSE has unacceptably high false-positive rates in poorly educated and lower socioeconomics subgroups.[34,35] Mild cognitive impairment is characterized by memory or language problems that do not interfere with daily activities, but which can be detected by certain screening tests.[36] The prevalence and optimal screening instruments for mild cognitive impairment in the ED have not yet been identified.[23]

A recent ED-based diagnostic meta-analysis identified seven dementia screening instruments with diagnostic accuracy summarized in Table 57.1.[23] The Short Blessed Test (SBT) and Brief Alzheimer's Screen (BAS) also identified all cases of delirium.[37] Based on two European ED studies, the Abbreviated Mental Test (AMT-4) (Table 57.2) demonstrates the highest positive likelihood ratio to increase the probability of dementia in older

Table 57.1 Diagnostic test characteristics of SBT, BAS, SIS, and cAD8

Instrument (number of ED-based studies)	Positive likelihood ratio (95% CI)	Negative likelihood ratio (95% CI)
Abbreviated mental test-4 (2)	7.7 (3.5–17.1)	0.31 (0.10–0.90)
Brief Alzheimer's screen (1)	2.0 (1.6–2.2)	0.10 (0.02–0.28)
Caregiver AD8 (2)	2.5 (1.8–3.5)	0.39 (0.26–0.59)
Mini-Cog (1)	4.9 (2.4–8.3)	0.30 (0.10–0.62)
Ottawa 3DY (3)	2.3 (1.5–3.5)	0.17 (0.05–0.66)
Short blessed test* (3)	2.7 (2.0–3.6)	0.18 (0.09–0.39)
Six item screener (3)	3.5 (2.4–5.3)	0.39 (0.31–0.50)

* Short blessed test also called orientation-memory-concentration test, quick confusion scale, and the six-item cognitive impairment test.
Source: Data from [23].

Table 57.2 Abbreviated mental test-4

1. How old are you?
2. What is your date of birth?
3. What is the name of this place?
4. What year is this?
Any error is considered high risk for dementia

adults.[38,39] Although the BAS had the lowest negative likelihood ratio to decrease the probability of dementia, it is too complex for incorporation into routine ED screening. The Ottawa 3DY (Table 57.3) balances brevity and simplicity with a lower negative likelihood ratio, although the confidence intervals across three studies are wide.[37,40,41] Notably, highly educated patients can create false-negative ED dementia screening results, but the caregiver-administered AD8 (Table 57.4) does not rely upon objective patient evaluation and may be preferable in that population.[23] The testing threshold was discussed in Chapter 1 and is estimated to benefit patients with a pretest probability of 15–43%, which is within the range that the average older ED patient presents.[23]

Table 57.3 Ottawa 3DY

1. What day is today?	**Correct**			**Incorrect**		
2. What is the date?	**Correct**			**Incorrect**		
3. Spell "world" backward	Number correct					
	0	**1**	**2**	**3**	**4**	**5**
4. What year is this?	**Correct**			**Incorrect**		

A single incorrect response on any of these four items is consistent with cognitive impairment

Table 57.4 Caregiver AD8

If the patient has an accompanying reliable informant, they are asked the following questions
Has this patient displayed any of the following issues? Remember a "Yes" response indicates that you think there has been **a change in the last several years** caused by thinking and memory (cognitive) problems
1. Problems with judgment (example, falls for scams, bad financial decisions, buys gifts inappropriate for recipients)?
2. Reduced interest in hobbies/activities?
3. Repeats questions, stories, or statements?
4. Trouble learning how to use a tool, appliance, or gadget (VCR, computer, microwave, remote control)?
5. Forgets correct month or year?
6. Difficulty handling complicated financial affairs (for example, balancing checkbook, income taxes, paying bills)?
7. Difficulty remembering appointments?
8. Consistent problems with thinking and/or memory?

Each affirmative response is one-point. A score of ≥2 is considered high risk for cognitive impairment

Clinical question

In older ED patients at risk for cognitive dysfunction, what are the diagnostic test characteristics of bedside delirium screening instruments?
Delirium is a transient disorder of cognitive capabilities, which is a symptom of an acute illness, injury, or medication exposure. Delirium is a neurological emergency because it accelerates Alzheimer's-related cognitive decline,[42] increases hospital length of stay,[43] and increases mortality.[44] Delirium also impedes effective patient–physician communication in the ED.[45] The Diagnostic and Statistical Manual (5th revision) criteria to establish a diagnosis of delirium requires the documentation of an acute onset and fluctuating disturbance in attention with an accompanying change in cognition (memory, orientation, language) unexplained by a preexisting condition and associated with a likely physiological or toxicological stressor identifiable on history, physical exam, and laboratory evaluation.[46] In contrast, dementia has a gradual onset over months to years. Delirium descriptors include motor subtypes: hyperactive, hypoactive, and mixed. Hypoactive delirium predominates in the ED representing 92% of cases.[47] ED studies detect delirium in 8–30% of ED patients, but up to 87% of the time delirium is unrecognized and/or undocumented by ED nurses and physicians.[25,47,48] A scoping review recently summarized the diagnostic accuracy of ED delirium screening instruments (Table 57.5).[49] The ED identification and prevention of delirium is a key quality indicator,[50,51] although ED delirium prevention or amelioration research is virtually nonexistent.[49]

The Confusion Assessment Method (CAM) has been the most frequently evaluated screening instrument for delirium, but like the MMSE the CAM has never formally been validated in ED settings.[52,53] In one scoping review, 27 ED delirium-screening instruments were identified.[49] This review noted

Table 57.5 Summary diagnostic test characteristics of brief delirium screening instruments

	Number of trials	Positive likelihood ratio	Negative likelihood ratio
CAM	12	9.6	0.16
DOSS	2	5.2	0.10
GAR<7	1	65	0.06
MMSE<24	1	1.6	0.12
Nu-DESC>0	1	3.1	0.06

Table 57.6 Richmond agitation-sedation scale (RASS)

+3	**Very agitated** =pulls or removes tube(s) or catheter(s); aggressive
+2	**Agitated** =frequent nonpurposeful movement, fights ventilator
+1	**Restless** =anxious but movements not aggressive or vigorous
0	**Alert and calm** =no issues, all appearances, and interactions appear normal
−1	**Drowsy** =not alert, but awake; eye opening/voice contact is >10 seconds
−2	**Light sedation** =briefly awakens with eye contact to voice (<10 seconds)
−3	**Moderate sedation** =movement or eye opening to voice (but no eye contact)
−4	**Deep sedation** =no response to voice, but moves/opens eyes to physical stimulation
−5	**Unarousable** =no response to voice or physical stimulation
	Score other than 0 = delirium

that the Delirium Triage Screen (20-seconds) and Richmond Agitation Sedation Scale (1 minute, Table 57.6) demonstrated the briefest screening time, while the brief CAM (kappa = 0.87–0.88, Figure 57.1) had the highest inter-rater reliability. Another diagnostic meta-analysis of ED delirium instruments highlighted the 4 "A" test (4AT) (Table 57.7) as the superior instrument to rule in (positive likelihood ratio 8.3) or rule out (negative likelihood ratio 0.15) delirium.[54]

Clinical question

In older ED patients who have suffered a standing level fall which features of the history and physical exam most accurately predict future falls?

Falls are the leading cause of trauma-related mortality in older adults and the incidence of injurious falls is increasing.[55,56] Among community-dwelling older adults presenting to the ED for a nonfall related chief complaint, approximately 14% will fall within 6 months.[57] The rate of falling increases to 31% at 6 months for those in the ED for a fall-related complaint.[58] Geriatric fall risk screening in the ED is recommended by guidelines but inconsistently delivered due to a variety of patient, provider, and healthcare system factors.[5,60] ED physicians acknowledge the importance of secondary falls prevention, but cite inability to accurately risk stratify patients and time constraints as major barriers impeding that effort.[61] To be effective, ED-based falls prevention programs require patients willing to participate, multidisciplinary professional teams with reliable and continual communication streams, and dependable follow-up across socioeconomic strata.[62] However, the first barrier to overcome is identifying individuals at highest risk of falling and most likely to benefit from ED interventions to reduce injurious falls.[63]

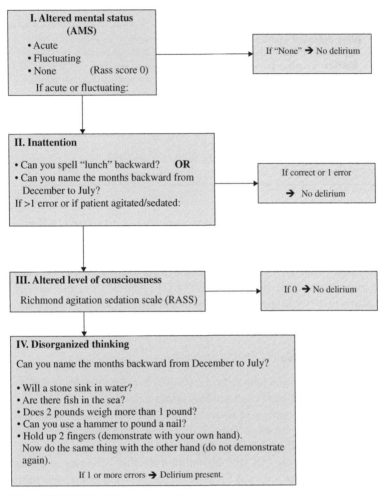

Figure 57.1 Brief confusion assessment method.

A systematic review of ED-based fall-risk screening, including individual risk factors and assessment instruments identified two prospectively derived decision aids summarized in Table 57.8.[64] Both risk assessment instruments more accurately identified low-risk (negative likelihood ratio range 0–0.44) than high-risk (positive likelihood ratio 1.3–3.8) community-dwelling older adults.[57,58] A wide range of individual risk factors such as self-reported prior falls or fall injuries, sense of imbalance, and polypharmacy failed to identify low- or high-risk fallers.[64] Secondary analysis of a secondary fall prevention

Table 57.7 4 assessment test (4AT)

---

[1] Alertness
This includes patients who may be markedly drowsy (e.g., difficult to rouse and/or obviously sleepy during assessment) or agitated/hyperactive. Observe the patient. If asleep, attempt to wake with speech or gentle touch on shoulder. Ask the patient to state their name and address to assist in rating.
Circle one
Normal (fully alert, but not agitated, throughout assessment) = 0
Mild sleepiness for <10 seconds after waking, then normal = 0
Clearly abnormal = 4

[2] AMT4
Age, date of birth, place (name of the hospital or building), current year
No mistakes = 0
One mistake = 1
Two or more mistakes/untestable = 2

[3] Attention
Ask the patient: "Please tell me the months of the year in backward order, starting in December." To assist initial understanding one prompt of "what is the month before December?" is permitted.
Months of the year backward Achieves 7 months or more correctly = 0
Starts but scores <7 months/refuses to start = 1
Untestable (cannot start because unwell, drowsy, inattentive) = 2

[4] Acute change or fluctuating course
Evidence of significant change or fluctuation in: alertness, cognition, other mental function (e.g., paranoia, hallucinations) arising over the last 2 weeks and still evident in the last 24 hours
No = 0
Yes = 4

Score Interpretation
4 or above:	Possible delirium ± cognitive impairment
1–3:	Possible cognitive impairment
0:	Delirium or cognitive impairment unlikely (but delirium still possible if [4] information incomplete)

---

randomized controlled trial initiated in British ED settings in higher risk populations identified past falls within the prior year, indoor falls, and inability to get up after a fall as predictors of future falls.[65] In addition, objective assessments of gait and balance including chair stand, raising feet while walking, and ability to turn 180° and return to chair did not identify low- or high-risk future fallers.[64] Other functional assessments commonly used outside ED settings such as Timed Up and Go and tandem walk do not predict short-term fall risk or ED/hospital returns.[66]

Table 57.8 ED-tested prediction instruments as predictors of 6-month fall risk

Finding	Sensitivity, % (95% CI)	Specificity, % (95% CI)	Positive LR (95% CI)	Negative LR (95% CI)
Carpenter score >1 Carpenter et al.[57]	93 (89–96)	61 (54–65)	2.40 (1.95–2.80)	0.11 (0.06–0.20)
Carpenter Score >2 Carpenter et al.[57]	100 (98–100)	22 (18–22)	1.30 (1.2–1.3)	0 (0–0.14)
Tiedemann Score >0 Tiedemann et al.[58]	80 (71–87)	46 (40–53)	1.48 (1.28–1.72)	0.44 (0.30–0.64)
Tiedemann Score >1 Tiedemann et al.[58]	75 (65–83)	62 (55–70)	2.00 (1.61–2.50)	0.40 (0.28–0.57)
Tiedemann Score >2 Tiedemann et al.[58]	61 (48–73)	84 (76–89)	3.76 (2.45–5.78)	0.46 (0.34–0.64)
Modified CAGE >0 Greenberg (2013)[59]	52 (34–39)	70 (59–80)	1.73 (1.07–2.81)	0.69 (0.47–1.01)

Source: Reproduced from [63] with permission from John Wiley and Sons Ltd.

Clinical question

Can older ED patients at risk for short-term adverse outcomes such as functional decline, hospitalization, or loss of independence be identified during the index episode of care?

Identifying the subset of older adults at highest risk for preventable adverse outcomes in the weeks and months following an ED visit is the holy grail of geriatric emergency medicine. For decades of health outcomes, researchers worked diligently to derive instruments like the Identification of Seniors at Risk (ISAR) and the Triage Risk Severity Tool.[67] Unfortunately, no individual risk factor, historical frailty construct, or ED decision aid accurately identifies low- or high-risk patients for any outcome at any threshold of "abnormal" (Table 57.9).[68] The Clinical Frailty Scale continues to undergo evaluation in ED settings as a viable predictor of 30-day mortality and hospitalization, but additional research linking more frail patients with resources to prevent unwanted outcomes is required.[69] The International Resident Assessment Instrument (interRAI) ED Screener is another risk-stratification instrument that does not accurately identify at-risk subsets of older adults.[70]

The barriers to deriving a sufficiently accurate risk-stratification instrument for "vulnerability" are myriad, including layers of unmeasured complexity at the level of the patient, ED, and health care system.[71,72] For example, prior research neglected to incorporate ED-validated assessments

Table 57.9 Current state of geriatric ED "vulnerability" instruments

Instrument	Year derived	Languages evaluated	Number of published ED accuracy studies	Outcomes predicted	LR+ range	LR- range
APOP	2018	Dutch	1	**90-day** functional decline or mortality	3.3	0.71
interRAI	2017	English French Flemish German Icelandic Portuguese	1	**30-day** Readmission	1.1	0.63
ISAR	1999	English, Spanish, Flemish	20	**90-day** Readmission	1.1	0.68
				30-day		
				ED returns	0.67–1.52	0.13–1.47
				Decline	1.09–1.45	0.45–0.62
				Readmission	0.86–1.18	0.38–1.32
				90-day		
				ED returns	0.84–1.34	0.49–1.47
				Decline	1.15–1.30	0.41–0.73
				Readmission	1.04–1.30	0.24–0.92
Rowland	1990	English	1	**6-month**		
				ED returns	1.28	0.94
				Readmission	1.35	0.93
Runciman	1996	English	1	**6-month**		
				ED returns	0.97	1.19
				Readmission	0.96	1.28

Silver Code	2010	English	1	**6-month** ED returns	1.15	0.73
				Readmission	1.19	0.65
TRST	2003	English	14	**30-day** ED returns	1.25–1.51	0.43–0.72
				Decline	1.11–1.58	0.46–0.74
				Readmission	0.94–1.57	0.48–1.13
				90-day ED returns	1.01–1.23	0.75–0.98
				Decline	0.94–1.58	0.42–1.10
				Readmission	1.16–1.22	0.51–0.73
Variables Indicative of Placement	2008	English	4	**30-day** Decline	1.11–3.55	0.58–0.65
				Readmission	0.93–1.12	0.77–1.48

Source: Reproduced from [66] with permission from John Wiley and Sons Ltd.

of dementia, delirium, or frailty.[23,49,69] In addition, observational study designs may underestimate the accuracy of these instruments because individual findings may prompt interventions that reduce the occurrence of the adverse outcomes via a "treatment paradox."[73] Tensions arise because current guidelines advocate using one or more of the imperfect instruments, while the next generation of "vulnerability" researchers seeks an intermediary strategy to advance accuracy while avoiding suboptimal contemporary ED care via paralysis by analysis (Figure 57.2).[5,67]

Comment

Screening older ED patients for dementia, delirium, falls, and overall vulnerability continues to evolve. An assumption of screening is that identification of individuals at high risk can trigger intervention(s) or referrals to reduce the occurrence of adverse outcomes. Interventional trials recently challenge this assumption.[74] For example, a large multicenter pragmatic randomized controlled trial to prevent falls failed to reduce fall injuries.[75] Similarly, studies evaluating ED interventions to prevent incident delirium or to reduce the duration/severity of prevalent delirium are virtually nonexistent.[49] Clearly, the humanistic response to these realities is not to abandon efforts to provide optimal care for aging adults by promoting therapeutic nihilism.[76] Many hypotheses remain untested and provide opportunities to improve evidence-based emergency care for older adults.

- Example 1: Delirium phenotypes beyond motor subtypes may exist that screening instruments detect with different accuracy and that respond to distinct preventative or therapeutic interventions.[49,77]
- Example 2: Similarly, linking fall risk assessment to real-world interventions may require incorporation of shared decision-making principles, harmonization of risk factor measures, and implementation science (Figure 57.3).[78]
- Example 3: General vulnerability assessments like ISAR or interRAI may require Utstein-style consensus on measures and outcomes to standardize research, while aligning risk assessment with preventable adverse outcomes.[70]

Aligning feasible ED geriatric syndrome screening with patient priorities and local resources continues to evolve in response to aging populations and increasing recognition of approaches to experience the experience and outcomes of emergency care.[79]

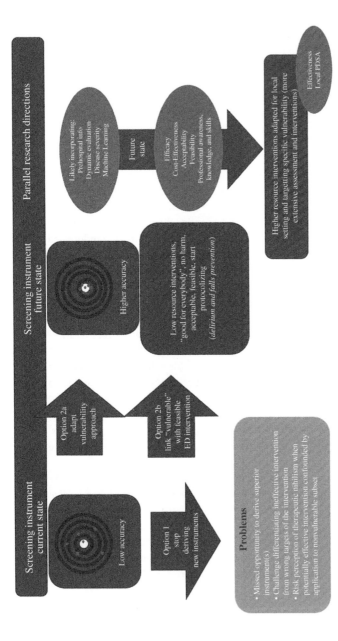

Figure 57.2 Approaches to advancing geriatric emergency department "vulnerability" screening research. Option #1 would cease efforts to derive more accurate instruments than currently exist to focus on hybrid-effectiveness research. Alternatively, Option 2a would adapt prior methods to derive "vulnerability" instruments that incorporate preemergency department data, dynamic re-evaluations throughout emergency department episode of care, social and system factors, and current disease severity – perhaps using disruptive innovation such as machine learning. Option 2b could occur simultaneously with 2a, while responding to risk identified by current imperfect instruments with widely available and generally acceptable interventions. More labor-intensive interventions like Comprehensive Geriatric Assessment would be reserved for high-resource settings or clinical research like Plan-Do-Study-Act (PDSA) cycles. (Reproduced from [66] with permission from John Wiley and Sons Ltd.)

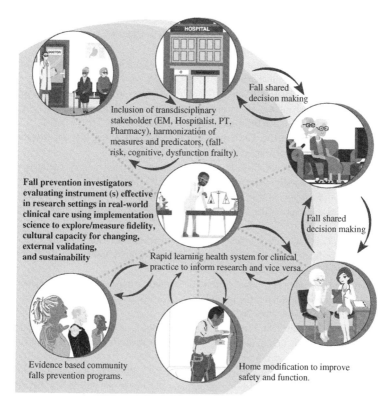

Inclusion of transdisciplinary stakeholder (EM, Hospitalist, PT, Pharmacy), harmonization of measures and predicators, (fall-risk, cognitive, dysfunction frailty).

Fall shared decision making

Fall prevention investigators evaluating instrument (s) effective in research settings in real-world clinical care using implementation science to explore/measure fidelity, cultural capacity for changing, external validating, and sustainability

Fall shared decision making

Rapid learning health system for clinical practice to inform research and vice versa.

Evidence based community falls prevention programs.

Home modification to improve safety and function.

Figure 57.3 This figure illustrates the real-world settings of falls prevention research moving forward: the outpatient clinic, the emergency department, the homes of older patients, the practice sites of nurse case managers, and physical therapists, the site which needs simple home modifications, and the community. Identifying effective fall prevention strategies in post-STRIDE research necessitates a multipronged approach incorporating implementation science principles and an evolving understanding of impactful shared decision-making. Transdisciplinary alignment and harmonization of fall-related definitions, screening instruments, and outcome measures while catalyzing impactful change can promote healthy skepticism while avoiding therapeutic nihilism and advance patient-centric fall prevention. Rapidly learning health systems can integrate incremental improvements from multiple settings to improve their research and clinical practice. (Reproduced from [75]/With permission from John Wiley and Sons.)

References

1. Colby SL, Ortman JM. The Baby Boom Cohort in the United States: 2012 to 2060. Population Estimates and Projections. United States Department of Commerce. https://www.census.gov/history/pdf/babyboomers-boc-2014.pdf. 2014. Accessed September 27, 2021.

2. Mackenbach JP, Valverde JR, Bopp M et al. Determinants of inequalities in life expectancy: An international comparative study of eight risk factors. *The Lancet Public Health.* 2019; 4(10): e529–37.

3. Chetty R, Stepner M, Abraham S et al. The association between income and life expectancy in the United States, 2001-2014. *JAMA.* 2016; 315(16): 1750–6.

4. Trucil DE, Lundebjerg NE, Busso DS. When it comes to older adults, language matters and is changing: American Geriatrics Society update on reframing aging style changes. *Journal of the American Geriatrics Society.* 2021; 69(1): 265–7.

5. Rosenberg M, Carpenter CR, Bromley M et al. Geriatric emergency department guidelines. *Annals of Emergency Medicine.* 2014; 63(5): e7–25.

6. Southerland LT, Lo AX, Biese K et al. Concepts in practice: Geriatric emergency departments. *Annals of Emergency Medicine.* 2020; 75(2): 162–70.

7. Pines JM, Edginton S, Aldeen AZ. What we can do to justify hospital investment in geriatric emergency departments. *Academic Emergency Medicine.* 2020; 27(10): 1074–6.

8. Lo AX, Carpenter CR. Balancing evidence and economics while adapting emergency medicine to the 21st century's geriatric demographic imperative. *Academic Emergency Medicine.* 2020; 27(10): 1070–3.

9. Hwang U, Dresden SM, Vargas-Torres C et al. Association of a geriatric emergency department innovation program with cost outcomes among medicare beneficiaries. *JAMA Network Open.* 2021; 4(3): e2037334.

10. Caterino JM, Kline DM, Leininger R et al. Nonspecific symptoms lack diagnostic accuracy for infection in older patients in the emergency department. *Journal of the American Geriatrics Society.* 2019; 67(3): 484–92.

11. Burkett E, Carpenter CR, Arendts G, Hullick C, Paterson DL, Caterino JM. Diagnosis of urinary tract infection in older persons in the emergency department: To pee or not to pee, that is the question. *Emergency Medicine Australasia.* 2019; 31(5): 856–62.

12. Carpenter CR, Arendts G, Hullick C, Nagaraj G, Cooper Z, Burkett E. Major trauma in the older patient: Evolving trauma care beyond management of bumps and bruises. *Emergency Medicine Australasia.* 2017; 29(4): 450–5.

13. Ostir GV, Schenkel SM, Berges IM, Kostelec T, Pimentel L. Cognitive health and risk of ED revisit in underserved older adults. *The American Journal of Emergency Medicine.* 2016; 34(10): 1973–6.

14. Kent T, Lesser A, Israni J, Hwang U, Carpenter C, Kelly KJ. 30-day emergency department revisit rates among older adults with documented dementia. *Journal of the American Geriatrics Society.* 2019; 67(11): 2254–9.

15. Nagaraj G, Hullick C, Arendts G, Burkett E, Hill KD, Carpenter CR. Avoiding anchoring bias by moving beyond 'mechanical falls' in geriatric emergency medicine. *Emergency Medicine Australasia.* 2018; 30(6): 843–50.

16. Nagaraj G, Burkett E, Hullick C, Carpenter CR, Arendts G. Is delirium the medical emergency we know least about? *Emergency medicine Australasia: EMA.* 2016; 28(4): 456–8.

17. Afonso-Argiles FJ, Meyer G, Stephan A et al. Emergency department and hospital admissions among people with dementia living at home or in nursing homes:

Results of the European RightTimePlaceCare project on their frequency, associated factors and costs. *BMC Geriatrics.* 2020; 20(1): 453.

18. Arendts G, Burkett E, Hullick C, Carpenter CR, Nagaraj G, Visvanathan R. Frailty, thy name is.... *Emergency Medicine Australasia.* 2017; 29(6): 712–6.

19. Southerland LT, Pearson S, Hullick C, Carpenter CR, Arendts G. Safe to send home? Discharge risk assessment in the emergency department. *Emergency Medicine Australasia.* 2019; 31(2): 266–70.

20. Inouye SK, Studenski S, Tinetti ME, Kuchel GA. Geriatric syndromes: Clinical, research, and policy implications of a core geriatric concept. *Journal of the American Geriatrics Society.* 2007; 55(5): 780–91.

21. Terrell KM, Hustey FM, Hwang U, Gerson LW, Wenger NS, Miller DK. Quality indicators for geriatric emergency care. *Academic Emergency Medicine.* 2009; 16(5): 441–9.

22. Hogan TM, Losman ED, Carpenter CR *et al.* Development of geriatric competencies for emergency medicine residents using an expert consensus process. *Academic Emergency Medicine.* 2010; 17(3): 316–24.

23. Carpenter CR, Banerjee J, Keyes D *et al.* Accuracy of dementia screening instruments in emergency medicine: A diagnostic meta-analysis. *Academic Emergency Medicine.* 2019; 26(2): 226–45.

24. Hustey FM, Meldon SW. The prevalence and documentation of impaired mental status in elderly emergency department patients. *Annals of Emergency Medicine.* 2002; 39(3): 248–53.

25. Elie M, Rousseau F, Cole M, Primeau F, McCusker J, Bellavance F. Prevalence and detection of delirium in elderly emergency department patients. *CMAJ.* 2000; 163(8): 977–81.

26. Ganz DA, Bao Y, Shekelle PG, Rubenstein LZ. Will my patient fall? *Journal of the American Medical Association.* 2007; 297(1): 77–86.

27. Carr DB. Commentary: The role of the emergency physician in older driver safety. *Annals of Emergency Medicine.* 2004; 43(6): 747–8.

28. Nerney MP, Chin MH, Jin L *et al.* Factors associated with older patients' satisfaction with care in an inner-city emergency department. *Annals of Emergency Medicine.* 2001; 38(2): 140–5.

29. Banerjee S, Samsi K, Petrie CD *et al.* What do we know about quality of life in dementia? A review of the emerging evidence on the predictive and explanatory value of disease specific measures of health related quality of life in people with dementia. *International Journal of Geriatric Psychiatry.* 2009; 24(1): 15–24.

30. Alzheimer's and Dementia Facts and Figures. Alzheimer's Association. https://www.alz.org/alzheimers-dementia/facts-figures. 2020. Accessed November 9, 2020.

31. Folstein MF, Folstein SE, McHugh PR. "Mini-mental state". A practical method for grading the cognitive state of patients for the clinician. *Journal of Psychiatric Research.* 1975; 12(3): 189–98.

32. Holsinger T, Deveau J, Boustani M, Williams JW. Does this patient have dementia? *Journal of the American Medical Association.* 2007; 297(21): 2391–404.

33. Nasreddine ZS, Phillips NA, Bédirian V *et al.* The montreal cognitive assessment, MoCA: A brief screening tool for mild cognitive impairment. *Journal of the American Geriatrics Society.* 2005; 53(4): 695–9.

34. Ihl R, Frölich L, Dierks T, Martin EM, Maurer K. Differential validity of psychometric tests in dementia of the Alzheimer type. *Psychiatry Research.* 1992; 44(2): 93–106.

35. Scazufca M, Almeida OP, Vallada HP, Tasse WA, Menezes PR. Limitations of the mini-mental state examination for screening dementia in a community with low socioeconomic status: Results from the Sao Paulo Ageing & Health Study. *European Archives of Psychiatry and Clinical Neuroscience.* 2009; 259(1): 8–15.

36. Morris JC. Mild cognitive impairment is early-stage Alzheimer disease: Time to revise diagnostic criteria. *Archives of Neurology.* 2006; 63(1): 15–6.

37. Carpenter CR, Bassett ER, Fischer GM, Shirshekan J, Galvin JE, Morris JC. Four sensitive screening tools to detect cognitive dysfunction in geriatric emergency department patients: Brief Alzheimer's Screen, Short Blessed Test, Ottawa 3DY, and the caregiver-completed AD8. *Academic Emergency Medicine: Official Journal of the Society for Academic Emergency Medicine.* 2011; 18(4): 374–84.

38. Schofield I, Stott DJ, Tolson D, McFadyen A, Monaghan J, Nelson D. Screening for cognitive impairment in older people attending accident and emergency using the 4-item abbreviated mental test. *European Journal of Emergency Medicine.* 2010; 17(6): 340–2.

39. Dyer AH, Briggs R, Nabeel S, O'Neill D, Kennelly SP. The abbreviated mental test 4 for cognitive screening of older adults presenting to the emergency department. *European Journal of Emergency Medicine.* 2017; 24(6): 417–22.

40. Wilding L, Eagles D, Molnar F *et al.* Prospective validation of the Ottawa 3DY scale by geriatric emergency management nurses to identify impaired cognition in older emergency department patients. *Annals of Emergency Medicine.* 2016; 67(2): 157–63.

41. Barbic D, Kim B, Salehmohamed Q, Kemplin K, Carpenter CR, Barbic SP. Diagnostic accuracy of the Ottawa 3DY and short blessed test to detect cognitive dysfunction in geriatric patients presenting to the emergency department. *BMJ Open.* 2018; 8(3): e019652.

42. Fong TG, Jones RN, Shi P *et al.* Delirium accelerates cognitive decline in Alzheimer disease. *Neurology.* 2009; 72(18): 1570–5.

43. Saravay SM, Kaplowitz M, Kurek J *et al.* How do delirium and dementia increase length of stay of elderly general medical inpatients? *Psychosomatics.* 2004; 45(3): 235–42.

44. Han JH, Shintani A, Eden S *et al.* Delirium in the emergency department: An independent predictor of death within 6 months. *Annals of Emergency Medicine.* 2010; 56(3): 244–52.e241.

45. Han JH, Bryce SN, Ely EW *et al.* The effect of cognitive impairment on the accuracy of the presenting complaint and discharge instruction comprehension in older emergency department patients. *Annals of Emergency Medicine.* 2011; 57(6): 662–71.e662.

46. European Delirium Association and American Delirium Society. The DSM-5 criteria, level of arousal and delirium diagnosis: Inclusiveness is safer. *BMC Medicine.* 2014; 12: 141.

47. Han JH, Zimmerman EE, Cutler N *et al.* Delirium in older emergency department patients: Recognition, risk factors, and psychomotor subtypes. *Academic Emergency Medicine.* 2009; 16(3): 193–200.

48. Lewis LM, Miller DK, Morley JE, Nork MJ, Lasater LC. Unrecognized delirium in ED geriatric patients. *The American Journal of Emergency Medicine.* 1995; 13(2): 142–5.

49. Carpenter CR, Hammouda N, Linton EA *et al.* Delirium prevention, detection, and treatment in emergency medicine settings: A geriatric emergency care applied research (GEAR) network scoping review and consensus statement. *Academic Emergency Medicine.* 2021; 28(1): 19–35.

50. Schnitker LM, Martin-Khan M, Burkett E, Beattie ERA, Jones RN, Gray LC. Process quality indicators targeting cognitive impairment to support quality of care for older people with cognitive impairment in emergency departments. *Academic Emergency Medicine.* 2015; 22(3): 285–98.

51. Schnitker LM, Martin-Khan M, Burkett E *et al.* Structural quality indicators to support quality of care for older people with cognitive impairment in emergency departments. *Academic Emergency Medicine.* 2015; 22(3): 273–84.

52. Inouye SK, van Dyck CH, Alessi CA, Balkin S, Siegal AP, Horwitz RI. Clarifying confusion: The confusion assessment method. A new method for detection of delirium. *Annals of Internal Medicine.* 1990; 113(12): 941–8.

53. Wong CL, Holroyd-Leduc J, Simel DL, Straus SE. Does this patient have delirium?: Value of bedside instruments. *Journal of the American Medical Association.* 2010; 304(7): 779–86.

54. Calf AH, Pouw MA, van Munster BC, Burgerhof JGM, de Rooij SE, Smidt N. Screening instruments for cognitive impairment in older patients in the emergency department: A systematic review and meta-analysis. *Age and Ageing.* 2021; 50(1): 105–12.

55. Albert M, McCaig LF, Ashman JJ. Emergency department visits by persons aged 65 and over: United States, 2009-2010. *NCHS Data Brief.* 2013; (130): 1–8.

56. Shankar KN, Liu SW, Ganz DA. Trends and characteristics of emergency department visits for fall-related injuries in older adults, 2003-2010. *The Western Journal of Emergency Medicine.* 2017; 18(5): 785–93.

57. Carpenter CR, Scheatzle MD, D'Antonio JA, Ricci PT, Coben JH. Identification of fall risk factors in older adult emergency department patients. *Academic Emergency Medicine.* 2009; 16(3): 211–9.

58. Tiedemann A, Sherrington C, Orr T *et al.* Identifying older people at high risk of future falls: Development and validation of a screening tool for use in emergency departments. *Emergency Medicine Journal.* 2013; 39(11): 918–22.

59. Greenberg MR, Nguyen MC, Porter BG, et al. Modified CAGE as a screening tool for mechanical fall risk assessment: A pilot survey. Annals of Emergency Medicine; 62: S107–S108.

60. Tirrell G, Sri-on J, Lipsitz LA, Camargo CA, Kabrhel C, Liu SW. Evaluation of older adult patients with falls in the emergency department: Discordance with national guidelines. *Academic Emergency Medicine*. 2015; 22(4): 461–7.

61. Davenport K, Cameron A, Samson M, Sri-on J, Liu SW. Fall prevention knowledge, attitudes, and behaviors: A survey of emergency providers. *The Western Journal of Emergency Medicine*. 2020; 21(4): 826–30.

62. Ganz DA, Alkema GE, Wu S. It takes a village to prevent falls: Reconceptualizing fall prevention and management for older adults. *Injury Prevention*. 2008; 14(4): 266–71.

63. Carpenter CR, Shah MN, Hustey FM, Heard K, Gerson LW, Miller DK. High yield research opportunities in geriatric emergency medicine: Prehospital care, delirium, adverse drug events, and falls. *The Journals of Gerontology. Series A, Biological Sciences and Medical Sciences*. 2011; 66(7): 775–83.

64. Carpenter CR, Avidan MS, Wildes T, Stark S, Fowler SA, Lo AX. Predicting geriatric falls following an episode of emergency department care: A systematic review. *Academic Emergency Medicine*. 2014; 21(10): 1069–82.

65. Close JCT, Hooper R, Glucksman E, Jackson SHD, Swift CG. Predictors of falls in a high risk population: Results from the prevention of falls in the elderly trial (PROFET). *Emergency Medicine Journal*. 2003; 20(5): 421–5.

66. Eagles D. Delirium in older emergency department patients. *CJEM: Canadian Journal of Emergency Medicine*. 2018; 80(6): 811–2.

67. Carpenter CR, Mooijaart SP. Geriatric screeners 2.0: Time for a paradigm shift in emergency department vulnerability research. *Journal of the American Geriatrics Society*. 2020; 68(7): 1402–5.

68. Carpenter CR, Shelton E, Fowler S *et al.* Risk factors and screening instruments to predict adverse outcomes for undifferentiated older emergency department patients: A systematic review and meta-analysis. *Academic Emergency Medicine*. 2015; 22(1): 1–21.

69. Kaeppeli T, Rueegg M, Dreher-Hummel T *et al.* Validation of the clinical frailty scale in an urban emergency department. *Annals of Emergency Medicine*. 2020; 76(3): 291–300.

70. Heeren P, Devriendt E, Wellens NIH *et al.* Old and new geriatric screening tools in a Belgian emergency department: A diagnostic accuracy study. *Journal of the American Geriatrics Society*. 2020; 68(7): 1454–61.

71. Hwang U, Carpenter C. Assessing geriatric vulnerability for post emergency department adverse outcomes: Challenges abound while progress is slow. *Emergency Medicine Journal*. 2016; 33(1): 2–3.

72. Carpenter CR, Émond M. Pragmatic barriers to assessing post-emergency department vulnerability for poor outcomes in an ageing society. *The Netherlands Journal of Medicine*. 2016; 74(8): 327–9.

73. Meyer G, Möhler R, Köpke S. Reducing waste in evaluation studies on fall risk assessment tools for older people. *Journal of Clinical Epidemiology*. 2018; 102: 139–43.

74. Hughes JM, Freiermuth CE, Shepherd-Banigan M *et al.* Emergency department interventions for older adults: A systematic review. *Journal of the American Geriatrics Society*. 2019; 67(7): 1516–25.

75. Bhasin S, Gill TM, Reuben DB *et al.* A randomized trial of a multifactorial strategy to prevent serious fall injuries. *The New England Journal of Medicine.* 2020; 383(2): 129–40.

76. Carpenter CR, Malone ML. Avoiding therapeutic nihilism from complex geriatric intervention "negative" trials: STRIDE lessons. *Journal of the American Geriatrics Society.* 2020; 68(12): 2752–6.

77. Kennedy M, Hwang U, Han JH. Delirium in the emergency department: Moving from tool-based research to system-wide change. *Journal of the American Geriatrics Society.* 2020; 68(5): 956–8.

78. Carpenter CR, Lo AX. Falling behind? Understanding implementation science in future emergency department management strategies for geriatric fall prevention. *Academic Emergency Medicine.* 2015; 22(4): 478–80.

79. Berning MJ, Silva LOJE, Suarez NE *et al.* Interventions to improve older adults' emergency department patient experience: A systematic review. *The American Journal of Emergency Medicine.* 2020; 38(6): 1257–69.

Chapter 58 **Skin and Soft Tissue Infections**

Ali S. Raja[1] and Fernanda Bellolio[2]

[1] Department of Emergency Medicine, Massachusetts General Hospital,
Harvard Medical School, Boston, MA, USA
[2] Department of Emergency Medicine, Mayo Clinic, Rochester, MN, USA

Highlights

- Skin and soft tissue infections are common reasons for presentation to the ED.
- While a history of cellulitis and the presence of a leg wound or ulcer can increase the odds of cellulitis, there are a number of mimics that make the diagnosis difficult to rule in or out.
- Point-of-care ultrasound has good diagnostic test accuracy and can confirm the diagnosis of abscess and differentiate from cellulitis.

Background

Skin and soft tissue infections are frequent reasons for visits to emergency departments (EDs); in the United States, approximately $3.7 billion of ambulatory care costs are expended on the estimated 14.5 million cases of cellulitis every year.[1] Nationally representative data from 2000 to 2015 demonstrated a rise in the incidence of outpatient visits for skin infections.[2]

The accurate diagnosis of cellulitis, erysipelas, and abscess is important – underdiagnosis can lead to infections progressing beyond their initial areas of presentation, and overdiagnosis can lead to unnecessary antibiotic use.[3–5] The risk of abscess formation increases with increasing prevalence of community-acquired methicillin-resistant *Staphylococcus aureus* strains.[6] The incidence of skin and soft tissue infection is twice that of urinary tract

---

Evidence-Based Emergency Care: Diagnostic Testing and Clinical Decision Rules, Third Edition.
Edited by Jesse M. Pines, Fernanda Bellolio, Christopher R. Carpenter, and Ali S. Raja.
© 2023 John Wiley & Sons Ltd. Published 2023 by John Wiley & Sons Ltd.

infections and 10-fold of that of pneumonia in patients aged 0–64 years. Among patients younger than 65 years, the incidence of skin infections is 49 cases/1000 person/year. Most skin and soft tissue infections (95%) are treated in the ED and ambulatory settings. Complications such as myositis, gangrene, and sepsis occurred in 0.9% and 16.9% of ambulatory-treated and inpatient-treated patients, respectively.[6] Please refer to Chapter 25 for Necrotizing Fasciitis and Chapter 31 for Sepsis.

Nevertheless, the diagnosis can be a difficult one; a recent narrative review listed 33 different mimics of cellulitis that may present with similar findings.[7] While antibiotic selection and the merits of various abscess drainage techniques are beyond the scope of this text, the two clinical questions below are relevant to almost every patient with potential cellulitis or abscess presenting to the ED.

Clinical question

Can history or physical exam accurately rule in or rule out cellulitis and abscess?
This question is fundamental to the diagnosis of skin and soft tissue infections. Cellulitis is typically described as a poorly demarcated area of erythema in a patient with fever, pain, warmth, and swelling, but these findings are all relatively insensitive and nonspecific.[1] A 2017 meta-analysis by Quirke *et al.*[8] included 6 studies and 2471 patients with nonpurulent leg cellulitis. From a total of 40 risk factors, several aspects of the history and physical exam increased the odds of developing cellulitis (Table 58.1). Local risk factors

Table 58.1 History and physical examination findings and risk of leg cellulitis

Finding	Odds ratio (95% CI)
Local factors	
Previous cellulitis	40.3 (22.6–71.9)
Previous ulcer	4.5 (1.6–12.5)
Previous surgery	2.7 (1.7–4.1)
Leg wound	19.1 (9.1–40.0)
Leg ulcer	13.7 (7.9–23.6)
Lymphedema or chronic edema	6.8 (3.5–13.3)
Excoriation	4.4 (2.7–7.1)
Tinea pedis causing toe-web disease	3.2 (1.9–5.3)
Systemic factors	
Diabetes mellitus	1.2 (0.9–4.5)
Obesity	2.0 (1.5–2.7)
Obesity (BMI > 25)	1.9 (1.3–2.8)
Obesity (BMI > 30)	2.4 (1.4–4.1)
Smoking (current or recent)	0.9 (0.7–1.2)
Alcohol consumption	1.1 (0.8–1.6)

Source: Data from [8].

were found to be more significantly related to nonpurulent cellulitis compared to systemic risk factors. Previous cellulitis, previous leg surgery, having a wound, ulcer, excoriation, toe intertrigo, and chronic leg edema were the most common factors. The authors reported that patients with diabetes were more likely to present with suppurative cellulitis from infected diabetic foot ulcers or wounds and may have been excluded from the systematic review. Also, the articles had to specifically report cellulitis affecting the lower extremities to be included.

Nevertheless, while the presence of these factors increased the odds of cellulitis, their absence cannot rule out the disease.

Clinical question

Can point-of-care ultrasound (POCUS) differentiate between cellulitis and abscess in ED patients?

The advent of POCUS use in the ED brought a new tool to the bedside for the diagnosis of soft tissue infections in ED patients. Ultrasound is involved in the diagnosis of many disease processes in this text, but its use for the evaluation of these superficial skin infections is one of the most common. The differentiation between cellulitis and abscess is especially important, as the latter needs drainage or aspiration, while the former can be treated with antibiotics (Figure 58.1).[9]

A number of studies have evaluated the use of ultrasound for the differentiation between cellulitis and abscess, and a 2017 meta-analysis by Barbic *et al.*[10] reviewed these data. A total of eight studies (including five from pediatric EDs and three from adult EDs) and 747 patients were included, and all were rated as good to excellent on quality assessment tool for diagnostic accuracy studies (QUADAS-2) criteria. Overall, ultrasound had a sensitivity of 96.2% (confidence interval [CI] 91.1–98.4%), a specificity of 82.9% (CI 60.4–93.9%), a LR+ of 5.6 (CI 2.2–14.6), and a LR− of 0.05 (CI 0.02–0.11). The diagnostic test accuracy on the pediatric population was a sensitivity of 93.9% (CI 84.8–97.7%) and specificity 82.9% (CI 34.2–97.9%), LR+ 5.5 (CI 0.9–33.9), and LR− 0.07 (CI 0.03–0.15). POCUS changed subsequent management in 14–27% of pediatric patients, and 17–56% of adult patients. POCUS changed management most often when there was uncertainty or equivocal physical exam findings. The authors concluded that the use of POCUS does help differentiate abscess from cellulitis in ED patients with skin and soft tissue infections.[10]

A more recent systematic review by Gottlieb *et al.* in 2020 included 14 studies (same eight studies included in Barbic *et al.* plus six more recent studies) and 2656 patients that received POCUS for the diagnosis of skin and soft tissue abscess. On meta-analysis POCUS was 94.6% sensitive

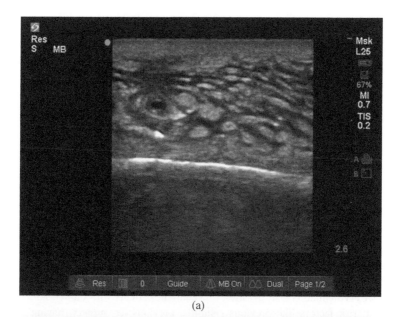

(a)

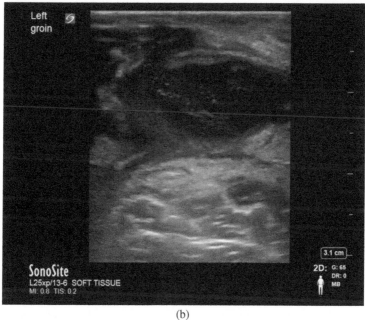

(b)

Figure 58.1 Ultrasound images of (a) cellulitis and (b) abscess. ((a,b) Courtesy of Hamid Shokoohi, MD, Massachusetts General Hospital.)

(CI 89.4–97.4%) and 85.4% specific (CI 78.9–90.2%), with a LR+ of 6.5 (CI 4.4–9.6) and LR– of 0.06 (CI 0.03–0.13). Among cases that were clinically unclear, POCUS was 91.9% sensitive (CI 77.5–97.4%) and 76.9% specific (CI 65.3–85.5%), with an LR+ of 4.0 (CI 2.5–6.3) and LR– of 0.11 (CI 0.03–0.32). Among adults, it was 98.7% sensitive (CI 95.3–99.8%) and 91.0% specific (CI 84.4–95.4%), LR+ of 10.9 (CI 6.2–19.2) and LR– of 0.01 (CI 0.001–0.06). Among children, POCUS was 89.9% sensitive (CI 81.8–94.6%) and 79.9% specific (CI 71.5–86.3%), LR+ of 4.5 (CI 3.1–6.4) and LR– of 0.13 (CI 0.07–0.23). POCUS was associated with management change in 10.3% of cases.[11]

Comment

This chapter highlights the difficulty in making the diagnosis of cellulitis in patients with suspected skin and soft tissue infections. While the presence of certain aspects of the history and physical examination can increase the odds of cellulitis, it can be difficult to rule out given its similarity to a number of other erythematous skin diseases, especially in patients with darker skin.[12] Local risk factors like previous cellulitis, previous leg surgery, having a wound, ulcer, excoriation, toe intertrigo, and chronic leg edema were the most common factors for nonpurulent cellulitis compared to systemic risk factors. Nevertheless, in the presence of cellulitis, POCUS can be used to differentiate between cellulitis and abscess, allowing for the drainage of the latter, when appropriate. Ultrasound is particularly helpful in equivocal cases, where the pretest probability is lower, and the posttest probability will increase or decrease beyond the treatment thresholds with the results of the ultrasound. (For more information review Chapter 3, Epidemiology and Statistics of Diagnostic Testing.)

References

1. Raff AB, Kroshinsky D. Cellulitis: A review. *Journal of the American Medical Association.* 2016; 316(3): 325–37.
2. Fritz SA, Shapiro DJ, Hersh AL. National trends in incidence of purulent skin and soft tissue infections in patients presenting to ambulatory and emergency department settings, 2000-2015. *Clinical Infectious Diseases.* 2020; 70(12): 2715–8.
3. Cross ELA, Jordan H, Godfrey R *et al.* Route and duration of antibiotic therapy in acute cellulitis: A systematic review and meta-analysis of the effectiveness and harms of antibiotic treatment. *Journal of Infection.* 2020; 81(4): 521–31.
4. Soper NS, Appukutty AJ, Paje D *et al.* Antibiotic overuse after discharge from medical short-stay units. *Infection Control and Hospital Epidemiology.* 2021: 1–4. doi: 10.1017/ice.2021.346.

5. Li DG, Xia FD, Khosravi H *et al.* Outcomes of early dermatology consultation for inpatients diagnosed with cellulitis. *JAMA Dermatology.* 2018; 154(5): 537–43.

6. Miller LG, Eisenberg DF, Liu H *et al.* Incidence of skin and soft tissue infections in ambulatory and inpatient settings, 2005-2010. *BMC Infectious Diseases.* 2015; 15: 362.

7. Long B, Gottlieb M. Diagnosis and management of cellulitis and abscess in the emergency department setting: An evidence-based review. *The Journal of Emergency Medicine.* 2022; 62(1): 16–27.

8. Quirke M, Ayoub F, McCabe A *et al.* Risk factors for nonpurulent leg cellulitis: A systematic review and meta-analysis. *The British Journal of Dermatology.* 2017; 177(2): 382–94.

9. Moran GJ, Abrahamian FM, LoVecchio F, Talan DA. Acute bacterial skin infections: Developments since the 2005 Infectious Diseases Society of America (IDSA) guidelines. *The Journal of Emergency Medicine.* 2013; 44(6): e397–412.

10. Barbic D, Chenkin J, Cho DD, Jelic T, Scheuermeyer FX. In patients presenting to the emergency department with skin and soft tissue infections what is the diagnostic accuracy of point-of-care ultrasonography for the diagnosis of abscess compared to the current standard of care? A systematic review and meta-analysis. *BMJ Open.* 2017; 7(1): e013688.

11. Gottlieb M, Avila J, Chottiner M, Peksa GD. Point-of-care ultrasonography for the diagnosis of skin and soft tissue abscesses: A systematic review and meta-analysis. *Annals of Emergency Medicine.* 2020; 76(1): 67–77.

12. Thakrar DB, Sultan MJ. Cellulitis: Diagnosis and differentiation. *Journal of Wound Care.* 2021; 30(12): 958–65.

Chapter 59 **Shared Decision-Making in Diagnostic Testing**

Fernanda Bellolio[1], Erik P. Hess[2]
and Christopher R. Carpenter[3]

[1] Department of Emergency Medicine, Mayo Clinic, Rochester, MN, USA
[2] Vanderbilt University, Nashville, TN, USA
[3] Department of Emergency Medicine, Washington University School of Medicine, St. Louis, MO, USA

Highlights

- Shared decision-making (SDM) is a collaborative process that allows patients and their clinicians to make healthcare decisions together, considering the best scientific evidence available, as well as the patient's values and preferences.
- Engaging in SDM provides patients the information they need to make decisions that affect their desired health outcomes.
- SDM in emergency medicine can improve the quality, safety, and outcomes of ED patients. SDM has been reported to improve patient satisfaction and reduce malpractice claims.
- Decision aids are evidence-based tools designed to increase patient understanding of medical options and possible outcomes, facilitate conversation between patients and clinicians, and improve patient engagement.

What is SDM?

Shared decision-making (SDM) is a conversational dynamic in which clinicians and patients discuss the best available evidence relevant to a medical decision.[1] It is a collaborative process that allows patients (in conjunction

---

Evidence-Based Emergency Care: Diagnostic Testing and Clinical Decision Rules, Third Edition.
Edited by Jesse M. Pines, Fernanda Bellolio, Christopher R. Carpenter, and Ali S. Raja.
© 2023 John Wiley & Sons Ltd. Published 2023 by John Wiley & Sons Ltd.

with their caregiver or care partner) and their clinicians to make healthcare decisions together, taking into account the best scientific evidence available, as well as the patient's values and preferences.

In SDM, both parties share information: the clinician offers evidence-based options and describes the potential harms and benefits of each choice, and the patient expresses his or her preferences and values. SDM is a key component of patient-centered care.[2, 3]

A patient's ability to engage in conversation and to understand the risks and benefits of diagnostic testing options is essential to effective SDM. In urban U.S. emergency departments (ED) the average health literacy is at a seventh grade level and that of rural EDs remains unquantified.[4, 5] Although an objective assessment of health literacy or numeracy is not routine in the ED (or any medical) settings, the clinician must elicit the patient's understanding of risks and benefits during the conversation to ensure patient comprehension.[6]

Key components of SDM include: (i) at least two participants (patient/care partner and provider); (ii) both parties share information; and (iii) work together to build consensus and reach agreement about the preferred option.[7]

Key steps of SDM include: (i) choice talk, let patients know that options are available; (ii) option talk, provide information about the options; (iii) decision talk, support the patient's preferences and decision.[8]

Patient involvement in the decision-making process includes:
(i) Recognizing that a decision is being made; (ii) feeling informed about options and outcomes; (iii) feeling clear about goals and preferences; (iv) being able to discuss goals and preferences with the clinician; (v) being involved in selecting tests and/or treatments.[9]

When is it appropriate to engage a patient in SDM?

There are often clinical scenarios in which more than one course of action is medically reasonable. Even in the chaotic ED in scenarios such as these, clinicians can engage patients in SDM.[10] SDM is appropriate for key decisions where there are multiple options equally supported by the weight of evidence. SDM is not appropriate when there are clinical pathways or scenarios in

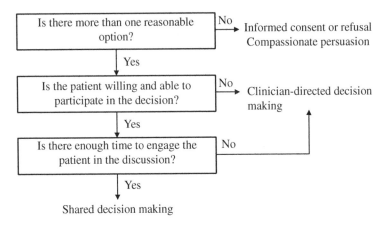

Figure 59.1 SDM appropriateness. (Adapted from [11].)

which there is clearly a single effective and appropriate decision, like, for example, obtaining an electrocardiogram (ECG) in a middle-aged patient presenting to the ED with acute retrosternal chest pain. (Figure 59.1)

> Considerations for SDM in diagnostic testing
> - What is the pretest probability of the disease?
> - Is there equipoise (i.e., both considerations are reasonable)?
> - What information is available to be used in the conversation?
> - Is there appropriate time, and when is the right time to engage the patient/care partner?
> - What are the diagnostic test characteristics necessary for SDM?
> - What are the benefits and harms of the diagnostic test?
> - Are there alternatives?
> - Is the patient/care partner interested and able to participate in SDM?

There are several factors to consider when determining the appropriateness of SDM for diagnostic testing:[6]

To engage in SDM we need to know the probability that the patient might have the disease. When available, clinical decision rules are a good tool to determine pretest probability (see Chapter 4). Tests that will not meaningfully alter the pretest probability should not be performed and therefore should not be considered as part of a SDM discussion. A situation in which the evidence clearly suggests an optimal diagnostic approach is different from a situation in which there is equipoise between two or more different diagnostic approaches. Of these only the second scenario is appropriate for SDM.[6]

Both benefits and harms of diagnostic tests as well as alternatives should be presented and contemplated in a way that patients can understand. Potential harms with imaging might include exposure to ionizing radiation, cost, and incidental findings that may lead to potentially harmful downstream testing.[12] Harms to the healthcare system at large (e.g., expensive, low-yield tests that contribute to the high cost of healthcare) should be considered. Clinicians may not consider SDM an option for situations in which there is only one testing option, but in these situations, there is still a decision to be made: to test or not to test.[6]

Why use SDM in EM?

Engaging patients in a SDM discussion provides patients the information they need to make decisions that affect their desired health outcomes. Patients want to be involved in decisions regarding their care and doing so respects their autonomy.[13, 14] SDM in emergency medicine (EM) can improve the quality, safety, and outcomes of ED patients. Evidence alone is never sufficient to make a clinical decision, and the better the quality of the available evidence, the higher quality of the decision. SDM has been reported to improve patient satisfaction[15] and reduce malpractice claims.[16, 17]

What are decision aids?

The process of SDM can occur informally, via conversation, or in a more standardized fashion using decision aids. Decision aids are evidence-based tools designed to increase patient understanding of medical options and possible outcomes, facilitate conversation between patients and clinicians, and improve patient engagement. These tools are developed for a particular decision-making context and identify the social, emotional, environmental, and cultural barriers that may need to be addressed for conversations to occur.[18] Decision aids increase patient involvement and patient–provider communication, improve patient knowledge and realistic perceptions of outcomes, and do not adversely affect health or patient satisfaction.[18] Decision aids are the most common tools used to support SDM in clinical encounters and have been shown to positively affect decisional quality[7] and increase knowledge when compared to usual care.[19]

SDM in clinical settings

SDM can be used in different clinical settings during the continuum of care including:

1. screening: breast cancer screening among women aged 40–49,[20] or prostate cancer screening among men aged 55–69 years[21];
2. adherence: a strategy to increase adherence to colorectal cancer screening[22];
3. therapy: selection of treatment for depression,[23] hypercholesterolemia,[24] osteoporosis,[25, 26] venous thromboembolism,[27] musculoskeletal pain in older adults,[28] and antibiotics for otitis media,[29] among others;
4. prognosis: to inform prognosis after emergent intubation in older adults[30];
5. diagnostic testing: to guide imaging utilization in head computed tomography (CT) in children with minor head trauma,[31] imaging for pulmonary embolism,[32] and lumbar puncture after negative cranial CT to rule out subarachnoid hemorrhage (SAH),[33–35] among others.

The goal of SDM is to ensure that patients are well informed, meaningfully involved in the decision-making process, and receive tests and treatments concordant with their goals.[9, 36] In this chapter, we focus our examples on the use of SDM for diagnostic testing. Tests are not perfect tools, and clinicians need to have a good understanding of the limitations of each test ordered. Clinicians should understand how to apply the results to the individual patient, and how a positive or negative test result alters the probability of having a specific diagnosis. As discussed in previous chapters, if a test will not change management, it should not be ordered unless there are extenuating circumstances.

Diagnostic testing is used to determine the presence or absence of a disease. The tests can be used to rule in or rule out a disease (see Chapters 1 and 3). As the "front porch" of the hospital straddled between inpatient and outpatient resources, as well as the safety net for an often frayed and inaccessible medical system, the focus of EM is often to definitively exclude threats to life. Ruling out worst-case scenarios has led to increasing rates of diagnostic test utilization without improved patient outcomes, as well as increased ED costs and incidental findings requiring further workup.[6, 12]

Reducing inappropriate utilization of advanced imaging is a research and public health priority.[12, 37, 38] Sharing the diagnostic test accuracy and associated health care utilization with patients is beneficial and appropriate. Translating validated risk estimates to practice and engaging patients in care decisions through SDM might tailor testing to disease risk in a way that is acceptable to patients, clinicians, and policymakers.[39, 40]

Examples of SDM for diagnostic testing

Chest pain

A common scenario for SDM of diagnostic testing is a 55-year-old patient with hypertension and diabetes mellitus presenting with 2 hours of chest pain. He has a normal ECG and negative initial troponin. Your plan is to repeat the troponin at 2 hours (if using high sensitivity troponin) or 3 hours (if using a fourth generation assay). Subsequently, there are several equivalent options such as observation unit admission for cardiology consultation, consideration of stress testing, overnight observation, or dismissal home.

You decide to use the history/ECG/age/risk factors/troponin (HEART) score pathway[41] and the patient has a moderate risk score (see Chapter 21). You decide to engage the patient in SDM to reach consensus on the best next step for this patient.

From the emergency physician's point of view, the decision regarding admission versus discharge for chest pain patients at moderate risk for acute coronary syndrome relies on the concern of missing acute myocardial infarction. From the patients' perspective, time spent in the ED and cost, are also concerns.

Hess *et al.* compared the effectiveness of SDM with usual care in choice of admission for observation and further cardiac testing or for referral for outpatient evaluation in patients with possible acute coronary syndrome. SDM facilitated by a decision aid increased patient knowledge and patient engagement, decreased decisional conflict, and did not affect trust in the physician. Use of the decision aid took an average of one additional minute of clinician time, decreased the rate of admission to an observation unit for advanced cardiac testing, and decreased cardiac stress testing within 30 days of the ED visit. There were no major adverse cardiovascular events (MACEs) related to SDM.[42]

Thunderclap headache

Patients presenting with a sudden onset, severe headache, and normal neurological exam represent a diagnostic challenge. Clinical decision rules exist to avoid missing potentially catastrophic diagnoses like SAH (see Chapter 46).[35] Less than 10% of patients with thunderclap headache are diagnosed with SAH, and no single characteristic of the history or physical exam is sufficient to rule in or rule out SAH.[33] A noncontrast CT of the head is extremely sensitive within the first 6 hours, and its sensitivity decreases over time.[34] Patients presenting after 6–12 hours of initial symptoms represent the ideal group for SDM regarding diagnostic testing. Lumbar puncture appears to benefit relatively few patients within a narrow pretest probability range.[33] CT angiography and no further testing are alternatives that need to be discussed with the patient.[43]

Head trauma

Another scenario is the care of a child with minor head trauma Parents want to be informed of the risks of tests their child might be exposed to.[44] There are clinical decision rules available to guide the use of diagnostic imaging in the case of children with head trauma (see Chapter 11).[45] These rules were incorporated into a decision aid and demonstrated the potential benefit of the use of the decision aid to facilitate SDM with parents of children with mild head trauma. A multicenter trial demonstrated increased parent knowledge, decreased decisional conflict, and increased involvement in decision-making. The decision aid did not reduce the CT rate but decreased health care utilization 7 days after injury.[31]

Similar to the example of SDM for imaging in head trauma, SDM could apply to many decisions around diagnostic testing. Engaging patients in SDM with respect to diagnostic imaging has been viewed as an essential component of evidence-based medicine.[46–49] For example, in a young patient with abdominal pain concerning for renal colic, the added diagnostic certainty to identify a nonobstructive kidney stone in which noninterventional symptom management is the next step, might not be worth the radiation risk, cost, and time associated with abdominal CT imaging.[50, 51] While clinicians who are unaccustomed to SDM may believe that patient satisfaction is always linked to more testing, this bias may be a fallacy in many situations.[52, 53] Even during times of emergency, many patients value inclusivity in decision-making.[54] For example, more than one-third of patients deferred imaging for pulmonary embolism based on low clinical probability and a D-dimer less than twice the normal threshold in a hypothetical scenario, suggesting that SDM was acceptable to patients and may decrease imaging for pulmonary embolism.[32]

The access and use of additional testing to help make a diagnosis can lead to overutilization, increased unnecessary cost, and incidental findings. SDM in diagnostic imaging can help mitigate the issue of overutilization.[49, 55] Diagnostic imaging has increased significantly over the last 15 years, and in a survey study emergency physicians reported that a significant proportion of advanced imaging studies were medically unnecessary, and likely obtained due to fear of litigation related to missing a low-probability diagnosis.[40]

Considerations for SDM

Factors to consider when engaging patients in SDM in the ED are the timing of the interventions, cost to patients and the health system, resource utilization (hospital admissions, return visits, imaging, laboratory tests, ED length of stay), and other circumstances such as language and cultural differences, vulnerable populations, low literacy, and numeracy.[56] Some decisions vary by practice setting (academic versus community versus private), as well as incentives (bundle payments) risk tolerance, and the availability of close follow-up.

SDM is applicable to vulnerable populations, and the use of accurate, group-specific data to inform risk estimates is recommended.[56] The differing circumstances, needs, and perspectives of each patient need to be considered when sharing decisions.[56]

Recommendations to improve health communication so that patients can participate in SDM include assessment of literacy, use of plain language at a fourth to sixth grade level, use of multiple forms of communication (written, oral, and visual), encouragement of questions, and confirmation of patient comprehension.[57] When providing numeric information, report probabilities in terms of numbers rather than percentages (e.g., 1 in 20 rather than 5%); keep the denominator consistent (e.g., do not change between 1 in 10 and 1 in 1000); and avoid discussing relative risk.[6]

Another consideration is the risk tolerance of patients and clinicians as discussed in Chapter 1. Individual clinician's risk tolerance may evolve over a career by increasing in relationship to recent bad outcomes. A potentially missed diagnosis, the medico-legal environment, hospital reimbursement systems, and incentives can affect risk tolerance.

Misconceptions about SDM

Although generations of physicians undoubtedly view their impactful interactions with patients during a health emergency as consummate and compassionate decision-making that is shared between the clinical team, patient, and family, the science of SDM is something more.[11, 58] Consequently, misconceptions about SDM are common. SDM is not synonymous with informed consent, which is a legal construct focused on the benefits and harms of individual approaches to a medical situation.[59] SDM melds patient's values and preferences with the balance of risks and benefits. Similarly, the motivation for SDM is not to save resources or deny care, but rather to ensure that medical or surgical decisions do not occur without the individual most affected to be fully informed and engaged – "nothing about me, without me." SDM is also not a substitute for clinician guidance to educate and counsel patients through complex scenarios and possible consequences amidst a sea of uncertainties. In other words, SDM is not a vehicle to offload malpractice risk of decisions to patients. Clinicians leveraging SDM are not abandoning patients to make decisions alone, but rather creating opportunities for patients to collaborate in the conversations to the extent they feel comfortable.[60] Finally, SDM is not a transformation of medicine into a restaurant buffet in which patients select from a menu of options without regard to futility or biological plausibility. Clinicians and patients will often require education and experience regarding what SDM is and what SDM is not as EM adapts to this evolving paradigm.

Barriers and facilitators of SDM

Barriers and facilitators of effective communication in SDM on diagnostic testing are displayed below. These barriers and facilitators may be influenced by patients' cultural background and health literacy.[6]

Barriers	Facilitators
Being in poor health	Limited debility and intact cognition
Cognitive impairment (e.g., dementia, intoxication)	Prior exposure to a similar process
Timing relative to the disease course (e.g., will the diagnostic test change management)	Physicians who effectively listen to patients, respect their concerns, and seek to understand individual needs
Power imbalance in the patient–clinician relationship	The presence of an advocate or caregiver
The desire to be a "good" patient and perceived benefits that might arise (e.g., lack of conflict in the encounter)	
Perception that there are "right" and "wrong" decisions Perceived unacceptability of asking the physician questions and raising options	

Source: Adapted from [6].

Summary

SDM can be beneficial for patients, providers, and healthcare systems and should be incorporated in clinical practice. Incorporating SDM for diagnostic decisions in the practice of EM provides the information needed for patients and clinicians to make decisions that affect patients' desired health outcomes. SDM in EM has the potential to improve quality, safety, and outcomes in ED patients, while potentially reducing overall healthcare costs by eliminating medical waste catalyzed by malalignment of patient priorities with test and treatment options.[61] In order to attain the full potential of SDM, medical educators will need to adapt,[62] decision aids for more common scenarios need to be developed,[63] meaningful and sustainable funding opportunities must accelerate,[64] and implementation science must be utilized.[65]

Online decision aid resources:

1. www.healthdecision.org, interactive decision aids for atrial fibrillation, osteoporosis, hypertension, breast and lung cancer screening.
2. https://www.ahrq.gov/, AHRQ provides decision aids designed for patients and providers for different topics.
3. http://optiongrid.org/, the Dartmouth Center for Shared Decision Making provides these decision grids that help people balance different decisions about screening and treatment decisions.
4. https://decisionaid.ohri.ca/azinvent.php, the Ottawa decision aid inventory provides a clearinghouse of decision aids on a variety of topics.
5. https://shareddecisions.mayoclinic.org/ Mayo Clinic Shared Decision Making National Resource Center.

References

1. Elwyn G, Laitner S, Coulter A, Walker E, Watson P, Thomson R. Implementing shared decision making in the NHS. *BMJ*. 2010; 341: c5146.
2. Institute_of_Medicine_(US)_Committee_on_Quality_of_Health_Care_in_ America. Formulating new rules to redesign and improve care. In: (US) NAP, editor. *Crossing the Quality Chasm: A New Health System for the 21st Century*. Washington (DC); 2001: 61–88.
3. Tzelepis F, Sanson-Fisher RW, Zucca AC, Fradgley EA. Measuring the quality of patient-centered care: Why patient-reported measures are critical to reliable assessment. *Patient Preference and Adherence*. 2015; 9: 831–5.
4. Carpenter CR, Kaphingst KA, Goodman MS, Lin MJ, Melson AT, Griffey RT. Feasibility and diagnostic accuracy of brief health literacy and numeracy screening instruments in an urban emergency department. *Academic Emergency Medicine*. 2014; 21(2): 137–46.
5. McNaughton C, Wallston KA, Rothman RL, Marcovitz DE, Storrow AB. Short, subjective measures of numeracy and general health literacy in an adult emergency department. *Academic Emergency Medicine*. 2011; 18(11): 1148–55.
6. Barrett TW, Rising KL, Bellolio MF et al. The 2016 Academic Emergency Medicine Consensus Conference, "Shared Decision Making in the Emergency Department: Development of a Policy-relevant Patient-centered Research Agenda" Diagnostic Testing Breakout Session Report. *Academic Emergency Medicine*. 2016; 23(12): 1354–61.
7. Charles C, Gafni A, Whelan T. Shared decision-making in the medical encounter: What does it mean? (or it takes at least two to tango). *Social Science & Medicine*. 1997; 44(5): 681–92.

8. Elwyn G, Frosch D, Thomson R *et al.* Shared decision making: A model for clinical practice. *Journal of General Internal Medicine.* 2012; 27(10): 1361–7.

9. Sepucha KR, Breslin M, Graffeo C, Carpenter CR, Hess EP. State of the science: Tools and measurement for shared decision making. *Academic Emergency Medicine.* 2016; 23(12): 1325–31.

10. Hess EP, Grudzen CR, Thomson R, Raja AS, Carpenter CR. Shared decision-making in the emergency department: Respecting patient autonomy when seconds count. *Academic Emergency Medicine.* 2015; 22(7): 856–64.

11. Probst MA, Kanzaria HK, Schoenfeld EM *et al.* Shared decisionmaking in the emergency department: A guiding framework for clinicians. *Annals of Emergency Medicine.* 2017; 70(5): 688–95.

12. Carpenter CR, Raja AS, Brown MD. Overtesting and the downstream consequences of overtreatment: Implications of "preventing overdiagnosis" for emergency medicine. *Academic Emergency Medicine.* 2015; 22(12): 1484–92.

13. Robey TE, Edwards K, Murphy MK. Barriers to computed tomography radiation risk communication in the emergency department: A qualitative analysis of patient and physician perspectives. *Academic Emergency Medicine.* 2014; 21(2): 122–9.

14. Schoenfeld EM, Kanzaria HK, Quigley DD *et al.* Patient preferences regarding shared decision making in the emergency department: Findings from a multisite survey. *Academic Emergency Medicine.* 2018; 25(10): 1118–28.

15. Schrager SB, Phillips G, Burnside E. A simple approach to shared decision making in cancer screening. *Family Practice Management.* 2017; 24(3): 5–10.

16. Durand MA, Moulton B, Cockle E, Mann M, Elwyn G. Can shared decision-making reduce medical malpractice litigation? A systematic review. *BMC Health Services Research.* 2015; 15: 167.

17. Schoenfeld EM, Mader S, Houghton C *et al.* The effect of shared decisionmaking on patients' likelihood of filing a complaint or lawsuit: A simulation study. *Annals of Emergency Medicine.* 2019; 74(1): 126–36.

18. Stacey D, Legare F, Col NF *et al.* Decision aids for people facing health treatment or screening decisions. *Cochrane Database of Systematic Reviews.* 2014; (1): CD001431.

19. Stacey D, Légaré F, Lewis K *et al.* Decision aids for people facing health treatment or screening decisions. *Cochrane Database of Systematic Reviews.* 2017; 4(4): CD001431.

20. U.S._Preventive_Services_Task_Force. Final Recommendation Statement - Breast Cancer: Screening. https://www.uspreventiveservicestaskforce.org/uspstf/document/RecommendationStatementFinal/breast-cancer-screening. 2016. Accessed September 5, 2022.

21. U.S._Preventive_Services_Task_Force. Final Recommendation Statement - Prostate Cancer: Screening. https://www.uspreventiveservicestaskforce.org/uspstf/document/RecommendationStatementFinal/prostate-cancer-screening. 2018. Accessed September 5, 2022.

22. Schroy PC 3rd, Emmons K, Peters E *et al.* The impact of a novel computer-based decision aid on shared decision making for colorectal cancer screening: A randomized trial. *Medical Decision Making.* 2011; 31(1): 93–107.

23. LeBlanc A, Herrin J, Williams MD et al. Shared decision making for antidepressants in primary care: A cluster randomized trial. *JAMA Internal Medicine*. 2015; 175(11): 1761–70.

24. Mann DM, Ponieman D, Montori VM, Arciniega J, McGinn T. The statin choice decision aid in primary care: a randomized trial. *Patient Education and Counseling*. 2010; 80(1): 138–40.

25. Montori VM, Shah ND, Pencille LJ et al. Use of a decision aid to improve treatment decisions in osteoporosis: The osteoporosis choice randomized trial. *The American Journal of Medicine*. 2011; 124(6): 549–56.

26. Watts NB, Manson JE. Osteoporosis and fracture risk evaluation and management: Shared decision making in clinical practice. *Journal of the American Medical Association*. 2017; 317(3): 253–4.

27. Barnes GD, Izzo B, Conte ML, Chopra V, Holbrook A, Fagerlin A. Use of decision aids for shared decision making in venous thromboembolism: A systematic review. *Thrombosis Research*. 2016; 143: 71–5.

28. Holland WC, Hunold KM, Mangipudi SA, Rittenberg AM, Yosipovitch N, Platts-Mills TF. A prospective evaluation of shared decision-making regarding analgesics selection for older emergency department patients with acute musculoskeletal pain. *Academic Emergency Medicine*. 2016; 23(3): 306–14.

29. Spiro DM, Tay KY, Arnold DH, Dziura JD, Baker MD, Shapiro ED. Wait-and-see prescription for the treatment of acute otitis media: A randomized controlled trial. *Journal of the American Medical Association*. 2006; 296(10): 1235–41.

30. Ouchi K, Jambaulikar GD, Hohmann S et al. Prognosis after emergency department intubation to inform shared decision-making. *Journal of the American Geriatrics Society*. 2018; 66(7): 1377–81.

31. Hess EP, Homme JL, Kharbanda AB et al. Effect of the head computed tomography choice decision aid in parents of children with minor head trauma: A cluster randomized trial. *JAMA Network Open*. 2018; 1(5): e182430.

32. Geyer BC, Xu M, Kabrhel C. Patient preferences for testing for pulmonary embolism in the ED using a shared decision-making model. *The American Journal of Emergency Medicine*. 2014; 32(3): 233–6.

33. Carpenter CR, Hussain AM, Ward MJ et al. Spontaneous subarachnoid hemorrhage: A systematic review and meta-analysis describing the diagnostic accuracy of history, physical examination, imaging, and lumbar puncture with an exploration of test thresholds. *Academic Emergency Medicine*. 2016; 23(9): 963–1003.

34. Dubosh NM, Bellolio MF, Rabinstein AA, Edlow JA. Sensitivity of early brain computed tomography to exclude aneurysmal subarachnoid hemorrhage: A systematic review and meta-analysis. *Stroke*. 2016; 47(3): 750–5.

35. Perry JJ, Stiell IG, Sivilotti ML et al. Clinical decision rules to rule out subarachnoid hemorrhage for acute headache. *Journal of the American Medical Association*. 2013; 310(12): 1248–55.

36. Barry MJ. Involving patients in medical decisions: How can physicians do better? *Journal of the American Medical Association*. 1999; 282(24): 2356–7.

37. Cheng AHY, Campbell S, Chartier LB et al. Choosing Wisely Canada(R): Five tests, procedures and treatments to question in emergency medicine. *CJEM*. 2017; 19(S2): S9–17.

38. Dorsett M, Cooper RJ, Taira BR, Wilkes E, Hoffman JR. Bringing value, balance and humanity to the emergency department: The right care top 10 for emergency medicine. *Emergency Medicine Journal.* 2020; 37(4): 240–5.

39. Hogan TM, Richmond NL, Carpenter CR *et al.* Shared decision making to improve the emergency care of older adults: A research agenda. *Academic Emergency Medicine.* 2016; 23(12): 1386–93.

40. Hess EP, Marin J, Mills A. Medically unnecessary advanced diagnostic imaging and shared decision-making in the emergency department: Opportunities for future research. *Academic Emergency Medicine.* 2015; 22(4): 475–7.

41. Backus BE, Six AJ, Kelder JC *et al.* A prospective validation of the HEART score for chest pain patients at the emergency department. *International Journal of Cardiology.* 2013; 168(3): 2153–8.

42. Hess EP, Hollander JE, Schaffer JT *et al.* Shared decision making in patients with low risk chest pain: Prospective randomized pragmatic trial. *BMJ.* 2016; 355: i6165.

43. Akhter M, Chen SP. Vascular emergencies and shared decision-making in patients with thunderclap headache. *Academic Emergency Medicine.* 2016; 23(10): 1194–5.

44. Hull A, Friedman T, Christianson H, Moore G, Walsh R, Wills B. Risk acceptance and desire for shared decision making in pediatric computed tomography scans: A survey of 350. *Pediatric Emergency Care.* 2015; 31(11): 759–61.

45. Kuppermann N, Holmes JF, Dayan PS *et al.* Identification of children at very low risk of clinically-important brain injuries after head trauma: A prospective cohort study. *Lancet.* 2009; 374(9696): 1160–70.

46. Nievelstein RA, Frush DP. Should we obtain informed consent for examinations that expose patients to radiation? *AJR. American Journal of Roentgenology.* 2012; 199(3): 664–9.

47. Picano E. Informed consent and communication of risk from radiological and nuclear medicine examinations: How to escape from a communication inferno. *BMJ.* 2004; 329(7470): 849–51.

48. Earnest F, Swensen SJ, Zink FE. Respecting patient autonomy: Screening at CT and informed consent. *Radiology.* 2003; 226(3): 633–4.

49. Marin JR, Grudzen CR. Emergency physician radiation risk communication: A role for shared decision-making. *Academic Emergency Medicine.* 2014; 21(2): 211–3.

50. Schoenfeld EM, Shieh MS, Pekow PS, Scales CD Jr, Munger JM, Lindenauer PK. Association of patient and visit characteristics with rate and timing of urologic procedures for patients discharged from the emergency department with renal colic. *JAMA Network Open.* 2019; 2(12): e1916454.

51. Moore CL, Carpenter CR, Heilbrun ME *et al.* Imaging in suspected renal colic: Systematic review of the literature and multispecialty consensus. *Annals of Emergency Medicine.* 2019; 74(3): 391–9.

52. Fatovich DM. The inverted U curve and emergency medicine: Overdiagnosis and the law of unintended consequences. *Emergency Medicine Australasia.* 2016; 28(4): 480–2.

53. Keijzers G, Cullen L, Egerton-Warburton D, Fatovich DM. Don't just do something, stand there! The value and art of deliberate clinical inertia. *Emergency Medicine Australasia.* 2018; 30(2): 273–8.

54. Wright Nee Blackwell R, Skolnik PJ, Skolnik DM, Grudzen C. "From tears to transparency: A conversation can change an outcome. A conversation can change a life": Reflections from patient advocates. *Academic Emergency Medicine.* 2016; 23(12): 1337–9.

55. Epstein RM, Franks P, Shields CG *et al.* Patient-centered communication and diagnostic testing. *Annals of Family Medicine.* 2005; 3(5): 415–21.

56. Castaneda-Guarderas A, Glassberg J, Grudzen CR *et al.* Shared decision making with vulnerable populations in the emergency department. *Academic Emergency Medicine.* 2016; 23(12): 1410–6.

57. Griffey RT, McNaughton CD, McCarthy DM *et al.* Shared decision making in the emergency department among patients with limited health literacy: Beyond slower and louder. *Academic Emergency Medicine.* 2016; 23(12): 1403–9.

58. Kanzaria HK, Brook RH, Probst MA, Harris D, Berry SH, Hoffman JR. Emergency physician perceptions of shared decision-making. *Academic Emergency Medicine.* 2015; 22(4): 399–405.

59. Lindor RA, Kunneman M, Hanzel M, Schuur JD, Montori VM, Sadosty AT. Liability and informed consent in the context of shared decision making. *Academic Emergency Medicine.* 2016; 23(12): 1428–33.

60. Hargraves I, LeBlanc A, Shah ND, Montori VM. Shared decision making: The need for patient-clinician conversation, not just information. *Health Affairs.* 2016; 35(4): 627–9.

61. Oshima Lee E, Emanuel EJ. Shared decision making to improve care and reduce costs. *The New England Journal of Medicine.* 2013; 368(1): 6–8.

62. Chen EH, Kanzaria HK, Itakura K, Booker-Vaughns J, Yadav K, Kane BG. The role of education in the implementation of shared decision making in emergency medicine: A research agenda. *Academic Emergency Medicine.* 2016; 23(12): 1362–7.

63. Melnick ER, Probst MA, Schoenfeld E *et al.* Development and testing of shared decision making interventions for use in emergency care: A research agenda. *Academic Emergency Medicine.* 2016; 23(12): 1346–53.

64. Dodd KW, Berman A, Brown J *et al.* Funding research in emergency department shared decision making: A summary of the 2016 academic emergency medicine consensus conference panel discussion. *Academic Emergency Medicine.* 2016; 23(12): 1340–5.

65. Kanzaria HK, Booker-Vaughns J, Itakura K *et al.* Dissemination and implementation of shared decision making into clinical practice: A research agenda. *Academic Emergency Medicine.* 2016; 23(12): 1368–79.

Chapter 60 Cognitive Biases and Mitigation Strategies in Emergency Diagnosis

John Bedolla[1] and Jesse M. Pines[2,3]

[1] Department of Surgery and Perioperative Care, Dell Medical School, University of Texas, Austin, TX, USA
[2] US Acute Care Solutions, Canton, OH, USA
[3] Department of Emergency Medicine, Drexel University, Philadelphia, PA, USA

Highlights

- Cognitive biases play a significant role in medical errors.
- Human cognition is susceptible to cognitive bias when the balance between fast mental heuristics and deliberate thought is altered in favor of fast automatic decisions.
- Some cognitive biases are more important than others in emergency medicine.
- Specific interventions can reduce the effects of most common cognitive biases.

Introduction

Emergency medical decision-making is a complex process and requires intense use of multiple brain functions. Human brain function has a performance envelope, performance limits, and failure modes. Cognitive biases are failure modes that negatively impact clinical reasoning, increase medical errors, and compromise patient safety.[1-23] Fortunately, cognitive biases are well understood and amenable to mitigation. This chapter focuses on the cognitive biases most salient to emergency medicine and mitigation strategies to reduce their effect in clinical practice.

Evidence-Based Emergency Care: Diagnostic Testing and Clinical Decision Rules, Third Edition.
Edited by Jesse M. Pines, Fernanda Bellolio, Christopher R. Carpenter, and Ali S. Raja.
© 2023 John Wiley & Sons Ltd. Published 2023 by John Wiley & Sons Ltd.

Scope of the problem

Cognitive bias is estimated to play a part in 36–77% of diagnostic errors.[4,5] Clinical reasoning is a complex task learned over many years and is learned as a self-aware and self-critical process that mitigates bias.[6,7] Nonetheless, difficult diagnostic scenarios, personal factors, and operational stressors can defeat the bias-mitigating effects of medical training and result in medical error.[8–13]

Dual processing, executive function, and cognitive errors

Kahnemann and Tversky,[14] human thinking is modeled as dual process: System 1 and System 2. System 1 is the default: it is fast, automatic, and works through heuristics and instinct. System 2 is slow, effortful, and expensive in terms of mental energy required. System 2 gets recruited only when necessary. However, System 1 is remarkably efficient but susceptible to errors. For example, System 1 reasoning can be erroneously influenced by emotion, fatigue, intrinsic cognitive biases, and personality.[15] System 2 prevents System 1 errors, but there is a limit on how frequently it can be recruited without slowing down or exhausting the clinician's cognitive apparatus. A long and complex resuscitation of a critically ill patient is an example of a case that calls on System 2 for a prolonged period. The heavy System 2 utilization often leaves the physician mentally depleted for some time afterward (Figure 60.1).

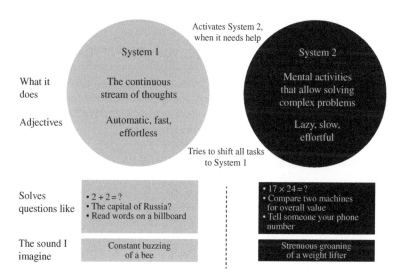

Figure 60.1 Dual-process decision model. (Adapted from [15].)

The medical encounter is a series of complex tasks, and executive function assigns cognitive resources to complete them. For each emergency medical visit, there is an ideal balanced allocation of System 1 and System 2 resources to achieve both efficiency and safety. It is theorized that System 1 runs automatically in the background, constantly and uncritically inputting into executive function. Executive function then judges if and how much System 2 thinking is needed to achieve the optimal balance. Most of the time executive function equilibrates this process well.

Cognitive errors occur when executive function's equilibrating process is overpowered, bypassed, suppressed, or de-calibrated.[16] Most cognitive biases overpower the equilibration process by amplifying the force and salience of System 1 input.[14,17] Executive function can also be de-calibrated or suppressed by operational stressors, burnout, sleep deprivation, fatigue, and deconditioning.[17,18] Operational stressors, personal stressors, or just being too busy for a prolonged period can leave the clinician too exhausted to recruit System 2.[19-21] In this setting, for example, in the Libby Zion case, the clinician can default to automatic and uncritical responses with catastrophic results.

Prospect theory

Humans do not experience negative and positive consequences equally. Kahneman and Tversky[22] show negative experiences are more salient than equivalent positive experiences. This is termed "loss aversion." For example, the negative feeling around losing 1 dollar is 2.6× larger than the positive experience of gaining 1 dollar.[22] By nature of the relationship between the amygdala, hippocampus, and limbic system, negative experiences are instinctually more salient than positive ones. From the perspective of evolutionary psychology, it's not hard to see how cognitive mechanisms that prompt animals to avoid previously negative experiences are associated with better survival, thus retaining the encoding genes over generations. For clinicians, the memory of a missed diagnosis is more painful and more salient than the memory of a good catch is pleasant and long-lasting.[23]

Uncertainty and risk

Humans are not innately adept at quantifying risk but do respond to risk thresholds.[24] Human beings are generally risk-avoidant. Humans also experience uncertainty as a risk. The aversion to uncertainty is called ambiguity aversion. The following example illustrates the difference. Avoiding a snake is risk aversion. Avoiding a pile of leaves because you're not sure there's no snake in it is ambiguity aversion. Human beings will often prefer to take on a small known risk to avoid complete (on Knightian) uncertainty. Compare the evaluation of chest pain, where the most common conditions, acute coronary syndrome (ACS)[25] and pulmonary embolism (PE),[26,27] which have well-worked pathways. By contrast, in the evaluation of dizziness in an elderly patient, where a myriad of conditions could be causative, the workup tends to be highly variable.[28] Next time you work with a clinician who is slow to pick up a dizziness chart, or tends to do extensive workups or each, realize it is most likely due to ambiguity aversion.[29,30]

Mitigation strategies

Cognitive errors can be reduced with debiasing strategies, cognitive best practices, attention to global mental function, and by engineering the emergency department (ED) to support and protect executive function. Below we focus on debiasing strategies and cognitive best practices.[31-44]

Debiasing strategies and cognitive best practices aim at decreasing bias and diagnostic error.[45] Below, we discuss the following categories: bias inoculation, cognitive best practices, mental workflow debiasing, traditional debiasing strategies, best practices, nudge, forcing strategies, and bias-specific interventions.

Bias inoculation includes education about bias and has been shown to enhance self-awareness and has been shown to decrease the effects of bias.[32] Education can take many forms, including selected readings, experiential review of cases in case conference, departmental meetings, mortality and morbidity conferences, and simulations. The most effective educational experiences are likely to be experiential.[46]

Cognitive best practices and mental workflow debiasing techniques include self-checking, structured data collection, Diagnostic Time Out, and the "Not Yet Diagnosed" strategy. Mindful self-reflection during the medical encounter activates System 2 thinking to decrease bias effects and enhance reliability.[39] Structured data collection is a debiasing technique and the history/ECG/age/risk factors/troponin (HEART) score is an example of structured data collection, which with routine practice can become much more proficient, and in the setting of time constraints, also quicker.[47,48] Structured data collection ensures that a core set of information is obtained for better decision-making. A thorough history and physical examination is another example of structured data collection.[49] A Diagnostic Time Out is a brief cognitive pause performed before making critical decisions. A Diagnostic Time Out enhances reliability by giving the clinician mental space to activate System 2, respool, review, and reflect on the clinician encounter and make sure no missing data, bias, or other error is present.

"Not Yet Diagnosed" is a strategy of reserving a final diagnosis until all the data is obtained and the clinician has had time for a Diagnostic Time Out. However, one controlled trial exploring diagnostic error did not demonstrate any medical error reduction with System 1 versus System 2 thinking.[50] At first these structured and reflective practices can result in slower decision-making, which can be a major problem in the time-constrained setting of the ED; however, with practice, the speed and quality of decision-making improve.[51-53]

Traditional strategies and best practices start with the classic history and physical examination. When well performed, this remains one of the best debiasing techniques available in emergency medicine. A well-performed history and physical examination serve as one debiasing technique. The key is to avoid shortcuts and extract the full value from the data and the process. The differential diagnosis is a classic tool for ensuring that several probabilities are considered before making a diagnosis. Life-long learning in evidence-based practices enhances System 2 thinking and provides a statistical framework to make sound decisions.[54] "Rule out worst case": considering the worst-case scenario for a chief complaint activates System 2 thinking. Checklists ensure that crucial elements of the encounter are performed prior to disposition.[55] Colleague consultation, when available, is among the most valuable strategies for ensuring reliability.[56-58]

Nudges and forcing strategies include "Until Proven Otherwise," prompts, soft stops, and hard stops are also debiasing techniques. "Until Proven Otherwise" is a traditional forcing strategy that helps disprove the presence of a serious diagnosis. Examples include "chest pain and neurological symptoms equal aortic dissection until proven otherwise," and "scrotal pain in a young male is torsion until proven otherwise." Care should be exercised in using this strategy with clinicians who have low-risk tolerance, because it may lead to over-testing. Prompts and soft stops: the electronic health record (EHR) can enhance the diagnostic process with soft stops. For example, if a patient is febrile and tachycardic, the EHR can pop up a sepsis screening alert. However, alerts should be used judiciously, as pop alert fatigue can occur. Pop-up fatigue can itself cause errors and has been shown to be serious issue in EHR design.[59,60] If not used carefully, EHR prompts can decrease patient safety by creating inefficiencies.[61] Hard stops are usually departmental policies that engage System 2 thinking before proceeding. Examples include Discharge Time Out, mandatory rechecks of abnormal vital signs, and mandatory checklists.[62,63]

Current evidence suggests that debiasing techniques are effective in bias reduction. Current research suggests that debiasing training can significantly reduce bias and enhance diagnostic decision-making.[64,65]

Prominent cognitive biases and interventions

Based on national claims analysis data one review identified the cognitive biases most salient to emergency medicine, with mitigation strategies for each type (Table 60.1).[3,4] However, most of these recommendations are theoretical, lack compelling proof-of-concept in real-world emergency medicine, and are thereby criticized by some experts as "myths of general thinking skills."[66]

Premature closure

Premature closure occurs when the information obtained in the first few seconds or minutes of the encounter points firmly in the direction of a particular diagnosis, and other probabilities are discarded without further contemplation. With premature closure the clinician fails to obtain a full picture, including information relevant to other possibilities – this is called an "unpacking error."

The fast pace, various operational stressors, and frequent interruptions of the ED can abbreviate the history and physical exam, creating an obstacle to System 2 recruitment.[67] Operational stressors (workload, patient acuity, and patient complexity) also deplete mental resources, with decreased executive function and recruitment of System 2 thinking.[68–70]

Premature closure occurs most commonly in the data acquisition phase of the medical encounter. Synthesis is often flawed because crucial data points are not obtained. Once started, it is difficult to reverse as there is a sunk cost bias (see below) against going back and asking more questions once critical decisions are made. As an example, a patient with chest pain has ST depression on electrocardiogram (ECG). The clinician sees typical coronary pain with dyspnea and does not inquire about travel history or PE risk factors. Cardiac enzymes are elevated, and the patient is taken urgently to the catheterization lab. Shortly before needle insertion, the patient dies from a massive pulmonary embolus.

Along with most common diseases, there are less common but still significant mimics. The key to finding the mimics is to avoid cutting short the standard structured history and physical exam. Every major chief complaint has one most common severe cause and 2–3 less common causes. As time and acuity permit, the clinician should screen for mimics through a complete history of present illness, augmented with the previous medical history, recent events, and a review of systems targeted to the body area involved and 2–3 proximal body systems. Time permitting, it is important to do a minimum standard every time and not skip too many steps because one feels like the diagnosis is clinched.

Table 60.1 Debiasing strategies

Strategy	Purpose	Examples of potential biases addressed
History and physical exam	Systematic gathering of data	Unpacking principle ascertainment bias
Differential diagnosis	Promotes consideration of diagnostic possibilities other than the most likely	Anchoring and adjustment Search satisficing Premature diagnostic closure Availability representativeness confirmation bias
"Not yet diagnosed" strategy	Keeps open diagnostic possibilities	Premature closure diagnostic momentum confirmation bias
Clinical prediction rules	Forces scientific, statistical assessment of signs and symptoms and uses other data to develop numerical probabilities of a disease outcome	Base rate fallacy errors of reasoning errors in estimating possibilities
Evidence-based medicine	Establishes an imperative for objective scientific data to support decision-making	Many biases
Checklists	Ensures specific, important issues have been considered, especially under conditions of complexity, stress, and fatigue	Anchoring and adjustment availability Memory failures
Mnemonics	Protects against memory failures ensuring a full differential diagnosis is considered	Availability Anchoring and adjustment premature closure
Pitfalls	Alerts inexperienced clinicians to predictable failures	Many biases
Rule out worst-case scenarios	Ensures the most serious condition in a particular clinical setting is not missed	Anchoring and adjustment premature diagnostic closure
Until proven otherwise	Ensures a particular diagnosis cannot be made unless other specific diagnoses have been excluded	Anchoring confirmation bias diagnostic momentum premature closure
Caveats	Offers discipline-specific warnings to ensure important rules are followed to avoid missing significant conditions	Many biases
Red flags	Salient, specific signs and symptoms in the context of commonly presenting conditions to avoid missing serious conditions	Anchoring confirmation bias diagnostic momentum premature closure

Source: Adapted from [4].

Before disposition, a brief cognitive pause to stop and think, a "Discharge Time Out" is warranted. In the Discharge Time Out, the clinician should mobilize System 2 to briefly respool the key elements of the clinical exams, and labs of tests and compare the "fit" of the final diagnosis to the overall picture.[63,71,72]

Satisficing, also called "search satisficing," can lead to premature closure. Satisficing occurs when the clinician settles on the first diagnosis that fits "well enough" with the clinical scenario. Example: settling on a positive urinalysis as the cause of altered mental status in an older patient. Confirmation bias occurs when the clinician looks for information that confirms the original impression and ignores data that does not.[73]

Diagnostic momentum

Diagnostic momentum[2] occurs when a patient receives an early label or diagnosis that continues uncritically through the episode of care and inhibits consideration of other possibilities. Diagnostic momentum differs from premature closure in that it is more of a passive uncritical acceptance of early information and often involves a social dimension of the influence of other clinicians' early opinions and framing of the clinical picture. Diagnostic momentum can start even before the patient arrives in the ED or as late as well into the hospital admission.[74]

The following case illustrates diagnostic momentum. A 6-year-old boy is sent from a clinic for "appendicitis." The exam reveals minimal discomfort in the right lower quadrant and labs and ultrasound are negative. The child is sent home and returns the next with torsion and a nonsalvageable right testicle. In this case, the diagnostic momentum led the clinician to focus solely on ruling appendicitis in or out.

Diagnostic momentum can be mitigated with strategies that help the clinician keep open to other possibilities. These include the differential diagnosis, the Discharge Time Out, and considering the worst-case scenario. In this case, one of the worst-case scenarios in right lower quadrant pain in young boys is testicular torsion.

Anchoring

Anchoring is often incorrectly defined in the medical literature as a "hanging one's hat" on a diagnosis. More precisely, anchoring is an inappropriate setting of the *range of possibilities* based on early information. It is not the same thing as a premature closure, but it can lead to premature closure by narrowing the range of possibilities to be considered.[75,76]

The following case illustrates anchoring. A clinician sees a young, healthy patient with no medical problems and pneumonia who does not look "toxic." Based on this early information, the clinician can correctly estimate that the patient is likely to do well–this is not anchoring. But when the clinician ignores a persistent tachycardia or other signs of sepsis because the patient looks well, the clinician has anchored on the patient's age, health, and appearance, and not considered sepsis within the range of probabilities.

It is appropriate to generate an early clinical Gestalt. The clinician should readjust the differential as well as the expected disease severity as new information appears. But clinicians can fail to readjust when they are rushed, under stress, or do not review and rethink before dispositioning the patient. Anchoring usually begins at the data acquisition phase. It negatively affects synthesis, and it commonly affects follow-up to labs and testing and can adversely affect the disposition decision. "I know he was tachycardic at discharge, but he looked good."

A discharge time out is a quick mental pause to recruit System 2, assemble all the original and new data obtained in the encounter, and review to make sure the picture still fits together. It is an excellent strategy to de-anchor. The key is to be willing to consider alternative to one's early impression if there is contradictory data.[77] Any data that does not fit with the original impression should be taken seriously, and the clinician should be willing to rethink the initial impression. If any element is far outside the norm, the clinician should consider if the whole case might outline usual heuristics and expectations. Following the example of a young, healthy patient with pneumonia who looks well, if there is persistent tachycardia at discharge, the clinician must recruit System 2 and deliberately consider that the patient might have occult sepsis.[78,79] This does mean one should question every single assumption or diagnosis – there is simply no time or sufficient mental resources to do that. It does mean one should open to new information and re-examine when the information does not fit the original impression.[80]

Availability heuristic and recency effect

The availability heuristic relates to a salient memory and the recency effect. In both, a memory that is more immediately recalled can cause the clinician to overestimate the likelihood of a particular diagnosis.[81–83]

Emotion and memory are tied together through the amygdala and hippocampus interaction. Furthermore, humans feel adverse outcomes more acutely than equivalent positive outcomes.[22] This effect is drastically increased in medicine, where bad outcomes can be catastrophic. It is also the case that recent memories are easier to recall and use, especially if they are vivid.

The availability heuristic and recency most affect the synthesis stage. The recency or vividness of a recalled outcome skews the synthesis, generally toward over-estimating the probability of a diagnosis or outcome.

The following case illustrates the availability heuristic. A clinician recently has a missed subdural hemorrhage in a patient with minimal trauma and not on anticoagulants. The clinician subsequently orders a head computed tomography (CT) on all patients with even minimal trauma because the memory is vivid. "I do CT all of them because that one time I got burned." The availability heuristic is contagious, and a single "bad case" can alter how all clinicians function in a local milieu.[81] The recency effect can also be individual or social. A single recent unusual case can lead to over-screening for the disease. For example, one clinician diagnoses Kawasaki's Disease, and then all the other clinicians in the group start over-screening for it.

The socialization of learning at the local level is a valuable intervention. Peer discussion of unusual cases and bad outcomes can motivate clinicians to generate a more balanced picture of the most expected outcomes and the community standard of care.

The Dunning–Kruger effect and overconfidence

The Dunning–Kruger effect is where marginal performers overestimate their ability.[84–86] Thanks to highly selective entry and prolonged high-quality training, few clinicians suffer from the Dunning–Kruger effect. But in selected scenarios, clinicians can make diagnostic errors by being overconfident in their ability to screen and manage rare and unusual conditions. It is simply not possible for any clinician to be 100% reliable in diagnosing and managing rare, subtle, and rapidly progressive diseases such as aortic dissection and Fournier's gangrene.

The expectation of high performance in rare and catastrophic diseases is self-imposed, as well as imposed by memorable models in popular culture such as "House MD." The overestimation of ability with rare diseases manifests throughout the clinical encounter. From the beginning, the clinician may think that it is within his clinical reach to detect rare and catastrophic outcomes. Going through the data acquisition phase, the clinician may believe that a routine history and exam will screen for rare and catastrophic conditions. In the synthesis phase, the clinician can easily mistake the "absence of evidence" for "evidence of absence" for rare and catastrophic conditions.

The following case illustrates overconfidence. A clinician sees a patient with chest pain and does not perform a structured clinical screening for aortic dissection because his "gut" does not tell him the patient may have an aortic dissection. The clinician does not ask if the pain is migratory or tearing or sudden and does not check pulses. Aortic dissection presents with a full set of typical symptoms and features in only in about 1/3 of patients (see Chapter 42). The patient did not present with a vivid picture of aortic dissection, and overconfidence leads the clinician to admit for evaluation of cardiac ischemia without further clinical screening to aortic dissection. About 12 hours into the admission, an undiagnosed partial dissection proceeds to full rupture, and the patient dies almost instantly. A brief structured clinical screening, including palpation of peripheral pulses and further investigation into the character of the pain is often all that is necessary to show "due diligence" in excluding aortic dissection, and no further testing is needed if the clinical screening is negative.[87]

Experience and recruitment of System 2 thinking do not reliably avoid misses in rare and catastrophic conditions. These conditions defy usual patterns, and their rarity means the average clinician will only see a handful of such cases in 2–3 decades of practice. There is also a downside to over-screening for rare and catastrophic conditions. Testing for diseases with a very low prevalence can yield many more false positives than true positives, leading to further overtesting.[88–90] The best approach is to structure the routine H and P with few additional elements that screen for rare and catastrophic conditions. For example, every patient with dizziness should be queried about diplopia and ataxia and receive a comprehensive neurological exam to detect posterior circulation stroke.[91–93] Every patient with chest pain should have radial and femoral arteries palpated for inequalities and queried if the pain is migratory.

Base rate neglect

Base rate neglect is an innate predisposition to weigh the likelihood of a diagnosis independent of its prevalence in the population of interest, or risk in the individual.[94,95] The base rate fallacy can play out on the low end or the high end of prevalence. On the low end of prevalence/risk, the base rate fallacy can lead to "zebra hunting," over-testing, and overdiagnosis.[96] Base rate neglect is influenced by previous clinical experience with rare outcomes or unusual presentation, especially if emotionally salient.

The following case illustrates neglect of low prevalence. A clinician sees an 18-year-old patient with sore throat and shortness of breath, no medical of family history, fever, and tachycardia to 120 bpm. On exam, the oropharynx is inflamed. Concerned the shortness of breath and tachycardia indicate a PE, the clinician orders a D-dimer, which is elevated. Thus, reinforced by the concern for PE, the clinician orders a CT pulmonary angiogram. During the procedure, the patient suffers a severe reaction with flushing and severe shortness of breath, requiring aggressive treatment to avoid intubation. The patient is observed overnight, where a throat swab confirms group A Streptococcus Pyogenes pharyngitis (Chapter 27).

On the high end of prevalence/risk, base rate neglect can lead to underdiagnosis. The following case illustrates neglect of a high base rate. A clinician sees a 60-year-old male with right lower quadrant pain. On exam, the patient has a low-grade fever and right quadrant tenderness to palpation. The white blood cell count is also elevated at 16,000/HPF (high power field). The CT is read as normal with no signs of appendicitis, and the clinician interprets this as ruling out appendicitis. The patient is discharged with abdominal precautions and returns the next septic with a ruptured appendix. After a rocky hospital course, he recovers and is discharged.

Base rate neglect and errors of statistical inference can interact synergistically to produce unfavorable outcome. Most commonly this occurs because clinicians are not naturally adept at understanding the effect of prevalence on test performance – that is, the difference between sensitivity/specificity and negative predictive value (NPV)/positive predictive value (PPV).[96]

In the low prevalence example, a more statistically aware interpretation would have helped the clinician know the positive D-dimer had a very low PPV for PE. In the high prevalence/risk example, the clinician took the sensitivity of negative CT abdomen and pelvis as also having a high NPV, and thus thought appendicitis had been ruled out.

Base rate neglect can be mitigated by diagnostic time-outs, greater attention to the performance features of frequently ordered tests, and a statistically aware approach to the effect of prevalence on PPV and NPV. Other names for this bias include neglect of prior probability and base rate fallacy.

Sunk cost bias

The sunk cost bias manifests bias increasing investment and unwillingness to abandon a position choice, or investment even when the evidence shows it was incorrect. The sunk cost bias is also known as irrational escalation and escalation of commitment.[97]

The sunk cost fallacy is most likely to affect the clinician at the time of disposition.[98] Ideally, a clinician should reconsider the diagnosis and all the available data before making a final diagnosis and disposition decision.[99] In addition to time pressure, the clinician has some emotional and reputational investment in not changing the diagnosis or disposition at the end. Reputationally, no clinician wants to be known as one who changes their mind frequently ("a flip-flopper") or as indecisive.

The following case illustrates the sunk cost bias. A clinician picks up a patient with abdominal pain. The RN (registered nurse) tells the clinician the patient is a frequent flyer and workups are always negative. This information is not conveyed neutrally – through tone and facial expression, the RN conveys irritation with the patient. The clinician thus becomes invested early in trying to avoid a CT scan. The physical exam and labs are normal, and the clinician readies the patient for discharge. The patient's exam is unchanged but now a mild tachycardia is present. For the reasons above, the clinician is too invested in the decision to change course and discharges the patient. The patient returns 2 days later septic from ruptured appendicitis but survives after a rocky course.

The sunk cost bias suppresses executive function and System 2 thinking. Executive function and System 2 thinking can be prompted by a Diagnostic Time Out. In the Diagnostic Time Out, the clinician should mobilize System 2 to briefly respool the key elements of the clinical exams, and labs of tests and compare the "fit" of the final diagnosis to the overall picture. In "Red Flag" functions, warning signs such as tachycardia at discharge, pain out of proportion to exam, and transient hypotension prompt reflection and Diagnostic Time Out. Forcing functions (also called behavior shaping constraints), such as mandatory time-outs, mandatory completion of early warning sign (EWS) Score when tachycardia is present, and policies against discharging patients with tachycardia are also effective for prevention of this and other biases.[100]

Ambiguity aversion

Ambiguity aversion manifests as a preference for known risks versus unknown risks. In the medical setting, ambiguity aversion can cause excessive testing or lead to a forced diagnosis that does not fit well but gives the impression of low risk.[101]

The following case illustrates ambiguity aversion. A 25-year-old female patient is seen for generalized abdominal pain and 1–2 loose bowel movements. The pain does not localize, labs are normal, and pregnancy is negative. Fearful of not providing a definitive answer, the clinician diagnoses the patient with "gastroenteritis," and discharges her. Despite worsening pain and 1–2 more loose bowel movements, she stays home, expecting her gastroenteritis to resolve. She is brought in by her roommate 3 days later after collapsing. She is found to be septic with a ruptured appendix.

The negative effects of ambiguity aversion can be mitigated by allowing for open-ended diagnoses such as "abdominal pain" when no diagnosis is clear. This approach requires a certain amount of risk tolerance and may require more explanation to the patient, but it diminishes the barrier to reconsideration of the diagnosis. The "Not Yet Diagnosed" strategy may also be effective.

Comment

Medical decision-making is complex and calls upon many of the clinician's mental resources.[102] Naturally present predispositions embedded in System 1, called cognitive biases, can lead to diagnostic error. The most prominent cognitive biases in emergency medicine are premature closure, diagnostic momentum, anchoring, availability heuristic, overconfidence, base rate neglect, sunk cost bias, and ambiguity aversion. Cognitive bias research continues to expand medical educator and quality improvement experts' ability to mitigate bias and reduce diagnostic error. Minimizing diagnostic error logically depends upon a thorough history and physical examination, but ED time constraints, operational flow expectations, frequent interruptions, and contemporary EHR documentation requirements are barriers to the idealistic bedside evaluation. Other strategizes include specific debiasing techniques that remain largely theoretical without demonstrable improvement improving patient safety by reducing diagnostic or decisional errors. Other approaches are intended to enhance reliability when making choices in the setting of uncertainty. By understanding the cognitive psychology of clinical decision-making, clinicians can claim more complete autonomy, agency, and reliability in the ED to optimize patient safety by reducing preventable medical error.

Notes

1 Libby Zion was an 18-year-old college student who died after an overdose. Her death was attributed to medical error caused by impaired cognition secondary to the extremely long resident work hours which were considered essential to training at the time. The landmark court case, concluded in 1995, sparked internal reforms as well as the Libby Zion Law which imposed legal limits on resident work hours.

2 The bandwagon effect is related to diagnostic momentum. The bandwagon effect is said to occur when one clinician makes a diagnosis early on multiple other clinicians adopt uncritically.

References

1. Kane B, Carpenter C. Chapter 17: Cognition and decision making. In: Fondahn E, De Fer TM, Lane M, Vannucci A, editors. *Washington manual of patient safety and quality improvement*. Philadelphia (PA): Lippincott Williams & Wilkins; 2016.

2. Antonacci AC, Dechario SP, Antonacci C *et al.* Cognitive bias impact on management of postoperative complications, medical error, and standard of care. *The Journal of Surgical Research.* 2021; 258: 47–53.
3. Saposnik G, Redelmeier D, Ruff C, Tobler P. Cognitive biases associated with medical decisions: A systematic review. *BMC Medical Informatics and Decision Making.* 2016; 16(1): 1–14.
4. Croskerry P, Cosby K, Graber M, Singh H. *Diagnosis: Interpreting the shadows.* London: CRC Press; 2017. doi: 10.1201/9781315116334.
5. Graber M. The incidence of diagnostic error in medicine. *BMJ Quality and Safety.* 2013; 22(Suppl 2): ii21–7.
6. Sinek S, editor. *The infinite game.* London: Penguin; 2019.
7. Carse J, editor. *Finite and infinite games.* New York: Simon and Schuster; 2011.
8. Croskerry P, Sinclair D. Emergency medicine: A practice prone to error? *CJEM.* 2001; 3(04): 271–6.
9. Croskerry P. The importance of cognitive errors in diagnosis and strategies to minimize them. *Academic Medicine.* 2003; 78(8): 775–80.
10. Norman G, Eva K. Diagnostic error and clinical reasoning. *Medical Education.* 2010; 44(1): 94–100.
11. Saleh J, Marais K. Highlights from the early (and pre-) history of reliability engineering. *Reliability Engineering and System Safety.* 2006; 91(2): 249–56.
12. Buschman T, Siegel M, Roy J, Miller E. Neural substrates of cognitive capacity limitations. *Proceedings of the National Academy of Sciences of the United States of America.* 2011; 108(27): 11252–5.
13. Silvagni S, Napoletano L, Graziani I, Le Blaye P, Rognin L. Concept for Human Performance Envelope. https://www.futuresky-safety.eu/wp-content/uploads/2015/12/FSS_P6_DBL_D6.1-Concept-for-Human-Performance-Envelope_v2.0.pdf. 2022. Accessed January 6, 2022.
14. Kahneman D, editor. *Thinking, Fast and Slow.* New York: Farrar, Straus and Giroux; 2011.
15. Campbell S, Croskerry P, Bond W. Profiles in patient safety: A "perfect storm" in the emergency department. Journal of Academic Emergency Medicine. 2007; 14(8): 743–9.
16. Croskerry P. Critical thinking and reasoning in emergency medicine. In: Croskerry P, Cosby KS, Schenkel SM, Wears RL, editors. *Patient Safety in Emergency Medicine.* Philadelphia (PA): Lippincott Williams & Wilkins; 2009: 213–8.
17. Norman G, Monteiro S, Sherbino J, Ilgen J, Schmidt H, Mamede S. The causes of errors in clinical reasoning. *Academic Medicine.* 2017; 92(1): 23–30.
18. Malenka RC, Nestler EJ, Hyman SE. Higher cognitive function and behavioral control. In: Sydor A, Brown RY, editors. *Molecular neuropharmacology: A foundation for clinical neuroscience.* New York: McGraw-Hill Medical; 2009: 313–21.
19. Croskerry P. Clinical cognition and diagnostic error: Applications of a dual process model of reasoning. *Advances in Health Sciences Education.* 2009; 14(S1): 27–35.
20. Norman G. Dual processing and diagnostic errors. *Advances in Health Sciences Education.* 2009; 14(S1): 37–49.

21. McCall T. The impact of long working hours on resident physicians. *The New England Journal of Medicine*. 1988; 318(12): 775–8.

22. Kahneman D, Tversky A. Prospect theory: An analysis of decision under risk. *Econometrica*. 1979; 47(2): 263–92.

23. Kahneman D, Slovic P, Tversky A, editors. *Judgment under uncertainty: Heuristics and biases*. 1st ed. Cambridge: Cambridge University Press; 1982.

24. Brush JE Jr, Lee M, Sherbino J, Taylor-Fishwick JC, Norman G. Effect of teaching bayesian methods using learning by concept vs learning by example on medical students' ability to estimate probability of a diagnosis: A randomized clinical trial. *JAMA Network Open*. 2019; 2(12): e1918023.

25. Tomaszewski C, Nestler D, Shah K *et al*. Clinical policy: Critical issues in the evaluation and management of emergency department patients with suspected non-ST-elevation acute coronary syndromes. *Annals of Emergency Medicine*. 2018; 72(5): e65–106.

26. Reid MC, Lane DA, Feinstein AR. Academic calculations versus clinical judgments: Practicing physicians' use of quantitative measures of test accuracy. *The American Journal of Medicine*. 1998; 104(4): 374–80.

27. Wolf SJ, Hahn SA, Nentwich L, Raja A, Silvers S, Brown M. Clinical policy: Critical issues in the evaluation and management of adult patients presenting to the emergency department with suspected acute venous thromboembolic disease. *Annals of Emergency Medicine*. 2018; 71(5): e59–109.

28. Edlow JA. Managing patients with acute episodic dizziness. *Annals of Emergency Medicine*. 2018; 72(5): 602–10.

29. Al-Najjar N, Weinstein J. The ambiguity aversion literature: A critical assessment. *Economics and Philosophy*. 2009; 25(3): 249–84.

30. Al-Najjar N. A Bayesian framework for the precautionary principle. *The Journal of Legal Studies*. 2015; 44(S2): S337–65.

31. Hartigan S, Brooks M, Hartley S, Miller R, Santen S, Hemphill R. Review of the basics of cognitive error in emergency medicine: Still no easy answers. *The Western Journal of Emergency Medicine*. 2020; 21(6): 125–31.

32. Lambe K, O'Reilly G, Kelly B, Curristan S. Dual-process cognitive interventions to enhance diagnostic reasoning: A systematic review. *BMJ Quality and Safety*. 2016; 25(10): 808–20.

33. Ludolph R, Schulz P. Debiasing health-related judgments and decision making: A systematic review. *Medical Decision Making*. 2017; 38(1): 3–13.

34. Croskerry P. Diagnostic failure: A cognitive and affective approach. In: Henriksen K, Battles JB, Marks ES *et al.*, editors. *Advances in patient safety: From research to implementation (Volume 2: Concepts and methodology)*. Rockville (MD): Agency for Healthcare Research and Quality (US); 2005. https://www.ncbi.nlm.nih.gov/books/NBK20487/.

35. Mirhoseini S, Hassanein K, Head M, Watter S. User performance in the face of IT interruptions: The role of executive functions. In: Davis FD, Riedl R, vom Brocke J, Léger P-M, Randolph AB, Fischer T, editors. *Information systems and neuroscience*. Cham: Springer; 2020: 41–51.

36. Foroughi CK, Malihi P, Boehm-Davis DA. Working memory capacity and errors following interruptions. *Journal of Applied Research in Memory and Cognition.* 2016; 5(4): 410–4.
37. Henneman EA, Marquard JL, Nicholas C *et al.* The stay S.A.F.E. strategy for managing interruptions reduces distraction time in the simulated clinical setting. *Critical Care Nursing Quarterly.* 2018; 41(2): 215–23.
38. Jha AP, Stanley EA, Kiyonaga A, Wong L, Gelfand L. Examining the protective effects of mindfulness training on working memory capacity and affective experience. *Emotion.* 2010; 10(1): 54–64.
39. Croskerry P. From mindless to mindful practice — cognitive bias and clinical decision making. *The New England Journal of Medicine.* 2013; 368(26): 2445–8.
40. Burgess D, Beach M, Saha S. Mindfulness practice: A promising approach to reducing the effects of clinician implicit bias on patients. *Patient Education and Counseling.* 2017; 100(2): 372–6.
41. Venditti EG. Avoiding diagnostic fixation errors: A person-focused approach to human factors analysis. In: Zimmerman DL, Osborn-Harrison DG, editors. *Person-focused health care management: A foundational guide for health care managers.* New York: Springer Publishing Company; 2016: 203–10.
42. Westbrook JI, Raban MZ, Walter SR, Douglas H. Task errors by emergency physicians are associated with interruptions, multitasking, fatigue and working memory capacity: A prospective, direct observation study. *BMJ Quality and Safety.* 2018; 27(8): 655–63.
43. Walter SR, Raban MZ, Dunsmuir WTM, Douglas HE, Westbrook JI. Emergency doctors' strategies to manage competing workload demands in an interruptive environment: An observational workflow time study. *Applied Ergonomics.* 2017; 58: 454–60.
44. Lim D, Mosinski N, Perfetti J, Powers E, Augustine J. Optimizing Emergency Department Workspace to Promote Wellness - Page 2 of 4 - ACEP Now. ACEP Now. https://www.acepnow.com/article/optimizing-emergency-department-workspace-to-promote-wellness/2/?singlepage=1. 2019. Accessed January 6, 2022.
45. Prakash S, Sladek RM, Schuwirth L. Interventions to improve diagnostic decision making: A systematic review and meta-analysis on reflective strategies. *Medical Teacher.* 2018; 41(5): 517–24.
46. Monteiro SD, Sherbino J, Patel A, Mazzetti I, Norman GR, Howey E. Reflecting on diagnostic errors: Taking a second look is not enough. *Journal of General Internal Medicine.* 2015; 30(9): 1270–4.
47. Gershon CA, Yagapen AN, Lin A, Yanez D, Sun BC. Inter-rater reliability of the HEART score. *Academic Emergency Medicine.* 2019; 26(5): 552–5.
48. Laureiro-Martinez D. Cognitive control capabilities, routinization propensity, and decision-making performance. *Organization Science.* 2014; 25(4): 1111–33.
49. Osler W. An address on the medical clinic: A retrospect and a forecast: Delivered before the Abernethian Society, St. Bartholomew's Hospital, London, December 4th, 1913. *BMJ.* 1914; 1(2766): 10–6.

50. Norman G, Sherbino J, Dore K *et al.* The etiology of diagnostic errors: A controlled trial of system 1 versus system 2 reasoning. *Academic Medicine.* 2014; 89(2): 277–84.
51. Karelaia N, Jochen R. Improving decision making through mindfulness. In: Reb J, Paul WBA, editors. *Mindfulness in organizations: Foundations, research, and applications.* Cambridge: Cambridge University Press; 2015: 256–84.
52. Im S, Marder M, Imbriano G, Sussman T, Mohanty A. Effects of a brief mindfulness-based attentional intervention on threat-related perceptual decision-making. *Mindfulness.* 2021; 12(4): 959–69.
53. Kane A. Mindfulness and Developing Decision Making. https://www.workpsychologyhub.co.uk/wp-content/uploads/2017/03/White-Paper-Mindfulness-and-Decision-Making.pdf. 2022. Accessed January 6, 2022.
54. Carpenter CR, Kane BG, Carter M, Lucas R, Wilbur LG, Graffeo CS. Incorporating evidence-based medicine into resident education: A CORD survey of faculty and resident expectations. *Academic Emergency Medicine.* 2010; 17(Suppl 2): S54–61.
55. Rising KL, Powell RE, Cameron KA *et al.* Development of the uncertainty communication checklist: A patient-centered approach to patient discharge from the emergency department. *Academic Medicine.* 2020; 95(7): 1026–34.
56. Pizzi L, Goldfarb N, Nash D. Crew resource management and its applications in medicine. In: Shojania KG, Duncan BW, McDonald KM, Wachter RM, Markowitz AJ, editors. *Making health care safer: A critical analysis of patient safety practices.* Vol. 44. Evidence report/technology assessment (summary). Maryland, USA: Agency for Healthcare Research and Quality, Rockville; 2001: 511–9.
57. Weinberg A, Ullian L, Richards W, Cooper P. Informal advice- and information-seeking between physicians. *Journal of Medical Education.* 1981; 56(3): 174–80.
58. Reijnders U, Bakker K, Schuitmaker I, Dorn T. Does peer consultation between forensic physicians reduce inter-doctor variation when issuing medical death certifications? *Journal of Forensic and Legal Medicine.* 2021; 81: 102187.
59. Bravo-Lillo C, Cranor L, Komanduri S, Schechter S, Sleeper M. Harder to ignore? Revisiting pop-up fatigue and approaches to prevent it. Paper presented at: 10th Symposium On Usable Privacy and Security; July 9–11, 2014; MenloPark, CA.
60. van der Sijs H. Errors related to alert fatigue. In: Agrawal A, editor. *Safety of health IT.* Cham: Springer; 2016: 41–54.
61. Salwei M, Carayon P, Hoonakker P *et al.* Workflow integration analysis of a human factors-based clinical decision support in the emergency department. *Applied Ergonomics.* 2021; 97: 103498.
62. Treadwell J, Lucas S, Tsou A. Surgical checklists: A systematic review of impacts and implementation. *BMJ Quality and Safety.* 2013; 23(4): 299–318.
63. Gao M, Martin P, Motal J *et al.* A multidisciplinary discharge timeout checklist improves patient education and captures discharge process errors. *Quality Management in Health Care.* 2018; 27(2): 63–8.
64. Morewedge CK, Yoon H, Scopelliti I, Symborski C, Korris J, Kassam K. Debiasing decisions: Improved decision making with a single training intervention. *Policy Insights From the Behavioral and Brain Sciences.* 2015; 2(1): 129–40.

65. Sellier A, Scopelliti I, Morewedge C. Debiasing training improves decision making in the field. *Psychological Science.* 2019; 30(9): 1371–9.
66. Monteiro S, Sherbino J, Sibbald M, Norman G. Critical thinking, biases and dual processing: The enduring myth of generalisable skills. *Medical Education.* 2019; 54(1): 66–73.
67. Monteiro S, Sherbino J, Ilgen J *et al.* Disrupting diagnostic reasoning. *Academic Medicine.* 2015; 90(4): 511–7.
68. US Marine Corps. Combat and operational stress control. Marine Corps Reference Publication (MCRP) 6-11C and Navy Tactics, Techniques, and Procedures (NTTP) 1-15M. Washington, DC: Dept. of the Navy, Headquarters, U.S. Marine Corps; 2010.
69. Baumeister RF, Faber JE, Wallace HM. Coping and ego depletion: Recovery after the coping process. In: Snyder CR, editor. *Coping: The psychology of what works.* New York: Oxford University Press; 1999: 50–69.
70. Chen M, Chen L, Yan X, Yu Z, Fang Y, Yu Y. Investigating the nonlinear effect of ego depletion on safety compliance: The moderating role of rumination. *Journal of Safety Research.* 2018; 67: 27–35.
71. Beardsley JR, Schomberg R, Heatherly S, Williams B. Implementation of a standardized discharge time-out process to reduce prescribing errors at discharge. *Hospital Pharmacy.* 2013; 48(1): 39–47.
72. Koethe L, Vanderhoef M. Improving transitional care in rural health using a standardized discharge time-out process. http://hdl.handle.net/10755/20745. 2020. Accessed January 7, 2022.
73. Pines J. Profiles in patient safety: Confirmation bias in emergency medicine. *Academic Emergency Medicine.* 2006; 13(1): 90–4.
74. Ryan W. Diagnostic momentum error. In: Raz M, Pouryahya P, editors. *Decision making in emergency medicine.* Singapore: Springer; 2021: 117–22.
75. Nagaraj G, Hullick C, Arendts G, Burkett E, Hill K, Carpenter C. Avoiding anchoring bias by moving beyond 'mechanical falls' in geriatric emergency medicine. *Emergency Medicine Australasia.* 2018; 30(6): 843–50.
76. Richie M, Josephson SA. Quantifying heuristic bias: Anchoring, availability, and representativeness. *Teaching and Learning in Medicine.* 2017; 30(1): 67–75.
77. Mamede S, Schmidt HG, Rikers R. Diagnostic errors and reflective practice in medicine. *Journal of Evaluation in Clinical Practice.* 2007; 13(1): 138–45.
78. Lawson AE, Daniel ES. Inferences of clinical diagnostic reasoning and diagnostic error. *Journal of Biomedical Informatics.* 2011; 44(3): 402–12.
79. Graber ML, Franklin N, Gordon R. Diagnostic error in internal medicine. *Archives of Internal Medicine.* 2005; 165(13): 1493–9.
80. Stanton N, Wong W, Gore J, Sevdalis N, Strub M. Critical thinking. *Theoretical Issues in Ergonomics Science.* 2011; 12(3): 204–9.
81. Ly DP. The influence of the availability heuristic on physicians in the emergency department. *Annals of Emergency Medicine.* 2021; 78(5): 650–7.
82. Mamede S, van Gog T, van den Berge K *et al.* Effect of availability bias and reflective reasoning on diagnostic accuracy among internal medicine residents. *Journal of the American Medical Association.* 2010; 304(11): 1198–203.

83. van den Berge K, Mamede S. Cognitive diagnostic error in internal medicine. *European Journal of Internal Medicine*. 2013; 24(6): 525–9.
84. Rahmani M. Medical trainees and the Dunning–Kruger effect: When they don't know what they don't know. *Journal of Graduate Medical Education*. 2020; 12(5): 532–4.
85. Tan LT. Innovations in continuing professional development — countering the Dunning–Kruger effect. *Clinical Oncology*. 2011; 23(10): 659–61.
86. Prozesky DR, Molwantwa M, Nkomazana O, Kebaetse M. Intern preparedness for the CanMEDS roles and the Dunning-Kruger effect: A survey. *BMC Medical Education*. 2019; 19(1): 422.
87. Strayer RJ, Shearer PL, Hermann LK. Screening, evaluation, and early management of acute aortic dissection in the ED. *Current Cardiology Reviews*. 2012; 8(2): 152–7.
88. Carpenter CR, Raja AS, Brown MD. Overtesting and the downstream consequences of overtreatment: Implications of "preventing overdiagnosis" for emergency medicine. *Academic Emergency Medicine*. 2015; 22(12): 1484–92.
89. Diamandis EP, Li M. The side effects of translational omics: Overtesting, overdiagnosis, overtreatment. *Clinical Chemistry and Laboratory Medicine (CCLM)*. 2016; 54(3): 389–96.
90. O'Sullivan JW, Albasri A, Nicholson B *et al*. Overtesting and undertesting in primary care: A systematic review and meta-analysis. *BMJ Open*. 2018; 8(2): e018557.
91. Barnett HJM. A modern approach to posterior circulation ischemic stroke. *Archives of Neurology*. 2002; 59(3): 359–60.
92. Runchey S, McGee S. Does this patient have a hemorrhagic stroke? *Journal of the American Medical Association*. 2010; 303(22): 2280–6.
93. Siniscalchi A, Sztajzel R, Malferrari G, Gallelli L. The National Institutes of Health Stroke Scale: Its role in patients with posterior circulation stroke. *Hospital Topics*. 2017; 95(4): 79–81.
94. Morgenstern J. Base rate neglect. In: Raz M, Pouryahya P, editors. *Decision making in emergency medicine*. Singapore: Springer; 2021: 59–63.
95. Thompson C. Clinical experience as evidence in evidence-based practice. *Journal of Advanced Nursing*. 2003; 43(3): 230–7.
96. Kuklin B. Probability misestimates in medical care. Arkansas Law Review. 2006; 59(3): 527–54.
97. Braverman JA, Blumenthal-Barby JS. Assessment of the sunk-cost effect in clinical decision-making. *Social Science & Medicine*. 2012; 75(1): 186–92.
98. Coleman MD. Sunk cost and commitment to medical treatment. *Current Psychology*. 2010; 29(2): 121–34.
99. Hafenbrack AC, Kinias Z, Barsade SG. Debiasing the mind through meditation: Mindfulness and the sunk cost bias. *Psychological Science*. 2014; 25(2): 369–76.
100. Sehgal NL, Fox M, Sharpe BA, Vidyarthi AR, Blegen M, Wachter RM. Critical conversations: A call for a nonprocedural "time out". *Journal of Hospital Medicine*. 2011; 6(4): 225–30.

101. Han PKJ, Williams A, Haskins A *et al.* Individual differences in aversion to ambiguity regarding medical tests and treatments: Association with cancer screening cognitions. *Cancer Epidemiology, Biomarkers & Prevention.* 2014; 23(12): 2916–23.

102. Sandhu H, Carpenter C, Freeman K, Nabors S, Olson A. Clinical decisionmaking: Opening the black box of cognitive reasoning. *Annals of Emergency Medicine.* 2006; 48(6): 713–9.

Chapter 61 **Diagnosis in Telemedicine**

John Bedolla[1] and Jesse M. Pines[2,3]

[1] Department of Surgery and Perioperative Care, Dell Medical School, University of Texas, Austin, TX, USA
[2] US Acute Care Solutions, Canton, OH, USA
[3] Department of Emergency Medicine, Drexel University, Philadelphia, PA, USA

Highlights

- The use of telemedicine increased dramatically after the onset of the COVID-19 pandemic.
- Given current trends, telemedicine is likely here to stay.
- Understanding the benefits and limitations of diagnosis in telemedicine is important.
- The limitations of telemedicine include the lack of an ability to perform multiple parts of the physical examination, and obtain laboratory and imaging information.
- Peripheral tools can increase the fidelity of the telemedicine encounter.
- Specific complaints in emergency care are more or less amenable to telemedicine diagnosis.

The first wave of the coronavirus 2019 (COVID-19) pandemic (2020–early 2021) spurred a massive increase in telemedicine utilization.[1,2] The COVID-19 pandemic made the remote medical evaluation more appealing to patients, hospitals, and clinicians.[3,4] It also broke down the two most important barriers to adoption: reimbursement and regulatory constraints.[5–7] At the time of this writing, the United States is in the fifth wave of the COVID pandemic, which will likely spur adoption of telemedicine further.[5]

However, telemedicine is not only increasing due to the COVID-19 pandemic. Prior to the pandemic, several use cases for telemedicine had been developed and were in place, such as tele-stroke, tele-intensive care (ICU), tele-neonatology, and tele-emergency department (ED). Going forward, there are multiple forces that ensure telemedicine will play an increasing role in acute care. Patients voice a strong preference for telemedicine as a convenient way to take care of chronic and even acute medical needs. Insurers see telemedicine as a way to drive down costs. Regulators and physician leaders think telemedicine will increase access to underserved populations and decrease the barrier to entry for medical care for all patients. Physicians also voice greater acceptance and satisfaction with telemedicine as an option in their practice profile.[8]

This revolution in medicine, in which the physician sees the patient not in person but remotely, was not directed by an academic study or detailed long-term planning. Instead, rapid advances in the quality, security, and cost of two-way audiovisual technology made it possible for telemedicine to be adopted rapidly in the setting of favorable market forces and a disruptive pandemic.[9] For the individual clinician and the physician leader this presents a reversal of the normal adoption process for new medical processes.[10] Optimally, medical processes are adopted only after academic studies show their efficacy.[11] Regardless, market forces, patient preference, and improving technology all ensure that telemedicine will continue to grow.

Emergency groups and clinicians who want to stay relevant in the changing ecosystem need to understand how the emergency telemedicine encounter is similar to, and differs from, the in-person emergency encounter. There are fundamental differences in the raw clinical data that can be obtained in the two encounter types, and understanding these differences is essential to utilizing telemedicine.

Emergency groups and clinicians must therefore ask themselves a series of strategic questions to decide not *if* telemedicine is going to be part of their practice profile but rather *how* to adapt to telemedicine and ensure that it is used in the populations, settings, and for clinical conditions where they can provide the best care for their patients. In this chapter, we pose and answer what we consider to be the important strategic questions for the clinician or clinician leader considering adoption of telemedicine.

The Society for Academic Emergency Medicine (SAEM) addressed Telehealth in emergency medicine (EM) at the 2020 consensus conference.[12] The authors reached consensus on evidence to support the feasibility of telehealth to improve health care access to acute, unscheduled care in a variety of settings and conditions. According to the report, they found that telemedicine has been shown to improve care efficiency including lower length of stays and decreased transfer rates. Yet, the authors report the lack of objective and controlled studies describing benefits to patient-level or population-level health outcomes. Telemedicine is a tool that can potentially mitigate disparities in access, and better understanding of how telehealth influences patient's access and health outcomes in rural and underserved settings are needed. The consensus group created a list of priorities and future research agenda available in Table 61.1.

Table 61.1 Research questions for telehealth in emergency care

Educational needs and outcomes
Competencies and training
1. What are the core competencies in telehealth common to all providers, regardless of role, specialty, or training?
2. What gaps in current EM training exist to adapt practice to telehealth?
3. In patient–provider telehealth, what are components of video-based physical examinations?

Educational approaches
4. What educational experiences and instructional modalities are effective to teach telehealth in EM?
5. How do we train ED providers in virtual presence for patient-to-provider and provider-to-provider telehealth?
6. What are the best ways to integrate telehealth into EM training?
7. How do we train interprofessional teams in EM to deliver collaborative telehealth care?

Health care access
Patient- and population-level outcomes
8. How does access to emergency telehealth vary by patient or population characteristics?
9. When improved access from telehealth, what are patient-level and population-level outcomes?
10. What are the costs and cost-effectiveness of telehealth from the patient and system perspective, and what is best way assess the value of increased access versus excessive utilization?

Quality of care delivery
11. Among the underserved, how are disparities in emergency care impacted by telehealth?

Outcomes of telehealth programs
12. What are the barriers and facilitators of implementation of ED telehealth such as payment models or care delivery systems?

Process measures in telehealth
13. What lessons have been learned from expansions of telehealth during the COVID-19 pandemic?
14. What are the barriers and facilitators to improving access and quality for underserved populations using telehealth?

(Continued)

Table 61.1 (*Continued*)

Quality/safety

15. How can telehealth be used to improve transitions of care?
16. When should the quality and safety of telehealth be compared to in-person care and when should it be compared to "no care"?
17. In what clinical conditions, populations, and settings do emergency telehealth improve patient and process outcomes?

Facilitating research

18. How should telehealth be used for EM research, including recruitment, informed consent, reducing attrition, and data collection?
19. What populations require special considerations as in EM telehealth research and what are the barriers for engaging these populations in studies?

Workforce

20. How effective can telehealth for hospitals, particularly rural and critical access, who face trouble staffing with board-certified EM physicians?
21. What types of training should be required for practicing providers?
22. What kinds of staffing are best suited for emergency telehealth in different settings (e.g., advanced practice provider [APP] versus physician, rural versus urban, etc.)?
23. What kinds of staffing and systems are needed to ensure provider efficiency in emergency telehealth?

Source: Adapted from [12].

Does the telemedicine evaluation have the same fidelity as the in-person evaluation?

No. Compared with the in-person evaluation, the telemedicine evaluation provides less perceptual information to the clinician. In the telemedicine evaluation smell and touch are not possible. Relative to the human eye, which can instantaneously scan and focus wherever the clinician directs attention, similar functions of computer and phone cameras are slow and limited. The human eye is equivalent to a 50-millimeter lens, but most teleconferencing cameras are a wider lens which, relative to the human eye, has a spherical, or "fisheye" distortion. For practical purposes, the limit of resolution of the human eye is about 8K (e.g. a horizontal resolution of 8000 pixels). At either end of the telemedicine encounter, the resolution is usually limited to standard definition (SD) or high definition (HD), which are much lower than 8K. The refresh rate of the human eye is 1000/second or 1000 Hz. By contrast, the standard refresh rate of computer screens is 30 Hz.[13-16] Many subtle emotional micro-expressions and cues happen at 1/100 of a second or faster, far beyond the ability of the video to pick up and limiting the ability of the clinician to pick up on some subtle cues.[17-21] Additionally, without special equipment, the telemedicine visual inspection is from a single camera, precluding accurate depth perception. The color spectrum of the camera and computer screen are also compressed compared with natural vision.[22,23]

Microphones can pick up higher and lower frequency sounds than the human ear, but they are inferior in most other ways. Human hearing is three-dimensional meaning the human brain stem uses subtle differences in timing and character of the sound in the right versus left ear different ear to generate an "image" of the space and the objects in it. While this is not a high-resolution ability in humans, it is largely lost in the telemedicine format. Like the human eye can zoom and focus, the human ear has an ability to focus on sound in a particular direction and pitch – this is called the "cocktail party effect" and allows the human ear to pick up conversation even in a complex environment. By contrast, the microphone picks up all sounds with the same affinity.[24]

Can you obtain a reliable history of present illness, past history, family history, and social history in the telemedicine format?

There are no head-to-head studies comparing the quality and reliability of the in person versus telemedicine history taking in emergency care. There are studies in several disciplines which indirectly compare the quality of history taking by focusing on endpoints intuitively related to the quality of the history taking. In the surgical and anesthesia literature, the endpoint of canceled or delayed surgery has been compared in telemedicine and in-person presurgical screening. The rate of surgical cancelation due to inadequate or missing elements of the history is close to the same independently if the patient was seen through telemedicine or in person.[25-27] Mullen-Fortino et al.[28] performed a retrospective review of 361 patients with telemedicine presurgical evaluations and 7442 patients with in-person presurgical evaluations and similar rates of cancelation (0% telemedicine versus 1.1% for in-person). In neurology, there are several head-to-head comparisons of clinical efficacy in conditions which require extensive history taking.[29-32] Müller et al.[33] randomized 409 patients to telemedicine versus in-person management of nonacute headaches and found no differences in treatment compliance or patient satisfaction, but did find that rural patients in the telemedicine group had less frequent headache visits at 3-month follow-up. There is also a robust body of literature showing the noninferiority of telepsychiatry with in-person psychiatry – a discipline in which the history is the essential evaluation.[34-36]

Besides the microphone and camera, what other peripheral tools are available to increase the amount of perceptual information available to the clinician?

Telemedicine software platforms fall under the Food and Drug Administration (FDA) regulation as medical devices.[37] The regulation extends to software applications (apps) that might yield information that could be critical and require acute intervention. Examples include apps that connect to electrocardiogram (ECG) equipment, measure physiologic parameters used in diagnosis, calibrate cochlear implants, connect to bedside monitors that transfer data to doctors or nurses, altar pump infusion rates, or amplify sounds from electronic stethoscopes. The FDA generally encourages innovation and has taken a hands-off approach to most software apps, except when the app provides a diagnosis or attempts to substitute for the clinician's judgment.[38] A recent example was the removal of the Visibly Online Refractive Vision Test, which was judged to provide diagnostic information while excluding the clinician.[39] However, devices or apps used synchronously in the telemedicine encounter to enhance the amount of perceptual information, such as high-resolution cameras, ophthalmoscopes, or otoscope apps or devices, are largely unregulated and will likely remain so in the setting of a continuing pandemic.

Most tools designed to increase the amount of perceptual information available to the clinician are not stand-alone devices. Rather, they are apps the patient can install on a mobile phone or desktop computer. These apps use the native functionality of the device to deliver added information synchronously to the clinician. Examples include eye and retinal visualization apps, middle ear, intranasal and oropharyngeal, visualization apps, skin magnification apps, and stethoscope apps.[40]

Some stand-alone peripherals are available such as electronic stethoscopes, tele-ophthalmoscopes, video-otoscopes, electronic dermatoscopes, digital endoscopes, and electronic scales.[41,42] The primary target customer for these peripherals are clinics, EDs, and hospitals for specialty consultation rather than consumers, due to expense and setup complexity.[43–48] These devices do allow for specialty consultation, such as telestroke, teleophthalmology, second opinions, enhanced resident supervision, and teletriage. Most regular telemedicine encounters are still mediated through computers or mobile devices equipped with a camera, visual display, audio input, and audio output.

Can wearable devices enhance the telemedicine encounter?

Consumer-driven wearables for personal and sports use have become commonplace. Examples include smart watches, shirts with built-in electronic connected hardware, connected jewelry, smartphone apps, eyeglasses, earbuds, and headbands. These devices can deliver cardiac rhythms, step counts, sleep cycles, respiratory rate, accelerometry data, location, distances, temperature, respiratory rate, oxygen saturation, blood pressure, and skin plethysmography data.[49-51] Aggregate data from millions of these devices are useful at the population level for limited patient-specific apps, such as adherence to home quarantine. Yet for making patient-specific clinical decisions, four problems arise: (i) consumer devices are not reliable enough to make high-risk decisions, (ii) few of these devices are FDA approved, (iii) there are no reference standards for consumer devices, and (iv) the makers of these devices have largely treated these medical functionalities as marketing tools and not as true medical devices, and consequently few have been tested to a medical standard of reliability. Studies have shown that, outside of the laboratory setting, they are less reliable for measuring heart rate, step-counting, activity, sleep, and other health measures.[52-58] Consumer wearable devices may enhance the telemedicine encounter, but they do not add information that would be considered medically reliable. They should be used with caution in the telemedicine encounter when they are not FDA approved.[59]

Can patients accurately measure their own vital signs?

There is published evidence that people without medical training can be directed in real time to obtain a reliable measure of heart rate.[60,61] However, accuracy does appear to diminish with advancing age due to age-related decline in finger sensitivity.[62] Accuracy of temperature taking appears to be primarily related to the device used. Since there are no reference standards for consumer-level thermometers, measurements should be used with caution. Automated blood pressure devices have a reasonable high reliability; however, there is a wide range of reliability in nonvalidated devices. Operator error is also common, and therefore, it is probably best to observe the patient while the self-measurement takes place. It is best to know the brand and price of the blood pressure device to get a sense of how accurate it is. There are few studies on the reliability of oxygen saturation using consumer devices.[63-68] Measurement of respiratory rate is unreliable by most methods. It is often inaccurate even in the hands of professionals because they are noncompliant with waiting a full minute to measure the respiratory rate. It is therefore unlikely that self-measured respiratory rate is reliable.[69-73]

Can you assess dyspnea in the telemedicine format?

One pediatric study included 148 patients and 135 paired observations and reported interclass coefficient rating of 0.95 (confidence interval [CI] 0.93–0.96) showing high concordance between telemedicine and in-person assessment of dyspnea. The Roth Score, which involves having the patient count to 30 as rapidly as possible and noting the highest number has been shown to be reliable in one small study of 93 patients. The Roth Score was shown to be valuable in the assessment of dyspnea in 500 patients with suspected COVID-19.[74-76]

Can the National Institute of Health Stroke Scale (NIHSS) be performed in the telemedicine format?

Telemedicine administration of the National Institute of Health Stroke Scale (NIHSS) appears to generate reliable results. Investigators have compared the in person and the telemedicine exam directly and found a strong positive correlation. In a study of 174 patients receiving an in-person NIHSS versus a telemedicine NIHSS, 2% of telemedicine consultations could not be completed and the telemedicine NIHSS were concordant 88% of the time for a $\kappa = 0.73$.[77] Another study found high or moderate agreement with all elements except ataxia, which was poor.[78] Compared with in-person NIHSS for tissue plasminogen activator (tPA) or thrombolysis, the telemedicine exam results in equal sometimes faster administration times. The use of telemedicine consultation was also associated with a higher rate of tPA administration in remote locations. Of note, the NIHSS in all these studies is used in a consultative role, not as the only neurological exam performed.[79,80] Considering the high stakes and liability involved in stroke care, the telemedicine administered NIHSS remains a consultative rather than stand-alone modality. For the emergency clinician in-person administration of the NIHSS by the emergency clinician or the neurologist remains the gold standard, and tele-neurological evaluation is valuable for confirmation and consultation.[81-83]

Can a psychiatric assessment be done in the telemedicine format?

Psychiatric assessment lends itself well to the telemedicine format and has been shown to be effective in multiple studies and meta-analyses,[84-88] including among pediatric patients.[89]

A systematic review of the use of telepsychiatry in depression found that patient satisfaction is equivalent to or higher than face-to-face interventions. Both telemedicine and control groups had improvement on depressive symptoms. Despite the increased cost upfront for telemedicine due to the technology required, telemedicine would eventually be more cost-effective due to reducing travel expenses.[90] Another systematic review regarding the use of telepsychiatry in geriatric patients found that tele mental health is feasible and well accepted when used in inpatient areas and nursing homes for consultation, cognitive testing assessments, dementia diagnosis and treatment, depression management, and psychotherapy.[91] This systematic review found that the main barrier to broader implementation of telemedicine for geriatric patients was Medicare reimbursement, limiting the development of telemedicine programs in the pre-COVID era. Many older adults have mobility problems or difficulties finding a care partner to take them to appointments, and home-based telemedicine services would allow for better access to care.

A systematic review of telemedicine for older adults with dementia during COVID-19 found that telemedicine was a feasible approach for cognitive and mental health assessments (e.g., Montreal Cognitive Assessment [MoCA], focused assessment with sonography for trauma [FAST], etc. – see Chapter 57). Telemedicine appears effective in connecting persons living with dementia and their health care providers while reducing travel difficulties or challenges.[92] A qualitative study on emergency physician's perspective on using telehealth with older adults found that telemedicine gained acceptability among ED physicians and provided options to patients who may have otherwise deferred care.[93]

Can orthopedic injuries be reliably assessed in the telemedicine format?

Telemedicine has been used effectively for trauma consultation and as a substitute for follow-up office fracture care visits.[94-96] For acute care of minor injuries, there is a high degree of concordance between in-person and telemedicine visits, with similar rates of radiographic utilization and similar miss rates. Researchers have noted that visual inspection, capillary refill, color, and goniometry are sensitive and accurate in the telemedicine format. Patients can also palpate their own injury while being watched and can point out areas of tenderness. The rate of X-ray utilization and the rate of "misses," defined as an injury assessed to not need an X-ray, but subsequently found to be a fracture, were similar to in person and in both scenarios' complications were very low. Clearly, interventions such as splinting cannot be performed by the clinician in the telemedicine format, but the patient can be instructed in methods of home care, including premade splints and wraps.[97-99]

Can a patient self-assess abdominal tenderness to palpation?

Abdominal tenderness by telemedicine requires patient self-assessment, and to date, there is little evidence that patients can accurately self-assess tenderness. There is one case report and one small laboratory study using smartphone accelerometry to assess tenderness; otherwise, trials or good evidence exists to date to show that abdominal tenderness can be adequately assessed in the telemedicine format. While that does not mean that abdominal pain is entirely out of the reach of telemedicine evaluation, it does mean that a key element of the exam – the assessment of tenderness – is not accessible in the telemedicine format currently.[100,101]

What is the risk of serious misdiagnosis in the telemedicine format for other common acute emergency department chief complaints?

The table below describes specific chief complaints, whether they are low, medium, or high risk from a clinical perspective, and the authors' assessment of the risk of telemedicine for the encounter with accompanying references.

Chief complaint	Low risk	Medium risk	High risk	Rationale/References
Abdominal pain			X	The clinician cannot assess abdominal tenderness, percussion, or auscultation.[102,103] Special tools to assess tenderness are not available in the standard telemedicine format, and the usefulness of adjuncts such as accelerometers is not well established.[98,99]
Upper respiratory symptoms	X			CENTOR criteria, oxygen saturation monitors are inexpensive and widely available. Diagnosis, treatment, and quality measures for telemedicine are highly concordant with in-person visits.[104, 105] The rate of inappropriate antibiotic prescribing is somewhat higher with telemedicine.[106]
Sprains/ strains	X			Visual inspection and referral for X-ray can be accomplished. Clinical effectiveness of telemedicine is similar to in-person.[92–94,107]
Soft tissue injury	X			Visual inspection is reliable and referral for X-ray can be accomplished.[92–94]
Nontraumatic chest pain			X	History taking is reliable, but key components, such as palpation of pulses, auscultation of murmurs, the pulmonary exam, ECG and Troponin cannot be obtained in the direct-to-consumer (DTC) telemedicine format.[108,109]
Back pain		X		Many elements of the back and lumbar plexus can be done by telemedicine, but gaps exist in sensation and reflexes. Deficits and lateralizing signs can be subtle.[110–112]

Chief complaint	Low risk	Medium risk	High risk	Rationale/References
Lower urinary tract symptoms	X			History is reliable and referral for outpatient UA can be accomplished. The rate of inappropriate antibiotic prescribing is higher with telemedicine.[104]
Skin and soft tissue infections	X			Skin examination has good reliability and fidelity by telemedicine. There is good concordance between in-person and telemedicine assessment of severity, disposition, and indications for antibiotics.[105,113-115]
Headache			X	Chronic headache care by telemedicine is reliable and as rated by neurologists who care for patients with chronic headache syndromes and has been shown to be noninferior to in-person visits.[33,116-118] Regarding acute headache, key physical exam features such as blood pressure, nuchal rigidity, and special reflexes cannot be obtained and therefore it is very difficult to assess risk for rare but high-risk conditions such as meningitis, vertebral artery dissection, and subarachnoid hemorrhage.[119,120]
Nontraumatic extremity and soft tissue pain		X		Cellulitis, rashes, skin changes, and rheumatologic diseases can be well assessed in the telemedicine format.[104,111-113] Rare catastrophic conditions such as necrotizing fasciitis, compartment syndrome, and acute vascular insufficiency cannot be well assessed without palpation, though it is expected the extreme level of pain associated with these conditions would prompt referral to the ED.
Lower respiratory symptoms	X			Auscultation with a wireless stethoscope is not available with the standard telemedicine format.[121] Dyspnea, however, can be relatively well assessed in the telemedicine format.[74-76] Meta-analysis shows antibiotics are generally prescribed more often in telemedicine visits compared with in-person visits.[122] Some of these large studies are not granular enough to detect if there were more pneumonias missed by telemedicine or in-person visit, or bouncebacks, or admissions.[103]

(Continued)

Chief complaint	Low risk	Medium risk	High risk	Rationale/References
Nontraumatic joint pain	X			In the assessment of nontraumatic joint pain, the history is essential, and can be reliably obtained. Joints can be visually inspected for color, range of motion, and swelling. Thus, studies of tele rheumatology consultations and management show a high degree of concordance between telemedicine and in person assessment.[105,123–125]
Dental or jaw pain	X			Visual inspection of the oral cavity and jaw can be reliably performed in the telemedicine format. Studies show a high degree of concordance for common dental conditions seen in the ED.[126–128]
Nausea and vomiting		X		Telemedicine has not been studied as a stand-alone modality for nausea and vomiting, but it can be a valuable adjunct for prehospital care.[129]
Chronic obstructive pulmonary disease (COPD) and asthma		X		Although the standard telemedicine format does not allow for auscultation of the lungs, and therefore the exact cause of dyspnea is difficult to ascertain, through visual cues and the patient's self-report, severity of the dyspnea can be reliably estimated.[73,74] Dyspnea can also be quantified with the Roth Score.[75]
Other gastrointestinal (GI) symptoms		X		A variety of GI conditions are commonly treated on intercontinental flights through telemedicine, and studies show diversions are rare, and in nondiverted flights deteriorations are rare. The inability to perform an abdominal exam is a significant limitation.[130,131]
Limb fractures	X			Visual inspection of limbs for signs of fractures, such as swelling, deformity, and decreased range of motion is reliable. Tele-orthopedics delivers similar results to in-person examinations.[105,132] Certain joints and bones, such as the hip and scaphoid bone, do not lend themselves to visual-only examination. Likewise, knee instability likely cannot be well assessed in the telemedicine format.
Ear pain		X		The canal and tympanic membrane cannot be assessed in the standard telemedicine format. As with in-person evaluation, there is high variability in diagnosis and treatment.[133]
Alcohol-related		X		Visual cues to acute intoxication can be mixed. However, alcohol counseling through telemedicine has been shown to be noninferior to in-person counseling.[134,135]

What is the malpractice landscape for telemedicine?

In the 1990s and early 2000s, there was a great deal of concern for malpractice risk around telemedicine. To date, however, malpractice risk appears to be very low. Two recent studies querying Lexis Nexis malpractice cases related to DTC telemedicine found no reported cases. To date, the largest medicolegal risk is violation of statutes, rather than involvement in civil torts or claims. However, the view that telemedicine is low risk should be tempered by the fact that (i) claims lag 1–2 years behind practice, and (ii) the COVID-19 pandemic has closed courts temporarily and resulted in temporary protection from malpractice claims.[136–138]

Can telehealth address disparities?

Beyond the improved access to psychiatry services and care for older adults discussed earlier in this chapter, the Patient-Centered Outcomes Research Institute (PCORI) has funded 89 comparative effectiveness studies in telehealth, of which 41 assessed the use of telehealth to improve outcomes for populations at risk for health disparities. A scoping review of these 41 studies reported the use of different technologies including mobile devices (71%), web-based interventions (73%), real-time videoconferencing (37%), remote patient monitoring (20%), and asynchronous electronic transmission interventions (10%). These studies targeted racial and ethnic minorities, people living in rural areas, and low socioeconomic status, low health literacy, or disabilities.[139] The review highlighted the importance of patient-centered design, cultural tailoring of telehealth solutions, delivering telehealth through trusted intermediaries, partnering with payers to expand telehealth reimbursement, and ensuring confidential sharing of private information. Best practices in telehealth implementation include delivery of telehealth through trusted intermediaries, close partnership with payers to facilitate reimbursement and sustainability, and safeguards to ensure patient-guided confidential sharing of personal health information.

In EM, telehealth has been associated with improved access to consultation from specialists in rural or under-resourced settings and has been associated with improvements in metrics such as length of stay, reduced transfers, increased discharges, improved costs, and similar quality of care. Cost is one of the most frequently cited barriers for telehealth development in rural EDs. There is limited data on the role and adoption of telemedicine in non-English speaking populations and those with low health literacy; or how social determinants of health, race, and ethnicity affect access to telemedicine.

So far, we have mostly focused on DTC use of telemedicine; however, other uses include the provider-to-provider use of telemedicine in the hospital setting. Several hospitals were providing tele-stroke among other services like tele-ICU, tele-neonatology, tele-obstetrics (tele-OB), and tele ED while integrating community hospitals into new larger health care systems. For example, some health systems have adapted the ED staffing in lower volumes EDs, and advance practice provider (nurse practitioner or physician assistant) can access to a board-certified emergency physician as needed for higher acuity cases, including resuscitations, febrile infants, procedural sedation, intubations, and point-of-care ultrasound (POCUS) among others, increasing diagnostic accuracy and assisting with referrals, or decreasing transfers as appropriate.[140,141] Other uses include the use of telemedicine by paramedics and prehospital providers including the emergency triage, treat, and transport (ET3) program use of telemedicine to facilitate initiation of care in the waiting room, among other uses.[142-144] This is a rapidly evolving field, and the reimbursement and regulation adjustments during the pandemic allowed this process to progress at a much faster rate.

Conclusions

Research to date has mixed results for the accuracy, efficacy, and impact of telehealth services, and a research agenda has been proposed to provide the scientific basis to guide the development of telehealth in EM. Patients, payors, and health care institutions look for ways to provide increased access to high-quality care at decreased costs, and the accelerated use of telehealth during the pandemic has led to the implementation of modalities and processes that need the development of simultaneous research opportunities to evaluate its impact.

From the statistical point of view, most studies on telemedicine are single arm and only report feasibility. Among those that compare two interventions, most are designed as noninferiority studies, aiming to show that telemedicine is not inferior to usual care. In a systematic review, several studies claimed to be noninferiority studies, but less than one-half of those tested for statistical differences as a proxy of noninferiority.[145]

Compared with the in-person encounter, the information obtainable in the telemedicine encounter is constrained. The visual and auditory data available to the clinician in the telemedicine encounter are low fidelity, and haptic data (i.e. three-dimensional touch) is completely absent. Nonetheless, there is a significant subset of ED chief complaints that can be safely and effectively managed with telemedicine because the quantitative difference in information does result in qualitative difference in the assessment and care of the patient. There are ED chief complaints which can be managed with a low threshold for referral to the ED because sometimes the haptic data and higher fidelity of the in-person exam are needed to rule out dangerous conditions. Finally, there is a subset of encounters which at minimum require the higher fidelity and haptics of the in-person exam.

References

1. Betancourt JA, Rosenberg MA, Zevallos A, Brown JR, Mileski M. The impact of COVID-19 on telemedicine utilization across multiple service lines in the United States. *Healthcare.* 2020; 8(4): 380.
2. Mann DM, Chen J, Chunara R, Testa PA, Nov O. COVID-19 transforms health care through telemedicine: Evidence from the field. *Journal of the American Medical Informatics Association.* 2020; 27(7): 1132–5.
3. Miner H, Fatehi A, Ring D, Reichenberg JS. Clinician telemedicine perceptions during the COVID-19 pandemic. *Telemedicine Journal and E-Health.* 2021; 27(5): 508–12.
4. Ramaswamy A, Yu M, Drangsholt S *et al.* Patient satisfaction with telemedicine during the COVID-19 pandemic: Retrospective cohort study. *Journal of Medical Internet Research.* 2020; 22(9): e20786.
5. Kichloo A, Albosta M, Dettloff K *et al.* Telemedicine, the current COVID-19 pandemic and the future: A narrative review and perspectives moving forward in the USA. *Family Medicine and Community Health.* 2020; 8(3): e000530.
6. Rockwell KL, Gilroy AS. Incorporating telemedicine as part of COVID-19 outbreak response systems. *The American Journal of Managed Care.* 2020; 26(4): 147–8.
7. Lee NT, Karsten J, Roberts J. Removing regulatory barriers to telehealth before and after COVID-19. Brookings Institution; 2020.
8. American College of Emergency Physician (ACEP). Emergency Telemedicine Section. Telehealth in Emergency Medicine: A Primer. https://www.acep.org/globalassets/uploads/uploaded-files/acep/membership/sections-of-membership/telemd/acep-telemedicine-primer.pdf. 2014. Accessed January 2022.
9. Ansary AM, Martinez JN, Scott JD. The virtual physical exam in the 21st century. *Journal of Telemedicine and Telecare.* 2021; 27(6): 382–92.
10. Länsisalmi H, Kivimäki M, Aalto P, Ruoranen R. Innovation in healthcare: A systematic review of recent research. *Nursing Science Quarterly.* 2006; 19(1): 66–72.
11. Margarete A, Bigelow B. Presenting structural innovation in an institutional environment: Hospitals' use of impression management. *Administrative Science Quarterly.* 2000; 45(3): 494–522.
12. Hayden EM, Davis C, Clark S *et al.* Society for Academic Emergency Medicine 2020 Consensus Conference. Telehealth in emergency medicine: A consensus conference to map the intersection of telehealth and emergency medicine. *Academic Emergency Medicine.* 2021; 28(12): 1452–74.

13. Eastham M. Resolution: Photography and the human eye. *Rock Art Research.* 2011; 28(1): 128.

14. Roschelle J. Choosing and using video equipment for data collection. In: Kelly AE, Lesh R, editors. *Handbook of research design in mathematics and science education.* New York, NY: Routledge; 2000: 709–29.

15. Inoué S. Physiological characteristics of the eye. In: *Video microscopy.* Boston (MA): Springer; 1986.

16. Inoué S. *Video microscopy.* Boston (MA): Springer; 2013.

17. Cameras v. Human Eye. https://www.cambridgeincolour.com/tutorials/cameras-vs-human-eye.htm. Accessed February 6, 2022.

18. Kreis S. Megapixels and human recognition of resolution. *The Physics Teacher.* 2008; 46(5): 304–5.

19. Skorka O, Joseph D. Toward a digital camera to rival the human eye. *Journal of Electronic Imaging.* 2011; 20(3): 033009.

20. Egamberdiev K. Eyes and lenses: A comparison and differences. *Journal of Multimedia Information System.* 2016; 3(2): 43–6.

21. What is the Resolution of the Human Eye in Megapixels? https://www.forbes.com/sites/quora/2016/10/06/what-is-the-resolution-of-the-human-eye-in-megapixels/?sh=54cdafd05912. Accessed February 6, 2022.

22. Tachakra S. Depth perception in telemedical consultations. *Telemedicine Journal and E-Health.* 2001; 7(2): 77–85.

23. Tachakra S. Colour perception in telemedicine. *Journal of Telemedicine and Telecare.* 1999; 5(4): 211–9.

24. Foley D. Binaural Hearing Vs. Microphone "Hearing" and the Human Ear, 2012. https://www.acousticfields.com/binaural-hearing-vs-microphone-hearing/. Accessed February 6, 2022.

25. Applegate RL 2nd, Gildea B, Patchin R et al. Telemedicine pre-anesthesia evaluation: A randomized pilot trial. *Telemedicine Journal and E-Health.* 2013; 19(3): 211–6.

26. Rogers G. Using telemedicine for pediatric preanesthesia evaluation: A pilot project. *Journal of Perianesthesia Nursing.* 2020; 35(1): 3–6.

27. Kamdar NV, Huverserian A, Jalilian L et al. Development, implementation, and evaluation of a telemedicine preoperative evaluation initiative at a Major Academic Medical Center. *Anesthesia and Analgesia.* 2020; 131(6): 1647–56.

28. Mullen-Fortino M, Rising KL, Duckworth J, Gwynn V, Sites FD, Hollander JE. Presurgical assessment using telemedicine technology: Impact on efficiency, effectiveness, and patient experience of care. *Telemedicine Journal and E-Health.* 2019; 25(2): 137–42.

29. Bekkelund SI, Müller KI. Video consultations in medication overuse headache. A randomized controlled trial. *Brain and Behavior.* 2019; 9(7): e01344.

30. Friedman DI, Rajan B, Seidmann A. A randomized trial of telemedicine for migraine management. *Cephalalgia.* 2019; 39(12): 1577–85.

31. Spina E, Tedeschi G, Russo A et al. Telemedicine application to headache: A critical review. *Neurological Sciences.* 2022; 43(6): 3795–801.

32. Qubty W, Patniyot I, Gelfand A. Telemedicine in a pediatric headache clinic: A prospective survey. *Neurology.* 2018; 90(19): e1702–5.
33. Müller KI, Alstadhaug KB, Bekkelund SI. Telemedicine in the management of non-acute headaches: A prospective, open-labelled non-inferiority, randomised clinical trial. *Cephalalgia.* 2017; 37(9): 855–63.
34. Egede LE, Acierno R, Knapp RG *et al.* Psychotherapy for depression in older veterans via telemedicine: A randomised, open-label, non-inferiority trial. *Lancet Psychiatry.* 2015; 2(8): 693–701.
35. Fortney JC, Pyne JM, Mouden SB *et al.* Practice-based versus telemedicine-based collaborative care for depression in rural federally qualified health centers: A pragmatic randomized comparative effectiveness trial. *The American Journal of Psychiatry.* 2013; 170(4): 414–25.
36. Luxton DD, Pruitt LD, Wagner A, Smolenski DJ, Jenkins-Guarnieri MA, Gahm G. Home-based telebehavioral health for U.S. military personnel and veterans with depression: A randomized controlled trial. *Journal of Consulting and Clinical Psychology.* 2016; 84(11): 923–34.
37. Changes to Existing Medical Software Policies Resulting from Section 3060 of the 21st Century Cures Act. https://www.fda.gov/regulatory-information/search-fda-guidance-documents/changes-existing-medical-software-policies-resulting-section-3060-21st-century-cures-act. Accessed February 2, 2022.
38. Crico C, Renzi C, Graf N *et al.* mHealth and telemedicine apps: In search of a common regulation. *Ecancermedicalscience.* 2018; 12: 853.
39. Janos E, Zegarelli B Telemedicine Platform Recalled Over Failure to Obtain Pre-Market Clearance or Approval from FDA. https://www.jdsupra.com/legalnews/telemedicine-platform-recalled-over-77581/. Accessed February 6, 2022.
40. Haleem A, Javaid M, Singh RP, Suman R. Telemedicine for healthcare: Capabilities, features, barriers, and applications. *Sensors International.* 2021; 2: 100117.
41. Bashi N, Karunanithi M, Fatehi F, Ding H, Walters D. Remote monitoring of patients with heart failure: An overview of systematic reviews. *Journal of Medical Internet Research.* 2017; 19(1): e18.
42. Satou GM, Rheuban K, Alverson D *et al.* Telemedicine in pediatric cardiology: A scientific statement from the American Heart Association. *Circulation.* 2017; 135(11): e648–78.
43. Fierson WM, Capone A Jr, American Academy of Pediatrics Section on Ophthalmology; American Academy of Ophthalmology, American Association of Certified Orthoptists. Telemedicine for evaluation of retinopathy of prematurity. *Pediatrics.* 2015; 135(1): e238–54.
44. Rathi S, Tsui E, Mehta N, Zahid S, Schuman JS. The current state of teleophthalmology in the United States. *Ophthalmology.* 2017; 124(12): 1729–34.
45. Biagio L, Swanepoel de W, Adeyemo A, Hall JW 3rd, Vinck B. Asynchronous video-otoscopy with a telehealth facilitator. *Telemedicine Journal and E-Health.* 2013; 19(4): 252–8.
46. Lundberg T, Biagio de Jager L, Swanepoel W, Laurent C. Diagnostic accuracy of a general practitioner with video-otoscopy collected by a health care facilitator

compared to traditional otoscopy. *International Journal of Pediatric Otorhinolaryngology.* 2017; 99: 49–53.

47. Ferrándiz L, Ojeda-Vila T, Corrales A *et al.* Internet-based skin cancer screening using clinical images alone or in conjunction with dermoscopic images: A randomized teledermoscopy trial. *Journal of the American Academy of Dermatology.* 2017; 76(4): 676–82.

48. Ohta H, Kawashima M. Technical feasibility of patient-friendly screening and treatment of digestive disease by remote control robotic capsule endoscopes via the internet. *Annual International Conference of the IEEE Engineering in Medicine and Biology Society.* 2014; 2014: 7001–4.

49. Cosoli G, Scalise L, Poli A, Spinsante S. Wearable devices as a valid support for diagnostic excellence: Lessons from a pandemic going forward. *Health and Technology.* 2021; 11(3): 673–5.

50. Pépin JL, Bruno RM, Yang RY *et al.* Wearable activity trackers for monitoring adherence to home confinement during the COVID-19 pandemic worldwide: Data aggregation and analysis. *Journal of Medical Internet Research.* 2020; 22(6): e19787.

51. Fuller D, Colwell E, Low J *et al.* Reliability and validity of commercially available wearable devices for measuring steps, energy expenditure, and heart rate: Systematic review. *JMIR mHealth and uHealth.* 2020; 8(9): e18694.

52. Evenson KR, Goto MM, Furberg RD. Systematic review of the validity and reliability of consumer-wearable activity trackers. *International Journal of Behavioral Nutrition and Physical Activity.* 2015; 12: 159.

53. Wen D, Zhang X, Liu X, Lei J. Evaluating the consistency of current mainstream wearable devices in health monitoring: A comparison under free-living conditions. *Journal of Medical Internet Research.* 2017; 19(3): e68.

54. Dooley EE, Golaszewski NM, Bartholomew JB. Estimating accuracy at exercise intensities: A comparative study of self-monitoring heart rate and physical activity wearable devices. *JMIR mHealth and uHealth.* 2017; 5(3): e34.

55. Gillinov S, Etiwy M, Wang R *et al.* Variable accuracy of wearable heart rate monitors during aerobic exercise. *Medicine and Science in Sports and Exercise.* 2017; 49(8): 1697–703.

56. Wang R, Blackburn G, Desai M *et al.* Accuracy of wrist-worn heart rate monitors. *JAMA Cardiology.* 2017; 2(1): 104–6.

57. Reddy RK, Pooni R, Zaharieva DP *et al.* Accuracy of wrist-worn activity monitors during common daily physical activities and types of structured exercise: Evaluation study. *JMIR mHealth and uHealth.* 2018; 6(12): e10338.

58. Ramesh J, Solatidehkordi Z, Aburukba R, Sagahyroon A. Atrial fibrillation classification with smart wearables using short-term heart rate variability and deep convolutional neural networks. *Sensors (Basel).* 2021; 21(21): 7233.

59. Soon S, Svavarsdottir H, Downey C, Jayne DG. Wearable devices for remote vital signs monitoring in the outpatient setting: An overview of the field. *BMJ Innovations.* 2020; 6(2): 55–71.

60. Da Silva SP. Validity and reliability of a classroom heart-rate collection procedure, with application for assessing arousal related to test anticipation. *Psychology Learning and Teaching.* 2021; 11(2): 186–93.

61. Sedlock KRG, Fitzgerald PI, Tahamont MV, Schneider DA. Accuracy of subject-palpated carotid pulse after exercise. *The Physician and Sportsmedicine*. 1982; 11(4): 106–16.

62. Takeshima N, Brechue WF, Ueya S, Tanaka K. Age-related decreases in finger sensitivity can produce error in palpated heart-rate determination. *Journal of Aging and Physical Activity*. 2000; 8(2): 120–8.

63. Frommelt T, Ott C, Hays V. Accuracy of different devices to measure temperature. *Medsurg Nursing*. 2008; 17(3): 171–82.

64. Jung MH, Kim GH, Kim JH *et al*. Reliability of home blood pressure monitoring: In the context of validation and accuracy. *Blood Pressure Monitoring*. 2015; 20(4): 215–20.

65. Nasothimiou EG, Tzamouranis D, Rarra V, Roussias LG, Stergiou GS. Diagnostic accuracy of home vs. ambulatory blood pressure monitoring in untreated and treated hypertension. *Hypertension Research*. 2012; 35(7): 750–5.

66. Ringrose JS, Polley G, McLean D, Thompson A, Morales F, Padwal R. An assessment of the accuracy of home blood pressure monitors when used in device owners. *American Journal of Hypertension*. 2017; 30(7): 683–9.

67. Stryker T, Wilson M, Wilson TW. Accuracy of home blood pressure readings: Monitors and operators. *Blood Pressure Monitoring*. 2004; 9(3): 143–7.

68. Whiting P, Elwenspoek M. Accuracy of Self-Monitoring Heart Rate, Respiratory Rate and Oxygen Saturation in Patients with Symptoms Suggestive of Covid Infection. National Institute for Health Research and University of Bristol. https://arc-w.nihr.ac.uk/Wordpress/wp-content/uploads/2020/04/BNSSG-COV.10-COVID-19-report-1_4_2020_-1-1.pdf/. 2020. Accessed February 4, 2022.

69. Liu H, Allen J, Zheng D, Chen F. Recent development of respiratory rate measurement technologies. *Physiological Measurement*. 2019; 40(7): 07TR01.

70. Ansermino JM, Dumont G, Ginsburg AS. How uncertain is our reference standard for respiratory rate measurement? *American Journal of Respiratory and Critical Care Medicine*. 2019; 199(8): 1036–7.

71. Drummond GB, Fischer D, Arvind DK. Current clinical methods of measurement of respiratory rate give imprecise values. *ERJ Open Research*. 2020; 6(3): 00023–2020.

72. Latten GHP, Spek M, Muris JWM, Cals JWL, Stassen PM. Accuracy and interobserver-agreement of respiratory rate measurements by healthcare professionals, and its effect on the outcomes of clinical prediction/diagnostic rules. *PLoS One*. 2019; 14(10): e0223155.

73. Lim WS, Carty SM, Macfarlane JT *et al*. Respiratory rate measurement in adults – how reliable is it? *Respiratory Medicine*. 2002; 96(1): 31–3.

74. Gattu R, Scollan J, DeSouza A, Devereaux D, Weaver H, Agthe AG. Telemedicine: A reliable tool to assess the severity of respiratory distress in children. *Hospital Pediatrics*. 2016; 6(8): 476–82.

75. Chorin E, Padegimas A, Havakuk O *et al*. Assessment of respiratory distress by the Roth Score. *Clinical Cardiology*. 2016; 39(11): 636–9.

76. Accorsi TAD, Amicis K, Brígido ARD *et al*. Assessment of patients with acute respiratory symptoms during the COVID-19 pandemic by telemedicine: Clinical features and impact on referral. *Einstein (Sao Paulo)*. 2020; 18: eAO6106.

77. Shafqat S, Kvedar JC, Guanci MM, Chang Y, Schwamm LH. Role for telemedicine in acute stroke. Feasibility and reliability of remote administration of the NIH stroke scale. *Stroke.* 1999; 30(10): 2141–5.
78. Wu TC, Parker SA, Jagolino A *et al.* Telemedicine can replace the neurologist on a mobile stroke unit. *Stroke.* 2017; 48(2): 493–6.
79. Handschu R, Littmann R, Reulbach U *et al.* Telemedicine in emergency evaluation of acute stroke: Interrater agreement in remote video examination with a novel multimedia system. *Stroke.* 2003; 34(12): 2842–6.
80. Taqui A, Cerejo R, Itrat A *et al.* Reduction in time to treatment in prehospital telemedicine evaluation and thrombolysis. *Neurology.* 2017; 88(14): 1305–12.
81. Demaerschalk BM, Vegunta S, Vargas BB, Wu Q, Channer DD, Hentz JG. Reliability of real-time video smartphone for assessing National Institutes of Health Stroke Scale scores in acute stroke patients. *Stroke.* 2012; 43(12): 3271–7.
82. Bowry R, Parker SA, Yamal JM *et al.* Time to decision and treatment with tPA (tissue-type plasminogen activator) using telemedicine versus an onboard neurologist on a mobile stroke unit. *Stroke.* 2018; 49(6): 1528–30.
83. Amorim E, Shih MM, Koehler SA *et al.* Impact of telemedicine implementation in thrombolytic use for acute ischemic stroke: The University of Pittsburgh Medical Center telestroke network experience. *Journal of Stroke and Cerebrovascular Diseases.* 2013; 22(4): 527–31.
84. Amarendran V, George A, Gersappe V, Krishnaswamy S, Warren C. The reliability of telepsychiatry for a neuropsychiatric assessment. *Telemedicine Journal and E-Health.* 2011; 17(3): 223–5.
85. Hubley S, Lynch SB, Schneck C, Thomas M, Shore J. Review of key telepsychiatry outcomes. *World Journal of Psychiatry.* 2016; 6(2): 269–82.
86. Chipps J, Brysiewicz P, Mars M. Effectiveness and feasibility of telepsychiatry in resource constrained environments? A systematic review of the evidence. *African Journal of Psychiatry.* 2012; 15(4): 235–43.
87. Hyler SE, Gangure DP, Batchelder ST. Can telepsychiatry replace in-person psychiatric assessments? A review and meta-analysis of comparison studies. *CNS Spectrums.* 2005; 10(5): 403–13.
88. Chakrabarti S. Usefulness of telepsychiatry: A critical evaluation of videoconferencing-based approaches. *World Journal of Psychiatry.* 2015; 5(3): 286–304.
89. Mitra A, Veerakone R, Li K, Nix T, Hashikawa A, Mahajan P. Telemedicine in paediatric emergency care: A systematic review. *Journal of Telemedicine and Telecare.* 2021: 1357633X211010106.
90. Guaiana G, Mastrangelo J, Hendrikx S, Barbui C. A systematic review of the use of telepsychiatry in depression. *Community Mental Health Journal.* 2021; 57(1): 93–100.
91. Gentry MT, Lapid MI, Rummans TA. Geriatric telepsychiatry: Systematic review and policy considerations. *The American Journal of Geriatric Psychiatry.* 2019; 27(2): 109–27.
92. Elbaz S, Cinalioglu K, Sekhon K *et al.* A systematic review of telemedicine for older adults with dementia during COVID-19: An alternative to in-person health services? *Frontiers in Neurology.* 2021; 12: 761965.

93. Davoodi NM, Chen K, Zou M *et al.* Emergency physician perspectives on using telehealth with older adults during COVID-19: A qualitative study. *Journal of the American College of Emergency Physicians Open.* 2021; 2(5): e12577.

94. Latifi R. Telemedicine for trauma and emergency care management. In: Latifi R, Doarn CR, Merrell RC, editors. *Telemedicine, telehealth and telepresence.* Switzerland: Springer International Publishing; 2020: 293–305.

95. Smith AJ, Pfister BF, Woo EWY *et al.* Safe and rapid implementation of telemedicine fracture clinics: The impact of the COVID-19 pandemic. *ANZ Journal of Surgery.* 2020; 90(11): 2237–41.

96. Asiri A, AlBishi S, AlMadani W, ElMetwally A, Househ M. The use of telemedicine in surgical care: A systematic review. *Acta Informatica Medica.* 2018; 26(3): 201–6.

97. Benger JR, Noble SM, Coast J, Kendall JM. The safety and effectiveness of minor injuries telemedicine. *Emergency Medicine Journal.* 2004; 21(4): 438–45.

98. Mair F, Ferguson J. More patients with minor injuries could be seen by telemedicine. *Journal of Telemedicine and Telecare.* 2008; 14(3): 132–4.

99. Beach M, Goodall I, Miller P. Evaluating telemedicine for minor injuries units. *Journal of Telemedicine and Telecare.* 2000; 6(Suppl 1): S90–2.

100. Nachum S, Stern ME, Greenwald PW, Sharma R. Use of physician-guided patient self-examination to diagnose appendicitis: A telemedicine case report. *Telemedicine Journal and E-Health.* 2019; 25(8): 769–71.

101. Myers DR, Weiss A, Rollins MR, Lam WA. Towards remote assessment and screening of acute abdominal pain using only a smartphone with native accelerometers. *Scientific Reports.* 2017; 7(1): 12750.

102. Gorincour G, Monneuse O, Ben Cheikh A *et al.* Management of abdominal emergencies in adults using telemedicine and artificial intelligence. *Journal of Visceral Surgery.* 2021; 158(3S): S26–31.

103. Pappan N, Benkhadra R, Papincak D *et al.* Values and limits of telemedicine: A case report. *SN Comprehensive Clinical Medicine.* 2021; 3(1): 317–9.

104. Shi Z, Mehrotra A, Gidengil CA, Poon SJ, Uscher-Pines L, Ray KN. Quality of care for acute respiratory infections during direct-to-consumer telemedicine visits for adults. *Health Affairs.* 2018; 37(12): 2014–23.

105. Ray KN, Martin JM, Wolfson D *et al.* Antibiotic prescribing for acute respiratory tract infections during telemedicine visits within a pediatric primary care network. *Academic Pediatrics.* 2021; 21(7): 1239–43.

106. Mehrotra A, Paone S, Martich GD, Albert SM, Shevchik GJ. A comparison of care at e-visits and physician office visits for sinusitis and urinary tract infection. *JAMA Internal Medicine.* 2013; 173(1): 72–4.

107. Tachakra S, Lynch M, Newson R *et al.* A comparison of telemedicine with face-to-face consultations for trauma management. *Journal of Telemedicine and Telecare.* 2000; 6(Suppl 1): S178–81.

108. Scalvini S, Zanelli E, Conti C *et al.* Assessment of prehospital chest pain using telecardiology. *Journal of Telemedicine and Telecare.* 2002; 8(4): 231–6.

109. Brunetti ND, Amodio G, De Gennaro L *et al.* Telecardiology applied to a region-wide public emergency health-care service. *Journal of Thrombosis and Thrombolysis.* 2009; 28(1): 23–30.

110. Piche J, Butt BB, Ahmady A, Patel R, Aleem I. Physical examination of the spine using telemedicine: A systematic review. *Global Spine Journal.* 2021; 11(7): 1142–7.

111. Laskowski ER, Johnson SE, Shelerud RA et al. The telemedicine musculoskeletal examination [published correction appears in Mayo Clin Proc. 2020 Oct;95(10):2299]. *Mayo Clinic Proceedings.* 2020; 95(8): 1715–31.

112. Lovecchio F, Riew GJ, Samartzis D et al. Provider confidence in the telemedicine spine evaluation: Results from a global study. *European Spine Journal.* 2021; 30(8): 2109–23.

113. Korman AM, Kroshinsky D, Raff AB et al. A survey-based study of diagnostic and treatment concordance in standardized cases of cellulitis and pseudocellulitis via teledermatology. *Journal of the American Academy of Dermatology.* 2020; 82(5): 1221–3. doi: 10.1016/j.jaad.2019.09.084.

114. Keller JJ, Johnson JP, Latour E. Inpatient teledermatology: Diagnostic and therapeutic concordance among a hospitalist, dermatologist, and teledermatologist using store-and-forward teledermatology. *Journal of the American Academy of Dermatology.* 2020; 82(5): 1262–7. doi: 10.1016/j.jaad.2020.01.030.

115. Barbieri JS, Nelson CA, James WD et al. The reliability of teledermatology to triage inpatient dermatology consultations. *JAMA Dermatology.* 2014; 150(4): 419–24.

116. Müller KI, Alstadhaug KB, Bekkelund SI. Acceptability, feasibility, and cost of telemedicine for nonacute headaches: A randomized study comparing video and traditional consultations. *Journal of Medical Internet Research.* 2016; 18(5): e140.

117. Noutsios CD, Boisvert-Plante V, Perez J, Hudon J, Ingelmo P. Telemedicine applications for the evaluation of patients with non-acute headache: A narrative review. *Journal of Pain Research.* 2021; 14: 1533–42.

118. Müller KI, Alstadhaug KB, Bekkelund SI. A randomized trial of telemedicine efficacy and safety for nonacute headaches. *Neurology.* 2017; 89(2): 153–62.

119. Minen MT, Szperka CL, Kaplan K et al. Telehealth as a new care delivery model: The headache provider experience. *Headache.* 2021; 61(7): 1123–31.

120. Hatcher-Martin JM, Adams JL, Anderson ER et al. Telemedicine in neurology: Telemedicine Work Group of the American Academy of Neurology update. *Neurology.* 2020; 94(1): 30–8.

121. Noda A, Saraya T, Morita K et al. Evidence of the sequential changes of lung sounds in COVID-19 pneumonia using a novel wireless stethoscope with the telemedicine system. *Internal Medicine.* 2020; 59(24): 3213–6.

122. Han SM, Greenfield G, Majeed A, Hayhoe B. Impact of remote consultations on antibiotic prescribing in primary health care: Systematic review. *Journal of Medical Internet Research.* 2020; 22(11): e23482.

123. Piovesan DM, Busato VB, da Silveira RG et al. Quality of referrals to a rheumatology service before and after implementation of a triage system with telemedicine support. *Advances in Rheumatology.* 2021; 61(1): 47.

124. Bateman J, Cleaton N. Managing patients using telerheumatology: Lessons from a pandemic. *Best Practice & Research. Clinical Rheumatology.* 2021; 35(1): 101662.

125. El Aoufy K, Melis MR, Bellando Randone S *et al.* The positive side of the coin: Sars-Cov-2 pandemic has taught us how much Telemedicine is useful as standard of care procedure in real life. *Clinical Rheumatology.* 2022; 41(2): 573–9.

126. Miladinović M, Mladenović D, Mihailović B *et al.* Evaluation of telemedicine in the management of dentogenous infections. *Vojnosanitetski Pregled.* 2013; 70(6): 569–75.

127. Alabdullah JH, Daniel SJ. A systematic review on the validity of teledentistry. *Telemedicine Journal and E-Health.* 2018; 24(8): 639–48.

128. Queyroux A, Saricassapian B, Herzog D *et al.* Accuracy of teledentistry for diagnosing dental pathology using direct examination as a gold standard: Results of the Tel-e-dent study of older adults living in nursing homes. *Journal of the American Medical Directors Association.* 2017; 18(6): 528–32.

129. Champagne-Langabeer T, Langabeer JR, Roberts KE *et al.* Telehealth impact on primary care related ambulance transports. *Prehospital Emergency Care.* 2019; 23(5): 712–7.

130. Peterson DC, Martin-Gill C, Guyette FX *et al.* Outcomes of medical emergencies on commercial airline flights. *The New England Journal of Medicine.* 2013; 368(22): 2075–83.

131. Bagshaw M. Telemedicine in British Airways. *Journal of Telemedicine and Telecare.* 1996; 2(Suppl 1): 36–8.

132. Buvik A, Bugge E, Knutsen G, Småbrekke A, Wilsgaard T. Quality of care for remote orthopaedic consultations using telemedicine: A randomised controlled trial. *BMC Health Services Research.* 2016; 16(1): 483.

133. Shah AC, Badawy SM. Telemedicine in pediatrics: Systematic review of randomized controlled trials. *JMIR Pediatrics and Parenting.* 2021; 4(1): e22696.

134. King SC, Richner KA, Tuliao AP, Kennedy JL, McChargue DE. A comparison between telehealth and face-to-face delivery of a brief alcohol intervention for college students. *Substance Abuse.* 2020; 41(4): 501–9.

135. Byaruhanga J, Atorkey P, McLaughlin M *et al.* Effectiveness of individual real-time video counseling on smoking, nutrition, alcohol, physical activity, and obesity health risks: Systematic review. *Journal of Medical Internet Research.* 2020; 22(9): e18621.

136. Fogel AL, Kvedar JC. Reported cases of medical malpractice in direct-to-consumer telemedicine. *Journal of the American Medical Association.* 2019; 321(13): 1309–10.

137. Fogel AL, Lacktman NM, Kvedar JC. Skin cancer telemedicine medical malpractice risk. *JAMA Dermatology.* 2021; 157(7): 870–1.

138. Telemedicine and Malpractice Claims. https://www.hg.org/legal-articles/telemedicine-and-malpractice-claims-55323. Accessed February 6, 2022.

139. Bailey JE, Gurgol C, Pan E *et al.* Early patient-centered outcomes research experience with the use of telehealth to address disparities: Scoping review. *Journal of Medical Internet Research.* 2021; 23(12): e28503.

140. Marsh-Feiley G, Eadie L, Wilson P. Telesonography in emergency medicine: A systematic review. *PLoS One.* 2018; 13(5): e0194840.

141. Salerno A, Tupchong K, Verceles AC, McCurdy MT. Point-of-care teleultra-sound: A systematic review. *Telemedicine Journal and E-Health.* 2020; 26(11): 1314–21.

142. Winburn AS, Brixey JJ, Langabeer J 2nd, Champagne-Langabeer T. A systematic review of prehospital telehealth utilization. *Journal of Telemedicine and Telecare.* 2018; 24(7): 473–81.

143. Emergency Triage, Treat, and Transport (ET3) Model. https://innovation.cms. gov/innovation-models/et3. Accessed February 6, 2022.

144. Osmanlliu E, Gagnon I, Weber S, Bach CQ, Turnbull J, Seguin J. The waiting room assessment to virtual emergency department pathway: Initiating video-based telemedicine in the pediatric emergency department. *Journal of Telemedicine and Telecare.* 2022; 28(6): 452–7.

145. Kummervold PE, Johnsen JA, Skrøvseth SO, Wynn R. Using noninferiority tests to evaluate telemedicine and e-health services: Systematic review. *Journal of Medical Internet Research.* 2012; 14(5): e132.

Chapter 62 **Diagnosing COVID-19**

Christopher R. Carpenter[1] and Jesse M. Pines[2,3]

[1] Department of Emergency Medicine, Washington University School of Medicine, St. Louis, MO, USA
[2] US Acute Care Solutions, Canton, OH, USA
[3] Department of Emergency Medicine, Drexel University, Philadelphia, PA, USA

Highlights

- Clinical signs and symptoms are neither sensitive nor specific in diagnosing COVID-19 infections.
- Interleukin-6, C-reactive protein, and lymphocyte are the most accurate routine labs for the diagnosis of COVID-19 but they demonstrate low sensitivity and specificity, rendering them inadequate to rule in or rule out COVID-19 in isolation.
- Real-time reverse transcription polymerase chain reaction (rRT-PCR) is more sensitive than antigen tests to diagnose COVID-19.
- False-negative rRT-PCR results are not uncommon and can occur for many reasons related to sample collection, viral load, and stage of COVID-19.
- Computed tomography is the imaging modality studied most frequently, but may not be superior to experienced sonographer's point-of-care ultrasound.

Background

A novel viral respiratory pathogen emerged in December 2019 called severe acute respiratory syndrome coronavirus 2 (SARS-CoV-2) with the corresponding illness called coronavirus disease (COVID-19). COVID-19 became a potentially life-threatening viral infection for a significant portion of the population and millions of people died worldwide during the 2 years.

Evidence-Based Emergency Care: Diagnostic Testing and Clinical Decision Rules, Third Edition.
Edited by Jesse M. Pines, Fernanda Bellolio, Christopher R. Carpenter, and Ali S. Raja.
© 2023 John Wiley & Sons Ltd. Published 2023 by John Wiley & Sons Ltd.

The global pandemic catalyzed economic stress and exposed geopolitical divisions, while scientists grappled with emerging diagnostic, prognostic, and therapeutic approaches at an unprecedented pace. Amidst the backdrop of this generational catastrophe, the existential foundations of evidence-based medicine described in Chapters 2 and 3 were challenged as never before with a rush to reporting at a pace that created an accelerating avalanche of unreviewed or inadequately peer-reviewed research and placed an increased onus on clinicians to display healthy skepticism and concomitant clinical agility.[1]

Before the science of COVID-19 prognosis or therapeutics could evolve, accurate and readily available diagnostic tests were required. In February 2020, the United States Food and Drug Administration issued an emergency use authorization (EUA) enabling Centers for Disease Control-qualified labs to perform COVID-19 testing. Over 100 EUAs were issued for commercial COVID-19 assays over the next year as the emergency department (ED) served simultaneously as a societal safety net for routine emergencies, a rapid testing and disposition site, and a lynchpin for epidemic surveillance (Figure 62.1).[2] While clinicians managed intermittent waves of symptomatic

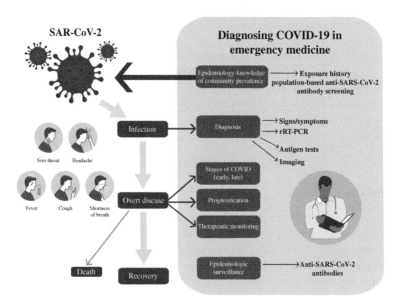

Figure 62.1 Diagnosing COVID-19 in the ED requires awareness of exposure history and symptom duration. Test results can guide both diagnosis and prognosis. COVID-19 testing can also be used as a screening test for patient clustering during admission to reduce hospital spread. (Reproduced from [2]/With permission of John Wiley & Sons.)

and asymptomatic exposed patients amidst a sea of diagnostic and management recommendations and protocols that changed frequently, decision-making was further complicated by shortages of personal protective equipment and test assays.

Clinical question

Can clinical signs and symptoms or routine labs accurately distinguish COVID-19 from other respiratory viral infection?
An emergency medicine-focused diagnostic scoping review in the early months of the pandemic identified few studies quantifying the accuracy or reliability of history and physical exam for diagnosing COVID-19.[2] Few studies reported sensitivity or specificity and none adhered to the Standards for Reporting of Diagnostic Accuracy (STARD) reporting standards for history and physical exam.[3] Hypogeusia (positive likelihood ratio [LR+] 7.1, negative likelihood ratio [LR–] 0.38) and hyposmia (LR+ 5.3, LR– 0.61) better ruled in COVID-19 than ruled out the diagnosis.[4] Subsequently, a Cochrane diagnostic accuracy systematic review identified studies evaluating 27 signs and systems categorized as general, respiratory, gastrointestinal, and cardiovascular.[5] In general, signs and symptoms had higher specificity and sensitivity of less than 50%. Therefore, COVID-19 infections often present with different constellations of symptoms, rather than having a classic clinical presentation. The five findings with sensitivity greater than 50% and LR+ >5 in at least one study included fever, myalgia or arthralgia, fatigue, and headache. Studies that examined clinical features enrolled hospitalized patients or patients presenting to the hospital rather than presumably healthier outpatient cohorts. Therefore, spectrum bias likely increased observed sensitivity as discussed in Chapter 6.[6] Both the Cochrane review and the emergency medicine scoping review concluded that signs and symptoms alone were inadequate to rule in or rule out COVID-19 – and that future history/physical exam research needed to adhere to STARD guidelines.[2,5] The inaccuracy of history/physical exam alone to rule in or rule out COVID-19 in the ED suggests that in scenarios with clinician suspicion for SARS-CoV-2 based on epidemiological grounds (i.e., high population prevalence or community test positivity rate), adopting a liberal testing strategy is preferred to detect a high proportion of infections in clinical settings.

A separate Cochrane review evaluated 21 studies that included 14,126 COVID-19 patients and 55,585 non-COVID-19 patients that quantified the diagnostic accuracy of 67 labs routinely available in most hospitals.[7] Only three of the labs had summary sensitivity and specificity over 50%: increase in interleukin-6, increase in C-reactive protein, and lymphocyte count

Table 62.1 Routine labs with highest accuracy for COVID-19

Lab	Number of studies / Level of certainty	Summary sensitivity (%)	Median specificity (%)
Interleukin-6	4 Very low	73	58
C-reactive protein	14 Very low	66	44
Lymphocyte count	13 Low	64	53

Source: Data from [7].

decrease (Table 62.1). Other tests based on low-certainty evidence demonstrated less accuracy, including white blood cell count, increase neutrophil percentage, decrease platelet count, liver function tests, and procalcitonin. None of these labs are sufficient to rule in or rule out COVID-19.

Clinical question

Which COVID-19 molecular or antigen test most accurately diagnoses the presence or absence of SARS-CoV-2?

Real-time reverse transcription polymerase chain reaction (rRT-PCR, a molecular test) has become the criterion standard for the presence or absence of COVID-19 across clinical and imaging studies. The rRT-PCR tests provide a qualitative detection of SARS-CoV-2 nucleic acid. In the United States, the CDC-developed rRT-PCR detects two separate regions of the SARS-CoV-2 nucleocapsid gene (N1 and N2) with the virus considered present (a positive test) when amplification of both N1 and N2 are detected and absent when neither N1 nor N2 is detected. An inconclusive test represents detection of only one nucleocapsid gene. False-negative rRT-PCR results are common, so clinicians and researchers using this test as a criterion standard should include patient's exposure risk, epidemiological risk based on community prevalence, and clinical and imaging findings when interpreting the accuracy of this result. Unfortunately, most early COVID-19 diagnostic studies did not incorporate these factors when reporting rRT-PCR results. Table 62.2 provides common causes of false-negative rRT-PCR results.[2] COVID-19 test samples in the ED were most commonly nasopharyngeal, but oropharyngeal sputum sampling is about 3% less sensitive.[8] Blood and urine are inadequate specimens for rRT-PCR because SARS-CoV-2 is not present in those body compartments.[9]

Table 62.2 Common causes of false negative rRT-PCR

Lab handling (heat inactivation)
Limit of detection (RNA particle detection)
Mutations in the probe target
Sampling procedure (training, fidelity, patient cooperation)
Selective virus replication (patient variability, disease severity variability)
Specimen sampled (NP, OP, saliva, sputum, BAL, stool)
Test kit quality
Timing of sampling in course of disease

RNA = ribonucleic acid; NP = nasopharyngeal; OP = oropharyngeal;
BAL = bronchoalveolar lavage.
Source: Reproduced from [2]/With permission of John Wiley & Sons.

Table 62.3 Comparative accuracy of antigen and rRT-PCR for COVID-19

Diagnostic tests	Number of evaluations (samples)	SARS-CoV-2 prevalence (%)	Sensitivity (95% CI)	Specificity (95% CI)
Antigen tests	8 (943)	63	56% (30–80)	99.5% (98–99.9)
Shenzhen Bioeasy Ag assay	2 (238)	68	90% (84–94)	100% (95–100)
Coris BioConcept	2 (466)	48	54% (48–61)	99.6% (98–99.9)
Molecular tests	13 (2255)	52	95% (87–98)	99% (97–99.5)
ID NOW	5 (1003)	49	77% (73–80)	99.6% (98–99.9)
Xpert Xpress	6 (919)	52	99.4% (98–99.8)	97% (91–99)

Source: Adapted from [10].

Antigen tests designed to detect SARS-CoV-2 nucleocapsid protein antigens from nasopharyngeal specimens emerged months after the initial rRT-PCR tests. Hospital labs intermittently experienced inadequate supplies of rRT-PCR reagents during the waves of COVID-19 and some sites relied upon antigen tests as a necessary replacement. In comparing rRT-PCR tests and antigen tests that provide results in less than 2-hours after obtaining the specimen, a Cochrane diagnostic accuracy review summarized 18 studies evaluating antigen tests or molecular tests (Table 62.3).[11] Most of these study designs were at risk for spectrum bias and incorporation bias, which can skew observed sensitivity and specificity upward.[6,10] Across studies, antigen tests were just as specific as molecular tests but usually far less sensitive. The United States Food and Drug Administration recommended that negative antigen results "be treated as presumptive and confirmed with a molecular assay, if necessary for patient management."[12]

Clinical question

Can imaging (chest X-ray, ultrasound, or computed tomography [CT]) accurately identify the presence or absence of COVID-19?

Chest X-ray is the most widely available and generally well-accepted first-line imaging choice to evaluate patients with respiratory symptoms and concern for COVID-19. Early diagnostic research only reported sensitivity, which ranged from 33% to 60% excluding one outlier at 100%.[2] A subsequent Cochrane diagnostic accuracy review of three studies and 1243 participants demonstrated a similarly wide range of sensitivities and an even wider range of specificities (Table 62.4).[13]

The same Cochrane review quantified the accuracy of ultrasound to diagnose COVID-19 pneumonia based on one study of inpatients that provided no details on who obtained/interpreted the sonographic images.[13,14] In addition, the case-control study had unclear risk of spectrum bias, differential verification bias, and incorporation bias, all threats to study validity.[6] Two subsequent studies of point-of-care ultrasound (POCUS) by nonradiologist physicians demonstrated similarly impressive accuracy. Peyrony *et al.* evaluated 391 patients with suspected COVID-19, reporting LR+ 7.1 (confidence interval [CI] 2.8–18.1) for the presence of bilateral B-lines on lung ultrasonography. They also noted that the absence of high clinical probability determined by the emergency physician in conjunction with the absence of bilateral B-lines demonstrated LR– 0.33 (CI 0.15–0.45).[15] Lieveld *et al.* evaluated 187 patients referred to Internal Medicine with suspected COVID-19. Internists certified in point-of-care sonography performed by or supervised the ultrasounds. Lung ultrasound was similar to CT for the diagnosis of COVID-19 pneumonia (POCUS LR+ 4.5 versus CT LR+ 4.9, POCUS LR– 0.12 versus CT LR– 0.14).[16]

Table 62.4 Imaging accuracy for diagnosing COVID-19 pneumonia

Lab	Number of studies Patients	Sensitivity	Specificity
CXR	3 1243	Range 57–89%	Range 11–89%
US	1 100	97%	62%
CT	31 8014	Range 57–100% Pooled 89%	Range 0–96% Pooled 61%

Source: Adapted from [13].

CT findings suggestive of COVID-19 include often-bilateral ground glass opacity and predominantly peripheral findings without associated mediastinal adenopathy or pleural effusions. In the early months of the pandemic with uncertain rRT-PCR accuracy or limited access to these molecular tests, some advocated for CT as a first-line approach to diagnose COVID-19 instead of or in addition to rRT-PCR.[17,18] The logic was that if CT alone or in combination with rRT-PCR reduced false negatives, propagation of the virus across populations could be mitigated more quickly. However, widespread use of CT as a first-line COVID-19 diagnostic approach would increase medical radiation exposure to many patients, accelerate healthcare spending as economies struggled to overcome the strains of a global pandemic, expose radiology technicians to the virus, and delay CT access to others as recommended cleaning times exceeded 30-minutes.[2,19] Since no cure exists and care is supportive for noncritically ill individuals, obtaining diagnostic certainty about the presence or absence of COVID-19 pneumonia via CT is unlikely to benefit most patients individually. Consequently, the British Society of Thoracic Imaging recommended against routine CT when rRT-PCR is positive and instead to consider CT when the initial rRT-PCR is negative to identify coexisting diseases or potential COVID-19 complications.[20] Some hospitals subsequently developed clinical protocols to guide decisions about CT ordering.[21]

With these caveats about the potential benefits and harms of CT for the diagnosis of COVID-19, the Cochrane review noted more research and potentially less biased research for CT as compared with chest X-ray or ultrasound. CT demonstrated sensitivity and specificity similar to ultrasound and superior to chest X-ray.[13] In the near future, lower dose CTs and technology may reduce the potential harms of CT while improving diagnostic accuracy. Low dose CT reduces the medical radiation exposure without significantly decreasing sensitivity or specificity.[22] Artificial intelligence can increase the sensitivity and specificity of radiologist's accuracy for COVID-19 pneumonia.[23]

Comments

Acknowledging the fluid nature of COVID-19 diagnostic, prognostic, and therapeutic research in the first years of the pandemic, the American College of Emergency Physicians (ACEP) created an interactive and continually updated "COVID-19 ED Management Tool."[24,25] Although the ACEP tool did not focus on diagnostic testing, the recommendations did provide a living document by which lab and imaging decisions to guide COVID-19 prognosis could be better understood. In terms of the presence or absence of SARS-CoV-2 in an individual patient, rRT-PCR quickly became the most widely accepted and readily available criterion standard. Diagnostic research exploring the optimal specimen site and collection method, as well as the potential roles for antigen or antibody testing continued to emerge at the time of this book's publication. Currently, rRT-PCR testing should be considered based on local COVID-19 prevalence and interpreted with the understanding that false positives are far less common than false negatives. Neither history/physical exam nor imaging results should be used to rule in or rule out the presence of COVID-19 pneumonia. Imaging should be used as an adjunct to identify complications associated with COVID-19 such as severe pneumonia or venous thromboembolism.

The societal strife and economic hardships caused by the global pandemic of COVID-19 strained the real-world application of evidence-based diagnostics. The pace of manuscript submissions to journals worldwide accelerated significantly, but the vast majority of published research did not cite or adhere to STARD reporting guidelines.[3,26] One consequence was large volumes of COVID-19 diagnostic manuscripts that neglected the basic design constructs of diagnostic research described in the first six chapters of this textbook. For example, some early manuscripts did not explicitly report the criterion standard they used, while others did not justify or contemplate their reference standard. Thoughtful and pragmatic contemplation about more convincing criterion standards were lacking but have been proposed (Table 62.5).[2]

The implications of false-positive and false-negative results were often underemphasized in COVID-19 diagnostic testing research.[2,27] Since COVID-19 occurred in multiple waves at different times across geographic regions combined with the reality that false-positive and false-negative rates vary with disease prevalence (see Chapter 6), the interpretation of test results like rRT-PCR was most meaningful with an understanding of the current local COVID-19 prevalence.[2] One diagnostic accuracy scoping review

Table 62.5 Proposed COVID-19 criterion standard

Expert consensus months after acute illness, including
• Exposure history
• Symptoms
• Laboratory tests
• rRT-PCR
• Imaging
• Serology
• Viral cultures

Source: Reproduced from [2]/With permission of John Wiley & Sons.

Table 62.6 Test result interpretation relative to COVID-19 prevalence

Pre-test probability when TP = FP
[(1/sensitivity) ÷ ((1/sensitivity)+(1/(1 − specificity)))]

Pre-test probability when FN = TN
[(1/(1 − sensitivity) ÷ ((1/(1 − sensitivity)+(1/specificity)))]

Source: Adapted from [2].

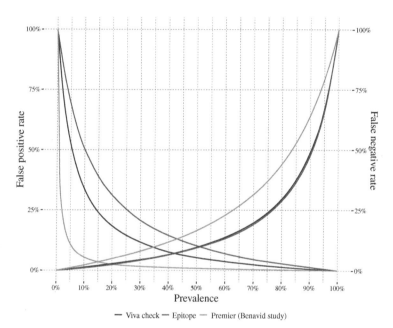

Figure 62.2 Association of COVID-19 prevalence with false-positive and false-negative serology results. (Reproduced from [2]/With permission of John Wiley & Sons.)

manipulated Bayes Theorem (see Chapter 3) to define prevalence thresholds where a positive result was more likely a false positive than a true positive and vice versa a threshold where a negative result was more likely false negative than true negative (Table 62.6).[2] As an example, Whitman *et al.*[28] reported a sensitivity of 90.9% and specificity of 81.8% for a COVID-19 antibody test, so using Table 62.6 the probability at which a positive result is equally likely to be a true positive as a false positive is 10% (Figure 62.2). If the pretest probability of COVID-19 (or local COVID-19 prevalence) is less than 10% then a positive test is more likely a false positive than a true positive.[2]

Future COVID-19 researchers should adhere to STARD reporting standards in order to provide clarity into potential diagnostic biases and enhance reproducibility.[6,29] Clinical investigators are deriving and validating decision aids based on constellations of history, physical exam, imaging, or laboratory findings to improve bedside decision-making when access to molecular tests are intermittently disrupted and concerns about false negatives persist.[30] Additional decision aids are being developed to evaluate COVID-19 severity at a point in time and predict likelihood of decompensation requiring critical care in the days to follow.[31] Ultimately, these diagnostic and prognostic decision aids could be the foundation of shared decision-making resources to help patients and families interpret test results within the contexts of their work, home situation, and societal exposure risks during the era of a global pandemic.[2]

References

1. Carley S, Horner D, Body R, Mackway-Jones K. Evidence-based medicine and COVID-19: What to believe and when to change. *Emergency Medicine Journal.* 2020; 37: 572–5.
2. Carpenter CR, Mudd PA, West CP, Wilber E, Wilber ST. Diagnosing COVID-19 in the emergency department: A scoping review of clinical examinations, laboratory tests, imaging accuracy, and biases. *Academic Emergency Medicine.* 2020; 27: 653–70.
3. Simel DL, Rennie D, Bossuyt PM. The STARD statement for reporting diagnostic accuracy studies: Application to the history and physical examination. *Journal of General Internal Medicine.* 2008; 23: 768–74.
4. Benezit F, Le Turnier P, Declerck C et al. Utility of hyposmia and hypogeusia for the diagnosis of COVID-19. *The Lancet Infectious Diseases.* 2020; 20: 1014–5.
5. Struyf T, Deeks JJ, Dinnes J et al. Signs and symptoms to determine if a patient presenting in primary care or hospital outpatient settings has COVID-19 disease. *Cochrane Database of Systematic Reviews.* 2020; 7: CD013665.
6. Kohn MA, Carpenter CR, Newman TB. Understanding the direction of bias in studies of diagnostic test accuracy. *Academic Emergency Medicine.* 2013; 20: 1194–206.
7. Stegeman I, Ochodo EA, Guleid F et al. Routine laboratory testing to determine if a patient has COVID-19. *Cochrane Database of Systematic Reviews.* 2020; 11: CD013787.
8. Bastos ML, Perlman-Arrow S, Menzies D, Campbell JR. The sensitivity and costs of testing for SARS-CoV-2 infection with saliva versus nasopharyngeal swabs: A systematic review and meta-analysis. *Annals of Internal Medicine.* 2021; 174: 501–10.
9. Xie C, Jiang L, Huang G et al. Comparison of different samples for 2019 novel coronavirus detection by nucleic acid amplification tests. *International Journal of Infectious Diseases.* 2020; 93: 264–7.

10. Carpenter CR. Rapid antigen and molecular tests had varied sensitivity and ≥97% specificity for detecting SARS-CoV-2 infection. *Annals of Internal Medicine.* 2020; 173: JC69.

11. Dinnes J, Deeks JJ, Adriano A *et al.* Rapid, point-of-care antigen and molecular-based tests for diagnosis of SARS-CoV-2 infection. *Cochrane Database of Systematic Reviews.* 2020; 8: CD013705.

12. FDA. Coronavirus (COVID-19) Update: FDA Authorizes First Antigen Test to Help in the Rapid Detection of the Virus that Causes COVID-19 in Patients. https://www.fda.gov/news-events/press-announcements/coronavirus-covid-19-update-fda-authorizes-first-antigen-test-help-rapid-detection-virus-causes. 2020. Accessed June 2, 2020.

13. Islam N, Salameh JP, Leeflang MM *et al.* Thoracic imaging tests for the diagnosis of COVID-19. *Cochrane Database of Systematic Reviews.* 2020; 11: CD013639.

14. Bar S, Lecourtois A, Diouf M *et al.* The association of lung ultrasound images with COVID-19 infection in an emergency room cohort. *Anaesthesia.* 2020; 75: 1620–5.

15. Peyrony O, Marbeuf-Gueye C, Truong V *et al.* Accuracy of emergency department clinical findings for diagnosis of coronavirus disease 2019. *Annals of Emergency Medicine.* 2020; 76: 405–12.

16. Lieveld AWE, Kok B, Schuit FH *et al.* Diagnosing COVID-19 pneumonia in a pandemic setting: Lung ultrasound versus CT (LUVCT) - a multicentre, prospective, observational study. *ERJ Open Research.* 2020; 6: 00539–2020.

17. Chen X, Tang Y, Mo Y *et al.* A diagnostic model for coronavirus disease 2019 (COVID-19) based on radiological semantic and clinical features: A multi-center study. *European Radiology.* 2020; 30(9): 4893–902.

18. Feng H, Liu Y, Lv M, Zhong J. A case report of COVID-19 with false negative RT-PCR test: Necessity of chest CT. *Japanese Journal of Radiology.* 2020; 38: 409–10.

19. Raptis CA, Hammer MM, Short RG *et al.* Chest CT and coronavirus disease (COVID-19): A critical review of the literature to date. *AJR American Journal of Roentgenology.* 2020; 215(4): 839–42.

20. Nair A, Rodrigues JCL, Hare S *et al.* A British Society of Thoracic Imaging statement: Considerations in designing local imaging diagnostic algorithms for the COVID-19 pandemic. *Clinical Radiology.* 2020; 75: 329–34.

21. Tavare AN, Braddy A, Brill S *et al.* Managing high clinical suspicion COVID-19 inpatients with negative RT-PCR: A pragmatic and limited role for thoracic CT. *Thorax.* 2020; 75(7): 537–8.

22. Schulze-Hagen M, Hübel C, Meier-Schorers M *et al.* Low-dose chest CT for the diagnosis of COVID-19—A systematic, prospective comparison with PCR. *Deutsches Ärzteblatt International.* 2020; 117: 389–95.

23. Bai HX, Wang R, Xiong Z *et al.* AI augmentation of radiologist performance in distinguishing COVID-19 from pneumonia of other etiology on chest CT. *Radiology.* 2020; 296(3): E156–65.

24. American College of Emergency Physicians. COVID-19 ED Management Tool. https://www.acep.org/corona/COVID-19-alert/covid-19-articles/covid-19-ED-management-tool-now-available/. 2021. Accessed September 29, 2021.

25. Steel PAD, Carpenter CR, Fengler B, Cantrill S, Schneider S. Calculated decisions: ACEP ED COVID-19 management tool. *Emergency Medicine Practice.* 2021; 23: CD1–6.
26. Bossuyt PMM, Reitsma JB, Bruns DE *et al.* STARD 2015: An updated list of essential items for reporting diagnostic accuracy studies. *BMJ.* 2015; 351: h5527.
27. West CP, Montori VM, Sampathkumar P. COVID-19 testing: The threat of false-negative results. *Mayo Clinic Proceedings.* 2020; 95: 1127–9.
28. Whitman JD, Hiatt J, Mowery CT, *et al.* Test performance evaluation of SARS-CoV-02 serological assays. medRxiv;2020:04.25.20074856.
29. Carpenter CR, Meizel Z. Overcoming the tower of babel in medical science by finding the "EQUATOR": Research reporting guidelines. *Academic Emergency Medicine.* 2017; 24: 1030–3.
30. Kline JA, Pettit KL, Kabrhel C, Courtney DM, Nordenholz KE, Camargo CA. Multicenter registry of United States emergency department patients tested for SARS-CoV-2. *Journal of the American College of Emergency Physicians Open.* 2020; 1: 1341–8.
31. Wynants L, Van Calster B, Bonten MMJ *et al.* Prediction models for diagnosis and prognosis of covid-19 infection: Systematic review and critical appraisal. *BMJ (Clinical Research Ed.).* 2020; 369: m1328.

Index

Note: Page numbers in *italics* refer to Figures; those in **bold** to Tables

Evidence-Based Emergency Care: Diagnostic Testing and Clinical Decision Rules, Third Edition.
Edited by Jesse M. Pines, Fernanda Bellolio, Christopher R. Carpenter, and Ali S. Raja.
© 2023 John Wiley & Sons Ltd. Published 2023 by John Wiley & Sons Ltd.